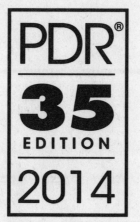

PDR® 35 EDITION 2014

PDR®

for Nonprescription Drugs

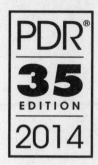

PDR® 35 EDITION 2014

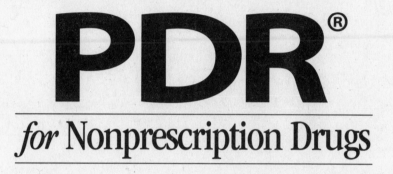

PDR®
for Nonprescription Drugs

Executive Chairman: Edward Fotsch, MD

President: Richard C. Altus

Chief Medical Officer: Salvatore Volpe, MD, FAAP, FACP, CHCQM

Executive Vice President and Chief Financial Officer: Gary Lubin

Chief Technology Officer: David Cheng

Senior Vice President, Operations: Dawn Carfora

Senior Vice President, Sales: Jeffrey Davis

Senior Vice President, Corporate Development & General Counsel: Andrew Gelman

Senior Vice President, Marketing & Business Line Management: Barbara Senich, BSN, MBA, MPH

Vice President, Clinical & Regulatory Solutions: Mukesh Mehta, DPh, MBA, RPh

Director, Clinical Services: Sylvia Nashed, PharmD

Manager, Clinical Databases and Services: Christine Sunwoo, PharmD

Associate Manager, Clinical Content Development: Anila Patel, PharmD

Senior Drug Information Specialist: Pauline Lee, PharmD

Drug Information Specialists: Vanessa DeAlmeida, PharmD; Demyana Farag, PharmD; Kristine Mecca, PharmD; Autri Sajedeen, PharmD

Managing Clinical Editor: Julia Tonelli, MD

Medical Editor: Christa Mary Kronick, MA

Director, Marketing: Kim Marich

Manager, Corporate Communications: Thomas W. Eck

Manager, Art Department: Livio Udina

Senior Director, Content Operations & Manufacturing: Jeffrey D. Schaefer

Associate Director, Manufacturing & Distribution: Thomas Westburgh

Senior Production Manager, PDR: Steven Maher

Project Manager, Fulfillment: Gary Lew

Web Operations and Customer Service Manager: Lee Reynolds

ISBN: 978-1-56363-827-5

FOREWORD TO THE 35ᵀᴴ EDITION

About PDR Network, LLC

As the nation's leading aggregator and distributor of drug labeling information, product safety alerts, and pharmaceutical Risk Evaluation and Mitigation Strategy (REMS) programs, PDR Network® is committed to ensuring that prescribers have access to the right information at the point of prescribing. This information is distributed across channels through the PDR® suite of digital and print services, which includes the *Physicians' Desk Reference®* (*PDR®*), the most highly trusted drug information reference available in the U.S., now available in multiple book formats; PDR interactive drug services for Electronic Health Record (EHR) systems; PDR.net®, the Internet home of PDR; *mobile*PDR®; and PDR Drug Alerts, the only specialty-specific service that provides electronic delivery of FDA-approved Drug Alerts to physicians and other healthcare professionals.

By improving communication of important medication information and FDA-approved Drug Alerts, PDR Network's unique services enhance patient safety and may help to reduce medical liability.

For more information or to sign up for electronic PDR Drug Alerts, visit PDR.net.

About PDR® for Nonprescription Drugs (NPD), 35ᵗʰ Edition

NPD is the true over-the-counter (OTC) companion to the *PDR*. It is the premier source for information on the most commonly used OTC medications. These include analgesics, cough and cold preparations, fever reducers, and more. The 2014 *NPD* offers physicians, residents, and medical students invaluable, easily accessible content. *NPD* is a source for OTC drugs and contains manufacturer names, product names, indications and usage, drug warnings, and comparison tables for quick, at-a-glance dosing and ingredient information.

NPD is published annually by PDR Network, LLC. In organizing and presenting the material in *NPD*, PDR Network does not warrant or guarantee any of the products described, or perform any independent analysis in connection with any of the product information contained herein. PDR Network does not assume, and expressly disclaims, any obligation to obtain and include any information other than that provided to it by the manufacturers. It should be understood that by making this material available, PDR Network is not advocating the use of any product described herein, nor is PDR Network responsible for the use of any product, or the misuse of any product, due to content or typographical error. Additional information on any product may be obtained from the manufacturer.

Other Resources from PDR

PDR® for Nonprescription Drugs enters its 35ᵗʰ year as part of the products and services of PDR Network, LLC, the leading distributor of medical product labeling, FDA-approved Drug Alerts, and REMS program communications. PDR Network products and services include:

Physicians' Desk Reference®, the most trusted drug information reference. To ensure that clinicians have the most current available information at their fingertips, PDR Network's Drug Information Service for active prescribers also provides:

PDR Updates, a quick reference designed to make prescribers aware of labeling changes, including newly approved labeling, that have occurred since the publication of *PDR*. Distributed every other month, each one lists changes that have occurred in the past 60 days. These updates and the full product information can be viewed at **PDR.net/Updates**.

PDR eDrug Updates, monthly electronic newsletters that provide specialty-specific drug information, including FDA alerts, new drug approvals, and labeling changes that have occurred in the past 30 days. To sign up for this free e-newsletter, send an email to customerservice@pdr.net.

Electronic PDR Resources

PDR.net

PDR.net, a web portal designed specifically for healthcare professionals, provides trusted, professional drug information, including full FDA-approved labeling as well as concise point-of-care drug information. **PDR.net** provides prescribers with online access to the authoritative drug information they need to support their treatment decisions.

mobilePDR

*mobile*PDR provides the only source for FDA-approved full product labeling and concise point-of-care drug information from the PDR database directly on a mobile device. Prescribing information on more than 2,400 drugs, full-color product images, and weekly updates provide up-to-date drug information. *mobile*PDR is free for U.S.-based MDs, DOs, NPs, and PAs in full-time patient practice and can be downloaded from PDR.net. *mobile*PDR is available for all major mobile platforms.

PDR Drug Alerts

FDA-approved Drug Alerts are delivered electronically to physicians and other prescribers who register to receive them at PDR.net, through participating medical societies, or by returning the verification form distributed with complimentary copies of *PDR*. By ensuring that this service is used exclusively for the rapid delivery of **PDR Drug Alerts**—not advertising or marketing—PDR Network fulfills FDA guidance for electronic delivery of alerts, improves patient safety, and may help to reduce liability.

Electronic Health Records

PDR BRIEF

PDR BRIEF offers an intuitive dashboard of full labeling information and provider resources surfacing within your EHR system to support your treatment decisions within your workflow. **PDR BRIEF** is activated when a medication is selected to ensure you have the most current full prescribing information, label updates, boxed warnings, patient education, financial support, and adherence resources available.

PDR®+ for Patients

PDR+ for Patients drug education guides are designed to help patients understand the drugs prescribed by their physician. Available in your EHR workflow, the guides are easy to hand out during an office visit or automatically send to the Patient Portal. By addressing potential concerns early on and sharing **PDR+ for Patients**, physicians can help their patients start and stay on therapy.

PDR® Search

PDR Search delivers an unparalleled interactive and searchable drug database of drug labeling and safety and product support information. **PDR Search** supplies full drug prescribing information and prescribing summaries with access to FDA and PDR Drug Alerts, as well as patient education, financial support, and adherence resources directly through your EHR application.

Patient Financial Support

PDR® Pharmacy Discount Card

This free program provides patients with access to medications at discounted prices, helping them save up to 75% on their prescriptions at more than 60,000 pharmacies nationwide. PDR Network distributes this program via healthcare provider offices, allowing them to share the program with their patients directly. The program is offered at no cost to participating providers or their patients who benefit from it. If you are not already enrolled, call 800 232-7379 or visit PDR.net/PharmacyDiscountCard.

A wide range of other prescribing references and clinical decision publications are also available.

For more information on the growing family of PDR Network products, please call toll-free 800-232-7379; fax 201-722-2680; or visit PDRbooks.com.

CONTENTS

HOW TO USE THIS BOOK

The 2014 edition of *PDR® for Nonprescription Drugs* features a user-friendly format designed to help you find the information you need as quickly and easily as possible. In addition to the index, you can go directly to a specific **Product Comparison Table** to find the relevant OTC products for a particular condition.

The **Product Name Index** provides the page number of each product in the Nonprescription Drug Information section. Listings appear alphabetically by brand name.

NONPRESCRIPTION DRUG INFORMATION
Organized alphabetically by product name. The product labeling in this section includes brand-name OTC products marketed for home use. **Please keep in mind that the product information included herein is valid as of press time (November 2013).** Additional information, as well as updates to the product labeling, can be obtained from the manufacturer.

PRODUCT COMPARISON TABLES
Each therapeutic category or condition is organized alphabetically. Brand names within each table are also listed alphabetically. These tables provide a quick and easy way to compare the active ingredients and dosages of common brand-name OTC products.

NONPRESCRIPTION DRUG INFORMATION

This section presents information on nonprescription products marketed for home use by consumers.

The descriptions of over-the-counter (OTC) products in this section reflect the manufacturers' information, as included in the product labeling provided to consumers. Those descriptions are designed to provide the information necessary for informed use by consumers, including, when applicable, active ingredients, uses (indications), specific warnings (including when a product should not be used under any circumstances), when it is appropriate to consult a doctor or pharmacist, substances or activities to avoid, dosage instructions, inactive ingredients, and other pertinent facts about each product.

The function of the Publisher is solely the compilation, organization, and distribution of this information. The descriptions seen here include all information made available by the manufacturer. The Publisher does not warrant or guarantee any product described herein, and does not perform any independent analysis of the information provided. Inclusion of a product in this book does not represent an endorsement, and the Publisher does not advocate the use of any product listed.

A+D DIAPER RASH CREAM (dimethicone and zinc oxide)

MSD Consumer Care, Inc.

DRUG FACTS

Active Ingredient(s)	Purpose(s)
Dimethicone 1%	Diaper Rash Cream
Zinc Oxide 10%	Diaper Rash Cream

USES
- helps treat and prevent diaper rash
- protects minor skin irritation due to diaper rash and helps seal out wetness

WARNINGS
For external use only
When using this product
- do not get into eyes

DO NOT USE
- with any other drug containing acetaminophen (prescription or nonprescription). If you are not sure whether a drug contains acetaminophen, ask a doctor or pharmacist.
- if you are allergic to acetaminophen or any of the inactive ingredients in this product

ASK A DOCTOR BEFORE USE IF THE USER
- has liver disease
- takes the blood thinning drug warfarin

STOP USE AND ASK A DOCTOR IF
- condition worsens
- symptoms last more than 7 days or clear up and occur again within a few days

Keep out of reach of children.
If swallowed, get medical help or contact a Poison Control Center right away.

DIRECTIONS
- change wet and soiled diapers promptly
- cleanse the diaper area, and allow to dry
- apply cream liberally as often as necessary, with each diaper change, especially at bedtime or anytime when exposure to wet diapers may be prolonged

OTHER INFORMATION
- store between 20°C to 25°C (68° to 77°F)

INACTIVE INGREDIENTS
aloe barbadensis extract, benzyl alcohol, coconut oil, cod liver oil (contains vitamin A & Vitamin D), fragrance, glyceryl oleate, light mineral oil, ozokerite, paraffin, propylene glycol, sorbitol, synthetic beeswax, water

A AND D ORIGINAL (lanolin and petrolatum)

MSD Consumer Care, Inc.

DRUG FACTS

Active Ingredient(s)	Purpose(s)
Lanolin 15.5%	Diaper rash ointment
Petrolatum 53.4%	Skin Protectant

USES
- helps treat and prevent diaper rash
- temporarily protects minor:
  - cuts
  - scrapes
  - burns
- temporarily protects and helps relieve chapped, chafed or cracked skin and lips
- protect chafed skin due to diaper rash and helps seal out wetness

WARNINGS
For external use only

WHEN USING THIS PRODUCT
- do not get into eyes

STOP USE AND ASK A DOCTOR IF
- condition worsens
- symptoms last more than 7 days or clear up and occur again within a few days

DO NOT USE ON
- deep or puncture wounds
- animal bites
- serious burns

Keep out of reach of children. If swallowed, get medical help or contact a Poison Control Center right away.

DIRECTIONS
- **for skin protectant use** apply as needed
- **for diaper rash use:**
  - change wet and soiled diapers promptly
  - cleanse the diaper area, and allow to dry
  - apply ointment liberally as often as necessary, with each diaper change, especially at bedtime or anytime when exposure to wet diapers may be prolonged

OTHER INFORMATION
store between 20°C to 25 °C (68° to 77°F)

INACTIVE INGREDIENTS
cod liver oil (contains vitamin A & vitamin D), fragrance, light mineral oil, microcrystalline wax, paraffin

ABREVA (docosanol)

GlaxoSmithKline Consumer Healthcare LP

Active Ingredient(s)
Docosanol 10%

Purpose(s)
Cold sore/fever blister treatment

USES
- treats cold sores/fever blisters on the face or lips
- shortens healing time and duration of symptoms:
  - tingling, pain, burning, and/or itching

WARNINGS
For external use only

DO NOT USE
- if you are allergic to any ingredient in this product

WHEN USING THIS PRODUCT
- apply only to affected areas
- do not use in or near the eyes
- avoid applying directly inside your mouth

- do not share this product with anyone. This may spread infection.

STOP USE AND ASK A DOCTOR IF
- your cold sore gets worse or the cold sore is not healed within 10 days

Keep out of reach of children.
If swallowed, get medical help or contact a poison control center right away.

DIRECTIONS
- **adults and children 12 years or over:**
  - wash hands before and after applying cream
  - apply to affected area on face or lips at the first sign of cold sore/fever blister (tingle).
  - early treatment ensures the best results
  - rub in gently but completely
  - use 5 times a day until healed
- **children under 12 years:** ask a doctor

OTHER INFORMATION
- store at 20°-25°C (68°-77°F)
- do not freeze

INACTIVE INGREDIENTS
benzyl alcohol, light mineral oil, propylene glycol, purified water, sucrose distearate, sucrose stearate

QUESTIONS OR COMMENTS?
call toll-free **1-877-709-3539** (English/Spanish) weekdays
visit us at **www.abreva.com**
Distributed for **Avanir Pharmaceuticals** by
GlaxoSmithKline Consumer Healthcare, L.P.
Moon Twp, PA 15108
Made in Germany
© 2008 GlaxoSmithKline. 27675PA

INFANTS ADVIL CONCENTRATED DROPS
(ibuprofen)

Pfizer Consumer Healthcare

DRUG FACTS

Active Ingredient(s) (in each 1.25 mL)
Ibuprofen 50 mg (NSAID)*
*nonsteroidal anti-inflammatory drug

Purpose(s)
Fever reducer/Pain reliever

USES
temporarily:
- reduces fever
- relieves minor aches and pains due to the common cold, flu, headaches and toothaches

WARNINGS
Allergy alert:
Ibuprofen may cause a severe allergic reaction, especially in people allergic to aspirin. Symptoms may include:
- hives
- facial swelling
- asthma (wheezing)
- shock
- skin reddening
- rash
- blisters

If an allergic reaction occurs, stop use and seek medical help right away.

Stomach bleeding warning:
This product contains an NSAID which may cause severe stomach bleeding. The chance is higher if the child:
- has had stomach ulcers or bleeding problems
- takes a blood thinning (anticoagulant) or steroid drug
- takes other drugs containing prescription or nonprescription an NSAIDs [aspirin, ibuprofen, naproxen, or others]
- takes more or for a longer time than directed

DO NOT USE
- if the child has ever had an allergic reaction to any other pain reliever/fever reducer
- right before or after heart surgery

ASK A DOCTOR BEFORE USE IF
- stomach bleeding warning applies to the child
- child has problems or serious side effects from taking pain relievers or fever reducers
- child has a history of stomach problems, such as heartburn
- child has high blood pressure, heart disease, liver cirrhosis, kidney disease, or asthma
- child has not been drinking fluids
- child has lost a lot of fluid due to vomiting or diarrhea
- child is taking a diuretic

ASK A DOCTOR OR PHARMACIST BEFORE USE IF THE CHILD IS
- under a doctor's care for any serious condition
- taking any other drug

WHEN USING THIS PRODUCT
- take with food or milk if stomach upset occurs
- the risk of heart attack or stroke may increase if you use more than directed or for longer than directed

STOP USE AND ASK A DOCTOR IF
- the child feels faint, vomits blood, or has bloody or black stools. These are signs of stomach bleeding.
- stomach pain or upset gets worse or lasts
- the child does not get any relief within first day (24 hours) of treatment
- fever or pain gets worse or lasts more than 3 days
- redness or swelling is present in the painful area
- any new symptoms appear

Keep out of reach of children.
In case of overdose, get medical help or contact a Poison Control Center right away.

DIRECTIONS
- **this product does not contain directions or complete warnings for adult use**
- **do not give more than directed**
- **shake well before using**
- find right dose on chart below. If possible, use weight to dose; otherwise use age.
- repeat dose every **6-8 hours**, if needed
- do not use more than **4 times a day**
- measure with the dosing device provided. Do not use with any other device.

Dosing Chart

Weight (lb)	Age (mos)	Dose (mL)
under 6 mos ask a doctor		
12-17 lb	6-11 mos	1.25 mL
18-23 lb	12-23 mos	1.875 mL

OTHER INFORMATION
- one dose lasts 6-8 hours
- store at 20-25°C (68-77°F)
- see bottom of box for lot number and expiration date

INACTIVE INGREDIENTS
acetic acid, artificial flavor, butylated hydroxytoluene, carboxymethylcellulose sodium, citric acid monohydrate, edetate disodium, glycerin, microcrystalline cellulose, polysorbate 80, propylene glycol, purified water, sodium benzoate, sorbitol solution, sucrose, xanthan gum

QUESTIONS OR COMMENTS?
Call toll-free **1-800-88-ADVIL** or ask your pharmacist, doctor or health care professional
For most recent product information, visit www.Advil.com.

JUNIOR STRENGTH ADVIL CHEWABLE TABLETS (ibuprofen)

Pfizer Consumer Healthcare

DRUG FACTS

Active Ingredient(s) (in each tablet)
Ibuprofen 100 mg (NSAID)*
*nonsteroidal anti-inflammatory drug

Purpose(s)
Fever Reducer/Pain reliever

USES
temporarily:
- reduces fever
- relieves minor aches and pains due to the common cold, flu, sore throat, headaches and toothaches

WARNINGS
Allergy alert:
Ibuprofen may cause a severe allergic reaction, especially in people allergic to aspirin. Symptoms may include:
- hives
- facial swelling
- asthma (wheezing)
- shock
- skin reddening
- rash
- blisters

If an allergic reaction occurs, stop use and seek medical help right away.

Stomach bleeding warning:
This product contains an NSAID, which may cause severe stomach bleeding. The chance is higher if the child
- has had stomach ulcers or bleeding problems
- takes a blood thinning (anticoagulant) or steroid drug
- takes other drugs containing prescription or nonprescription NSAIDs [aspirin, ibuprofen, naproxen, or others]
- takes more or for a longer time than directed

Sore throat warning:
Severe or persistent sore throat or sore throat accompanied by high fever, headache, nausea, and vomiting may be serious. Consult doctor promptly. Do not use more than 2 days or administer to children under 3 years of age unless directed by doctor.

DO NOT USE
- if the child has ever had an allergic reaction to any other pain reliever/fever reducer
- right before or after heart surgery

ASK A DOCTOR BEFORE USE IF
- stomach bleeding warning applies to the child
- child has problems or serious side effects from taking pain relievers or fever reducers
- child has a history of stomach problems, such as heartburn
- child has high blood pressure, heart disease, liver cirrhosis, kidney disease, or asthma
- child has not been drinking fluids
- child has lost a lot of fluid due to vomiting or diarrhea
- child is taking a diuretic

ASK A DOCTOR OR PHARMACIST BEFORE USE IF THE CHILD IS
- under a doctor's care for any serious condition
- taking any other drug

WHEN USING THIS PRODUCT
- take with food or milk if stomach upset occurs
- the risk of heart attack or stroke may increase if you use more than directed or for longer than directed

STOP USE AND ASK A DOCTOR IF
- child experiences any of the following signs of stomach bleeding:
  - feels faint
  - vomits blood
  - has bloody or black stools
  - has stomach pain that does not get better
- child does not get any relief within first day (24 hours) of treatment
- fever or pain gets worse or lasts more than 3 days
- redness or swelling is present in the painful area
- any new symptoms appear

Keep out of reach of children
In case of overdose, get medical help or contact a Poison Control Center right away.

DIRECTIONS
- **this product does not contain directions or complete warnings for adult use**
- **do not give more than directed**
- find right dose on chart below. If possible, use weight to dose; otherwise use age.
- repeat dose every **6-8 hours**, if needed
- do not use more than **4 times a day**

Dosing Chart		
Weight (lb)	**Age (yr)**	**Dose (tablets)**
under 48 lb	under 6 yr	ask a doctor
48-59 lb	6-8 yr	2 tablets
60-71 lb	9-10 yr	2 1/2 tablets
72-95 lb	11yr	3 tablets

OTHER INFORMATION
- **Phenylketonurics**: contains phenylalanine 4.2 mg per tablet
- one dose lasts 6-8 hours
- store at 20-25°C (68-77°F)
- see side of box for lot number and expiration date

INACTIVE INGREDIENTS
aspartame, cellacefate, colloidal silicon dioxide, D&C red no. 30 aluminum lake, FD&C blue no. 2 aluminum lake, gelatin, magnesium stearate, mannitol, microcrystalline cellulose, natural and artificial flavors, sodium starch glycolate

QUESTIONS OR COMMENTS?
call toll free **1-800-88-ADVIL** or ask your pharmacist, doctor or health care professional

JUNIOR STRENGTH ADVIL TABLETS
(ibuprofen)

Pfizer Consumer Healthcare

DRUG FACTS

Active Ingredient(s) (in each tablet)
Ibuprofen 100 mg (NSAID)*
*nonsteroidal anti-inflammatory drug

Purpose(s)
Fever reducer/Pain reliever

USES
temporarily:
• reduces fever
• relieves minor aches and pains due to the common cold, flu, sore throat, headaches and toothaches

WARNINGS
Allergy alert:
Ibuprofen may cause a severe allergic reaction, especially in people allergic to aspirin. Symptoms may include:
• hives
• facial swelling
• asthma (wheezing)
• shock
• skin reddening
• rash
• blisters

If an allergic reaction occurs, stop use and seek medical help right away.

Stomach bleeding warning:
This product contains an NSAID, which may cause severe stomach bleeding. The chance is higher if the child
• has had stomach ulcers or bleeding problems
• takes a blood thinning (anticoagulant) or steroid drug
• takes other drugs containing prescription or nonprescription NSAIDs [aspirin, ibuprofen, naproxen, or others]
• takes more or for a longer time than directed

Sore throat warning:
Severe or persistent sore throat or sore throat accompanied by high fever, headache, nausea, and vomiting may be serious. Consult doctor promptly. Do not use more than 2 days or administer to children under 3 years of age unless directed by doctor.

DO NOT USE
• if the child has ever had an allergic reaction to any other pain reliever/fever reducer
• right before or after heart surgery

ASK A DOCTOR BEFORE USE IF
• stomach bleeding warning applies to the child
• child has problems or serious side effects from taking pain relievers or fever reducers
• child has a history of stomach problems, such as heartburn
• child has high blood pressure, heart disease, liver cirrhosis, kidney disease, or asthma
• child has not been drinking fluids
• child has lost a lot of fluid due to vomiting or diarrhea
• child is taking a diuretic

ASK A DOCTOR OR PHARMACIST BEFORE USE IF THE CHILD IS
• under a doctor's care for any serious condition
• taking any other drug

WHEN USING THIS PRODUCT
• take with food or milk if stomach upset occurs
• the risk of heart attack or stroke may increase if you use more than directed or for longer than directed

STOP USE AND ASK A DOCTOR IF
• child experiences any of the following signs of stomach bleeding:
  • feels faint
  • vomits blood
  • has bloody or black stools
  • has stomach pain that does not get better
• child does not get any relief within first day (24 hours) of treatment
• fever or pain gets worse or lasts more than 3 days
• redness or swelling is present in the painful area
• any new symptoms appear

Keep out of reach of children
In case of overdose, get medical help or contact a Poison Control Center right away.

DIRECTIONS
• **this product does not contain directions or complete warnings for adult use**
• **do not give more than directed**
• find right dose on chart below. If possible, use weight to dose; otherwise use age.
• repeat dose every **6-8 hours**, if needed
• do not use more than **4 times a day**

Dosing Chart		
Weight (lb)	Age (yr)	Dose (tablets)
under 48 lb	under 6 yr	ask a doctor
48-71 lb	6-10 yr	2 tablets
72-95 lb	11 yr	3 tablets

OTHER INFORMATION
• one dose lasts 6-8 hours
• store at 20-25°C (68-77°F)
• avoid excessive heat above 40°C (104°F)
• see side of box for lot number and expiration date

INACTIVE INGREDIENTS
acetylated monoglycerides, carnauba wax, colloidal silicon dioxide, corn starch, croscarmellose sodium, methylparaben, microcrystalline cellulose, pharmaceutical glaze, pharmaceutical ink, povidone, pregelatinized starch, propylparaben, sodium benzoate, stearic acid, sucrose, synthetic iron oxides, titanium dioxide

QUESTIONS OR COMMENTS?
call toll free **1-800-88-ADVIL** or ask your pharmacist, doctor or health care professional

---

ADVIL (ibuprofen)
Pfizer Consumer Healthcare

DRUG FACTS

Active Ingredient(s)

Advil Tablets (in each tablet)
Ibuprofen 200 mg (NSAID)*
*nonsteroidal anti-inflammatory drug

Advil Caplets (in each caplet)
Ibuprofen 200 mg (NSAID)*
*nonsteroidal anti-inflammatory drug

Advil Gel Caplets (in each gel caplet)
Ibuprofen 200 mg (NSAID)*
*nonsteroidal anti-inflammatory drug

Purpose(s)
Pain reliever/Fever reducer

USES
- temporarily relieves minor aches and pains due to:
  - headache
  - toothache
  - backache
  - menstrual cramps
  - the common cold
  - muscular aches
  - minor pain of arthritis
- temporarily reduces fever

WARNINGS
Allergy alert:
Ibuprofen may cause a severe allergic reaction, especially in people allergic to aspirin. Symptoms may include:
- hives
- facial swelling
- asthma (wheezing)
- shock
- skin reddening
- rash
- blisters

If an allergic reaction occurs, stop use and seek medical help right away.

Stomach bleeding warning:
This product contains an NSAID, which may cause severe stomach bleeding. The chance is higher if you
- are age 60 or older
- have had stomach ulcers or bleeding problems
- take a blood thinning (anticoagulant) or steroid drug
- take other drugs containing prescription or non-prescription NSAIDs [aspirin, ibuprofen, naproxen, or others]
- have 3 or more alcoholic drinks every day while using this product
- take more or for a longer time than directed

DO NOT USE
- if you have ever had an allergic reaction to any other pain reliever/fever reducer
- right before or after heart surgery

ASK A DOCTOR BEFORE USE IF
- stomach bleeding warning applies to you
- you have problems or serious side effects from taking pain relievers or fever reducers
- you have a history of stomach problems, such as heartburn
- you have high blood pressure, heart disease, liver cirrhosis, kidney disease, or asthma
- you are taking a diuretic

ASK A DOCTOR OR PHARMACIST BEFORE USE IF YOU ARE
- under a doctor's care for any serious condition
- taking aspirin for heart attack or stroke, because ibuprofen may decrease this benefit of aspirin
- taking any other drug

WHEN USING THIS PRODUCT
- take with food or milk if stomach upset occurs
- the risk of heart attack or stroke may increase if you use more than directed or for longer than directed

STOP USE AND ASK A DOCTOR IF
- you experience any of the following signs of stomach bleeding:
  - feel faint
  - vomit blood
  - have bloody or black stools
  - have stomach pain that does not get better
- pain gets worse or lasts more than 10 days
- fever gets worse or lasts more than 3 days
- redness or swelling is present in the painful area
- any new symptoms appear

If pregnant or breast-feeding,
ask a health professional before use. It is especially important not to use ibuprofen during the last 3 months of pregnancy unless definitely directed to do so by a doctor because it may cause problems in the unborn child or complications during delivery.

Keep out of reach of children.
In case of overdose, get medical help or contact a Poison Control Center right away.

DIRECTIONS
Advil Tablets
- **do not take more than directed**
- **the smallest effective dose should be used**
- adults and children 12 years and over: take 1 tablet every 4 to 6 hours while symptoms persist
- if pain or fever does not respond to 1 tablet, 2 tablets may be used
- do not exceed 6 tablets in 24 hours, unless directed by a doctor
- children under 12 years: ask a doctor

Advil Caplets
- **do not take more than directed**
- **the smallest effective dose should be used**
- adults and children 12 years and over: take 1 caplet every 4 to 6 hours while symptoms persist
- if pain or fever does not respond to 1 caplet, 2 caplets may be used
- do not exceed 6 caplets in 24 hours, unless directed by a doctor
- children under 12 years: ask a doctor

Advil Gel Caplets
- **do not take more than directed**
- **the smallest effective dose should be used**
- adults and children 12 years and over: take 1 gel caplet every 4 to 6 hours while symptoms persist
- if pain or fever does not respond to 1 gel caplet, 2 gel caplets may be used
- do not exceed 6 gel caplets in 24 hours, unless directed by a doctor
- children under 12 years: ask a doctor

OTHER INFORMATION
- read all warnings and directions before use. Keep carton.
- store at 20-25°C (68-77°F)
- avoid excessive heat above 40°C (104°F)

INACTIVE INGREDIENTS
Advil Tablets
acetylated monoglycerides, colloidal silicon dioxide, corn starch, croscarmellose sodium, methylparaben, microcrystalline cellulose, pharmaceutical glaze, pharmaceutical ink, povidone, pregelatinized starch, propylparaben, sodium benzoate, sodium lauryl sulfate, stearic acid, sucrose, synthetic iron oxide, titanium dioxide, white wax

Advil Caplets
acetylated monoglycerides, colloidal silicon dioxide, corn starch, croscarmellose sodium, methylparaben, microcrystalline cellulose, pharmaceutical glaze, pharmaceutical ink, povidone, pregelatinized starch, propylparaben, sodium benzoate, sodium lauryl sulfate, stearic acid, sucrose, synthetic iron oxide, titanium dioxide, white wax

Advil Gel Caplets
colloidal silicon dioxide, corn starch, croscarmellose sodium, FD&C red no. 40, FD&C yellow no. 6, fractionated coconut oil, gelatin, glycerin, hypromellose, pharmaceutical ink, pregelatinized starch, propyl gallate, purified water, sodium

lauryl sulfate, stearic acid, synthetic iron oxides, titanium dioxide, triacetin

QUESTIONS OR COMMENTS?
call toll free **1-800-88-ADVIL**

ADVIL ALLERGY & CONGESTION RELIEF
(chlorpheniramine maleate, ibuprofen, and phenylephrine HCl)

Pfizer Consumer Healthcare

DRUG FACTS

Active Ingredient(s) (in each tablet)	Purpose(s)
Chlorpheniramine Maleate 4mg	Antihistamine
Ibuprofen 200 mg (NSAID)*	Pain reliever/fever reducer
Phenylephrine HCl 10 mg	Nasal decongestant
*nonsteroidal anti-inflammatory drug	

USES
temporarily relieves these symptoms associated with hay fever or other upper respiratory allergies, and the common cold:
- runny nose
- itchy, watery eyes
- itching of the nose or throat
- sneezing
- nasal congestion
- sinus pressure
- headache
- minor body aches and pains
- fever
- reduces swelling of the nasal passages
- temporarily restores freer breathing through the nose

WARNINGS
Allergy alert
Ibuprofen may cause a severe allergic reaction, especially in people allergic to aspirin. Symptoms may include:
- hives
- facial swelling
- asthma (wheezing)
- shock
- skin reddening
- rash
- blisters

If an allergic reaction occurs, stop use and seek medical help right away.

Stomach bleeding warning
This product contains an NSAID, which may cause severe stomach bleeding. The chance is higher if you:
- are age 60 or older
- have had stomach ulcers or bleeding problems
- take a blood thinning (anticoagulant) or steroid drug
- take other drugs containing prescription or nonprescription NSAIDs [aspirin, ibuprofen, naproxen, or others]
- have 3 or more alcoholic drinks every day while using this product
- take more or for a longer time than directed

DO NOT USE
- in children under 12 years of age because this product contains too much medication for children under this age
- if you have ever had an allergic reaction to any other pain reliever/fever reducer
- right before or after heart surgery

- if you are now taking a prescription monoamine oxidase inhibitor (MAOI) (certain drugs for depression, psychiatric, or emotional conditions, or Parkinson's disease), or for 2 weeks after stopping the MAOI drug. If you do not know if your prescription drug contains an MAOI, ask a doctor or pharmacist before taking this product

ASK A DOCTOR BEFORE USE IF
- you have a breathing problem such as emphysema or chronic bronchitis
- stomach bleeding warning applies to you
- you have problems or serious side effects from taking pain relievers or fever reducers
- you have a history of stomach problems, such as heartburn
- you have high blood pressure, heart disease, liver cirrhosis, kidney disease, asthma, thyroid disease, diabetes or have trouble urinating due to an enlarged prostate gland
- you are taking a diuretic

ASK A DOCTOR OR PHARMACIST BEFORE USE IF YOU ARE
- under a doctor's care for any serious condition
- taking sedatives or tranquilizers
- taking any other product that contains phenylephrine, chlorpheniramine or any other nasal decongestant or antihistamine
- taking aspirin for heart attack or stroke, because ibuprofen may decrease this benefit of aspirin
- taking any other drug

WHEN USING THIS PRODUCT
- take with food or milk if stomach upset occurs
- the risk of heart attack or stroke may increase if you use more than directed or for longer than directed
- avoid alcoholic drinks
- be careful when driving a motor vehicle or operating machinery
- drowsiness may occur
- alcohol, sedatives, and tranquilizers may increase drowsiness
- may cause excitability especially in children

STOP USE AND ASK A DOCTOR IF
you experience any of the following signs of stomach bleeding:
- feel faint
- vomit blood
- have bloody or black stools
- have stomach pain that does not get better
- pain gets worse or lasts more than 7 days
- fever gets worse or lasts more than 3 days
- nasal congestion lasts for more than 7 days
- redness or swelling is present in the painful area
- you get nervous, dizzy, or sleepless
- symptoms continue or get worse
- any new symptoms appear

If pregnant or breast-feeding, ask a health professional before use. It is especially important not to use ibuprofen during the last 3 months of pregnancy unless definitely directed to do so by a doctor because it may cause problems in the unborn child or complications during delivery.
Keep out of reach of children. In case of overdose, get medical help or contact a Poison Control Center right away.

DIRECTIONS
do not take more than directed
adults and children 12 years of age and over:
- take 1 tablet every 4 hours while symptoms persist.
- do not use more than 6 tablets in any 24-hour period unless directed by a doctor

children under 12 years of age: do not use because this product contains too much medication for children under this age

OTHER INFORMATION
read all warnings and directions before use. Keep carton.

store at 20 -25°C (68 -77°F).
Avoid excessive heat above 40°C (104°F).

INACTIVE INGREDIENTS
acesulfame potassium, artificial flavors, carnauba wax, colloidal silicon dioxide, corn starch, croscarmellose sodium, glycerin, glyceryl behenate, hypromellose, lactic acid, lecithin, maltodextrin, medium-chain triglycerides, microcrystalline cellulose, pharmaceutical ink, polydextrose, polyvinyl alcohol, pregelatinized starch, propyl gallate, silicon dioxide, sucralose, synthetic iron oxide, talc, titanium dioxide, triacetin, xanthan gum

QUESTIONS OR COMMENTS?
Call weekdays from **9 AM to 5 PM EST** toll free at **1-800-88-ADVIL**

ADVIL ALLERGY SINUS (chlorpheniramine maleate, ibuprofen, and pseudoephedrine HCl)
Pfizer Consumer Healthcare

DRUG FACTS

Active Ingredient(s) (in each caplet)
Chlorpheniramine maleate 2 mg
Ibuprofen 200 mg (NSAID)*
Pseudoephedrine HCl 30 mg
*nonsteroidal anti-inflammatory drug

Purpose(s)
Antihistamine
Pain reliever/fever reducer
Nasal decongestant

USES
temporarily relieves these symptoms associated with hay fever or other upper respiratory allergies, and the common cold:
- runny nose
- itchy, watery eyes
- itching of the nose or throat
- sneezing
- nasal congestion
- sinus pressure
- headache
- minor aches and pains
- fever

WARNINGS
Allergy alert:
Ibuprofen may cause a severe allergic reaction, especially in people allergic to aspirin. Symptoms may include:
- hives
- facial swelling
- asthma (wheezing)
- shock
- skin reddening
- rash
- blisters

If an allergic reaction occurs, stop use and seek medical help right away.

Stomach bleeding warning:
This product contains an NSAID, which may cause severe stomach bleeding. The chance is higher if you:
- are age 60 or older
- have had stomach ulcers or bleeding problems
- take a blood thinning (anticoagulant) or steroid drug
- take other drugs containing prescription or nonprescription NSAIDs [aspirin, ibuprofen, naproxen, or others]
- have 3 or more alcoholic drinks every day while using this product
- take more or for a longer time than directed

DO NOT USE
- in children under 12 years of age
- if you have ever had an allergic reaction to any other pain reliever/fever reducer
- right before or after heart surgery
- if you are now taking a prescription monoamine oxidase inhibitor (MAOI) (certain drugs for depression, psychiatric, or emotional conditions, or Parkinson's disease), or for 2 weeks after stopping the MAOI drug. If you do not know if your prescription drug contains an MAOI, ask a doctor or pharmacist before taking this product.

ASK A DOCTOR BEFORE USE IF
- you have a breathing problem such as emphysema or chronic bronchitis
- stomach bleeding warning applies to you
- you have problems or serious side effects from taking pain relievers or fever reducers
- you have a history of stomach problems, such as heartburn
- you have high blood pressure, heart disease, liver cirrhosis, kidney disease, asthma, thyroid disease, diabetes, glaucoma, or trouble urinating due to an enlarged prostate gland
- you are taking a diuretic

ASK A DOCTOR OR PHARMACIST BEFORE USE IF YOU ARE
- under a doctor's care for any serious condition
- taking sedatives or tranquilizers
- taking any other product that contains pseudoephedrine, chlorpheniramine or any other nasal decongestant or antihistamine
- taking aspirin for heart attack or stroke, because ibuprofen may decrease this benefit of aspirin
- taking any other drug

WHEN USING THIS PRODUCT
- take with food or milk if stomach upset occurs
- the risk of heart attack or stroke may increase if you use more than directed or for longer than directed
- avoid alcoholic drinks
- be careful when driving a motor vehicle or operating machinery
- drowsiness may occur
- alcohol, sedatives, and tranquilizers may increase drowsiness

STOP USE AND ASK A DOCTOR IF
- you experience any of the following signs of stomach bleeding:
  - feel faint
  - vomit blood
  - have bloody or black stools
  - have stomach pain that does not get better
- fever gets worse or lasts more than 3 days
- nasal congestion lasts for more than 7 days
- redness or swelling is present in the painful area
- you get nervous, dizzy, or sleepless
- symptoms continue or get worse
- any new symptoms appear

If pregnant or breast-feeding,
ask a health professional before use. It is especially important not to use ibuprofen during the last 3 months of pregnancy unless definitely directed to do so by a doctor because it may cause problems in the unborn child or complications during delivery.

Keep out of reach of children.
In case of overdose, get medical help or contact a Poison Control Center right away.

DIRECTIONS
- **do not take more than directed**
- **the smallest effective dose should be used**
- adults: take 1 caplet every 4-6 hours while symptoms persist.

- do not take more than 6 caplets in any 24-hour period, unless directed by a doctor
- children under 12 years of age: do not use

OTHER INFORMATION
- read all warnings and directions before use. Keep carton.
- store at 20-25°C (68-77°F)
- avoid excessive heat above 40°C (104°F)

INACTIVE INGREDIENTS
carnauba wax, colloidal silicon dioxide, corn starch, croscarmellose sodium, FD&C red no. 40 aluminum lake, FD&C yellow no. 6 aluminum lake, glyceryl behenate, hypromellose, microcrystalline cellulose, pharmaceutical ink, polydextrose, polyethylene glycol, pregelatinized starch, propylene glycol, silicon dioxide, titanium dioxide

QUESTIONS OR COMMENTS?
Call weekdays from **9 AM to 5 PM EST** at **1-800-88-ADVIL**

ADVIL COLD AND SINUS (ibuprofen and pseudoephedrine HCl)
Pfizer Consumer Healthcare

DRUG FACTS
Active Ingredient(s) (in each liquid-filled capsule)
Solubilized ibuprofen equal to 200 mg ibuprofen (NSAID)*
(present as the free acid and potassium salt)
Pseudoephedrine HCl 30 mg
*nonsteroidal anti-inflammatory drug

Purpose(s)
Pain reliever/fever reducer
Nasal decongestant

USES
temporarily relieves these symptoms associated with the common cold or flu:
- headache
- fever
- sinus pressure
- nasal congestion
- minor body aches and pains

WARNINGS
Allergy alert:
Ibuprofen may cause a severe allergic reaction, especially in people allergic to aspirin. Symptoms may include:
- hives
- facial swelling
- asthma (wheezing)
- shock
- skin reddening
- rash
- blisters

If an allergic reaction occurs, stop use and seek medical help right away.

Stomach bleeding warning:
This product contains an NSAID, which may cause severe stomach bleeding. The chance is higher if you:
- are age 60 or older
- have had stomach ulcers or bleeding problems
- take a blood thinning (anticoagulant) or steroid drug
- take other drugs containing prescription or nonprescription NSAIDs [aspirin, ibuprofen, naproxen, or others]
- have 3 or more alcoholic drinks every day while using this product
- take more or for a longer time than directed

DO NOT USE
- in children under 12 years of age
- if you have ever had an allergic reaction to any other pain reliever/fever reducer
- right before or after heart surgery
- if you are now taking a prescription monoamine oxidase inhibitor (MAOI) (certain drugs for depression, psychiatric, or emotional conditions, or Parkinson's disease), or for 2 weeks after stopping the MAOI drug. If you do not know if your prescription drug contains an MAOI, ask a doctor or pharmacist before taking this product.

ASK A DOCTOR BEFORE USE IF
- stomach bleeding warning applies to you
- you have problems or serious side effects from taking pain relievers or fever reducers
- you have a history of stomach problems, such as heartburn
- you have high blood pressure, heart disease, liver cirrhosis, kidney disease, asthma, thyroid disease, diabetes or have trouble urinating due to an enlarged prostate gland
- you are taking a diuretic

ASK A DOCTOR OR PHARMACIST BEFORE USE IF YOU ARE
- under a doctor's care for any serious condition
- taking any other product that contains pseudoephedrine or any other nasal decongestant
- taking aspirin for heart attack or stroke, because ibuprofen may decrease this benefit of aspirin
- taking any other drug

WHEN USING THIS PRODUCT
- take with food or milk if stomach upset occurs
- the risk of heart attack or stroke may increase if you use more than directed or for longer than directed

STOP USE AND ASK A DOCTOR IF
- you experience any of the following signs of stomach bleeding:
  - feel faint
  - vomit blood
  - have bloody or black stools
  - have stomach pain that does not get better
- fever gets worse or lasts more than 3 days
- nasal congestion lasts for more than 7 days
- symptoms continue or get worse
- redness or swelling is present in the painful area
- you get nervous, dizzy, or sleepless
- any new symptoms appear

If pregnant or breast-feeding,
ask a health professional before use. It is especially important not to use ibuprofen during the last 3 months of pregnancy unless definitely directed to do so by a doctor because it may cause problems in the unborn child or complications during delivery.

Keep out of reach of children.
In case of overdose, get medical help or contact a Poison Control Center right away.

DIRECTIONS
- **do not take more than directed**
- **the smallest effective dose should be used**
- adults and children 12 years of age and over:
  - take 1 caplet every 4 to 6 hours while symptoms persist. If symptoms do not respond to 1 caplet, 2 caplets may be used.
  - do not use more than 6 caplets in any 24-hour period unless directed by a doctor
- children under 12 years of age: do not use

OTHER INFORMATION
- **each capsule contains:** potassium 20 mg
- store at 20-25°C (68-77°F). Avoid excessive heat above 40°C (104°F).
- read all warnings and directions before use. Keep carton.

INACTIVE INGREDIENTS
D&C yellow no. 10, FD&C red no. 40, fractionated coconut oil, gelatin, pharmaceutical ink, polyethylene glycol, potassium hydroxide, purified water, sorbitan, sorbitol

QUESTIONS OR COMMENTS?
Call toll free **1-800-88-ADVIL**

ADVIL CONGESTION RELIEF (ibuprofen and phenylephrine HCl)

Pfizer Consumer Healthcare

DRUG FACTS

Active Ingredient(s) (in each tablet)
Ibuprofen 200 mg (NSAID)*
Phenylephrine HCl 10 mg
* nonsteroidal anti-inflammatory drug

Purpose(s)
Pain reliever/fever reducer
Nasal decongestant

USES
- temporarily relieves these symptoms associated with the common cold or flu:
  - headache
  - fever
  - sinus pressure
  - nasal congestion
  - minor body aches and pains
- reduces swelling of the nasal passages
- temporarily restores freer breathing through the nose

WARNINGS
Allergy alert:
Ibuprofen may cause a severe allergic reaction, especially in people allergic to aspirin. Symptoms may include:
- hives
- facial swelling
- asthma (wheezing)
- shock
- skin reddening
- rash
- blisters

If an allergic reaction occurs, stop use and seek medical help right away.

Stomach bleeding warning:
This product contains an NSAID, which may cause severe stomach bleeding. The chance is higher if you:
- are age 60 or older
- have had stomach ulcers or bleeding problems
- take a blood thinning (anticoagulant) or steroid drug
- take other drugs containing prescription or nonprescription NSAIDs [aspirin, ibuprofen, naproxen, or others]
- have 3 or more alcoholic drinks every day while using this product
- take more or for a longer time than directed

DO NOT USE
- in children under 12 years of age because this product contains too much medication for children under this age
- if you have ever had an allergic reaction to any other pain reliever/fever reducer
- right before or after heart surgery
- if you are now taking a prescription monoamine oxidase inhibitor (MAOI) (certain drugs for depression, psychiatric, or emotional conditions, or Parkinson's disease), or for 2 weeks after stopping the MAOI drug. If you do not know if your prescription drug contains an MAOI, ask a doctor or pharmacist before taking this product.

ASK A DOCTOR BEFORE USE IF
- stomach bleeding warning applies to you
- you have problems or serious side effects from taking pain relievers or fever reducers
- you have a history of stomach problems, such as heartburn
- you have high blood pressure, heart disease, liver cirrhosis, kidney disease, asthma, thyroid disease, diabetes, or have trouble urinating due to an enlarged prostate gland
- you are taking a diuretic

ASK A DOCTOR OR PHARMACIST BEFORE USE IF YOU ARE
- under a doctor's care for any serious condition
- taking any other product that contains phenylephrine or any other nasal decongestant
- taking aspirin for heart attack or stroke, because ibuprofen may decrease this benefit of aspirin
- taking any other drug

WHEN USING THIS PRODUCT
- take with food or milk if stomach upset occurs
- the risk of heart attack or stroke may increase if you use more than directed or for longer than directed

STOP USE AND ASK A DOCTOR IF
- you experience any of the following signs of stomach bleeding:
  - feel faint
  - vomit blood
  - have bloody or black stools
  - have stomach pain that does not get better
- pain gets worse or lasts more than 7 days
- fever gets worse or lasts more than 3 days
- nasal congestion lasts for more than 7 days
- symptoms continue or get worse
- redness or swelling is present in the painful area
- you get nervous, dizzy, or sleepless
- any new symptoms appear

If pregnant or breast-feeding,
ask a health professional before use. It is especially important not to use ibuprofen during the last 3 months of pregnancy unless definitely directed to do so by a doctor because it may cause problems in the unborn child or complications during delivery.

Keep out of reach of children.
In case of overdose, get medical help or contact a Poison Control Center right away.

DIRECTIONS
- **do not take more than directed**
- adults and children 12 years of age and over:
  - take 1 tablet every 4 hours while symptoms persist.
  - do not use more than 6 tablets in any 24-hour period unless directed by a doctor
- children under 12 years of age: do not use because this product contains too much medication for children under this age

OTHER INFORMATION
- store at 20-25°C (68-77°F). Avoid excessive heat above 40°C (104°F).
- read all warnings and directions before use. Keep carton.

INACTIVE INGREDIENTS
acesulfame potassium, artificial flavor, carnauba wax, colloidal silicon dioxide, corn starch, croscarmellose sodium, glycerin, hypromellose, lactic acid, lecithin, maltodextrin, medium-chain triglycerides, microcrystalline cellulose, pharmaceutical ink, polydextrose, polyvinyl alcohol, pregelatinized starch, propyl gallate, sodium lauryl sulfate, stearic acid, sucralose, synthetic iron oxide, talc, titanium dioxide, triacetin, xanthan gum

QUESTIONS OR COMMENTS?
Call weekdays from **9 AM to 5 PM** toll free at **1-800-88-ADVIL**
For most recent product information, visit www.advil.com

ADVIL LIQUI-GELS (ibuprofen)
Pfizer Consumer Healthcare

DRUG FACTS

Active Ingredient(s) (in each capsule)
Solubilized ibuprofen equal to 200 mg ibuprofen (NSAID)*
(present as the free acid and potassium salt)
*nonsteroidal anti-inflammatory drug

Purpose(s)
Pain reliever/Fever reducer

USES
- temporarily relieves minor aches and pains due to:
  - headache
  - toothache
  - backache
  - menstrual cramps
  - the common cold
  - muscular aches
  - minor pain of arthritis
- temporarily reduces fever

WARNINGS
Allergy alert:
Ibuprofen may cause a severe allergic reaction, especially in people allergic to aspirin. Symptoms may include:
- hives
- facial swelling
- asthma (wheezing)
- shock
- skin reddening
- rash
- blisters

If an allergic reaction occurs, stop use and seek medical help right away.

Stomach bleeding warning:
This product contains an NSAID, which may cause severe stomach bleeding. The chance is higher if you
- are age 60 or older
- have had stomach ulcers or bleeding problems
- take a blood thinning (anticoagulant) or steroid drug
- take other drugs containing prescription or nonprescription NSAIDs [aspirin, ibuprofen, naproxen, or others]
- have 3 or more alcoholic drinks every day while using this product
- take more or for a longer time than directed

DO NOT USE
- if you have ever had an allergic reaction to any other pain reliever/fever reducer
- right before or after heart surgery

ASK A DOCTOR BEFORE USE IF
- stomach bleeding warning applies to you
- you have problems or serious side effects from taking pain relievers or fever reducers
- you have a history of stomach problems, such as heartburn
- you have high blood pressure, heart disease, liver cirrhosis, kidney disease, or asthma
- you are taking a diuretic

ASK A DOCTOR OR PHARMACIST BEFORE USE IF YOU ARE
- under a doctor's care for any serious condition
- taking aspirin for heart attack or stroke, because ibuprofen may decrease this benefit of aspirin
- taking any other drug

WHEN USING THIS PRODUCT
- take with food or milk if stomach upset occurs
- the risk of heart attack or stroke may increase if you use more than directed or for longer than directed

STOP USE AND ASK A DOCTOR IF
- you experience any of the following signs of stomach bleeding:
  - feel faint
  - vomit blood
  - have bloody or black stools
  - have stomach pain that does not get better
- pain gets worse or lasts more than 10 days
- fever gets worse or lasts more than 3 days
- redness or swelling is present in the painful area
- any new symptoms appear

If pregnant or breast-feeding,
ask a health professional before use. It is especially important not to use ibuprofen during the last 3 months of pregnancy unless definitely directed to do so by a doctor because it may cause problems in the unborn child or complications during delivery.

Keep out of reach of children.
In case of overdose, get medical help or contact a Poison Control Center right away.

DIRECTIONS
- **do not take more than directed**
- **the smallest effective dose should be used**
- adults and children 12 years and over: take 1 capsule every 4 to 6 hours while symptoms persist
- if pain or fever does not respond to 1 capsule, 2 capsules may be used
- do not exceed 6 capsules in 24 hours, unless directed by a doctor
- children under 12 years: ask a doctor

OTHER INFORMATION
- **each capsule contains:** potassium 20 mg
- read all warnings and directions before use. Keep carton.
- store at 20-25°C (68-77°F)
- avoid excessive heat above 40°C (104°F)

INACTIVE INGREDIENTS
FD&C green no. 3, gelatin, light mineral oil, pharmaceutical ink, polyethylene glycol, potassium hydroxide, purified water, sorbitan, sorbitol

QUESTIONS OR COMMENTS?
call toll free **1-800-88-ADVIL**

ADVIL MIGRAINE (ibuprofen)
Pfizer Consumer Healthcare

DRUG FACTS

Active Ingredient(s) (in each brown oval capsule)
Solubilized ibuprofen equal to 200 mg ibuprofen (NSAID)*
(present as the free acid and potassium salt)
*nonsteroidal anti-inflammatory drug

Purpose(s)
Pain reliever

USE
- treats migraine

WARNINGS
Allergy alert:
Ibuprofen may cause a severe allergic reaction, especially in people allergic to aspirin. Symptoms may include:

- hives
- facial swelling
- asthma (wheezing)
- shock
- skin reddening
- rash
- blisters

If an allergic reaction occurs, stop use and seek medical help right away.

Stomach bleeding warning:
This product contains an NSAID, which may cause severe stomach bleeding. The chance is higher if you
- are age 60 or older
- have had stomach ulcers or bleeding problems
- take a blood thinning (anticoagulant) or steroid drug
- take other drugs containing prescription or nonprescription NSAIDs [aspirin, ibuprofen, naproxen, or others]
- have 3 or more alcoholic drinks every day while using this product
- take more or for a longer time than directed

DO NOT USE
- if you have ever had an allergic reaction to any other pain reliever/fever reducer
- right before or after heart surgery

ASK A DOCTOR BEFORE USE IF
- you have never had migraines diagnosed by a health professional
- you have a headache that is different from your usual migraines
- you have the worst headache of your life
- you have fever and stiff neck
- you have headaches beginning after or caused by head injury, exertion, coughing or bending
- you have experienced your first headache after the age of 50
- you have daily headaches
- you have a migraine so severe as to require bed rest
- stomach bleeding warning applies to you
- you have problems or serious side effects from taking pain relievers or fever reducers
- you have a history of stomach problems, such as heartburn
- you have high blood pressure, heart disease, liver cirrhosis, kidney disease, or asthma
- you are taking a diuretic

ASK A DOCTOR OR PHARMACIST BEFORE USE IF YOU ARE
- under a doctor's care for any serious condition
- taking aspirin for heart attack or stroke, because ibuprofen may decrease this benefit of aspirin
- taking any other drug

WHEN USING THIS PRODUCT
- take with food or milk if stomach upset occurs
- the risk of heart attack or stroke may increase if you use more than directed or for longer than directed

STOP USE AND ASK A DOCTOR IF
- you experience any of the following signs of stomach bleeding:
  - feel faint
  - vomit blood
  - have bloody or black stools
  - have stomach pain that does not get better
- migraine headache pain is not relieved or gets worse after the first dose
- any new symptoms appear

If pregnant or breast-feeding,
ask a health professional before use. It is especially important not to use ibuprofen during the last 3 months of pregnancy unless definitely directed to do so by a doctor because it may cause problems in the unborn child or complications during delivery.

Keep out of reach of children.
In case of overdose, get medical help or contact a Poison Control Center right away.

DIRECTIONS
- **do not take more than directed**
- **the smallest effective dose should be used**

adults	take 2 capsules with a glass of water if symptoms persist of worsen, ask your doctor do not take more than 2 capsules in 24 hours, unless directed by a doctor
under 18 years of age	ask a doctor

OTHER INFORMATION
- **each capsule contains:** potassium 20 mg
- read all directions and warnings before use. Keep carton.
- store at 20-25°C (68-77°F)
- avoid excessive heat above 40°C (104°F)

INACTIVE INGREDIENTS
D&C yellow no. 10, FD&C green no. 3, FD&C red no. 40, gelatin, light mineral oil, pharmaceutical ink, polyethylene glycol, potassium hydroxide, purified water, sorbitan, sorbitol

QUESTIONS OR COMMENTS?
Call toll-free **1-800-88-ADVIL**

ADVIL PM CAPLETS (diphenhydramine citrate and ibuprofen)

Pfizer Consumer Healthcare

DRUG FACTS

Active Ingredient(s) (in each caplet)
Diphenhydramine citrate 38 mg
Ibuprofen 200 mg (NSAID)*
*nonsteroidal anti-inflammatory drug

Purpose(s)
Nighttime sleep-aid
Pain reliever

USES
- for relief of occasional sleeplessness when associated with minor aches and pains
- helps you fall asleep and stay asleep

WARNINGS
Allergy alert:
Ibuprofen may cause a severe allergic reaction, especially in people allergic to aspirin. Symptoms may include:
- hives
- facial swelling
- asthma (wheezing)
- shock
- skin reddening
- rash
- blisters

If an allergic reaction occurs, stop use and seek medical help right away.

Stomach bleeding warning:
This product contains an NSAID, which may cause severe stomach bleeding. The chance is higher if you
- are age 60 or older
- have had stomach ulcers or bleeding problems

- take a blood thinning (anticoagulant) or steroid drug
- take other drugs containing prescription or nonprescription NSAIDs [aspirin, ibuprofen, naproxen, or others]
- have 3 or more alcoholic drinks every day while using this product
- take more or for a longer time than directed

DO NOT USE
- if you have ever had an allergic reaction to any other pain reliever/fever reducer
- unless you have time for a full night's sleep
- in children under 12 years of age
- right before or after heart surgery
- with any other product containing diphenhydramine, even one used on skin
- if you have sleeplessness without pain

ASK A DOCTOR BEFORE USE IF
- stomach bleeding warning applies to you
- you have problems or serious side effects from taking pain relievers or fever reducers
- you have a history of stomach problems, such as heartburn
- you have high blood pressure, heart disease, liver cirrhosis, kidney disease, or asthma
- you are taking a diuretic
- you have a breathing problem such as emphysema or chronic bronchitis
- you have glaucoma
- you have trouble urinating due to an enlarged prostate gland

ASK A DOCTOR OR PHARMACIST BEFORE USE IF YOU ARE
- taking sedatives or tranquilizers, or any other sleep-aid
- under a doctor's care for any continuing medical illness
- taking any other antihistamines
- taking aspirin for heart attack or stroke, because ibuprofen may decrease this benefit of aspirin
- taking any other drug

WHEN USING THIS PRODUCT
- drowsiness will occur
- avoid alcoholic drinks
- do not drive a motor vehicle or operate machinery
- take with food or milk if stomach upset occurs
- the risk of heart attack or stroke may increase if you use more than directed or for longer than directed

STOP USE AND ASK A DOCTOR IF
- you experience any of the following signs of stomach bleeding:
  - feel faint
  - vomit blood
  - have bloody or black stools
  - have stomach pain that does not get better
- pain gets worse or lasts more than 10 days
- sleeplessness persists continuously for more than 2 weeks. Insomnia may be a symptom of a serious underlying medical illness.
- redness or swelling is present in the painful area
- any new symptoms appear

If pregnant or breast-feeding,
ask a health professional before use. It is especially important not to use ibuprofen during the last 3 months of pregnancy unless definitely directed to do so by a doctor because it may cause problems in the unborn child or complications during delivery.

Keep out of reach of children.
In case of overdose, get medical help or contact a Poison Control Center right away.

DIRECTIONS
- **do not take more than directed**
- adults and children 12 years and over: take 2 caplets at bedtime
- do not take more than 2 caplets in 24 hours

OTHER INFORMATION
- read all warnings and directions before use. Keep carton.
- store at 20-25°C (68-77°F)
- avoid excessive heat above 40°C (104°F)

INACTIVE INGREDIENTS
calcium stearate, carnauba wax, colloidal silicon dioxide, corn starch, croscarmellose sodium, FD&C blue no. 2 aluminum lake, glyceryl behenate, hypromellose, lactose monohydrate, microcrystalline cellulose, pharmaceutical ink, polydextrose, polyethylene glycol, pregelatinized starch, sodium lauryl sulfate, sodium starch glycolate, stearic acid, titanium dioxide

QUESTIONS OR COMMENTS?
Call weekdays 9 AM to 5 PM EST at **1-800-88-ADVIL**
For most recent product information, visit www.Advil.com.

ADVIL PM LIQUI-GELS (diphenhydramine HCI and ibuprofen)

Pfizer Consumer Healthcare

DRUG FACTS

Active Ingredient(s) (in each capsule)
Diphenhydramine hydrochloride 25 mg
Solubilized ibuprofen equal to 200 mg ibuprofen (NSAID)*
(present as the free acid and potassium salt)
*nonsteroidal anti-inflammatory drug

Purpose(s)
Nighttime sleep-aid
Pain reliever

USES
- for relief of occasional sleeplessness when associated with minor aches and pains
- helps you fall asleep and stay asleep

WARNINGS
Allergy alert:
Ibuprofen may cause a severe allergic reaction, especially in people allergic to aspirin. Symptoms may include:
- hives
- facial swelling
- asthma (wheezing)
- shock
- skin reddening
- rash
- blisters

If an allergic reaction occurs, stop use and seek medical help right away.

Stomach bleeding warning:
This product contains an NSAID, which may cause stomach bleeding. The chance is higher if you
- are age 60 or older
- have had stomach ulcers or bleeding problems
- take a blood thinning (anticoagulant) or steroid drug
- take other drugs containing prescription or nonprescription NSAIDs [aspirin, ibuprofen, naproxen, or others]
- have 3 or more alcoholic drinks every day while using this product
- take more or for a longer time than directed

DO NOT USE
- if you have ever had an allergic reaction to any other pain reliever/fever reducer
- unless you have time for a full night's sleep
- in children under 12 years of age
- right before or after heart surgery
- with any other product containing diphenhydramine, even one used on skin
- if you have sleeplessness without pain

ASK A DOCTOR BEFORE USE IF
- stomach bleeding warning applies to you
- you have problems or serious side effects from taking pain relievers or fever reducers
- you have a history of stomach problems, such as heartburn
- you have high blood pressure, heart disease, liver cirrhosis, kidney disease, or asthma
- you are taking a diuretic
- you have a breathing problem such as emphysema or chronic bronchitis
- you have glaucoma
- you have trouble urinating due to an enlarged prostate gland

ASK A DOCTOR OR PHARMACIST BEFORE USE IF YOU ARE
- taking sedatives or tranquilizers, or any other sleep-aid
- under a doctor's care for any continuing medical illness
- taking any other antihistamines
- taking aspirin for heart attack or stroke, because ibuprofen may decrease this benefit of aspirin
- taking any other drug

WHEN USING THIS PRODUCT
- drowsiness will occur
- avoid alcoholic drinks
- do not drive a motor vehicle or operate machinery
- take with food or milk if stomach upset occurs
- the risk of heart attack or stroke may increase if you use more than directed or for longer than directed

STOP USE AND ASK A DOCTOR IF
- you experience any of the following signs of stomach bleeding:
  - feel faint
  - vomit blood
  - have bloody or black stools
  - have stomach pain that does not get better
- pain gets worse or lasts more than 10 days
- sleeplessness persists continuously for more than 2 weeks. Insomnia may be a symptom of a serious underlying medical illness.
- redness or swelling is present in the painful area
- any new symptoms appear

If pregnant or breast-feeding,
ask a health professional before use. It is especially important not to use ibuprofen during the last 3 months of pregnancy unless definitely directed to do so by a doctor because it may cause problems in the unborn child or complications during delivery.

Keep out of reach of children.
In case of medical overdose, get medical help or contact a Poison Control Center right away.

DIRECTIONS
- **do not take more than directed**
- adults and children 12 years and over: take 2 capsules at bedtime
- do not take more than 2 capsules in 24 hours

OTHER INFORMATION
- **each capsule contains:** potassium 20 mg
- read all warnings and directions before use. Keep carton.
- store at 20-25°C (68-77°F)
- avoid excessive heat above 40°C (104°F)
- protect from light

INACTIVE INGREDIENTS
D&C red no. 33, FD&C blue no. 1, fractionated coconut oil, gelatin, pharmaceutical ink, polyethylene glycol, potassium hydroxide, purified water, sorbitan, sorbitol

QUESTIONS OR COMMENTS?
Call weekdays 9 AM to 5 PM EST at **1-800-88-ADVIL**

CHILDRENS ADVIL SUSPENSION (ibuprofen)
Pfizer Consumer Healthcare

DRUG FACTS

Active Ingredient(s) (in each 5 mL)
Ibuprofen 100 mg (NSAID)*
*nonsteroidal anti-inflammatory drug

Purpose(s)
Fever reducer/Pain reliever

USES
temporarily:
- reduces fever
- relieves minor aches and pains due to the common cold, flu, sore throat, headaches and toothaches

WARNINGS
Allergy alert:
Ibuprofen may cause a severe allergic reaction, especially in people allergic to aspirin. Symptoms may include:
- hives
- facial swelling
- asthma (wheezing)
- shock
- skin reddening
- rash
- blisters

If an allergic reaction occurs, stop use and seek medical help right away.

Stomach bleeding warning:
This product contains an NSAID, which may cause severe stomach bleeding. The chance is higher if the child
- has had stomach ulcers or bleeding problems
- takes a blood thinning (anticoagulant) or steroid drug
- takes other drugs containing prescription or nonprescription NSAIDs [aspirin, ibuprofen, naproxen, or others]
- takes more or for a longer time than directed

Sore throat warning:
Severe or persistent sore throat or sore throat accompanied by high fever, headache, nausea, and vomiting may be serious. Consult doctor promptly. Do not use more than 2 days or administer to children under 3 years of age unless directed by doctor.

DO NOT USE
- if the child has ever had an allergic reaction to any other pain reliever/fever reducer
- right before or after heart surgery

ASK A DOCTOR BEFORE USE IF
- stomach bleeding warning applies to the child
- child has problems or serious side effects from taking pain relievers or fever reducers
- child has a history of stomach problems, such as heartburn
- child has high blood pressure, heart disease, liver cirrhosis, kidney disease, or asthma
- child has not been drinking fluids
- child has lost a lot of fluid due to vomiting or diarrhea
- child is taking a diuretic

ASK A DOCTOR OR PHARMACIST BEFORE USE IF THE CHILD IS
- under a doctor's care for any serious condition
- taking any other drug

WHEN USING THIS PRODUCT
- take with food or milk if stomach upset occurs
- the risk of heart attack or stroke may increase if you use more than directed or for longer than directed

STOP USE AND ASK A DOCTOR IF
- child experiences any of the following signs of stomach bleeding:
  - feels faint
  - vomits blood
  - has bloody or black stools
  - has stomach pain that does not get better
- the child does not get any relief within first day (24 hours) of treatment
- fever or pain gets worse or lasts more than 3 days
- redness or swelling is present in the painful area
- any new symptoms appear

Keep out of reach of children.
In case of overdose, get medical help or contact a Poison Control Center right away.

DIRECTIONS
- **this product does not contain directions or complete warnings for adult use**
- **do not give more than directed**
- **shake well before using**
- find right dose on chart below. If possible, use weight to dose; otherwise use age.
- repeat dose every **6-8 hours**, if needed
- do not use more than **4 times a day**
- measure only with the dosing cup provided. Dosing cup to be used with Children's Advil Suspension only. Do not use with other products. Dose lines account for product remaining in cup due to thickness of suspension.

Dosing Chart

Weight (lb)	Age (yr)	Dose (tsp)
under 24 lb	under 2 yr	ask a doctor
24-35 lb	2-3 yr	1 tsp
36-47 lb	4-5 yr	1½ tsp
48-59 lb	6-8 yr	2 tsp
60-71 lb	9-10 yr	2½ tsp
72-95 lb	11 yr	3 tsp

OTHER INFORMATION
Children's Advil Suspension Fruit Flavor; Children's Advil Suspension Grape Flavor; Children's Advil Suspension White Grape Flavor; Children's Advil Bubblegum
- **each teaspoon contains:** sodium 3 mg
- one dose lasts 6-8 hours
- store at 20-25°C (68-77°F)
- see bottom of box for lot number and expiration date

Children's Advil Suspension Blue Raspberry Flavor
- **each teaspoon contains:** sodium 10 mg
- one dose lasts 6-8 hours
- store at 20-25°C (68-77°F)
- see bottom of box for lot number and expiration date

INACTIVE INGREDIENTS
Children's Advil Suspension Fruit Flavor
artificial flavors, carboxymethylcellulose sodium, citric acid monohydrate, edetate disodium, FD&C red no. 40, glycerin, microcrystalline cellulose, polysorbate 80, purified water, sodium benzoate, sorbitol solution, sucrose, xanthan gum

Children's Advil Suspension Grape Flavor
acetic acid, artificial flavor, butylated hydroxytoluene, carboxymethylcellulose sodium, citric acid monohydrate, edetate disodium, FD&C blue no.1, FD&C red no. 40, glycerin, microcrystalline cellulose, polysorbate 80, propylene glycol, purified water, sodium benzoate, sorbitol solution, sucrose, xanthan gum

Children's Advil Suspension Blue Raspberry Flavor
artificial and natural flavors, carboxymethylcellulose sodium, citric acid monohydrate, edetate disodium, FD&C blue no. 1, glycerin, microcrystalline cellulose, polysorbate 80, propylene glycol, purified water, sodium benzoate, sodium citrate, sorbitol solution, sucrose, xanthan gum

Children's Advil Suspension White Grape Flavor
acetic acid, artificial flavor, butylated hydroxytoluene, carboxymethylcellulose sodium, citric acid monohydrate, edetate disodium, glycerin, microcrystalline cellulose, polysorbate 80, propylene glycol, purified water, sodium benzoate, sorbitol solution, sucrose, xanthan gum

Children's Advil Suspension Bubblegum Flavor
carboxymethylcellulose sodium, citric acid monohydrate, edetate disodium, FD&C red no. 40, glycerin, microcrystalline cellulose, natural and artificial flavor, polysorbate 80, propylene glycol, purified water, sodium benzoate, sorbitol solution, sucrose, xanthan gum

QUESTIONS OR COMMENTS?
call toll-free **1-800-88-ADVIL** or ask your pharmacist, doctor or health care professional

AFTERBITE WITH ANTIHISTIMINE
(diphenhydramine hydrochloride)

Tender Corporation

Active Ingredient(s)
Diphenhydramine 2%

Purpose(s)
Topical Analgesic

USES
For temporary relief of pain and itching caused by
- insect bites
- minor burns
- minor skin irritation
- minor cuts and scrapes

WARNINGS
For external use only.

WHEN USING THIS PRODUCT
- do not get into eyes

DO NOT USE
on chicken pox, poison ivy, sunburn, large areas of the body, broken, blistered or oozing skin, more often than directed, or with any other product containing diphenhydramine, even one taken by mouth.

STOP USE AND ASK A DOCTOR IF
- condition worsens
- symptoms persist for more than 7 days or clear up and occur again within a few days.

Keep out of reach of children
If swallowed get medical help or contact a Poison Control Center right away. If in eyes flush with water for 15 minutes and call a doctor

DIRECTIONS
- Do not use more than directed
- **Adults and children 2 years and older** apply to the affected area not more than 3 to 4 times daily
- **Children under 2 years** ask a doctor
- For a bee sting, remove stinger before treatment

INACTIVE INGREDIENTS
ammonia, carbomer, glycerin, purified water, and tea tree oil

AIRBORNE CHEWABLES

Reckitt Benckiser LLC

DIRECTIONS
For adults and children 12 years and older: Chew 4 tablets per serving. Repeat as necessary; up to 12 tablets per day.

SUPPLEMENT FACTS
Serving Size 4 Chewable Tablets
Servings Per Container 8

Each Serving Contains	Amount Per Serving	%DV
Calories	19	
Total Carbohydrates	5 g	2%*
Vitamin A (as Retinyl Palmitate)	2000 IU	40 %
Vitamin C (as Ascorbic Acid)	1000 mg	1667 %
Vitamin E (as dl-Aplha Tocopheryl Acetate)	30 IU	100 %
Magnesium (as Oxide)	40 mg	10 %
Zinc (as Oxide)	8 mg	53 %
Selenium (as Sodium Selenite)	15 mcg	21 %
Manganese (as Sulfate)	3 mg	150 %
Herbal Extract Proprietary Blend	350 mg	†
Maltodextrin, Lonicera (flower), Forsythia (fruit) Schizonepeta (above-ground parts), Ginger (dried rhizome), Chinese Vitex (fruit), Isatis (root), Echinacea (above-ground parts)		
Amino Acids Blend	50 mg	†
Glutamine (as L-Glutamine), Lysine (as L-Lysine HCl)		
*Percent Daily Values are based on a 2,000 calorie diet.		
†Daily Value not established		

OTHER INGREDIENTS
dextrose, natural and artifical flavors, magnesium stearate, vegetable fibers, sucralose, silicon dioxide, FD&C red #40, FD&C blue #1.
Contains No Artificial Colors orPreservatives.
Store in a cool dry place.

AIRBORNE EFFERVESCENCE

Reckitt Benckiser LLC

SUPPLEMENT FACTS
Serving Size 1 Tablet

Each Serving Contains	Amount Per Serving	%DV
Calories	5	
Total Carbohydrates	1 g	<1%*
Vitamin A (as Retinyl Acetate)	2000 IU	40 %
Vitamin C (as Ascorbic Acid)	1000 mg	1667 %
Vitamin E (as dl-Aplha Tocopheryl Acetate)	30 IU	100 %
Riboflavin (as Riboflavin)	2.8 mg	165 %
Magnesium (as Oxide & Sulfate)	40 mg	10 %
Zinc (as Sulfate)	8 mg	53 %
Selenium (as Chelate)	15 mcg	21%
Manganese (as Gluconate)	3 mg	150%
Sodium (as Bicarbonate)	230 mg	10%
Potassium (as Bicarbonate)	75 mg	2 %
Herbal Extract Proprietary Blend	350 mg	†
Maltodextrin, Lonicera (flower), Forsythia (fruit), Schizonepeta (above-ground parts), Ginger (dried rhizome), Chinese Vitex (fruit), Isatis (root), Echinacea (above-ground parts)		
Amino Acids Blend	50 mg	†
Glutamine (as L-Glutamine), Lysine (as L-Lysine HCl)		
*Percent Daily Values are based on a 2,000 calorie diet.		
†Daily Value not established		

OTHER INGREDIENTS
sorbitol, citric acid, natural and artifical orange flavor, mineral oil, acesulfame potassium, sucralose.
Contains No Artificial Colors or Preservatives.

ALAVERT ALLERGY SINUS D-12 (loratadine and pseudoephedrine sulfate)

Wyeth Consumer Healthcare

DRUG FACTS

Active Ingredient(s) (in each tablet)
Loratadine 5 mg
Pseudoephedrine sulfate 120 mg

Purpose(s)
Antihistamine
Nasal decongestant

USES
- temporarily relieves these symptoms due to hay fever or other upper respiratory allergies:
  - runny nose
  - sneezing
  - itchy, watery eyes
  - itching of the nose or throat
- temporarily relieves nasal congestion due to the common cold, hay fever or other respiratory allergies
- reduces swelling of nasal passages
- temporarily relieves sinus congestion and pressure
- temporarily restores freer breathing through the nose

WARNINGS

DO NOT USE
- if you have ever had an allergic reaction to this product or any of its ingredients
- if you are now taking a prescription monoamine oxidase inhibitor (MAOI) (certain drugs for depression, psychiatric, or emotional conditions, or Parkinson's disease), or for 2 weeks after stopping the MAOI drug. If you do not know if your prescription drug contains an MAOI, ask a doctor or pharmacist before taking this product.

ASK A DOCTOR BEFORE USE IF YOU HAVE
- heart disease
- high blood pressure
- thyroid disease
- diabetes
- trouble urinating due to an enlarged prostate gland
- liver or kidney disease. Your doctor should determine if you need a different dose.

WHEN USING THIS PRODUCT
do not take more than directed.
Taking more than directed may cause drowsiness.

STOP USE AND ASK A DOCTOR IF
- an allergic reaction to this product occurs. Seek medical help right away.
- symptoms do not improve within 7 days or are accompanied by a fever
- nervousness, dizziness or sleeplessness occurs

If pregnant or breast-feeding,
ask a health professional before use.

Keep out of reach of children.
In case of overdose, get medical help or contact a Poison Control Center right away.

DIRECTIONS
- do not divide, crush, chew or dissolve the tablet

Age	Dose
adults and children 12 years and over	1 tablet every 12 hours; not more than 2 tablets in 24 hours
children under 12 years of age	ask a doctor
consumers with liver or kidney disease	ask a doctor

OTHER INFORMATION
- **each tablet contains:** calcium 30 mg
- store between 15° and 25°C (59° and 77°F)
- keep in a dry place

INACTIVE INGREDIENTS
croscarmellose sodium, dibasic calcium phosphate, hypromellose, lactose monohydrate, magnesium stearate, pharmaceutical ink, povidone, titanium dioxide

QUESTIONS OR COMMENTS?
Call weekdays from 9 AM to 5 PM EST at **1-800-ALAVERT** (**1-800-252-8378**)

ALAVERT ALLERGY BUBBLE GUM FLAVOR
(loratadine)

Pfizer Consumer Healthcare

DRUG FACTS

Active Ingredient(s) (in each tablet)
Loratadine 10 mg

Purpose(s)
Antihistamine

USES
temporarily relieves these symptoms due to hay fever or other upper respiratory allergies:
- runny nose
- sneezing
- itchy, watery eyes
- itching of the nose or throat

WARNINGS

DO NOT USE
if you have ever had an allergic reaction to this product or any of its ingredients

ASK A DOCTOR BEFORE USE IF YOU HAVE
liver or kidney disease. Your doctor should determine if you need a different dose.

WHEN USING THIS PRODUCT
do not use more than directed. Taking more than recommended may cause drowsiness.

STOP USE AND ASK A DOCTOR IF
an allergic reaction to this product occurs. Seek medical help right away.

If pregnant or breast-feeding,
ask a health professional before use.

Keep out of reach of children.
In case of overdose, get medical help or contact a Poison Control Center right away.

DIRECTIONS
- tablet melts in mouth. Can be taken with or without water.

Age	Dose
adults and children 6 years and over	1 tablet daily; do not use more than 1 tablet daily
children under 6	ask a doctor
consumers who have liver or kidney disease	ask a doctor

OTHER INFORMATION
- **Phenylketonurics:** Contains Phenylalanine 8.4 mg per tablet
- store at 20-25°C (68-77°F)
- keep in a dry place

INACTIVE INGREDIENTS
anhydrous citric acid, artificial and natural flavor, ascorbic acid, aspartame, colloidal silicon dioxide, crospovidone, ferric oxide, magnesium stearate, maltodextrin, mannitol, microcrystalline cellulose, modified starch, sodium bicarbonate

QUESTIONS OR COMMENTS?
call weekdays from 9 AM to 5 PM EST at **1-800-ALAVERT** (**1-800-252-8378**)

ALAVERT ALLERGY FRESH MINT & CITRUS BURST (loratadine)

Pfizer Consumer Healthcare

DRUG FACTS

Active Ingredient(s) (in each tablet)	Purpose(s)
Loratadine 10 mg	Antihistamine

USES
temporarily relieves these symptoms due to hay fever or other upper respiratory allergies:
- runny nose
- sneezing
- itchy, watery eyes
- itching of the nose or throat

WARNINGS

DO NOT USE
if you have ever had an allergic reaction to this product or any of its ingredients

ASK A DOCTOR BEFORE USE IF YOU HAVE
liver or kidney disease. Your doctor should determine if you need a different dose.

WHEN USING THIS PRODUCT
do not use more than directed. Taking more than recommended may cause drowsiness.

STOP USE AND ASK A DOCTOR IF
an allergic reaction to this product occurs. Seek medical help right away.
If pregnant or breast-feeding, ask a health professional before use.
Keep out of reach of children. In case of overdose, get medical help or contact a Poison Control Center right away.

DIRECTIONS
- tablet melts in mouth. Can be taken with or without water.

Age	Dose
adults and children 6 years and over	1 tablet daily; do not use more than 1 tablet daily
children under 6	ask a doctor
consumers who have liver or kidney disease	ask a doctor

OTHER INFORMATION
- **Phenylketonurics**: Contains Phenylalanine 8.4 mg per tablet
- store at 20-25°C (68-77°F)
- keep in a dry place

INACTIVE INGREDIENTS
Alavert Allergy Fresh Mint
anhydrous citric acid, aspartame, colloidal silicon dioxide, corn syrup solids, crospovidone, magnesium stearate, mannitol, microcrystalline cellulose, modified starch, natural and artificial flavors, sodium bicarbonate

Alavert Allergy Citrus Burst
anhydrous citric acid, aspartame, butylated hydroxyanisole, colloidal silicon dioxide, corn syrup solids, crospovidone, dextrin, ferric oxides, magnesium stearate, maltodextrin, mannitol, microcrystalline cellulose, modified starch, natural and artificial flavors, sodium bicarbonate

QUESTIONS OR COMMENTS?
call weekdays from 9 AM to 5 PM EST at **1-800-ALAVERT** (**1-800-252-8378**)

ALEVE CAPLETS (naproxen sodium)

Bayer HealthCare

DRUG FACTS

Active Ingredient(s) (in each caplet)	Purpose(s)
Naproxen sodium 220 mg (naproxen 200 mg) (NSAID)*	Pain reliever/fever reducer
*nonsteroidal anti-inflammatory drug	

USES
- temporarily relieves minor aches and pains due to:
  - minor pain of arthritis
  - muscular aches
  - backache
  - menstrual cramps
  - headache
  - toothache
  - the common cold
- temporarily reduces fever

WARNINGS
Allergy alert
Naproxen sodium may cause a severe allergic reaction, especially in people allergic to aspirin. Symptoms may include:
- hives
- facial swelling
- asthma (wheezing)
- shock
- skin reddening
- rash
- blisters

If an allergic reaction occurs, stop use and seek medical help right away.

Stomach Bleeding Warning
This product contains an NSAID, which may cause severe stomach bleeding. The chance is higher if you:
- are age 60 or older
- have had stomach ulcers or bleeding problems
- take a blood thinning (anticoagulant) or steroid drug
- take other drugs containing prescription or nonprescription NSAIDs (aspirin, ibuprofen, naproxen, or others)
- have 3 or more alcoholic drinks every day while using this product
- take more or for a longer time than directed

DO NOT USE
- if you have ever had an allergic reaction to any other pain reliever/fever reducer
- right before or after heart surgery

ASK A DOCTOR BEFORE USE IF
- the stomach bleeding warning applies to you
- you have a history of stomach problems, such as heartburn
- you have high blood pressure, heart disease, liver cirrhosis, or kidney disease
- you are taking a diuretic

- you have problems or serious side effects from taking pain relievers or fever reducers
- you have asthma

ASK A DOCTOR OR PHARMACIST BEFORE USE IF YOU ARE
- under a doctor's care for any serious condition
- taking any other drug

WHEN USING THIS PRODUCT
- take with food or milk if stomach upset occurs
- the risk of heart attack or stroke may increase if you use more than directed or for longer than directed

STOP USE AND ASK A DOCTOR IF
- you experience any of the following signs of stomach bleeding:
  - feel faint
  - vomit blood
  - have bloody or black stools
  - have stomach pain that does not get better
- pain gets worse or lasts more than 10 days
- fever gets worse or lasts more than 3 days
- you have difficulty swallowing
- it feels like the pill is stuck in your throat
- redness or swelling is present in the painful area
- any new symptoms appear

If pregnant or breast-feeding, ask a health professional before use. It is especially important not to use naproxen sodium during the last 3 months of pregnancy unless definitely directed to do so by a doctor because it may cause problems in the unborn child or complications during delivery.
Keep out of reach of children. In case of overdose, get medical help or contact a Poison Control Center right away.

DIRECTIONS
- **do not take more than directed**
- **the smallest effective dose should be used**
- drink a full glass of water with each dose

Adults and Children 12 years and older
- take 1 caplet every 8 to 12 hours while symptoms last
- for the first dose you may take 2 caplets within the first hour
- do not exceed 2 caplets in any 8- to 12-hour period
- do not exceed 3 caplets in a 24-hour period

Children under 12 years
- ask a doctor

OTHER INFORMATION
- **each caplet contains:** sodium 20 mg
- store at 20-25°C (68-77°F). Avoid high humidity and excessive heat above 40°C (104°F).

INACTIVE INGREDIENTS
FD&C blue #2 lake, hypromellose, magnesium stearate, microcrystalline cellulose, polyethylene glycol, povidone, talc, titanium dioxide

QUESTIONS OR COMMENTS?
1-800-395-0689 (Mon-Fri 9AM - 5PM EST) or www.aleve.com

ALEVE GELCAPS (naproxen sodium)
Bayer HealthCare

DRUG FACTS

Active Ingredient(s) (in each tablet)	Purpose(s)
Naproxen sodium 220 mg (naproxen 200 mg) (NSAID)*	Pain reliever/fever reducer
*nonsteroidal anti-inflammatory drug	

USES
- temporarily relieves minor aches and pains due to:
  - minor pain of arthritis
  - muscular aches
  - backache
  - menstrual cramps
  - headache
  - toothache
  - the common cold
- temporarily reduces fever

WARNINGS
Allergy alert: Naproxen sodium may cause a severe allergic reaction, especially in people allergic to aspirin. Symptoms may include:
- hives
- facial swelling
- asthma (wheezing)
- shock
- skin reddening
- rash
- blisters

If an allergic reaction occurs, stop use and seek medical help right away.
Stomach Bleeding Warning:
This product contains an NSAID, which may cause severe stomach bleeding. The chance is higher if you:
- are age 60 or older
- have had stomach ulcers or bleeding problems
- take a blood thinning (anticoagulant) or steroid drug
- take other drugs containing prescription or nonprescription NSAIDs (aspirin, ibuprofen, naproxen, or others)
- have 3 or more alcoholic drinks every day while using this product
- take more or for a longer time than directed

DO NOT USE
- if you have ever had an allergic reaction to any other pain reliever/fever reducer
- right before or after heart surgery

ASK A DOCTOR BEFORE USE IF
- the stomach bleeding warning applies to you
- you have a history of stomach problems, such as heartburn
- you have high blood pressure, heart disease, liver cirrhosis, or kidney disease
- you are taking a diuretic
- you have problems or serious side effects from taking pain relievers or fever reducers
- you have asthma

ASK A DOCTOR OR PHARMACIST BEFORE USE IF YOU ARE
- under a doctor's care for any serious condition
- taking any other drug

WHEN USING THIS PRODUCT
- take with food or milk if stomach upset occurs

- the risk of heart attack or stroke may increase if you use more than directed or for longer than directed

STOP USE AND ASK A DOCTOR IF
- you experience any of the following signs of stomach bleeding:
  - feel faint
  - vomit blood
  - have bloody or black stools
  - have stomach pain that does not get better
- pain gets worse or lasts more than 10 days
- fever gets worse or lasts more than 3 days
- you have difficulty swallowing
- it feels like the pill is stuck in your throat
- redness or swelling is present in the painful area
- any new symptoms appear

If pregnant or breast-feeding, ask a health professional before use. It is especially important not to use naproxen sodium during the last 3 months of pregnancy unless definitely directed to do so by a doctor because it may cause problems in the unborn child or complications during delivery.
Keep out of reach of children. In case of overdose, get medical help or contact a Poison Control Center right away.

DIRECTIONS
- **do not take more than directed**
- **the smallest effective dose should be used**
- drink a full glass of water with each dose

Adults and Children 12 years and older
- take 1 tablet every 8 to 12 hours while symptoms last
- for the first dose you may take 2 tablets within the first hour
- do not exceed 2 tablets in any 8- to 12-hour period
- do not exceed 3 tablets in a 24-hour period

Children under 12 years
- ask a doctor

OTHER INFORMATION
- **each tablet contains:** sodium 20 mg
- store at 20-25°C (68-77°F). Avoid high humidity and excessive heat above 40°C (104°F).

INACTIVE INGREDIENTS
D&C yellow #10 aluminum lake, edetate disodium, edible ink, FD&C blue #1, FD&C yellow #6 aluminum lake, gelatin, glycerin, hypromellose, magnesium stearate, microcrystalline cellulose, polyethylene glycol, povidone, stearic acid, talc, titanium dioxide

QUESTIONS OR COMMENTS?
1-800-395-0689 (Mon-Fri 9AM - 5PM EST) or www.aleve.com

ALEVE LIQUID GELS (naproxen sodium)
Bayer HealthCare

DRUG FACTS

Active Ingredient(s) (in each capsule)	Purpose(s)
Naproxen sodium 220 mg (naproxen 200 mg) (NSAID)*	Pain reliever/fever reducer
*nonsteroidal anti-inflammatory drug	

USES
- temporarily relieves minor aches and pains due to:
  - minor pain of arthritis
  - muscular aches
  - backache
  - menstrual cramps
  - headache
  - toothache
  - the common cold
- temporarily reduces fever

WARNINGS
Allergy alert
Naproxen sodium may cause a severe allergic reaction, especially in people allergic to aspirin. Symptoms may include:
- hives
- facial swelling
- asthma (wheezing)
- shock
- skin reddening
- rash
- blisters

If an allergic reaction occurs, stop use and seek medical help right away.

Stomach Bleeding Warning
This product contains an NSAID, which may cause severe stomach bleeding. The chance is higher if you:
- are age 60 or older
- have had stomach ulcers or bleeding problems
- take a blood thinning (anticoagulant) or steroid drug
- take other drugs containing prescription or nonprescription NSAIDs (aspirin, ibuprofen, naproxen, or others)
- have 3 or more alcoholic drinks every day while using this product
- take more or for a longer time than directed

DO NOT USE
- if you have ever had an allergic reaction to any other pain reliever/fever reducer
- right before or after heart surgery

ASK A DOCTOR BEFORE USE IF
- the stomach bleeding warning applies to you
- you have a history of stomach problems, such as heartburn
- you have high blood pressure, heart disease, liver cirrhosis, or kidney disease
- you are taking a diuretic
- you have problems or serious side effects from taking pain relievers or fever reducers
- you have asthma

ASK A DOCTOR OR PHARMACIST BEFORE USE IF YOU ARE
- under a doctor's care for any serious condition
- taking any other drug

WHEN USING THIS PRODUCT
- take with food or milk if stomach upset occurs
- the risk of heart attack or stroke may increase if you use more than directed or for longer than directed

STOP USE AND ASK A DOCTOR IF
- you experience any of the following signs of stomach bleeding:
  - feel faint
  - vomit blood
  - have bloody or black stools
  - have stomach pain that does not get better
- pain gets worse or lasts more than 10 days
- fever gets worse or lasts more than 3 days
- redness or swelling is present in the painful area
- any new symptoms appear
- you have difficulty swallowing
- it feels like the capsule is stuck in your throat

If pregnant or breast-feeding, ask a health professional before use. It is especially important not to use naproxen sodium during the last 3 months of pregnancy unless definitely directed to do so by a doctor because it may cause problems in the unborn child or complications during delivery.

Keep out of reach of children. In case of overdose, get medical help or contact a Poison Control Center right away.

DIRECTIONS
- **do not take more than directed**
- **the smallest effective dose should be used**
- drink a full glass of water with each dose
- if taken with food, this product may take longer to work

Adults and Children 12 years and older
- take 1 capsule every 8 to 12 hours while symptoms last
- for the first dose you may take 2 capsules within the first hour
- do not exceed 2 capsules in any 8- to 12-hour period
- do not exceed 3 capsules in a 24-hour period

Children under 12 years
- ask a doctor

OTHER INFORMATION
- **each capsule contains:** sodium 20 mg
- store at 20-25°C (68-77°F) avoid high humidity and excessive heat above 40°C (104°F).
- read all directions and warnings before use. Keep carton.

INACTIVE INGREDIENTS
FD&C blue #1, gelatin, glycerin, lactic acid, mannitol, pharmaceutical ink, polyethylene glycol, povidone, propylene glycol, purified water, sorbitan, sorbitol

QUESTIONS OR COMMENTS?
1-800-395-0689 (Mon-Fri 9AM - 5PM EST) or www.aleve.com

ALEVE (naproxen sodium) tablets, 220 mg (nsaid) pain reliever/fever reducer

Bayer HealthCare

DRUG FACTS

Active Ingredient(s) (in each caplet)	Purpose(s)
Naproxen sodium 220 mg (naproxen 200 mg) (NSAID)*	Pain reliever/fever reducer

USES
temporarily relieves minor aches and pains due to:
- minor pain of arthritis
- muscular aches
- backache
- menstrual cramps
- headache
- toothache
- the common cold
- temporarily reduces fever

WARNINGS
Allergy alert
Naproxen sodium may cause a severe allergic reaction, especially in people allergic to aspirin.
Symptoms may include:
- hives
- facial swelling
- asthma (wheezing)
- shock
- skin reddening
- rash
- blisters

If an allergic reaction occurs, stop use and seek medical help right away.

Stomach bleeding warning:
This product contains an NSAID, which may cause severe stomach bleeding. The chance is higher if you:
- are age 60 or older
- have had stomach ulcers or bleeding problems
- take a blood thinning (anticoagulant) or steroid drug
- take other drugs containing prescription or nonprescription NSAIDs(aspirin, ibuprofen, naproxen, or others)
- have 3 or more alcoholic drinks every day while using this product

take more or for a longer time than directed

DO NOT USE
- if you have ever had an allergic reaction to any other pain reliever/fever reducer
- right before or after heart surgery

ASK A DOCTOR BEFORE USE IF
- the stomach bleeding warning applies to you
- you have a history of stomach problems, such as heartburn
- you have high blood pressure, heart disease, liver cirrhosis, or kidney disease
- you are taking a diuretic
- you have problems or serious side effects from taking pain relievers or
- fever reducers
- you have asthma

ASK A DOCTOR OR PHARMACIST BEFORE USE IF
- under a doctor's care for any serious condition
- taking any other drug

WHEN USING THIS PRODUCT
- take with food or milk if stomach upset occurs
- the risk of heart attack or stroke may increase if you use more than directed or for longer than directed

STOP USE AND ASK A DOCTOR IF
- you experience any of the following signs of stomach bleeding:
- feel faint
- vomit blood
- have bloody or black stools
- have stomach pain that does not get better
- pain gets worse or lasts more than 10 days
- fever gets worse or lasts more than 3 days
- you have difficulty swallowing or it feels like the pill is stuck in your throat
- redness or swelling is present in the painful area
- any new symptoms appear

If pregnant or breast-feeding, ask a health professional before use. It is especially important not to use naproxen sodium during the last 3 months of pregnancy unless definitely directed to do so by a doctor because it may cause problems in the unborn child or complications during delivery. Keep out of reach of children. In case of overdose, get medical help or contact a Poison Control Center right away.

DIRECTIONS
- do not take more than directed
- the smallest effective dose should be used
- drink a full glass of water with each dose

Adults and children 12 years and older: **take 1 tablet every 8 to 12 hours while symptoms last**
- for the first dose you may take 2 tablets within the first hour
- do not exceed 2 tablets in any 8- to 12-hour period
- do not exceed 3 tablets in a 24-hour period

Children under 12 years: ask a doctor

OTHER INFORMATION
- **each tablet contains: sodium 20 mg**
- store at 20-25°C (68-77°F).
- Avoid high humidity and excessive heat above 40°C (104°F).

INACTIVE INGREDIENTS
FD&C blue #2 lake, hypromellose, magnesium stearate, microcrystalline cellulose, polyethylene glycol, povidone, talc, titanium dioxide

QUESTIONS OR COMMENTS?
1-800-395-0689 (Mon -Fri 9AM - 5PM EST) or www.aleve.com

ALEVE - D SINUS & COLD CAPLETS
(naproxen sodium and pseudoephedrine hydrochloride)
Bayer HealthCare

DRUG FACTS

Active Ingredient(s) (in each caplet)	Purpose(s)
Naproxen sodium 220 mg (naproxen 200 mg) (NSAID)*	Pain reliever/fever reducer
Pseudoephedrine HCl 120 mg, extended-release	Nasal decongestant
*nonsteroidal anti-inflammatory drug	

USES
temporarily relieves these cold, sinus, and flu symptoms:
- sinus pressure
- minor body aches and pains
- headache
- nasal and sinus congestion (promotes sinus drainage and restores freer breathing through the nose)
- fever

WARNINGS
Allergy alert
Naproxen sodium may cause a severe allergic reaction, especially in people allergic to aspirin. Symptoms may include:
- hives
- facial swelling
- asthma (wheezing)
- shock
- skin reddening
- rash
- blisters

If an allergic reaction occurs, stop use and seek medical help right away.

Stomach bleeding warning
This product contains an NSAID, which may cause severe stomach bleeding. The chance is higher if you:
- are age 60 or older
- have had stomach ulcers or bleeding problems
- take a blood thinning (anticoagulant) or steroid drug
- take other drugs containing prescription or nonprescription NSAIDs (aspirin, ibuprofen, naproxen, or others)
- have 3 or more alcoholic drinks every day while using this product
- take more or for a longer time than directed

DO NOT USE
- if you have ever had an allergic reaction to any other pain reliever/fever reducer
- right before or after heart surgery
- if you are now taking a prescription monoamine oxidase inhibitor (MAOI) (certain drugs for depression, psychiatric, or emotional conditions, or Parkinson's disease), or for 2 weeks after stopping the MAOI drug. If you do not know if your prescription drug contains an MAOI, ask a doctor or pharmacist before taking this product.
- in children under 12 years of age

ASK A DOCTOR BEFORE USE IF
- the stomach bleeding warning applies to you
- you have a history of stomach problems, such as heartburn
- you have high blood pressure, heart disease, liver cirrhosis, or kidney disease
- you are taking a diuretic
- you have problems or serious side effects from taking pain relievers or fever reducers
- you have
  - asthma
  - diabetes
  - thyroid disease
  - trouble urinating due to an enlarged prostate gland

ASK A DOCTOR OR PHARMACIST BEFORE USE IF YOU ARE
- under a doctor's care for any serious condition
- taking any other drug

WHEN USING THIS PRODUCT
- take with food or milk if stomach upset occurs
- the risk of heart attack or stroke may increase if you use more than directed or for longer than directed

STOP USE AND ASK A DOCTOR IF
- you experience any of the following signs of stomach bleeding:
  - feel faint
  - vomit blood
  - have bloody or black stools
  - have stomach pain that does not get better
- redness or swelling is present in the painful area
- any new symptoms appear
- fever gets worse or lasts more than 3 days
- you have difficulty swallowing or the caplet feels stuck in your throat
- you get nervous, dizzy, or sleepless
- nasal congestion lasts more than 7 days

If pregnant or breast-feeding, ask a health professional before use. It is especially important not to use naproxen sodium during the last 3 months of pregnancy unless definitely directed to do so by a doctor because it may cause problems in the unborn child or complications during delivery.
Keep out of reach of children. In case of overdose, get medical help or contact a Poison Control Center right away.

DIRECTIONS
- **do not take more than directed**
- **the smallest effective dose should be used**
- **swallow whole;** do not crush or chew
- **drink a full glass of water with each dose**
- adults and children 12 years and older: **1 caplet every 12 hours;** do not take more than 2 caplets in 24 hours
- children under 12 years: do not use

OTHER INFORMATION
- **each caplet contains:** sodium 22 mg
- store at 20-25°C (68-77°F)
- store in a dry place

INACTIVE INGREDIENTS
colloidal silicon dioxide, hypromellose, lactose monohydrate, magnesium stearate, microcrystalline cellulose, polyethylene glycol, polysorbate 80, povidone, talc, titanium dioxide

QUESTIONS OR COMMENTS?
1-800-986-0369 (Mon-Fri 9AM - 5PM EST) or www.AleveD.com

ALEVE - D SINUS & HEADACHE CAPLETS
(naproxen sodium and pseudoephedrine hydrochloride)

Bayer HealthCare

DRUG FACTS

Active Ingredient(s) (in each caplet)	Purpose(s)
Naproxen sodium 220 mg (naproxen 200 mg) (NSAID)*	Pain reliever/fever reducer
Pseudoephedrine HCl 120 mg, extended-release	Nasal decongestant
*nonsteroidal anti-inflammatory drug	

USES
temporarily relieves these cold, sinus, and flu symptoms:
- sinus pressure
- minor body aches and pains
- headache
- nasal and sinus congestion (promotes sinus drainage and restores freer breathing through the nose)
- fever

WARNINGS
Allergy alert
Naproxen sodium may cause a severe allergic reaction, especially in people allergic to aspirin. Symptoms may include:
- hives
- facial swelling
- asthma (wheezing)
- shock
- skin reddening
- rash
- blisters

If an allergic reaction occurs, stop use and seek medical help right away.

Stomach bleeding warning
This product contains an NSAID, which may cause severe stomach bleeding. The chance is higher if you:
- are age 60 or older
- have had stomach ulcers or bleeding problems
- take a blood thinning (anticoagulant) or steroid drug
- take other drugs containing prescription or nonprescription NSAIDs (aspirin, ibuprofen, naproxen, or others)
- have 3 or more alcoholic drinks every day while using this product
- take more or for a longer time than directed

DO NOT USE
- if you have ever had an allergic reaction to any other pain reliever/fever reducer
- right before or after heart surgery
- if you are now taking a prescription monoamine oxidase inhibitor (MAOI) (certain drugs for depression, psychiatric, or emotional conditions, or Parkinson's disease), or for 2 weeks after stopping the MAOI drug. If you do not know if your prescription drug contains an MAOI, ask a doctor or pharmacist before taking this product.
- in children under 12 years of age

ASK A DOCTOR BEFORE USE IF
- the stomach bleeding warning applies to you
- you have a history of stomach problems, such as heartburn
- you have high blood pressure, heart disease, liver cirrhosis, or kidney disease
- you are taking a diuretic
- you have problems or serious side effects from taking pain relievers or fever reducers
- you have
- asthma
- diabetes
- thyroid disease
- trouble urinating due to an enlarged prostate gland

ASK A DOCTOR OR PHARMACIST BEFORE USE IF YOU ARE
- under a doctor's care for any serious condition
- taking any other drug

WHEN USING THIS PRODUCT
- take with food or milk if stomach upset occurs
- the risk of heart attack or stroke may increase if you use more than directed or for longer than directed

STOP USE AND ASK A DOCTOR IF
- you experience any of the following signs of stomach bleeding:
  - feel faint
  - vomit blood
  - have bloody or black stools
  - have stomach pain that does not get better
- redness or swelling is present in the painful area
- any new symptoms appear
- fever gets worse or lasts more than 3 days
- you have difficulty swallowing or the caplet feels stuck in your throat
- you get nervous, dizzy, or sleepless
- nasal congestion lasts more than 7 days

If pregnant or breast-feeding, ask a health professional before use. It is especially important not to use naproxen sodium during the last 3 months of pregnancy unless definitely directed to do so by a doctor because it may cause problems in the unborn child or complications during delivery.
Keep out of reach of children. In case of overdose, get medical help or contact a Poison Control Center right away.

DIRECTIONS
- **do not take more than directed**
- **the smallest effective dose should be used**
- **swallow whole;** do not crush or chew
- **drink a full glass of water with each dose**
- adults and children 12 years and older: **1 caplet every 12 hours;** do not take more than 2 caplets in 24 hours
- children under 12 years: do not use

OTHER INFORMATION
- **each caplet contains:** sodium 22 mg
- store at 20-25°C (68-77°F)
- store in a dry place

INACTIVE INGREDIENTS
colloidal silicon dioxide, hypromellose, lactose monohydrate, magnesium stearate, microcrystalline cellulose, polyethylene glycol, polysorbate 80, povidone, talc, titanium dioxide

QUESTIONS OR COMMENTS?
1-800-986-0369 (Mon - Fri 9AM - 5PM EST) or www.AleveD.com

ALIGN PROBIOTIC SUPPLEMENT
Procter & Gamble

ALIGN SUPPLEMENT FACTS

Probiotic strain: Bifantis (*Bifidobacterium infantis* 35624), contains 1×10^9 colony-forming units (1 billion) (4 mg) when manufactured and provides an effective level of bacteria (1×10^7) until at least the "best buy" date, microcrystalline cellulose, hypromellose, sucrose, magnesium stearate, sodium caseinate, titanium dioxide, sodium citrate dihydrate, propyl gallate (antioxidant). Contains: Milk

DIRECTIONS
- Take one capsule per day.
- Store at room temperature.
- For best results, we recommend to keep capsules in original blister packaging until use.

WARNINGS
- Parental supervision is recommended for use of Align by children. We recommend that you keep Align out of the reach of children.

OTHER INFORMATION
- As with other probiotics, in the first few days of taking Align, some consumers have reported experiencing some gas and bloating. This may be temporary while your system is adjusting to Align. For more information, take a look at how the My Align Advisor® program can help you when you start taking Align.

QUESTIONS OR COMMENTS?
Call (800) 208-0112 or **contact us by email.**

ALKA-SELTZER XTRA STRENGTH (anhydrous citric acid, sodium bicarbonate, and aspirin)
Bayer HealthCare

DRUG FACTS

Active Ingredient(s) (in each tablet)	Purpose(s)
Anhydrous citric acid 1000 mg	Antacid
Aspirin 500 mg	Analgesic
Sodium bicarbonate (heat-treated) 1985 mg	Antacid

USES
for the relief of:
- heartburn, acid indigestion, and sour stomach when accompanied with headache or body aches and pains
- upset stomach with headache from overindulgence in food or drink
- headache, body aches, and pain alone

WARNINGS
Reye's syndrome: Children and teenagers should not use this medicine for chicken pox or flu symptoms before a doctor is consulted about Reye's syndrome, a rare but serious illness reported to be associated with aspirin.
Allergy alert: Aspirin may cause a severe allergic reaction which may include:
- hives
- facial swelling
- asthma (wheezing)
- shock

Alcohol warning: If you consume 3 or more alcoholic drinks every day, ask your doctor whether you should take aspirin or other pain relievers/fever reducers.
Aspirin may cause stomach bleeding.

DO NOT USE
if you are allergic to aspirin or any other pain reliever/fever reducer

ASK A DOCTOR BEFORE USE IF YOU HAVE
- asthma
- ulcers
- bleeding problems
- stomach problems that last or come back frequently, such as heartburn, upset stomach, or pain
- a sodium-restricted diet

ASK A DOCTOR OR PHARMACIST BEFORE USE IF YOU ARE
- presently taking a prescription drug. Antacids may interact with certain prescription drugs.
- taking a prescription drug for anticoagulation (blood thinning), diabetes, gout, or arthritis

WHEN USING THIS PRODUCT
do not exceed recommended dosage

STOP USE AND ASK A DOCTOR IF
- an allergic reaction occurs. Seek medical help right away.
- symptoms get worse or last more than 10 days
- redness or swelling is present
- ringing in the ears or loss of hearing occurs
- new symptoms occur

If pregnant or breast-feeding, ask a health professional before use. **It is especially important not to use aspirin during the last 3 months of pregnancy unless definitely directed to do so by a doctor because it may cause problems in the unborn child or complications during delivery.**
Keep out of reach of children. In case of overdose, get medical help or contact a Poison Control Center right away.

DIRECTIONS
- fully dissolve 2 tablets in 4 ounces of water before taking

adults and children 12 years and over	2 tablets every 6 hours, or as directed by a doctor	do not exceed 7 tablets in 24 hours
adults 60 years and over	2 tablets every 6 hours, or as directed by a doctor	do not exceed 3 tablets in 24 hours
children under 12 years	consult a doctor	

OTHER INFORMATION
- **each tablet contains:** sodium 588 mg
- store at room temperature. Avoid excessive heat.
- Alka-Seltzer Extra Strength in water contains principally the antacid sodium citrate and the analgesic sodium acetylsalicylate

INACTIVE INGREDIENTS
flavor

QUESTIONS OR COMMENTS?
1-800-986-0369 (Mon - Fri 9AM - 5PM EST) or www.alkaseltzer.com

ALKA-SELTZER FRUIT CHEWS (calcium carbonate)

Bayer HealthCare

DRUG FACTS

Active Ingredient(s) (in each chewable tablet)	Purpose(s)
Calcium carbonate 750 mg	Antacid

USES
- acid indigestion
- heartburn
- sour stomach
- upset stomach associated with these symptoms

WARNINGS
do not use if you have ever had an allergic reaction to this product or any of its ingredients

ASK A DOCTOR OR PHARMACIST BEFORE USE IF YOU ARE
presently taking a prescription drug. Antacids may interact with certain prescription drugs

WHEN USING THIS PRODUCT
- **do not take more than 10 chewable tablets in a 24-hour period**
- **do not use the maximum dosage of this product for more than 2 weeks except under the advice and supervision of a physician**
- **constipation may occur**
- **If pregnant or breast-feeding,** ask a health professional before use.
- **Keep out of reach of children.**

DIRECTIONS
- do not take more than 10 chewable tablets in a 24-hour period

adults and children 12 years and over	chew and swallow 1-2 chewable tablets every 2 to 4 hours as symptoms occur, or as directed by a doctor
children under 12 years	consult a doctor

OTHER INFORMATION
- **each chewable tablet contains:** calcium 300 mg
- contains FD&C Yellow No. 5 (tartrazine) as a color additive
- store at room temperature. Avoid humidity. Close cap tightly after use.

INACTIVE INGREDIENTS
acacia, beeswax, carmine, carnauba wax, citric acid, corn starch, corn syrup, DL-alpha tocopherol, FD&C blue #1 aluminum lake, FD&C red #40 aluminum lake, FD&C yellow #5 lake (tartrazine), FD&C yellow #6, FD&C yellow #6 aluminum lake, FD&C yellow #6 lake, flavors, hydrogenated coconut oil, medium chain triglycerides, methyl paraben, modified starch, phosphoric acid, pregelatinized modified starch, propyl paraben, propylene glycol, purified water, shellac, sodium benzoate, sorbic acid, sorbitol, soy lecithin, sucrose, titanium dioxide

QUESTIONS OR COMMENTS?
call **1-800-986-0369** (Mon – Fri 9AM – 5PM EST) or visit www.alkaseltzer.com

ALKA-SELTZER GOLD (anhydrous citric acid, potassium bicarbonate, and sodium bicarbonate)

Bayer HealthCare

Active Ingredient(s) (in each tablet).	Purpose(s)
Anhydrous citric acid 1000 mg	Antacid
Potassium bicarbonate 344 mg	Antacid
Sodium bicarbonate (heat-treated) 1050 mg	Antacid

USES
for the relief of:
- heartburn
- acid indigestion
- sour stomach

WARNINGS
Do not use if you have ever had an allergic reaction to this product or any of its ingredients

ASK A DOCTOR BEFORE USE IF YOU HAVE
- kidney disease
- a potassium or sodium-restricted diet

ASK A DOCTOR OR PHARMACIST BEFORE USE IF YOU ARE
presently taking a prescription drug. Antacids may interact with certain prescription drugs.
When using this product do not exceed recommended dosage

STOP USE AND ASK A DOCTOR
if you have taken the maximum dose for 2 weeks
If pregnant or breast-feeding, ask a health professional before use.
Keep out of reach of children.

DIRECTIONS
- fully dissolve tablets in 4 ounces of water before taking

adults and children 12 years and older
- 2 tablets every 4 hours as needed, or as directed by a doctor
- do not exceed 8 tablets in 24 hours

adults 60 years and over
- 2 tablets every 4 hours as needed, or as directed by a doctor
- do not exceed 6 tablets in 24 hours

Children under 12 years
- 1 tablet every 4 hours as needed, or as directed by a doctor
- do not exceed 4 tablets in 24 hours

OTHER INFORMATION
- **each tablet contains:** potassium 135 mg
- **each tablet contains:** sodium 309 mg
- store at room temperature. Avoid excessive heat
- this product does not contain aspirin
- Alka-Seltzer Gold in water contains principally the antacids sodium citrate and potassium citrate

INACTIVE INGREDIENTS
magnesium stearate, mannitol

QUESTIONS OR COMMENTS?
1-800-986-0369 (Mon - Fri 9AM - 5PM EST) or www.alkaseltzer.com

ALKA-SELTZER HEARTBURN (anhydrous citric acid and sodium bicarbonate)
Bayer HealthCare

DRUG FACTS

Active Ingredient(s) (in each tablet)	Purpose(s)
Anhydrous citric acid 1000 mg	Antacid
Sodium bicarbonate (heat-treated) 1940 mg	Antacid

USES
for the relief of
• heartburn
• acid indigestion
• upset stomach associated with these symptoms

WARNINGS

ASK A DOCTOR BEFORE USE IF YOU HAVE
a sodium-restricted diet

ASK A DOCTOR OR PHARMACIST BEFORE USE IF YOU ARE
presently taking a prescription drug. Antacids may interact with certain prescription drugs.

WHEN USING THIS PRODUCT
do not exceed recommended dosage

STOP USE AND ASK A DOCTOR IF
you have taken the maximum dose for 2 weeks
If pregnant or breast-feeding, ask a health professional before use.
Keep out of reach of children.

DIRECTIONS
• fully dissolve 2 tablets in 4 ounces of water before taking

adults and children 12 years and over	2 tablets every 4 hours as needed, or as directed by a doctor	do not exceed 8 tablets in 24 hours
adults 60 years and over	2 tablets every 4 hours as needed, or as directed by a doctor	do not exceed 4 tablets in 24 hours
children under 12 years	consult a doctor	

OTHER INFORMATION
• **each tablet contains:** sodium 575 mg
• **phenylketonurics:** contains phenylalanine 5.6 mg per tablet
• store at room temperature. Avoid excessive heat.
• Alka-Seltzer Heartburn in water contains the antacid sodium citrate as the principal active ingredient

INACTIVE INGREDIENTS
acesulfame potassium, aspartame, flavors, magnesium stearate, mannitol

QUESTIONS OR COMMENTS?
1-800-986-0369 (Mon - Fri 9AM - 5PM EST) or www.alkaseltzer.com

ALKA-SELTZER LEMON-LIME (anhydrous citric acid, aspirin, and sodium bicarbonate)
Bayer HealthCare

Active Ingredient(s) (in each tablet).	Purpose(s)
Anhydrous citric acid 1000 mg	Antacid
Aspirin 325 mg (NSAID)*	Analgesic
Sodium bicarbonate (heat-treated) 1700 mg	Antacid
*nonsteroidal anti-inflammatory drug	

USES
for the temporary relief of:
• heartburn, acid indigestion, and sour stomach when accompanied with headache or body aches and pains
• upset stomach with headache from overindulgence in food or drink
• pain alone (headache or body and muscular aches and pains)

WARNINGS
Reye's syndrome: Children and teenagers who have or are recovering from chicken pox or flu-like symptoms should not use this product. When using this product, if changes in behavior with nausea and vomiting occur, consult a doctor because these symptoms could be an early sign of Reye's syndrome, a rare but serious illness.
Allergy alert: Aspirin may cause a severe allergic reaction which may include:
• hives
• facial swelling
• asthma (wheezing)
• shock
Stomach bleeding warning: This product contains an NSAID, which may cause severe stomach bleeding. The chance is higher if you
• are age 60 or older
• have had stomach ulcers or bleeding problems
• take a blood thinning (anticoagulant) or steroid drug
• take other drugs containing prescription or nonprescription NSAIDs (aspirin, ibuprofen, naproxen, or others)
• have 3 or more alcoholic drinks every day while using this product
• take more or for a longer time than directed

DO NOT USE
if you are allergic to aspirin or any other pain reliever/fever reducer

ASK A DOCTOR BEFORE USE IF
• stomach bleeding warning applies to you
• you have a history of stomach problems, such as heartburn
• you have high blood pressure, heart disease, liver cirrhosis, or kidney disease
• you are taking a diuretic
• you have asthma
• you have a sodium-restricted diet

ASK A DOCTOR OR PHARMACIST BEFORE USE IF YOU ARE
• presently taking a prescription drug. Antacids may interact with certain prescription drugs.
• taking a prescription drug for diabetes, gout, or arthritis

WHEN USING THIS PRODUCT
do not exceed recommended dosage

STOP USE AND ASK A DOCTOR IF
- an allergic reaction occurs. Seek medical help right away.
- you experience any of the following signs of stomach bleeding
  - feel faint
  - vomit blood
  - have bloody or black stools
  - have stomach pain that does not get better
- symptoms get worse or last more than 10 days
- redness or swelling is present
- ringing in the ears or a loss of hearing occurs
- new symptoms occur

If pregnant or breast-feeding, ask a health professional before use. **It is especially important not to use aspirin during the last 3 months of pregnancy unless definitely directed to do so by a doctor because it may cause problems in the unborn child or complications during delivery.**
Keep out of reach of children. In case of overdose, get medical help or contact a Poison Control Center right away.

DIRECTIONS
- fully dissolve 2 tablets in 4 ounces of water before taking

adults and children 12 years and over
- 2 tablets every 4 hours, or as directed by a doctor
- do not exceed 8 tablets in 24 hours

adults 60 years and over
- 2 tablets every 4 hours, or as directed by a doctor
- do not exceed 4 tablets in 24 hours

children under 12 years
- consult a doctor

OTHER INFORMATION
- **each tablet contains:** sodium 504 mg
- Phenylketonurics: Contains Phenylalanine 9 mg Per Tablet
- store at room temperature. Avoid excessive heat.
- Alka-Seltzer Lemon Lime in water contains principally the antacid sodium citrate and the analgesic sodium acetylsalicylate

INACTIVE INGREDIENTS
aspartame, docusate sodium, flavor, povidone, sodium benzoate

QUESTIONS OR COMMENTS?
1-800-986-0369 (Mon - Fri 9AM - 5PM EST) or www.alkaseltzer.com

ALKA-SELTZER (citric acid, aspirin, and sodium bicarbonate)

Bayer HealthCare

Active Ingredient(s) (in each tablet).	Purpose(s)
Aspirin 325 mg	Analgesic
Citric acid 1000 mg	Antacid
Sodium bicarbonate (heat treated) 1916 mg	Antacid

Keep out of reach of children
In case of overdose, get medical help or contact a Poison Control Center right away.

USES
for the relief of:
- heartburn, acid indigestion, and sour stomach when accompanied with headache or body aches and pains
- upset stomach with headache from overindulgence in food or drink
- headache, body aches, and pain alone

WARNINGS
Reye's syndrome
Children and teenagers should not use this medicine for chicken pox or flu symptoms before a doctor is consulted about Reye's syndrome, a rare but serious illness reported to be associated with aspirin.

Allergy alert
Aspirin may cause a severe allergic reaction which may include:
- hives
- asthma (wheezing)

Alcohol warning: If you consume 3 or more alcoholic drinks every day, ask your doctor whether you should take aspirin or other pain relievers/fever reducers. Aspirin may cause stomach bleeding.

DIRECTIONS
- fully dissolve 2 tablets in 4 ounces of water before taking

adults and children 12 years and over
- 2 tablets every 4 hours, or as directed by a doctor
- do not exceed 8 tablets in 24 hours

adults 60 years and over
- 2 tablets every 4 hours, or as directed by a doctor
- do not exceed 4 tablets in 24 hours

children under 12 years
- consult a doctor

OTHER INFORMATION
- **each tablet contains:** sodium 567 mg
- store at room temperature. Avoid excessive heat.
- Alka-Seltzer in water contains principally the antacid sodium citrate and the analgesic sodium acetylsalicylate

INACTIVE INGREDIENTS
none

QUESTIONS OR COMMENTS?
1-800-986-0369 (Mon - Fri 9AM - 5PM EST) or www.alkaseltzer.com

ALKA-SELTZER PLUS ALLERGY
(diphenhydramine hydrochloride)

Bayer HealthCare

DRUG FACTS
Active Ingredient(s) (in each tablet)
Diphenhydramine hydrochloride 25 mg

Purpose(s)
Antihistamine

USES
- temporarily relieves these symptoms due to hay fever or other upper respiratory allergies:
  - runny nose
  - sneezing
  - itching of the nose or throat
  - itchy, watery eyes
- temporarily relieves these symptoms due to the common cold:
  - runny nose
  - sneezing

WARNINGS
Do not use to sedate children.

DO NOT USE
- with any other product containing diphenhydramine, even one used on the skin
- in children under 12 years of age

ASK A DOCTOR BEFORE USE IF YOU HAVE
- a breathing problem such as emphysema or chronic bronchitis
- difficulty in urination due to enlargement of the prostate gland
- glaucoma

ASK A DOCTOR OR PHARMACIST BEFORE USE IF YOU ARE
taking sedatives or tranquilizers

WHEN USING THIS PRODUCT
- may cause marked drowsiness
- avoid alcoholic drinks
- alcohol, sedatives, and tranquilizers may increase the drowsiness effect
- use caution when driving a motor vehicle or operating machinery
- excitability may occur, especially in children

If pregnant or breast-feeding, ask a health professional before use.
Keep out of reach of children. In case of overdose, get medical help or contact a Poison Control Center right away.

DIRECTIONS
- do not take more than the recommended dose
- adults and children 12 years and over: take 1 to 2 tablets every 4 to 6 hours. Do not exceed 12 tablets in 24 hours or as directed by a doctor
- children under 12 years: do not use

OTHER INFORMATION
- **each tablet contains:** calcium 20 mg
- store at controlled room temperature 15-30°C (59-86°F). Protect from light and moisture

INACTIVE INGREDIENTS
croscarmellose sodium, D&C red #27, dibasic calcium phosphate dihydrate, magnesium stearate, microcrystalline cellulose, polyethylene glycol, polyvinyl alcohol, talc, titanium dioxide

QUESTIONS OR COMMENTS?
1-800-986-0369
(Mon-Fri 9AM - 5PM EST) or www.alkaseltzerplus.com
Distributed by:
Bayer HealthCare LLC
Consumer Care
P.O. Box 1910
Morristown, NJ 07962-1910 USA

ALKA-SELTZER PLUS COLD FORMULA CHERRY BURST (aspirin, chlorpheniramine maleate, and phenylephrine bitartrate)
Bayer HealthCare

Active Ingredient(s) (in each tablet).	Purpose(s)
Aspirin 325 mg (NSAID)*	Pain reliever/fever reducer
Chlorpheniramine maleate 2 mg	Antihistamine
Phenylephrine bitartrate 7.8 mg	Nasal decongestant
*nonsteroidal anti-inflammatory drug	

USES
temporarily relieves these symptoms due to a cold:
- minor aches and pains
- headache
- runny nose
- nasal and sinus congestion
- sneezing
- sore throat

temporarily reduces fever

WARNINGS
Reye's syndrome: Children and teenagers who have or are recovering from chicken pox or flu-like symptoms should not use this product. When using this product, if changes in behavior with nausea and vomiting occur, consult a doctor because these symptoms could be an early sign of Reye's syndrome, a rare but serious illness.
Allergy alert:
Aspirin may cause a severe allergic reaction which may include:
- hives
- facial swelling
- asthma (wheezing)
- shock

Stomach bleeding warning: This product contains an NSAID, which may cause severe stomach bleeding. The chance is higher if you
- are age 60 or older
- have had stomach ulcers or bleeding problems
- take a blood thinning (anticoagulant) or steroid drug
- take other drugs containing prescription or nonprescription NSAIDs (aspirin, ibuprofen, naproxen, or others)
- have 3 or more alcoholic drinks every day while using this product
- take more or for a longer time than directed

Sore throat warning: If sore throat is severe, persists for more than 2 days, is accompanied or followed by fever, headache, rash, nausea, or vomiting, consult a doctor promptly. **Do not use to sedate children.**

DO NOT USE
- if you are allergic to aspirin or any other pain reliever/fever reducer
- if you are now taking a prescription monoamine oxidase inhibitor (MAOI) (certain drugs for depression, psychiatric, or emotional conditions, or Parkinson's disease), or for 2 weeks after stopping the MAOI drug. If you do not know if your prescription drug contains an MAOI, ask a doctor or pharmacist before taking this product.
- if you have ever had an allergic reaction to this product or any of its ingredients
- in children under 12 years of age

ASK A DOCTOR BEFORE USE IF

- stomach bleeding warning applies to you
- you have a history of stomach problems, such as heartburn
- you have high blood pressure, heart disease, liver cirrhosis, or kidney disease
- you are taking a diuretic
- you have
  - asthma
  - diabetes
  - thyroid disease
  - glaucoma
  - difficulty in urination due to enlargement of the prostate gland
  - a breathing problem such as emphysema or chronic bronchitis
  - a sodium-restricted diet

ASK A DOCTOR OR PHARMACIST BEFORE USE IF YOU ARE

- taking a prescription drug for
  - gout
  - diabetes
  - arthritis
- taking sedatives or tranquilizers

WHEN USING THIS PRODUCT

- **do not exceed recommended dosage**
- excitability may occur, especially in children
- you may get drowsy
- avoid alcoholic drinks
- alcohol, sedatives, and tranquilizers may increase drowsiness
- be careful when driving a motor vehicle or operating machinery

STOP USE AND ASK A DOCTOR IF

- an allergic reaction occurs. Seek medical help right away.
- you experience any of the following signs of stomach bleeding
  - feel faint
  - vomit blood
  - have bloody or black stools
  - have stomach pain that does not get better
- pain or nasal congestion gets worse or lasts more than 7 days
- fever gets worse or lasts more than 3 days
- redness or swelling is present
- new symptoms occur
- ringing in the ears or a loss of hearing occurs
- nervousness, dizziness, or sleeplessness occurs

If pregnant or breast-feeding, ask a health professional before use. **It is especially important not to use aspirin during the last 3 months of pregnancy unless definitely directed to do so by a doctor because it may cause problems in the unborn child or complications during delivery.**
Keep out of reach of children. In case of overdose, get medical help or contact a Poison Control Center right away.

DIRECTIONS

adults and children 12 years and over:
- take 2 tablets fully dissolved in 4 oz of water every 4 hours.
- do not exceed 8 tablets in 24 hours or as directed by a doctor.

children under 12 years:
- do not use

OTHER INFORMATION

- **each tablet contains:** sodium 476 mg
- Phenylketonurics: Contains Phenylalanine 10 mg Per Tablet
- store at room temperature. Avoid excessive heat.

INACTIVE INGREDIENTS

acesulfame potassium, anhydrous citric acid, aspartame, calcium silicate, dimethylpolysiloxane, docusate sodium, FD&C red #40, flavors, mannitol, povidone, sodium benzoate, sodium bicarbonate

QUESTIONS OR COMMENTS?
1-800-986-0369 (Mon - Fri 9AM - 5PM EST) or
www.alkaseltzerplus.com

ALKA-SELTZER PLUS COLD & COUGH FORMULA (acetaminophen, chlorpheniramine maleate, dextromethorphan hydrobromide, and phenylephrine hydrochloride)

Bayer HealthCare

Active Ingredient(s) (in each capsule).	Purpose(s)
Acetaminophen 325 mg	Pain reliever/fever reducer
Chlorpheniramine maleate 2 mg	Antihistamine
Dextromethorphan hydrobromide 10 mg	Cough suppressant
Phenylephrine hydrochloride 5 mg	Nasal decongestant

USES

- temporarily relieves these symptoms due to a cold or flu:
  - minor aches and pains
  - headache
  - nasal and sinus congestion
  - cough
  - runny nose
  - sneezing
  - sore throat
- temporarily reduces fever

WARNINGS

Liver warning
This product contains acetaminophen. Severe liver damage may occur if you take
- more than 12 capsules in 24 hours, which is the maximum daily amount
- with other drugs containing acetaminophen
- 3 or more alcoholic drinks every day while using this product

Sore throat warning
If sore throat is severe, persists for more than 2 days, is accompanied or followed by fever, headache, rash, nausea, or vomiting, consult a doctor promptly.
Do not use to sedate children.

DO NOT USE

- with any other drug containing acetaminophen (prescription or nonprescription). If you are not sure whether a drug contains acetaminophen, ask a doctor or pharmacist.
- if you are now taking a prescription monoamine oxidase inhibitor (MAOI) (certain drugs for depression, psychiatric, or emotional conditions, or Parkinson's disease), or for 2 weeks after stopping the MAOI drug. If you do not know if your prescription drug contains an MAOI, ask a doctor or pharmacist before taking this product.
- in children under 12 years of age

ASK A DOCTOR BEFORE USE IF YOU HAVE

- liver disease
- heart disease
- high blood pressure
- thyroid disease
- diabetes
- glaucoma
- cough with excessive phlegm (mucus)
- a breathing problem such as emphysema or chronic bronchitis

- difficulty in urination due to enlargement of the prostate gland
- persistent or chronic cough such as occurs with smoking, asthma, or emphysema

ASK A DOCTOR OR PHARMACIST BEFORE USE IF YOU ARE
- taking the blood thinning drug warfarin
- taking sedatives or tranquilizers

WHEN USING THIS PRODUCT
- **do not exceed recommended dosage**
- may cause marked drowsiness
- avoid alcoholic drinks
- alcohol, sedatives, and tranquilizers may increase drowsiness
- be careful when driving a motor vehicle or operating machinery
- excitability may occur, especially in children

STOP USE AND ASK A DOCTOR IF
- pain, cough, or nasal congestion gets worse or lasts more than 7 days
- fever gets worse or lasts more than 3 days
- redness or swelling is present
- new symptoms occur
- cough comes back or occurs with rash or headache that lasts. These could be signs of a serious condition.
- nervousness, dizziness, or sleeplessness occurs

If pregnant or breast-feeding, ask a health professional before use.
Keep out of reach of children. In case of overdose, get medical help or contact a Poison Control Center right away. Quick medical attention is critical for adults as well as for children even if you do not notice any signs or symptoms.

DIRECTIONS
do not take more than the recommended dose
adults and children 12 years and over:
- take 2 capsules with water every 4 hours.
- do not exceed 12 capsules in 24 hours or as directed by a doctor.

children under 12 years:
- do not use

OTHER INFORMATION
- store at room temperature. Avoid excessive heat.

INACTIVE INGREDIENTS
butylated hydroxyanisole, butylated hydroxytoluene, D&C red #33, FD&C blue #1, gelatin, glycerin, hypromellose, mannitol, polyethylene glycol 400, polyethylene glycol 600, povidone, propylene glycol, purified water, sorbitan, sorbitol, titanium dioxide

QUESTIONS OR COMMENTS?
1-800-986-0369 (Mon - Fri 9AM - 5PM EST) or www.alkaseltzerplus.com

ALKA-SELTZER PLUS DAY & NIGHT MULTI-SYMPTOM COLD & FLU FORMULA
(acetaminophen, dextromethorphan hydrobromide, doxylamine succinate, and phenylephrine hydrochloride)
Bayer HealthCare

Day Cold & Flu:

Active Ingredient(s) (in each capsule).	Purpose(s)
Acetaminophen 325 mg	Pain reliever/fever reducer
Dextromethorphan hydrobromide 10 mg	Cough suppressant
Phenylephrine hydrochloride 5 mg	Nasal decongestant

USES
- temporarily relieves these symptoms due to a cold or flu:
  - minor aches and pains
  - headache
  - cough
  - sore throat
  - nasal and sinus congestion
- temporarily reduces fever

WARNINGS
Liver warning: This product contains acetaminophen. Severe liver damage may occur if you take
- more than 10 capsules in 24 hours, which is the maximum daily amount for this product
- with other drugs containing acetaminophen
- 3 or more alcoholic drinks every day while using this product

Sore throat warning: If sore throat is severe, persists for more than 2 days, is accompanied or followed by fever, headache, rash, nausea, or vomiting, consult a doctor promptly.

DO NOT USE
- with any other drug containing acetaminophen (prescription or nonprescription). If you are not sure whether a drug contains acetaminophen, ask a doctor or pharmacist.
- if you are now taking a prescription monoamine oxidase inhibitor (MAOI) (certain drugs for depression, psychiatric, or emotional conditions, or Parkinson's disease), or for 2 weeks after stopping the MAOI drug. If you do not know if your prescription drug contains an MAOI, ask a doctor or pharmacist before taking this product.
- in children under 12 years of age

ASK A DOCTOR BEFORE USE IF YOU HAVE
- liver disease
- heart disease
- high blood pressure
- thyroid disease
- diabetes
- cough with excessive phlegm (mucus)
- difficulty in urination due to enlargement of the prostate gland
- persistent or chronic cough such as occurs with smoking, asthma, or emphysema

ASK A DOCTOR OR PHARMACIST BEFORE USE IF YOU ARE
taking the blood thinning drug warfarin

WHEN USING THIS PRODUCT
do not exceed recommended dosage

STOP USE AND ASK A DOCTOR IF
- pain, cough, or nasal congestion gets worse or lasts more than 7 days
- fever gets worse or lasts more than 3 days
- redness or swelling is present
- new symptoms occur
- cough comes back or occurs with rash or headache that lasts. These could be signs of a serious condition.
- nervousness, dizziness, or sleeplessness occurs

If pregnant or breast-feeding, ask a health professional before use.
Keep out of reach of children. In case of overdose, get medical help or contact a Poison Control Center right away. Quick medical attention is critical for adults as well as for children even if you do not notice any signs or symptoms.

DIRECTIONS
do not take more than the recommended dose
adults and children 12 years and over:
- take 2 capsules with water every 4 hours.
- do not exceed 12 capsules in 24 hours or as directed by a doctor

children under 12 years:
- do not use

OTHER INFORMATION
- store at room temperature. Avoid excessive heat.

INACTIVE INGREDIENTS
FD&C red #40, FD&C yellow #6, gelatin, glycerin, mannitol, polyethylene glycol 400, povidone, propylene glycol, purified water, shellac, simethicone, sorbitol sorbitan solution, titanium dioxide

QUESTIONS OR COMMENTS?
1-800-986-0369 (Mon - Fri 9AM - 5PM EST) or www.alkaseltzerplus.com

Night Cold & Flu:

Active Ingredient(s) (in each capsule).	Purpose(s)
Acetaminophen 325 mg	Pain reliever/fever reducer
Dextromethorphan hydrobromide 10 mg	Cough suppressant
Doxylamine succinate 6.25 mg	Antihistamine
Phenylephrine hydrochloride 5 mg	Nasal decongestant

USES
- temporarily relieves these symptoms due to a cold or flu:
  - minor aches and pains
  - headache
  - nasal and sinus congestion
  - cough
  - sore throat
  - runny nose
  - sneezing
- temporarily reduces fever

WARNINGS
Liver warning: This product contains acetaminophen. Severe liver damage may occur if you take
- more than 10 capsules in 24 hours, which is the maximum daily amount
- with other drugs containing acetaminophen
- 3 or more alcoholic drinks every day while using this product

Sore throat warning: If sore throat is severe, persists for more than 2 days, is accompanied or followed by fever, headache, rash, nausea, or vomiting, consult a doctor promptly.
Do not use to sedate children.

DO NOT USE
- with any other drug containing acetaminophen (prescription or nonprescription). If you are not sure whether a drug contains acetaminophen, ask a doctor or pharmacist.
- if you are now taking a prescription monoamine oxidase inhibitor (MAOI) (certain drugs for depression, psychiatric, or emotional conditions, or Parkinson's disease), or for 2 weeks after stopping the MAOI drug. If you do not know if your prescription drug contains an MAOI, ask a doctor or pharmacist before taking this product.
- in children under 12 years of age

ASK A DOCTOR BEFORE USE IF YOU HAVE
- liver disease
- heart disease
- high blood pressure
- thyroid disease
- diabetes
- glaucoma
- cough with excessive phlegm (mucus)
- a breathing problem such as emphysema or chronic bronchitis
- difficulty in urination due to enlargement of the prostate gland
- persistent or chronic cough such as occurs with smoking, asthma, or emphysema

ASK A DOCTOR OR PHARMACIST BEFORE USE IF YOU ARE
- taking the blood thinning drug warfarin
- taking sedatives or tranquilizers

WHEN USING THIS PRODUCT
- **do not exceed recommended dosage**
- may cause marked drowsiness
- avoid alcoholic drinks
- alcohol, sedatives, and tranquilizers may increase drowsiness
- be careful when driving a motor vehicle or operating machinery
- excitability may occur, especially in children

STOP USE AND ASK A DOCTOR IF
- pain, cough, or nasal congestion gets worse or lasts more than 7 days
- fever gets worse or lasts more than 3 days
- redness or swelling is present
- new symptoms occur
- cough comes back or occurs with rash or headache that lasts. These could be signs of a serious condition.
- nervousness, dizziness, or sleeplessness occurs

If pregnant or breast-feeding, ask a health professional before use.
Keep out of reach of children. In case of overdose, get medical help or contact a Poison Control Center right away. Quick medical attention is critical for adults as well as for children even if you do not notice any signs or symptoms.

DIRECTIONS
do not take more than the recommended dose
adults and children 12 years and over:
- take 2 capsules with water every 4 hours.
- do not exceed 10 capsules in 24 hours or as directed by a doctor.

children under 12 years:
- do not use

OTHER INFORMATION
- store at room temperature. Avoid excessive heat.

INACTIVE INGREDIENTS
D&C yellow #10, FD&C blue #1, gelatin, glycerin, mannitol, polyethylene glycol 400, povidone, propylene glycol, purified water, shellac, simethicone, sorbitan, sorbitol, titanium dioxide

QUESTIONS OR COMMENTS?
1-800-986-0369 (Mon - Fri 9AM - 5PM EST) or
www.alkaseltzerplus.com

ALKA-SELTZER PLUS DAY NON-DROWSY COLD AND FLU FORMULA (acetaminophen, dextromethorphan hydrobromide, and phenylephrine hydrochloride)

Bayer HealthCare

DRUG FACTS

Active Ingredient(s) (in each capsule)	Purpose(s)
Acetaminophen 325 mg	Pain reliever/fever reducer
Dextromethorphan hydrobromide 10 mg	Cough suppressant
Phenylephrine hydrochloride 5 mg	Nasal decongestant

USES
- temporarily relieves these symptoms due to a cold or flu:
  - minor aches and pains
  - headache
  - cough
  - sore throat
  - nasal and sinus congestion
- temporarily reduces fever

WARNINGS
Liver warning
This product contains acetaminophen. Severe liver damage may occur if you take
- more than 10 capsules in 24 hours, which is the maximum daily amount for this product
- with other drugs containing acetaminophen
- 3 or more alcoholic drinks every day while using this product

Sore throat warning
If sore throat is severe, persists for more than 2 days, is accompanied or followed by fever, headache, rash, nausea, or vomiting, consult a doctor promptly.

DO NOT USE
- with any other drug containing acetaminophen (prescription or nonprescription). If you are not sure whether a drug contains acetaminophen, ask a doctor or pharmacist.
- if you are now taking a prescription monoamine oxidase inhibitor (MAOI) (certain drugs for depression, psychiatric, or emotional conditions, or Parkinson's disease), or for 2 weeks after stopping the MAOI drug. If you do not know if your prescription drug contains an MAOI, ask a doctor or pharmacist before taking this product.
- in children under 12 years of age

ASK A DOCTOR BEFORE USE IF YOU HAVE
- liver disease
- heart disease
- high blood pressure
- thyroid disease
- diabetes
- cough with excessive phlegm (mucus)
- difficulty in urination due to enlargement of the prostate gland
- persistent or chronic cough such as occurs with smoking, asthma, or emphysema

ASK A DOCTOR OR PHARMACIST BEFORE USE IF YOU ARE
taking the blood thinning drug warfarin

WHEN USING THIS PRODUCT
do not exceed recommended dosage

STOP USE AND ASK A DOCTOR IF
- pain, cough, or nasal congestion gets worse or lasts more than 7 days
- fever gets worse or lasts more than 3 days
- redness or swelling is present
- new symptoms occur
- cough comes back or occurs with rash or headache that lasts. These could be signs of a serious condition.
- nervousness, dizziness, or sleeplessness occurs

If pregnant or breast-feeding, ask a health professional before use.
Keep out of reach of children. In case of overdose, get medical help or contact a Poison Control Center right away. Quick medical attention is critical for adults as well as for children even if you do not notice any signs or symptoms.

DIRECTIONS
- do not take more than the recommended dose
- adults and children 12 years and over: take 2 capsules with water every 4 hours. Do not exceed 10 capsules in 24 hours or as directed by a doctor
- children under 12 years: do not use

OTHER INFORMATION
- store at room temperature. Avoid excessive heat.

INACTIVE INGREDIENTS
FD&C red #40, FD&C yellow #6, gelatin, glycerin, mannitol, polyethylene glycol 400, povidone, propylene glycol, purified water, shellac, simethicone, sorbitol sorbitan solution, titanium dioxide

QUESTIONS OR COMMENTS?
1-800-986-0369 (Mon-Fri 9AM - 5PM EST) or
www.alkaseltzerplus.com
Distributed by:
Bayer HealthCare LLC
P.O. Box 1910 Morristown, NJ 07962-1910

ALKA-SELTZER PLUS DAY SEVERE COLD, COUGH & FLU (acetaminophen, dextromethorphan hydrobromide, and phenylephrine hydrochloride)

Bayer HealthCare

DRUG FACTS

Active Ingredient(s) (in each packet)	Purpose(s)
Acetaminophen 650 mg	Pain reliever/fever reducer
Dextromethorphan hydrobromide 20 mg	Cough Suppressant
Phenylephrine hydrochloride 10 mg	Nasal decongestant

USES
temporarily relieves these symptoms due to a cold or flu:
- minor aches and pains
- headache
- cough
- sore throat

- nasal and sinus congestion
- temporarily reduces fever

WARNINGS
Liver warning
This product contains acetaminophen. Severe liver damage may occur if you take
- more than 5 packets in 24 hours, which is the maximum daily amount for this product
- with other drugs containing acetaminophen
- 3 or more alcoholic drinks every day while using this product

Sore throat warning
If sore throat is severe, persists for more than 2 days, is accompanied or followed by fever, headache, rash, nausea, or vomiting, consult a doctor promptly.

DO NOT USE
- if you have ever had an allergic reaction to this product or any of its ingredients
- with any other drug containing acetaminophen (prescription or nonprescription). If you are not sure whether a drug contains acetaminophen, ask a doctor or pharmacist.
- if you are now taking a prescription monoamine oxidase inhibitor (MAOI) (certain drugs for depression, psychiatric, or emotional conditions, or Parkinson's disease), or for 2 weeks after stopping the MAOI drug. If you do not know if your prescription drug contains an MAOI, ask a doctor or pharmacist before taking this product.
- in children under 12 years of age

ASK A DOCTOR BEFORE USE IF YOU HAVE
- liver disease
- heart disease
- high blood pressure
- thyroid disease
- diabetes
- cough with excessive phlegm (mucus)
- difficulty in urination due to enlargement of the prostate gland
- persistent or chronic cough such as occurs with smoking, asthma, or emphysema
- a sodium-restricted diet

ASK A DOCTOR OR PHARMACIST BEFORE USE IF YOU ARE
- taking the blood thinning drug warfarin

WHEN USING THIS PRODUCT
do not exceed recommended dosage

STOP USE AND ASK A DOCTOR IF
- pain, cough, or nasal congestion gets worse or lasts more than 7 days
- fever gets worse or lasts more than 3 days
- redness or swelling is present
- new symptoms occur
- cough comes back or occurs with rash or headache that lasts. These could be signs of a serious condition.
- nervousness, dizziness, or sleeplessness occurs

If pregnant or breast-feeding, ask a health professional before use.
Keep out of reach of children. In case of overdose, get medical help or contact a Poison Control Center right away. Quick medical attention is critical for adults as well as for children even if you do not notice any signs or symptoms.

DIRECTIONS
- do not take more than the recommended dose
- take every 4 hours; do not exceed 5 packets in 24 hours or as directed by a doctor

- if using a microwave, add contents of one packet to 8 oz. of cool water; stir briskly before and after heating. Do not overheat.

adults and children 12 years and over	dissolve contents of one packet in 8 oz. hot water; sip while hot. Consume entire drink within 10-15 minutes
children under 12 years	do not use

OTHER INFORMATION
- **each packet contains:** potassium 5 mg and sodium 41 mg
- Phenylketonurics: Contains Phenylalanine 17 mg Per Packet
- store at room temperature

INACTIVE INGREDIENTS
acesulfame potassium, anhydrous citric acid, aspartame, colloidal silicon dioxide, FD&C blue #1, FD&C red #40, flavor, maltodextrin, pregelatinized starch, sodium citrate, sucrose, tribasic calcium phosphate

QUESTIONS OR COMMENTS?
Call **1-800-986-0369** (Mon-Fri 9AM - 5PM EST) or visit www.alkaseltzerplus.com

ALKA-SELTZER PLUS MUCUS & CONGESTION (dextromethorphan hydrobromide and guaifenesin)
Bayer HealthCare

Active Ingredient(s) (in each capsule)	Purpose(s)
Dextromethorphan hydrobromide 10 mg	Cough suppressant
Guaifenesin 200 mg	Expectorant

USES
- helps loosen phlegm (mucus) and thin bronchial secretions to rid the bronchial passageways of bothersome mucus and make coughs more productive
- temporarily relieves:
  - cough due to minor throat and bronchial irritation as may occur with a cold
  - the intensity of coughing
  - the impulse to cough to help you get to sleep

WARNINGS

DO NOT USE
- if you are now taking a prescription monoamine oxidase inhibitor (MAOI) (certain drugs for depression, psychiatric, or emotional conditions, or Parkinson's disease), or for 2 weeks after stopping the MAOI drug. If you do not know if your prescription drug contains an MAOI, ask a doctor or pharmacist before taking this product.
- if you have ever had an allergic reaction to this product or any of its ingredients
- in children under 12 years of age

ASK A DOCTOR BEFORE USE IF YOU HAVE
- cough with excessive phlegm (mucus)
- persistent or chronic cough such as occurs with smoking, asthma, chronic bronchitis, or emphysema

STOP USE AND ASK A DOCTOR IF
cough lasts more than 7 days, comes back, or is accompanied by a fever, rash, or persistent headache. These could be signs of a serious condition.
If pregnant or breast-feeding, ask a health professional before use.
Keep out of reach of children. In case of overdose, get medical help or contact a Poison Control Center right away.

DIRECTIONS
do not take more than the recommended dose
adults and children 12 years and over
• take 2 capsules every 4 hours
• do not exceed 12 capsules in 24 hours

children under 12 years
• do not use

OTHER INFORMATION
• store at room temperature. Avoid excessive heat.

INACTIVE INGREDIENTS
FD&C blue #1, FD&C red #40, gelatin, glycerin, hypromellose, mannitol, polyethylene glycol 400, polyethylene glycol 600, povidone, propylene glycol, purified water, sorbitan, sorbitol, titanium dioxide

QUESTIONS OR COMMENTS?
1-800-986-0369 (Mon - Fri 9AM - 5PM EST) or www.alkaseltzerplus.com

ALKA-SELTZER PLUS NIGHT COLD AND FLU FORMULA (acetaminophen, dextromethorphan hydrobromide, doxylamine succinate, and phenylephrine hydrochloride)
Bayer HealthCare

DRUG FACTS

Active Ingredient(s) (in each capsule)	Purpose(s)
Acetaminophen 325 mg	Pain reliever/fever reducer
Dextromethorphan hydrobromide 10 mg	Cough suppressant
Doxylamine succinate 6.25 mg	Antihistamine
Phenylephrine hydrochloride 5 mg	Nasal decongestant

USES
• temporarily relieves these symptoms due to a cold or flu:
  • minor aches and pains
  • headache
  • nasal and sinus congestion
  • cough
  • sore throat
  • runny nose
  • sneezing
• temporarily reduces fever

WARNINGS
Liver warning
This product contains acetaminophen. Severe liver damage may occur if you take
• more than 10 capsules in 24 hours, which is the maximum daily amount for this product
• with other drugs containing acetaminophen
• 3 or more alcoholic drinks every day while using this product

Sore throat warning
If sore throat is severe, persists for more than 2 days, is accompanied or followed by fever, headache, rash, nausea, or vomiting, consult a doctor promptly.
Do not use to sedate children.

DO NOT USE
• with any other drug containing acetaminophen (prescription or nonprescription). If you are not sure whether a drug contains acetaminophen, ask a doctor or pharmacist.
• if you are now taking a prescription monoamine oxidase inhibitor (MAOI) (certain drugs for depression, psychiatric, or emotional conditions, or Parkinson's disease), or for 2 weeks after stopping the MAOI drug. If you do not know if your prescription drug contains an MAOI, ask a doctor or pharmacist before taking this product.
• in children under 12 years of age

ASK A DOCTOR BEFORE USE IF YOU HAVE
• liver disease
• heart disease
• high blood pressure
• thyroid disease
• diabetes
• glaucoma
• cough with excessive phlegm (mucus)
• a breathing problem such as emphysema or chronic bronchitis
• difficulty in urination due to enlargement of the prostate gland
• persistent or chronic cough such as occurs with smoking, asthma, or emphysema

ASK A DOCTOR OR PHARMACIST BEFORE USE IF YOU ARE
• taking the blood thinning drug warfarin
• taking sedatives or tranquilizers

WHEN USING THIS PRODUCT
• **do not exceed recommended dosage**
• may cause marked drowsiness
• avoid alcoholic drinks
• alcohol, sedatives, and tranquilizers may increase drowsiness
• be careful when driving a motor vehicle or operating machinery
• excitability may occur, especially in children

STOP USE AND ASK A DOCTOR IF
• pain, cough, or nasal congestion gets worse or lasts more than 7 days
• fever gets worse or lasts more than 3 days
• redness or swelling is present
• new symptoms occur
• cough comes back or occurs with rash or headache that lasts. These could be signs of a serious condition.
• nervousness, dizziness, or sleeplessness occurs

If pregnant or breast-feeding, ask a health professional before use.
Keep out of reach of children. In case of overdose, get medical help or contact a Poison Control Center right away. Quick medical attention is critical for adults as well as for children even if you do not notice any signs or symptoms.

DIRECTIONS
• do not take more than the recommended dose
• adults and children 12 years and over: take 2 capsules with water every 4 hours.
  Do not exceed 10 capsules in 24 hours or as directed by a doctor.
• children under 12 years: do not use

OTHER INFORMATION
• store at room temperature. Avoid excessive heat.

INACTIVE INGREDIENTS
D&C yellow #10, FD&C blue #1, gelatin, glycerin, mannitol, polyethylene glycol 400, povidone, propylene glycol, purified water, shellac, simethicone, sorbitan, sorbitol, titanium dioxide

QUESTIONS OR COMMENTS?
1-800-986-0369 (Mon-Fri 9 - 5 EST) or www.alkaseltzerplus.com
Distributed by:
Bayer HealthCare LLC
P.O. Box 1910
Morristown, NJ 07962-1910

ALKA-SELTZER PLUS DAY & NIGHT COLD FORMULA (aspirin, dextromethorphan hydrobromide, doxylamine succinate, and phenylephrine bitartrate)

Bayer HealthCare

Active Ingredient(s) (in each tablet)	Purpose(s)
Aspirin 500 mg (NSAID)*	Pain reliever/fever reducer
Dextromethorphan hydrobromide 10 mg	Cough suppressant
Doxylamine succinate 6.25 mg	Antihistamine
Phenylephrine bitartrate 7.8 mg	Nasal decongestant
*nonsteroidal anti-inflammatory drug	

USES
- temporarily relieves these symptoms due to a cold:
  - minor aches and pains
  - headache
  - runny nose
  - sinus congestion and pressure
  - cough
  - sneezing
  - sore throat
  - nasal congestion
- temporarily reduces fever

WARNINGS
Reye's syndrome: Children and teenagers who have or are recovering from chicken pox or flu-like symptoms should not use this product. When using this product, if changes in behavior with nausea and vomiting occur, consult a doctor because these symptoms could be an early sign of Reye's syndrome, a rare but serious illness.
Allergy alert:
Aspirin may cause a severe allergic reaction which may include:
- hives
- facial swelling
- asthma (wheezing)
- shock

Stomach bleeding warning: This product contains an NSAID, which may cause severe stomach bleeding. The chance is higher if you
- are age 60 or older
- have had stomach ulcers or bleeding problems
- take a blood thinning (anticoagulant) or steroid drug
- take other drugs containing prescription or nonprescription NSAIDs (aspirin, ibuprofen, naproxen, or others)
- have 3 or more alcoholic drinks every day while using this product
- take more or for a longer time than directed

Sore throat warning: If sore throat is severe, persists for more than 2 days, is accompanied or followed by fever, headache, rash, nausea, or vomiting, consult a doctor promptly. **Do not use to sedate children.**

DO NOT USE
- if you are allergic to aspirin or any other pain reliever/fever reducer
- if you are now taking a prescription monoamine oxidase inhibitor (MAOI) (certain drugs for depression, psychiatric, or emotional conditions, or Parkinson's disease), or for 2 weeks after stopping the MAOI drug. If you do not know if your prescription drug contains an MAOI, ask a doctor or pharmacist before taking this product.
- in children under 12 years of age

ASK A DOCTOR BEFORE USE IF
- stomach bleeding warning applies to you
- you have a history of stomach problems, such as heartburn
- you have high blood pressure, heart disease, liver cirrhosis, or kidney disease
- you are taking a diuretic
- you have
  - asthma
  - diabetes
  - thyroid disease
  - glaucoma
  - cough with excessive phlegm (mucus)
  - a breathing problem such as emphysema or chronic bronchitis
  - difficulty in urination due to enlargement of the prostate gland
  - persistent or chronic cough such as occurs with smoking, asthma, or emphysema
  - a sodium-restricted diet

ASK A DOCTOR OR PHARMACIST BEFORE USE IF YOU ARE
- taking a prescription drug for
  - gout
  - diabetes
  - arthritis
- taking sedatives or tranquilizers

WHEN USING THIS PRODUCT
- **do not exceed recommended dosage**
- may cause marked drowsiness
- avoid alcoholic drinks
- alcohol, sedatives, and tranquilizers may increase drowsiness
- be careful when driving a motor vehicle or operating machinery
- excitability may occur, especially in children

STOP USE AND ASK A DOCTOR IF
- an allergic reaction occurs. Seek medical help right away.
- you experience any of the following signs of stomach bleeding
  - feel faint
  - vomit blood
  - have bloody or black stools
  - have stomach pain that does not get better
- pain, cough, or nasal congestion gets worse or lasts more than 7 days
- fever gets worse or lasts more than 3 days
- redness or swelling is present
- new symptoms occur
- ringing in the ears or a loss of hearing occurs
- cough comes back or occurs with rash or headache that lasts. These could be signs of a serious condition.
- nervousness, dizziness, or sleeplessness occurs

If pregnant or breast-feeding, ask a health professional before use. **It is especially important not to use aspirin during the last 3 months of pregnancy unless definitely directed to do so by a doctor because it may cause problems in the unborn child or complications during delivery.**
Keep out of reach of children. In case of overdose, get medical help or contact a Poison Control Center right away.

DIRECTIONS
adults and children 12 years and over:
• take 2 tablets fully dissolved in 4 oz of water at bedtime (may be taken every 4 to 6 hours).
• do not exceed 8 tablets in 24 hours or as directed by a doctor

children under 12 years:
• do not use

OTHER INFORMATION
• **each tablet contains:** sodium 474 mg
• Phenylketonurics: Contains Phenylalanine 5.6 mg Per Tablet
• store at room temperature. Avoid excessive heat.

INACTIVE INGREDIENTS
acesulfame potassium, anhydrous citric acid, aspartame, calcium silicate, dimethylpolysiloxane, docusate sodium, flavors, mannitol, povidone, sodium benzoate, sodium bicarbonate

QUESTIONS OR COMMENTS?
1-800-986-0369 (Mon - Fri 9AM - 5PM EST) or www.alkaseltzerplus.com

Do not take these products at the same time.

ALKA-SELTZER PLUS® DAY NON-DROWSY COLD EFFERVESCENT TABLETS

DRUG FACTS

Active Ingredient(s) (in each tablet)	Purpose(s)
Aspirin 325 Mg (NSAID) *	Pain reliever/fever reducer
Dextromethorphan hydrobromide 10 mg	Cough suppressant
Phenylephrine bitartrate 7.8 mg	Nasal decongestant
*nonsteroidal anti-inflammatory drug	

USES
• temporarily relieves these symptoms due to a cold with cough:
  • minor aches and pains
  • headache
  • cough
  • nasal and sinus congestion
  • sore throat
• temporarily reduces fever

WARNINGS
Reye's syndrome: Children and teenagers who have or are recovering from chicken pox or flu-like symptoms should not use this product. When using this product, if changes in behavior with nausea and vomiting occur, consult a doctor because these symptoms could be an early sign of Reye's syndrome, a rare but serious illness.

Allergy alert:
Aspirin may cause a severe allergic reaction, which may include:
• hives
• facial swelling
• asthma (wheezing)
• shock

Stomach bleeding warning: This product contains an NSAID, which may cause severe stomach bleeding. The chance is higher if you
• are age 60 or older
• have had stomach ulcers or bleeding problems
• take a blood thinning (anticoagulant) or steroid drug
• take other drugs containing prescription or nonprescription NSAIDs (aspirin, ibuprofen, naproxen, or others)

• have 3 or more alcoholic drinks every day while using this product
• take more or for a longer time than directed

Sore throat warning: If sore throat is severe, persists for more than 2 days, is accompanied or followed by fever, headache, rash, nausea, or vomiting, consult a doctor promptly.

DO NOT USE
• if you are allergic to aspirin or any other pain reliever/fever reducer
• if you are now taking a prescription monoamine oxidase inhibitor (MAOI) (certain drugs for depression, psychiatric, or emotional conditions, or Parkinson's disease), or for 2 weeks after stopping the MAOI drug. If you do not know if your prescription drug contains an MAOI, ask a doctor or pharmacist before taking this product.
• if you have ever had an allergic reaction to this product or any of its ingredients
• in children under 12 years of age

ASK A DOCTOR BEFORE USE IF
• stomach bleeding warning applies to you
• you have a history of stomach problems, such as heartburn
• you have high blood pressure, heart disease, liver cirrhosis, or kidney disease
• you are taking a diuretic
• you have
  • asthma
  • thyroid disease
  • diabetes
  • cough with excessive phlegm (mucus)
  • difficulty in urination due to enlargement of the prostate gland
  • persistent or chronic cough such as occurs with smoking, asthma, or emphysema
  • a sodium-restricted diet

ASK A DOCTOR OR PHARMACIST BEFORE USE IF YOU ARE
• taking a prescription drug for
  • gout
  • diabetes
  • arthritis

WHEN USING THIS PRODUCT
do not exceed recommended dosage

STOP USE AND ASK A DOCTOR IF
• an allergic reaction occurs. Seek medical help right away.
• you experience any of the following signs of stomach bleeding:
  • feel faint
  • vomit blood
  • have bloody or black stools
  • have stomach pain that does not get better
• pain, cough, or nasal congestion gets worse or lasts more than 7 days
• fever gets worse or lasts more than 3 days
• redness or swelling is present
• new symptoms occur
• ringing in the ears or loss of hearing occurs
• cough comes back or occurs with rash or headache that lasts. These could be signs of a serious condition.
• nervousness, dizziness, or sleeplessness occurs

If pregnant or breast-feeding, ask a health professional before use. **It is especially important not to use aspirin during the last three months of pregnancy unless definitely directed to do so by a doctor because it may cause problems in the unborn child or complications during delivery.**
Keep out of reach of children. In case of overdose, get medical help or contact a Poison Control Center right away.

DIRECTIONS

adults and children 12 years and over:	take 2 tablets fully dissolved in 4 oz of water every 4 hours. Do not exceed 8 tablets in 24 hours or as directed by a doctor.
children under 12 years	do not use

OTHER INFORMATION
- each tablet contains: sodium 416 mg
- phenylketonurics: Contains Phenylalanine 9 mg per tablet
- store at room temperature. Avoid excessive heat.

INACTIVE INGREDIENTS
acesulfame potassium, anhydrous citric acid, aspartame, calcium silicate, dimethylpolysiloxane, docusate sodium, flavors, mannitol, povidone, sodium benzoate, sodium bicarbonate

QUESTIONS OR COMMENTS?
1-800-986-0369 (Mon – Fri 9AM - 5PM EST) or www.alkaseltzerplus.com

---

ALKA-SELTZER PLUS NIGHT SEVERE COLD, COUGH & FLU (acetaminophen, diphenhydramine hydrochloride, and phenylephrine hydrochloride)
Bayer HealthCare

DRUG FACTS

Active Ingredient(s) (in each packet)	Purpose(s)
Acetaminophen 650 mg	Pain reliever/fever reducer
Diphenhydramine hydrochloride 25 mg	Antihistamine/cough suppressant
Phenylephrine hydrochloride 10 mg	Nasal decongestant

USES
temporarily relieves these symptoms due to a cold or flu:
- minor aches and pains
- headache
- cough
- sore throat
- nasal and sinus congestion
- runny nose
- sneezing
- itchy nose and throat
- itchy, watery eyes due to hay fever
- temporarily reduces fever

WARNINGS
Liver warning
This product contains acetaminophen. Severe liver damage may occur if you take
- more than 5 packets in 24 hours, which is the maximum daily amount for this product
- with other drugs containing acetaminophen
- 3 or more alcoholic drinks every day while using this product

Sore throat warning
If sore throat is severe, persists for more than 2 days, is accompanied or followed by fever, headache, rash, nausea, or vomiting, consult a doctor promptly.

Do not use to sedate children.

DO NOT USE
- if you have ever had an allergic reaction to this product or any of its ingredients
- with any other drug containing acetaminophen (prescription or nonprescription). If you are not sure whether a drug contains acetaminophen, ask a doctor or pharmacist.
- with any other product containing diphenhydramine, even one used on the skin
- if you are now taking a prescription monoamine oxidase inhibitor (MAOI) (certain drugs for depression, psychiatric, or emotional conditions, or Parkinson's disease), or for 2 weeks after stopping the MAOI drug. If you do not know if your prescription drug contains an MAOI, ask a doctor or pharmacist before taking this product.
- in children under 12 years of age

ASK A DOCTOR BEFORE USE IF YOU HAVE
- liver disease
- heart disease
- high blood pressure
- thyroid disease
- diabetes
- glaucoma
- cough with excessive phlegm (mucus)
- persistent or chronic cough such as occurs with smoking, asthma, or emphysema
- a breathing problem such as emphysema, asthma or chronic bronchitis
- difficulty in urination due to enlargement of the prostate gland

ASK A DOCTOR OR PHARMACIST BEFORE USE IF YOU ARE
- taking the blood thinning drug warfarin
- taking sedatives or tranquilizers

WHEN USING THIS PRODUCT
- **do not exceed recommended dosage**
- avoid alcoholic drinks
- marked drowsiness may occur
- alcohol, sedatives and tranquilizers may increase drowsiness
- be careful when driving a motor vehicle or operating machinery
- excitability may occur, especially in children

STOP USE AND ASK A DOCTOR IF
- pain, cough, or nasal congestion gets worse or lasts more than 7 days
- fever gets worse or lasts more than 3 days
- redness or swelling is present
- new symptoms occur
- cough comes back or occurs with rash or headache that lasts. These could be signs of a serious condition
- nervousness, dizziness, or sleeplessness

If pregnant or breast-feeding, ask a health professional before use.
Keep out of reach of children. In case of overdose, get medical help or contact a Poison Control Center right away. Quick medical attention is critical for adults as well as for children even if you do not notice any signs or symptoms.

DIRECTIONS
- do not take more than the recommended dose
- take every 4 hours; do not exceed 5 packets in 24 hours or as directed by a doctor
- if using a microwave, add contents of one packet to 8 oz. of cool water; stir briskly before and after heating; do not overheat

| adults and children 12 years and over | dissolve contents of one packet in 8 oz. hot water; sip while hot. Consume entire drink within 10-15 minutes. |
| children under 12 years | do not use |

OTHER INFORMATION
- **each packet contains:** potassium 10 mg and sodium 25 mg
- Phenylketonurics: Contains Phenylalanine 13 mg Per Packet
- store at room temperature

INACTIVE INGREDIENTS
acesulfame potassium, anhydrous citric acid, aspartame, colloidal silicon dioxide, D&C yellow #10, FD&C blue #1, FD&C red #40, flavors, maltodextrin, pregelatinized starch, sodium citrate, sucrose, tribasic calcium phosphate

QUESTIONS OR COMMENTS?
Call **1-800-986-0369** (Mon-Fri 9AM - 5PM EST) or visit www.alkaseltzerplus.com

ALKA-SELTZER PLUS ORANGE ZEST COLD FORMULA (aspirin, chlorpheniramine maleate, and phenylephrine bitartrate)
Bayer HealthCare

Active Ingredient(s) (in each tablet)	Purpose(s)
Aspirin 325 mg (NSAID)*	Pain reliever/fever reducer
Chlorpheniramine maleate 2 mg	Antihistamine
Phenylephrine bitartrate 7.8 mg	Nasal decongestant
*nonsteroidal anti-inflammatory drug	

USES
- temporarily relieves these symptoms due to a cold:
  - minor aches and pains
  - headache
  - runny nose
  - nasal and sinus congestion
  - sneezing
  - sore throat
- temporarily reduces fever

WARNINGS
Reye's syndrome: Children and teenagers who have or are recovering from chicken pox or flu-like symptoms should not use this product. When using this product, if changes in behavior with nausea and vomiting occur, consult a doctor because these symptoms could be an early sign of Reye's syndrome, a rare but serious illness.
Allergy alert:
Aspirin may cause a severe allergic reaction which may include:
- hives
- facial swelling
- asthma (wheezing)
- shock

Stomach bleeding warning: This product contains an NSAID, which may cause severe stomach bleeding. The chance is higher if you
- are age 60 or older
- have had stomach ulcers or bleeding problems
- take a blood thinning (anticoagulant) or steroid drug

- take other drugs containing prescription or nonprescription NSAIDs (aspirin, ibuprofen, naproxen, or others)
- have 3 or more alcoholic drinks every day while using this product
- take more or for a longer time than directed

Sore throat warning: If sore throat is severe, persists for more than 2 days, is accompanied or followed by fever, headache, rash, nausea, or vomiting, consult a doctor promptly. **Do not use to sedate children.**

DO NOT USE
- if you are allergic to aspirin or any other pain reliever/fever reducer
- if you are now taking a prescription monoamine oxidase inhibitor (MAOI) (certain drugs for depression, psychiatric, or emotional conditions, or Parkinson's disease), or for 2 weeks after stopping the MAOI drug. If you do not know if your prescription drug contains an MAOI, ask a doctor or pharmacist before taking this product.
- if you have ever had an allergic reaction to this product or any of its ingredients
- in children under 12 years of age

ASK A DOCTOR BEFORE USE IF
- stomach bleeding warning applies to you
- you have a history of stomach problems, such as heartburn
- you have high blood pressure, heart disease, liver cirrhosis, or kidney disease
- you are taking a diuretic
- you have
  - asthma
  - diabetes
  - thyroid disease
  - glaucoma
  - difficulty in urination due to enlargement of the prostate gland
  - a breathing problem such as emphysema or chronic bronchitis
  - a sodium-restricted diet

ASK A DOCTOR OR PHARMACIST BEFORE USE IF YOU ARE
- taking a prescription drug for
  - gout
  - diabetes
  - arthritis
- taking sedatives or tranquilizers

WHEN USING THIS PRODUCT
- **do not exceed recommended dosage**
- excitability may occur, especially in children
- you may get drowsy
- avoid alcoholic drinks
- alcohol, sedatives, and tranquilizers may increase drowsiness
- be careful when driving a motor vehicle or operating machinery

STOP USE AND ASK A DOCTOR IF
- an allergic reaction occurs. Seek medical help right away.
- you experience any of the following signs of stomach bleeding
  - feel faint
  - vomit blood
  - have bloody or black stools
  - have stomach pain that does not get better
- pain or nasal congestion gets worse or lasts more than 7 days
- fever gets worse or lasts more than 3 days
- redness or swelling is present
- new symptoms occur
- ringing in the ears or a loss of hearing occurs
- nervousness, dizziness, or sleeplessness occurs

If pregnant or breast-feeding, ask a health professional before use. **It is especially important not to use aspirin during the last 3 months of pregnancy unless definitely**

directed to do so by a doctor because it may cause problems in the unborn child or complications during delivery.

Keep out of reach of children. In case of overdose, get medical help or contact a Poison Control Center right away.

DIRECTIONS
adults and children 12 years and over:
- take 2 tablets fully dissolved in 4 oz of water every 4 hours.
- do not exceed 8 tablets in 24 hours or as directed by a doctor.

children under 12 years:
- do not use

OTHER INFORMATION
- **each tablet contains:** sodium 476 mg
- Phenylketonurics: Contains Phenylalanine 9 mg Per Tablet
- store at room temperature. Avoid excessive heat.

INACTIVE INGREDIENTS
acesulfame potassium, anhydrous citric acid, aspartame, calcium silicate, dimethylpolysiloxane, docusate sodium, FD&C red #40, FD&C yellow #6, flavors, mannitol, povidone, sodium benzoate, sodium bicarbonate

QUESTIONS OR COMMENTS?
1-800-986-0369 (Mon - Fri 9AM - 5PM EST) or www.alkaseltzerplus.com

---

ALKA-SELTZER PLUS SEVERE ALLERGY SINUS CONGESTION & HEADACHE LIQUID GELS (acetaminophen, doxylamine succinate, and phenylephrine hydrochloride)

Bayer HealthCare

DRUG FACTS

Active Ingredient(s) (in each capsule)	Purpose(s)
Acetaminophen 325 mg	Pain reliever-fever reducer
Doxylamine succinate 6.25 mg	Antihistamine
Phenylephrine hydrochloride 5 mg	Nasal decongestant

USES
- temporarily relieves these symptoms due to hay fever or other upper respiratory allergies
- runny nose
- sneezing
- itchy, watery eyes
- itching of the nose or throat
- nasal congestion
- sinus congestion and pressure
- headache
- minor aches and pains
- temporarily restores freer breathing through the nose
- temporarily reduces fever

WARNINGS
Liver warning
This product contains acetaminophen. Severe liver damage may occur if you take
- more than 10 capsules in 24 hours, which is the maximum daily amount for this product
- with other drugs containing acetaminophen
- 3 or more alcoholic drinks every day while using this product

Do not use to sedate children.

DO NOT USE
- with any other drug containing acetaminophen (prescription or nonprescription). If you are not sure whether a drug contains acetaminophen, ask a doctor or pharmacist.
- if you are now taking a prescription monoamine oxidase inhibitor (MAOI) (certain drugs for depression, psychiatric, or emotional conditions, or Parkinson's disease), or for 2 weeks after stopping the MAOI drug. If you do not know if your prescription drug contains an MAOI, ask a doctor or pharmacist before taking this product.
- if you have ever had an allergic reaction to this product or any of its ingredients
- in children under 12 years of age

ASK A DOCTOR BEFORE USE IF YOU HAVE
- liver disease
- heart disease
- high blood pressure
- thyroid disease
- diabetes
- glaucoma
- a breathing problem such as emphysema or chronic bronchitis
- difficulty in urination due to enlargement of the prostate gland

ASK A DOCTOR OR PHARMACIST BEFORE USE IF YOU ARE
- taking the blood thinning drug warfarin
- taking sedatives or tranquilizers

WHEN USING THIS PRODUCT
- **do not exceed recommended dosage**
- may cause marked drowsiness
- avoid alcoholic drinks
- alcohol, sedatives, and tranquilizers may increase drowsiness
- be careful when driving a motor vehicle or operating machinery
- excitability may occur, especially in children

STOP USE AND ASK A DOCTOR IF
- pain or nasal congestion gets worse or lasts more than 7 days
- fever gets worse or lasts more than 3 days
- redness or swelling is present
- new symptoms occur
- nervousness, dizziness, or sleeplessness occurs

If pregnant or breast-feeding, ask a health professional before use.

Keep out of reach of children. In case of overdose, get medical help or contact a Poison Control Center right away. Quick medical attention is critical for adults as well as for children even if you do not notice any signs or symptoms.

DIRECTIONS
- do not take more than the recommended dose

adults and children 12 years and over:	take 2 capsules with water every 4 hours. Do not exceed 10 capsules in 24 hours or as directed by a doctor.
children under 12 years	do not use

OTHER INFORMATION
- store at room temperature. Avoid excessive heat

INACTIVE INGREDIENTS
FD&C blue #1, gelatin, glycerin, mannitol, polyethylene glycol 400, povidone, propylene glycol, purified water, shellac, simethicone, sorbitan, sorbitol, titanium dioxide

QUESTIONS OR COMMENTS?
Call **1-800-986-0369** (Mon-Fri 9AM - 5PM EST) or visit
www.alkaseltzerplus.com

ALKA-SELTZER PLUS SEVERE COLD & FLU FORMULA (acetaminophen, chlorpheniramine maleate, dextromethorphan hydrobromide, and phenylephrine hydrochloride)

Bayer HealthCare

Active Ingredient(s) (in each tablet)	Purpose(s)
Acetaminophen 250 mg	Pain reliever/fever reducer
Chlorpheniramine maleate 2 mg	Antihistamine
Dextromethorphan hydrobromide 10 mg	Cough suppressant
Phenylephrine hydrochloride 5 mg	Nasal decongestant

USES
- temporarily relieves these symptoms due to a cold or flu:
  - minor aches and pains
  - headache
  - cough
  - sore throat
  - runny nose
  - sneezing
  - nasal and sinus congestion
- temporarily reduces fever

WARNINGS
Liver warning
This product contains acetaminophen. Severe liver damage may occur if you take
- more than 8 tablets in 24 hours, which is the maximum daily amount for this product with other drugs containing acetaminophen
- 3 or more alcoholic drinks every day while using this product

Sore throat warning
If sore throat is severe, persists for more than 2 days, is accompanied or followed by fever, headache, rash, nausea, or vomiting, consult a doctor promptly.
Do not use to sedate children

DO NOT USE
- with any other drug containing acetaminophen (prescription or nonprescription). If you are not sure whether a drug contains acetaminophen, ask a doctor or pharmacist.
- if you are now taking a prescription monoamine oxidase inhibitor (MAOI) (certain drugs for depression, psychiatric, or emotional conditions, or Parkinson's disease), or for 2 weeks after stopping the MAOI drug. If you do not know if your prescription drug contains an MAOI, ask a doctor or pharmacist before taking this product.
- in children under 12 years of age

ASK A DOCTOR BEFORE USE IF YOU HAVE
- liver disease
- heart disease
- high blood pressure
- thyroid disease
- diabetes
- glaucoma
- cough with excessive phlegm (mucus)
- a breathing problem such as emphysema or chronic bronchitis
- difficulty in urination due to enlargement of the prostate gland
- persistent or chronic cough such as occurs with smoking, asthma, or emphysema
- a sodium restricted diet

ASK A DOCTOR OR PHARMACIST BEFORE USE IF YOU ARE
- taking the blood thinning drug warfarin
- taking sedatives or tranquilizers

WHEN USING THIS PRODUCT
- **do not exceed recommended dosage**
- may cause marked drowsiness
- avoid alcoholic drinks
- alcohol, sedatives, and tranquilizers may increase drowsiness
- be careful when driving a motor vehicle or operating machinery
- excitability may occur, especially in children

STOP USE AND ASK A DOCTOR IF
- pain, cough, or nasal congestion gets worse or lasts more than 7 days
- fever gets worse or lasts more than 3 days
- redness or swelling is present
- new symptoms occur
- cough comes back or occurs with rash or headache that lasts. These could be signs of a serious condition.
- nervousness, dizziness, or sleeplessness occurs

If pregnant or breast-feeding, ask a health professional before use.
Keep out of reach of children. In case of overdose, get medical help or contact a Poison Control Center right away. Quick medical attention is critical for adults as well as for children even if you do not notice any signs or symptoms.

DIRECTIONS
- do not take more than the recommended dose
- adults and children 12 years and over:
  - take 2 tablets fully dissolved in 4 oz of water every 4 hours.
  - do not exceed 8 tablets in 24 hours or as directed by a doctor
- children under 12 years:
  - do not use

OTHER INFORMATION
- **each tablet contains:** sodium 416 mg
- Phenylketonurics: Contains Phenylalanine 5.6 mg Per Tablet
- store at room temperature. Avoid excessive heat.

INACTIVE INGREDIENTS
acesulfame potassium, anhydrous citric acid, aspartame, FD&C red #40, flavors, magnesium stearate, maltodextrin, mannitol, saccharin sodium, sodium bicarbonate

QUESTIONS OR COMMENTS?
1-800-986-0369 (Mon - Fri 9AM - 5PM EST) or www.alkaseltzerplus.com

ALKA-SELTZER PLUS SEVERE SINUS CONGESTION, ALLERGY, AND COUGH
(acetaminophen, dextromethorphan hydrobromide, doxylamine succinate, and phenylephrine hydrochloride)

Bayer HealthCare

DRUG FACTS

Active Ingredient(s) (in each capsule)	Purpose(s)
Acetaminophen 325 mg	Pain reliever/fever reducer
Dextromethorphan hydrobromide 10 mg	Cough suppressant
Doxylamine succinate 6.25 mg	Antihistamine
Phenylephrine hydrochloride 5 mg	Nasal decongestant

USES
- temporarily relieves these symptoms due to hay fever or other upper respiratory allergies:
  - runny nose
  - sneezing
  - itching of the nose or throat
  - itchy, watery eyes
- temporarily relieves these symptoms due to a cold
  - nasal congestion
  - sinus congestion and pressure
  - headache
  - minor aches and pains
  - cough
- temporarily reduces fever

WARNINGS
Liver warning
This product contains acetaminophen. Severe liver damage may occur if you take
- more than 10 capsules in 24 hours, which is the maximum daily amount for this product
- with other drugs containing acetaminophen
- 3 or more alcoholic drinks every day while using this product

Do not use to sedate children.

DO NOT USE
- with any other drug containing acetaminophen (prescription or nonprescription). If you are not sure whether a drug contains acetaminophen, ask a doctor or pharmacist.
- if you are now taking a prescription monoamine oxidase inhibitor (MAOI) (certain drugs for depression, psychiatric, or emotional conditions, or Parkinson's disease), or for 2 weeks after stopping the MAOI drug. If you do not know if your prescription drug contains an MAOI, ask a doctor or pharmacist before taking this product.
- in children under 12 years of age

ASK A DOCTOR BEFORE USE IF YOU HAVE
- liver disease
- heart disease
- high blood pressure
- thyroid disease
- diabetes
- glaucoma
- cough with excessive phlegm (mucus)
- a breathing problem such as emphysema or chronic bronchitis
- difficulty in urination due to enlargement of the prostate gland
- persistent or chronic cough such as occurs with smoking, asthma, or emphysema

ASK A DOCTOR OR PHARMACIST BEFORE USE IF YOU ARE
- taking the blood thinning drug warfarin
- taking sedatives or tranquilizers

WHEN USING THIS PRODUCT
- **do not exceed recommended dosage**
- may cause marked drowsiness
- avoid alcoholic drinks
- alcohol, sedatives, and tranquilizers may increase drowsiness
- be careful when driving a motor vehicle or operating machinery
- excitability may occur, especially in children

STOP USE AND ASK A DOCTOR IF
- pain, cough, or nasal congestion gets worse or lasts more than 7 days
- fever gets worse or lasts more than 3 days
- redness or swelling is present
- new symptoms occur
- cough comes back or occurs with rash or headache that lasts. These could be signs of a serious condition.
- nervousness, dizziness, or sleeplessness occurs

If pregnant or breast-feeding, ask a health professional before use.
Keep out of reach of children. In case of overdose, get medical help or contact a Poison Control Center right away. Quick medical attention is critical for adults as well as for children even if you do not notice any signs or symptoms.

DIRECTIONS
- do not take more than the recommended dose
- adults and children 12 years and over: take 2 capsules with water every 4 hours. Do not exceed 10 capsules in 24 hours or as directed by a doctor
- children under 12 years: do not use

OTHER INFORMATION
store at room temperature. Avoid excessive heat.

INACTIVE INGREDIENTS
D&C yellow #10, FD&C blue #1, gelatin, glycerin, mannitol, polyethylene glycol 400, povidone, propylene glycol, purified water, shellac, simethicone, sorbitan, sorbitol, titanium dioxide

QUESTIONS OR COMMENTS?
1-800-986-0369 (Mon-Fri 9AM - 5PM EST) or www.alkaseltzerplus.com

ALKA-SELTZER PLUS SEVERE SINUS CONGESTION AND COUGH DAY AND NIGHT (acetaminophen, dextromethorphan hydrobromide, phenylephrine hydrochloride, and doxylamine succinate)

Bayer HealthCare LLC and Consumer Care

Alka-Seltzer Plus® Severe Sinus Congestion & Cough Day Liquid Gels

DRUG FACTS

Active Ingredient(s) (in each capsule)	Purpose(s)
Acetaminophen 325 mg	Pain reliever/fever reducer
Dextromethorphan hydrobromide 10 mg	Cough suppressant
Phenylephrine hydrochloride 5 mg	Nasal decongestant

USES
- temporarily relieves these symptoms due to a cold or flu:
  - nasal congestion
  - sinus congestion and pressure
  - headache
  - minor aches and pains
  - cough
  - sore throat
- helps clear nasal passages and shrinks swollen membranes
- temporarily reduces fever

WARNINGS
Liver warning
This product contains acetaminophen. Severe liver damage may occur if you take
- more than 10 capsules in 24 hours, which is the maximum daily amount for this product
- with other drugs containing acetaminophen
- 3 or more alcoholic drinks every day while using this product

Sore throat warning
If sore throat is severe, persists for more than 2 days, is accompanied or followed by fever, headache, rash, nausea, or vomiting, consult a doctor promptly.

DO NOT USE
- with any other drug containing acetaminophen (prescription or nonprescription). If you are not sure whether a drug contains acetaminophen, ask a doctor or pharmacist.
- if you are now taking a prescription monoamine oxidase inhibitor (MAOI) (certain drugs for depression, psychiatric, or emotional conditions, or Parkinson's disease), or for 2 weeks after stopping the MAOI drug. If you do not know if your prescription drug contains an MAOI, ask a doctor or pharmacist before taking this product.
- in children under 12 years of age

ASK A DOCTOR BEFORE USE IF YOU HAVE
- liver disease
- heart disease
- high blood pressure
- thyroid disease
- diabetes
- cough with excessive phlegm (mucus)
- difficulty in urination due to enlargement of the prostate gland
- persistent or chronic cough such as occurs with smoking, asthma, or emphysema

ASK A DOCTOR OR PHARMACIST BEFORE USE IF YOU ARE
taking the blood thinning drug warfarin

WHEN USING THIS PRODUCT
do not exceed recommended dosage

STOP USE AND ASK A DOCTOR IF
- pain, cough, or nasal congestion gets worse or lasts more than 7 days
- fever gets worse or lasts more than 3 days
- redness or swelling is present
- new symptoms occur
- cough comes back or occurs with rash or headache that lasts. These could be signs of a serious condition.
- nervousness, dizziness, or sleeplessness occurs

If pregnant or breast-feeding, ask a health professional before use.
Keep out of reach of children. In case of overdose, get medical help or contact a Poison Control Center right away. Quick medical attention is critical for adults as well as for children even if you do not notice any signs or symptoms.

DIRECTIONS
- do not take more than the recommended dose
- adults and children 12 years and over: take 2 capsules with water every 4 hours. Do not exceed 10 capsules in 24 hours or as directed by a doctor
- children under 12 years: do not use

OTHER INFORMATION
- store at room temperature. Avoid excessive heat.

INACTIVE INGREDIENTS
FD&C blue #1, FD&C red #40, gelatin, glycerin, mannitol, polyethylene glycol 400, povidone, propylene glycol, purified water, shellac, simethicone, sorbitan, sorbitol, titanium dioxide

QUESTIONS OR COMMENTS?
1-800-986-0369 (Mon-Fri 9AM - 5PM EST) or www.alkaseltzerplus.com

Alka-Seltzer Plus® Severe Sinus Congestion & Cough Night Liquid Gels

DRUG FACTS

Active Ingredient(s) (in each capsule)	Purpose(s)
Acetaminophen 325 mg	Pain reliever/fever reducer
Dextromethorphan hydrobromide 10 mg	Cough suppressant
Doxylamine succinate 6.25 mg	Antihistamine
Phenylephrine hydrochloride 5 mg	Nasal decongestant

USES
- temporarily relieves these symptoms due to a cold or flu:
  - nasal congestion
  - sinus congestion and pressure
  - headache
  - minor aches and pains
  - cough
  - sore throat
  - runny nose
  - sneezing
- helps clear nasal passages and shrinks swollen membranes
- temporarily reduces fever

WARNINGS

Liver warning
This product contains acetaminophen. Severe liver damage may occur if you take
- more than 10 capsules in 24 hours, which is the maximum daily amount for this product
- with other drugs containing acetaminophen
- 3 or more alcoholic drinks every day while using this product

Sore throat warning
If sore throat is severe, persists for more than 2 days, is accompanied or followed by fever, headache, rash, nausea, or vomiting, consult a doctor promptly.
Do not use to sedate children.

DO NOT USE

- with any other drug containing acetaminophen (prescription or nonprescription). If you are not sure whether a drug contains acetaminophen, ask a doctor or pharmacist.
- if you are now taking a prescription monoamine oxidase inhibitor (MAOI) (certain drugs for depression, psychiatric, or emotional conditions, or Parkinson's disease), or for 2 weeks after stopping the MAOI drug. If you do not know if your prescription drug contains an MAOI, ask a doctor or pharmacist before taking this product.
- in children under 12 years of age

ASK A DOCTOR BEFORE USE IF YOU HAVE

- liver disease
- heart disease
- high blood pressure
- thyroid disease
- diabetes
- glaucoma
- cough with excessive phlegm (mucus)
- a breathing problem such as emphysema or chronic bronchitis
- difficulty in urination due to enlargement of the prostate gland
- persistent or chronic cough such as occurs with smoking, asthma, or emphysema

ASK A DOCTOR OR PHARMACIST BEFORE USE IF YOU ARE

- taking the blood thinning drug warfarin
- taking sedatives or tranquilizers

WHEN USING THIS PRODUCT

- **do not exceed recommended dosage**
- may cause marked drowsiness
- avoid alcoholic drinks
- alcohol, sedatives, and tranquilizers may increase drowsiness
- be careful when driving a motor vehicle or operating machinery
- excitability may occur, especially in children

STOP USE AND ASK A DOCTOR IF

- pain, cough, or nasal congestion gets worse or lasts more than 7 days
- fever gets worse or lasts more than 3 days
- redness or swelling is present
- new symptoms occur
- cough comes back or occurs with rash or headache that lasts. These could be signs of a serious condition.
- nervousness, dizziness, or sleeplessness occurs

If pregnant or breast-feeding, ask a health professional before use.
Keep out of reach of children. In case of overdose, get medical help or contact a Poison Control Center right away. Quick medical attention is critical for adults as well as for children even if you do not notice any signs or symptoms.

DIRECTIONS

- do not take more than the recommended dose
- adults and children 12 years and over: take 2 capsules with water every 4 hours. Do not exceed 10 capsules in 24 hours or as directed by a doctor.
- children under 12 years: do not use

OTHER INFORMATION

- store at room temperature. Avoid excessive heat.

INACTIVE INGREDIENTS

D&C yellow #10, FD&C blue #1, gelatin, glycerin, mannitol, polyethylene glycol 400, povidone, propylene glycol, purified water, shellac, simethicone, sorbitan, sorbitol, titanium dioxide

QUESTIONS OR COMMENTS?

1-800-986-0369 (Mon-Fri 9AM - 5PM EST) or
www.alkaseltzerplus.com
Distributed by:
Bayer HealthCare LLC
Consumer Care
P.O. Box 1910
Morristown, NJ 07962-1910 USA

ALKA-SELTZER PLUS SINUS FORMULA
(aspirin and phenylephrine bitartrate)
Bayer HealthCare

Active Ingredient(s) (in each tablet)	Purpose(s)
Aspirin 325 mg (NSAID)*	Pain reliever/fever reducer
Phenylephrine bitartrate 7.8 mg	Nasal decongestant
*nonsteroidal anti-inflammatory drug	

USES

- temporarily relieves these symptoms due to a cold:
  - minor aches and pains
  - headache
  - nasal congestion
  - sinus congestion and pressure
- temporarily reduces fever

WARNINGS

Reye's syndrome: Children and teenagers who have or are recovering from chicken pox or flu-like symptoms should not use this product. When using this product, if changes in behavior with nausea and vomiting occur, consult a doctor because these symptoms could be an early sign of Reye's syndrome, a rare but serious illness.
Allergy alert:
Aspirin may cause a severe allergic reaction which may include:
- hives
- facial swelling
- asthma (wheezing)
- shock

Stomach bleeding warning: This product contains an NSAID, which may cause severe stomach bleeding. The chance is higher if you
- are age 60 or older
- have had stomach ulcers or bleeding problems
- take a blood thinning (anticoagulant) or steroid drug
- take other drugs containing prescription or nonprescription NSAIDs (aspirin, ibuprofen, naproxen, or others)
- have 3 or more alcoholic drinks every day while using this product
- take more or for a longer time than directed

DO NOT USE
- if you are allergic to aspirin or any other pain reliever/fever reducer
- if you are now taking a prescription monoamine oxidase inhibitor (MAOI) (certain drugs for depression, psychiatric, or emotional conditions, or Parkinson's disease), or for 2 weeks after stopping the MAOI drug. If you do not know if your prescription drug contains an MAOI, ask a doctor or pharmacist before taking this product.
- in children under 12 years of age

ASK A DOCTOR BEFORE USE IF
- stomach bleeding warning applies to you
- you have a history of stomach problems, such as heartburn
- you have high blood pressure, heart disease, liver cirrhosis, or kidney disease
- you are taking a diuretic
- you have
  - asthma
  - thyroid disease
  - diabetes
  - difficulty in urination due to enlargement of the prostate gland
  - a sodium-restricted diet

ASK A DOCTOR OR PHARMACIST BEFORE USE IF YOU ARE
- taking a prescription drug for
  - gout
  - diabetes
  - arthritis

WHEN USING THIS PRODUCT
do not exceed recommended dosage

STOP USE AND ASK A DOCTOR IF
- an allergic reaction occurs. Seek medical help right away.
- you experience any of the following signs of stomach bleeding
  - feel faint
  - vomit blood
  - have bloody or black stools
  - have stomach pain that does not get better
- pain or nasal congestion gets worse or lasts more than 7 days
- fever gets worse or lasts more than 3 days
- redness or swelling is present
- new symptoms occur
- ringing in the ears or a loss of hearing occurs
- nervousness, dizziness, or sleeplessness occurs

If pregnant or breast-feeding, ask a health professional before use. **It is especially important not to use aspirin during the last 3 months of pregnancy unless definitely directed to do so by a doctor because it may cause problems in the unborn child or complications during delivery.**
Keep out of reach of children. In case of overdose, get medical help or contact a Poison Control Center right away.

DIRECTIONS
adults and children 12 years and over:
- take 2 tablets fully dissolved in 4 oz of water every 4 hours.
- do not exceed 8 tablets in 24 hours or as directed by a doctor.

children under 12 years:
- consult a doctor

OTHER INFORMATION
- **each tablet contains:** sodium 476 mg
- Phenylketonurics: Contains Phenylalanine 9 mg Per Tablet
- protect from excessive heat

INACTIVE INGREDIENTS
acesulfame potassium, anhydrous citric acid, aspartame, calcium silicate, dimethylpolysiloxane, docusate sodium, flavors, mannitol, povidone, sodium benzoate, sodium bicarbonate

QUESTIONS OR COMMENTS?
1-800-986-0369 (Mon - Fri 9AM - 5PM EST) or www.alkaseltzerplus.com

ALKA-SELTZER PLUS SPARKLING ORIGINAL COLD FORMULA (aspirin, chlorpheniramine maleate, and phenylephrine bitartrate)
Bayer HealthCare

Active Ingredient(s) (in each tablet)	Purpose(s)
Aspirin 325 mg (NSAID)*	Pain reliever/fever reducer
Chlorpheniramine maleate 2 mg	Antihistamine
Phenylephrine bitartrate 7.8 mg	Nasal decongestant
*nonsteroidal anti-inflammatory drug	

USES
- temporarily relieves these symptoms due to a cold:
  - minor aches and pains
  - headache
  - runny nose
  - nasal and sinus congestion
  - sneezing
  - sore throat
- temporarily reduces fever

WARNINGS
Reye's syndrome
Children and teenagers who have or are recovering from chicken pox or flu-like symptoms should not use this product. When using this product, if changes in behavior with nausea and vomiting occur, consult a doctor because these symptoms could be an early sign of Reye's syndrome, a rare but serious illness.

Allergy alert
Aspirin may cause a severe allergic reaction which may include:
- hives
- facial swelling
- asthma (wheezing)
- shock

Stomach bleeding warning
This product contains an NSAID, which may cause severe stomach bleeding. The chance is higher if you
- are age 60 or older
- have had stomach ulcers or bleeding problems
- take a blood thinning (anticoagulant) or steroid drug
- take other drugs containing prescription or nonprescription NSAIDs (aspirin, ibuprofen, naproxen, or others)
- have 3 or more alcoholic drinks every day while using this product
- take more or for a longer time than directed

Sore throat warning
If sore throat is severe, persists for more than 2 days, is accompanied or followed by fever, headache, rash, nausea, or vomiting, consult a doctor promptly.
Do not use to sedate children.

DO NOT USE

- if you are allergic to aspirin or any other pain reliever/fever reducer
- if you are now taking a prescription monoamine oxidase inhibitor (MAOI) (certain drugs for depression, psychiatric, or emotional conditions, or Parkinson's disease), or for 2 weeks after stopping the MAOI drug. If you do not know if your prescription drug contains an MAOI, ask a doctor or pharmacist before taking this product.
- if you have ever had an allergic reaction to this product or any of its ingredients
- in children under 12 years of age

ASK A DOCTOR BEFORE USE IF

- stomach bleeding warning applies to you
- you have a history of stomach problems, such as heartburn
- you have high blood pressure, heart disease, liver cirrhosis, or kidney disease
- you are taking a diuretic
- you have
  - asthma
  - diabetes
  - thyroid disease
  - glaucoma
  - difficulty in urination due to enlargement of the prostate gland
  - a breathing problem such as emphysema or chronic bronchitis
  - a sodium-restricted diet

ASK A DOCTOR OR PHARMACIST BEFORE USE IF YOU ARE

- taking a prescription drug for
  - gout
  - diabetes
  - arthritis
- taking sedatives or tranquilizers

WHEN USING THIS PRODUCT

- **do not exceed recommended dosage**
- excitability may occur, especially in children
- you may get drowsy
- avoid alcoholic drinks
- alcohol, sedatives, and tranquilizers may increase drowsiness
- be careful when driving a motor vehicle or operating machinery

STOP USE AND ASK A DOCTOR IF

- an allergic reaction occurs. Seek medical help right away.
- you experience any of the following signs of stomach bleeding
  - feel faint
  - vomit blood
  - have bloody or black stools
  - have stomach pain that does not get better
- pain or nasal congestion gets worse or lasts more than 7 days
- fever gets worse or lasts more than 3 days
- redness or swelling is present
- new symptoms occur
- ringing in the ears or a loss of hearing occurs
- nervousness, dizziness, or sleeplessness occurs

If pregnant or breast-feeding, ask a health professional before use. **It is especially important not to use aspirin during the last 3 months of pregnancy unless definitely directed to do so by a doctor because it may cause problems in the unborn child or complications during delivery.**
Keep out of reach of children. In case of overdose, get medical help or contact a Poison Control Center right away.

DIRECTIONS

adults and children 12 years and over:
- take 2 tablets fully dissolved in 4 oz of water every 4 hours.
- do not exceed 8 tablets in 24 hours or as directed by a doctor.

children under 12 years:
- do not use

OTHER INFORMATION

- **each tablet contains:** sodium 474 mg
- Phenylketonurics: Contains Phenylalanine 8.4 mg Per Tablet
- store at room temperature. Avoid excessive heat.

INACTIVE INGREDIENTS

acesulfame potassium, anhydrous citric acid, aspartame, calcium silicate, dimethylpolysiloxane, docusate sodium, flavors, mannitol, povidone, sodium benzoate, sodium bicarbonate

QUESTIONS OR COMMENTS?

1-800-986-0369 (Mon - Fri 9AM - 5PM EST) or www.alkaseltzerplus.com

CHILDRENS ALLEGRA ALLERGY ORAL SUSPENSION (fexofenadine hydrochloride)

Chattem, Inc.

DRUG FACTS

Active Ingredient(s)
(in each 5 mL teaspoonful)
Fexofenadine HCl 30 mg

Purpose(s)
Antihistamine

USES

temporarily relieves these symptoms due to hay fever or other upper respiratory allergies:
- runny nose
- sneezing
- itchy, water eyes
- itching of the nose or throat

WARNINGS

DO NOT USE

if you have ever had an allergic reaction to this product or any of its ingredients.

ASK A DOCTOR BEFORE USE IF YOU HAVE

kidney disease. Your doctor should determine if you need a different dose.

WHEN USING THIS PRODUCT

- do not take more than directed
- do not take at the same time as aluminum or magnesium antacids
- do not take with fruit juices (see Directions)

STOP USE AND ASK A DOCTOR IF

an allergic reaction to this product occurs. Seek medical help right away.

If pregnant or breast-feeding, ask a health professional before use.

Keep out of reach of children. In case of overdose, get medical help or contact a Poison Control Center right away.

DIRECTIONS

- shake well before using
- use only with enclosed dosing cup

adults and children 12 years of age and over	take 2 teaspoonfuls (10 mL) every 12 hours; do not take more than 4 teaspoonfuls (20 mL) in 24 hours
children 2 to under 12 years of age	take 1 teaspoonful (5 mL) every 12 hours; do not take more than 2 teaspoonfuls (10 mL) in 24 hours
children under 2 years of age	ask a doctor
adults 65 years of age and older	ask a doctor
consumers with kidney disease	ask a doctor

Note: teaspoonful = tsp

OTHER INFORMATION
- each 5 mL teaspoon contains: **sodium 18 mg**
- safety sealed: do not use if carton is opened or if printed foil inner seal on bottle is torn or missing
- store between 20° and 25°C (68° and 77°F)

INACTIVE INGREDIENTS
butylparaben, edetate disodium, flavor, poloxamer 407, propylene glycol, propylparaben, purified water, sodium phosphate dibasic heptahydrate, sodium phosphate monobasic monohydrate, sucrose, titanium dioxide, xanthan gum, xylitol

QUESTIONS OR COMMENTS?
call toll-free **1-800-633-1610** or www.allegra.com
The makers of Allegra® do not make
store brand products.
The trade dress of this Allegra® package is subject to trademark protection.
Dist. By: Chattem, Inc. (part of the sanofi-aventis Group), Chattanooga, TN 37409-0219 ©2010
Origin Canada 50094566

CHILDRENS ALLEGRA ALLERGY (fexofenadine hydrochloride)
Chattem, Inc.

Children's Allegra Allergy® - 12 HOUR

DRUG FACTS

Active Ingredient(s)
(in each tablet)
Fexofenadine HCl 30 mg

Purpose(s)
Antihistamine

USES
temporarily relieves these symptoms due to hay fever or other upper respiratory allergies:
- runny nose
- sneezing
- itchy, water eyes
- itching of the nose or throat

WARNINGS

DO NOT USE
if you have ever had an allergic reaction to this product or any of its ingredients.

ASK A DOCTOR BEFORE USE IF YOU HAVE
kidney disease. Your doctor should determine if you need a different dose.

WHEN USING THIS PRODUCT
- do not take more than directed
- do not take at the same time as aluminum or magnesium antacids
- do not take with fruit juices (see Directions)

STOP USE AND ASK A DOCTOR IF
an allergic reaction to this product occurs. Seek medical help right away.

If pregnant or breast-feeding,
ask a health professional before use.

Keep out of reach of children.
In case of overdose, get medical help or contact a Poison Control Center right away.

DIRECTIONS

adults and children 12 years of age and over	take two 30 mg tablets with water every 12 hours; do not take more than 4 tablets in 24 hours
children 6 to under 12 years of age	take one 30 mg tablet with water every 12 hours; do not take more than 2 tablets in 24 hours
children under 6 years of age	do not use
adults 65 years of age and older	ask a doctor
consumers with kidney disease	ask a doctor

OTHER INFORMATION
- safety sealed: do not use if carton is opened or if individual blister units are torn or opened
- store between 20° and 25°C (68° and 77°F)
- protect from excessive moisture

INACTIVE INGREDIENTS
colloidal silicone dioxide, croscarmellose sodium, hypromellose, iron oxide blends, magnesium stearate, microcrystalline cellulose, polyethylene glycol, povidone, pregelatinized starch, titanium dioxide

QUESTIONS OR COMMENTS?
call toll-free **1-800-633-1610** or www.allegra.com

Allegra Allergy® - 12 HOUR

DRUG FACTS

Active Ingredient(s)
(in each tablet)
Fexofenadine HCl 60 mg

Purpose(s)
Antihistamine

USES
temporarily relieves these symptoms due to hay fever or other upper respiratory allergies:
- runny nose
- sneezing
- itchy, water eyes
- itching of the nose or throat

WARNINGS

DO NOT USE
if you have ever had an allergic reaction to this product or any of its ingredients

ASK A DOCTOR BEFORE USE IF YOU HAVE
kidney disease. Your doctor should determine if you need a different dose.

WHEN USING THIS PRODUCT
- do not take more than directed
- do not take at the same time as aluminum or magnesium antacids
- do not take with fruit juices (see Directions)

STOP USE AND ASK A DOCTOR IF
an allergic reaction to this product occurs. Seek medical help right away.

If pregnant or breast-feeding, ask a health professional before use.

Keep out of reach of children. In case of overdose, get medical help or contact a Poison Control Center right away.

DIRECTIONS

adults and children 12 years of age and over	take one 60 mg tablet with water every 12 hours; do not take more than 2 tablets in 24 hours
children under 12 years of age	do not use
adults 65 years of age and older	ask a doctor
consumers with kidney disease	ask a doctor

OTHER INFORMATION
- safety sealed: do not use if carton is opened or if individual blister units are torn or opened
- store between 20° and 25°C (68° and 77°F)
- protect from excessive moisture

INACTIVE INGREDIENTS
colloidal silicone dioxide, croscarmellose sodium, hypromellose, iron oxide blends, magnesium stearate, microcrystalline cellulose, polyethylene glycol, povidone, pregelatinized starch, titanium dioxide

QUESTIONS OR COMMENTS?
call toll-free **1-800-633-1610** or www.allegra.com

Allegra Allergy® - 24 HOUR

DRUG FACTS

Active Ingredient(s)
(in each tablet)
Fexofenadine HCl 180 mg

Purpose(s)
Antihistamine

USES
temporarily relieves these symptoms due to hay fever or other upper respiratory allergies:
- runny nose
- sneezing
- itchy, water eyes
- itching of the nose or throat

WARNINGS

DO NOT USE
if you have ever had an allergic reaction to this product or any of its ingredients

ASK A DOCTOR BEFORE USE IF YOU HAVE
kidney disease. Your doctor should determine if you need a different dose.

WHEN USING THIS PRODUCT
- do not take more than directed
- do not take at the same time as aluminum or magnesium antacids
- do not take with fruit juices (see Directions)

STOP USE AND ASK A DOCTOR IF
an allergic reaction to this product occurs. Seek medical help right away.

If pregnant or breast-feeding, ask a health professional before use.

Keep out of reach of children. In case of overdose, get medical help or contact a Poison Control Center right away.

DIRECTIONS

adults and children 12 years of age and over	take one 180 mg tablet with water once a day; do not take more than 1 tablet in 24 hours
children under 12 years of age	do not use
adults 65 years of age and older	ask a doctor
consumers with kidney disease	ask a doctor

OTHER INFORMATION
- safety sealed: do not use if carton is opened or if printed foil inner seal on bottle is torn or missing
- store between 20° and 25°C (68° and 77°F)
- protect from excessive moisture

INACTIVE INGREDIENTS
colloidal silicone dioxide, croscarmellose sodium, hypromellose, iron oxide blends, magnesium stearate, microcrystalline cellulose, polyethylene glycol, povidone, pregelatinized starch, titanium dioxide

QUESTIONS OR COMMENTS?
call toll-free **1-800-633-1610** or www.allegra.com
The makers of Allegra® do not make store brand products. The trade dress of this Allegra® package is subject to trademark protection.
Dist. By: Chattem, Inc. (part of the sanofi-aventis Group), Chattanooga, TN 37409-0219 ©2010

CHILDRENS ALLEGRA ALLERGY-ODT
(fexofenadine hydrochloride)

Chattem, Inc.

DRUG FACTS

Active Ingredient(s)
(in each tablet)
Fexofenadine HCl 30 mg

Purpose(s)
Antihistamine

USES
temporarily relieves these symptoms due to hay fever or other upper respiratory allergies:
- runny nose
- sneezing
- itchy, water eyes
- itching of the nose or throat

WARNINGS

DO NOT USE
if you have ever had an allergic reaction to this product or any of its ingredients.

ASK A DOCTOR BEFORE USE IF YOU HAVE
kidney disease. Your doctor should determine if you need a different dose.

WHEN USING THIS PRODUCT
- do not take more than directed
- do not take at the same time as aluminum or magnesium antacids
- do not take with fruit juices (see Directions)

STOP USE AND ASK A DOCTOR IF
an allergic reaction to this product occurs. Seek medical help right away.

If pregnant or breast-feeding,
ask a health professional before use.

Keep out of reach of children.
In case of overdose, get medical help or contact a Poison Control Center right away.

DIRECTIONS
- place 1 tablet on tongue; tablet disintegrates, with or without water

adults and children 12 years of age and over	take 2 tablets every 12 hours on an empty stomach; do not take more than 4 tablets in 24 hours
children 6 to under 12 years of age	take 1 tablet every 12 hours on an empty stomach; do not take more than 2 tablets in 24 hours
children under 6 years of age	do not use
adults 65 years of age and older	ask a doctor
consumers with kidney disease	ask a doctor

OTHER INFORMATION
- each tablet contains: **sodium 5 mg**
- phenylketonurics: contains phenylalanine 5.3 mg per tablet
- safety sealed: do not use if carton is opened or if individual blister units are torn or opened
- store between 20° and 25°C (68° and 77°F)
- use tablet immediately after opening individual blister

INACTIVE INGREDIENTS
aspartame, citric acid anhydrous, crospovidone, flavors, magnesium stearate, mannitol, methacrylic acid copolymer, microcrystalline cellulose, povidone, sodium bicarbonate, sodium starch glycolate

QUESTIONS OR COMMENTS?
call toll-free **1-800-633-1610** or www.allegra.com

Dist. By: Chattem, Inc.(part of the sanofi-aventis Group), Chattanooga, TN 37409-0219 ©2010 50094020

ALLEGRA D 12 HOUR ALLERGY AND CONGESTION (fexofenadine hydrochloride and pseudoephedrine hydrochloride)
Chattem, Inc.

DRUG FACTS
Active Ingredient(s)
(in each tablet)
Fexofenadine HCl 60 mg

Purpose(s)
Antihistamine

Active Ingredient(s)
(in each tablet)
Pseudoephedrine HCl 120 mg

Purpose(s)
Nasal decongestant

USES
- temporarily relieves these symptoms due to hay fever or other
  - upper respiratory allergies:
  - runny nose
  - sneezing
  - nasal congestion
  - itchy, watery eyes
  - itching of the nose or throat
- reduces swelling of nasal passages
- temporarily relieves sinus congestion and pressure
- temporarily restores freer breathing through the nose

WARNINGS

DO NOT USE
- if you have ever had an allergic reaction to this product or any of its ingredients
- if you are now taking a prescription monoamine oxidase inhibitor (MAOI) (certain drugs for depression, psychiatric, or emotional conditions, or Parkinson's disease), or for 2 weeks after stopping the MAOI drug. If you do not know if your prescription drug contains an MAOI, ask a doctor or pharmacist before taking this product.
- if you have difficulty swallowing

ASK A DOCTOR BEFORE USE IF YOU HAVE
- heart disease
- thyroid disease
- glaucoma
- high blood pressure
- diabetes
- trouble urinating due to an enlarged prostate gland
- kidney disease. Your doctor should determine if you need a different dose.

WHEN USING THIS PRODUCT
- **do not take more than directed**
- do not take at the same time as aluminum or magnesium antacids
- do not take with fruit juices (see Directions)
- the tablet coating may be seen in the stool (this is normal). Continue to take as directed (see Directions).

STOP USE AND ASK A DOCTOR IF
- an allergic reaction to this product occurs. Seek medical help right away.

- symptoms do not improve within 7 days or are accompanied by a fever
- you get nervous, dizzy, or sleepless

If pregnant or breast-feeding,
ask a health professional before use.

Keep out of reach of children.
In case of overdose, get medical help or contact a Poison Control Center right away.

DIRECTIONS
- do not divide, crush, chew or dissolve the tablet; swallow tablet whole

adults and children 12 years of age and over	take 1 tablet with a glass of water every 12 hours on an empty stomach; do not take more than 2 tablets in 24 hours
children under 12 years of age	do not use
adults 65 years of age and older	ask a doctor
consumers with kidney disease	ask a doctor

OTHER INFORMATION
- safety sealed: do not use if carton is opened or if individual blister units are torn or opened
- store between 20° and 25°C (68° and 77°F)

INACTIVE INGREDIENTS
carnauba wax, colloidal silicon dioxide, croscarmellose sodium, hypromellose, magnesium stearate, microcrystalline cellulose, polyethylene glycol, pregelatinized starch, stearic acid

QUESTIONS OR COMMENTS?
call toll-free 1-800-633-1610 or www.allegra.com
Dist. By: Chattem, Inc. (part of the sanofi-aventis Group), Chattanooga, TN 37409-0219 ©2010 50094535

ALLEGRA-D 24 HOUR ALLERGY AND CONGESTION (fexofenadine hydrochloride and pseudoephedrine hydrochloride)

Chattem, Inc.

DRUG FACTS

Active Ingredient(s)
(in each tablet)
Fexofenadine HCl 180 mg

Purpose(s)
Antihistamine

Active Ingredient(s)
(in each tablet)
Pseudoephedrine HCl 240 mg

Purpose(s)
Nasal decongestant

USES
- temporarily relieves these symptoms due to hay fever or other upper respiratory allergies:
  - runny nose
  - sneezing
  - nasal congestion
  - itchy, watery eyes
  - itching of the nose or throat
- reduces swelling of nasal passages
- temporarily relieves sinus congestion and pressure
- temporarily restores freer breathing through the nose

WARNINGS

DO NOT USE
- if you have ever had an allergic reaction to this product or any of its ingredients
- if you are now taking a prescription monoamine oxidase inhibitor (MAOI) (certain drugs for depression, psychiatric, or emotional conditions, or Parkinson's disease), or for 2 weeks after stopping the MAOI drug. If you do not know if your prescription drug contains an MAOI, ask a doctor or pharmacist before taking this product.
- if you have difficulty swallowing

ASK A DOCTOR BEFORE USE IF YOU HAVE
- heart disease
- thyroid disease
- glaucoma
- high blood pressure
- diabetes
- trouble urinating due to an enlarged prostate gland
- kidney disease. Your doctor should determine if you need a different dose.

WHEN USING THIS PRODUCT
- **do not take more than directed**
- do not take at the same time as aluminum or magnesium antacids
- do not take with fruit juices (see Directions)
- the tablet coating may be seen in the stool (this is normal). Continue to take as directed (see Directions).

STOP USE AND ASK A DOCTOR IF
- an allergic reaction to this product occurs. Seek medical help right away.
- symptoms do not improve within 7 days or are accompanied by a fever
- you get nervous, dizzy, or sleepless

If pregnant or breast-feeding,
ask a health professional before use.

Keep out of reach of children.
In case of overdose, get medical help or contact a Poison Control Center right away.

DIRECTIONS
do not divide, crush, chew or dissolve the tablet; swallow tablet whole

adults and children 12 years of age and over	take 1 tablet with a glass of water every 24 hours on an empty stomach; do not take more than 1 tablet in 24 hours
children under 12 years of age	do not use
adults 65 years of age and older	ask a doctor
consumers with kidney disease	ask a doctor

OTHER INFORMATION
- each tablet contains: **sodium 33 mg**
- safety sealed: do not use if carton is opened or if individual blister units are torn or opened
- store between 20° and 25°C (68° and 77°F)

INACTIVE INGREDIENTS
acetone, black iron oxide, cellulose acetate, colloidal silicon dioxide, copovidone, croscarmellose sodium, FD&C blue #1 aluminum lake, glycerol triacetate, hypromellose, isopropyl

alcohol, magnesium stearate, methyl alcohol, methylene chloride, microcrystalline cellulose, polyethylene glycol, propylene glycol, povidone, sodium chloride, talc, titanium dioxide, water

QUESTIONS OR COMMENTS?
call toll-free 1-800-633-1610 or www.allegra.com
Dist. By: Chattem, Inc. (part of the sanofi-aventis Group), Chattanooga, TN 37409-0219 ©2010 50094540

BABY ANBESOL (benzocaine)
Wyeth Consumer Healthcare

DRUG FACTS

Active Ingredient(s)
Benzocaine 7.5%

Purpose(s)
Oral Anesthetic

USE
temporarily relieves sore gums due to teething in infants and children 4 months of age and older

WARNINGS
Allergy alert:
Do not use this product if you have a history of allergy to local anesthetics such as procaine, butacaine, benzocaine, or other "caine" anesthetics.

DO NOT USE
to treat fever and nasal congenstion. These are not symptoms of teething and may indicate the presence of infection. If these symptoms persist, consult your doctor.

WHEN USING THIS PRODUCT
• avoid contact with the eyes
• do not exceed recommended dosage
• do not use for more than 7 days unless directed by a doctor/dentist

STOP USE AND ASK A DOCTOR IF
• sore mouth symptoms do not improve in 7 days
• irritation, pain, or redness persists or worsens
• swelling, rash, or fever develops

Keep out of reach of children.
If more than used for pain is accidentally swallowed, get medical help or contact a Poison Control Center right away.

DIRECTIONS
• to open tube, cut tip of the tube on score mark with scissors
• children 4 months of age and older: apply to the affected area not more than 4 times daily or as directed by a doctor/dentist
• infants under 4 months of age: no recommended dosage or treatment except under the advice and supervision of a doctor/dentist.

OTHER INFORMATION
store at 20-25°C (68-77°F)

INACTIVE INGREDIENTS
artificial flavor, benzoic acid, carbomer 934P, D&C red no. 33, edetate disodium, FD&C blue no. 1, glycerin, methylparaben, polyethylene glycol, propylparaben, purified water, saccharin

QUESTIONS OR COMMENTS?
Call weekdays 9AM to 5PM EST at 1-888-797-5638

ANBESOL COLD SORE THERAPY (allantoin, benzocaine, camphor, and petrolatum)
Pfizer Consumer Healthcare

DRUG FACTS

Active Ingredient(s)
Allantoin 1%
Benzocaine 20%
Camphor 3%
White petrolatum 64.9%

Purpose(s)
Skin protectant
Fever blister/cold sore treatment
Fever blister/cold sore treatment
Skin protectant

USES
• temporarily relieves pain associated with fever blisters and cold sores
• relieves dryness and softens fever blisters and cold sores

WARNINGS
For external use only

Allergy alert:
Do not use this product if you have a history of allergy to local anesthetics such as procaine, butacaine, benzocaine, or other "caine" anesthetics.

DO NOT USE
over deep or puncture wounds, infections, or lacerations. Consult a doctor.

WHEN USING THIS PRODUCT
• avoid contact with the eyes
• do not exceed recommended dosage

STOP USE AND ASK A DOCTOR IF
• condition worsens
• symptoms persist for more than 7 days
• symptoms clear up and occur again within a few days

Keep out of reach of children.
If swallowed, get medical help or contact a Poison Control Center right away.

DIRECTIONS
• to open tube, cut tip of the tube on score mark with scissors
• adults and children 2 years of age and older: apply to the affected area not more than 3 to 4 times daily
• children under 12 years of age: adult supervision should be given in the use of this product
• children under 2 years of age: consult a doctor

OTHER INFORMATION
store at 20-25°C (68-77°F)

INACTIVE INGREDIENTS
aloe barbadenis leaf extract, benzyl alcohol, butylparaben, glyceryl monostearate, isocetyl stearate, menthol, methylparaben, mineral oil, propylparaben, sodium lauryl sulfate, vitamin E, white wax

QUESTIONS OR COMMENTS?
Call weekdays 9AM to 5PM EST at **1-888-797-5638**

ANBESOL (benzocaine)

Wyeth Consumer Healthcare

DRUG FACTS

Active Ingredient(s)

Anbesol Regular Strength Liquid and Gel
Benzocaine 10%

Anbesol Jr. Gel
Benzocaine 10%

Anbesol Maximum Strength Liquid and Gel
Benzocaine 20%

Purpose(s)
Oral Anesthetic

USES
- temporarily relieves pain associated with the following mouth and gum irritations:
  - toothache
  - sore gums
  - canker sores
  - braces
  - minor dental procedures
  - dentures

WARNINGS

Allergy alert
Do not use this product if you have a history of allergy to local anesthetics such as procaine, butacaine, benzocaine, or other "caine" anesthetics

WHEN USING THIS PRODUCT
- avoid contact with the eyes
- do not exceed recommended dosage
- do not use for more than 7 days unless directed by a doctor/dentist

STOP USE AND ASK A DOCTOR IF
- sore mouth symptoms do not improve in 7 days
- irritation, pain, or redness persists or worsens
- swelling, rash, or fever develops

Keep out of reach of children.
If more than used for pain is accidentally swallowed, get medical help or contact a Poison Control Center right away.

DIRECTIONS

Anbesol Regular and Maximum Strength Liquid
- adults and children 2 years of age and older:
  - wipe liquid on with cotton, or cotton swab, or fingertip
  - apply to the affected area up to 4 times daily or as directed by a doctor/dentist
- children under 12 years of age: adult supervision should be given in the use of this product
- children under 2 years of age: consult a doctor/dentist

Anbesol Regular and Maximum Strength Gel
- to open tube, cut tip of the tube on score mark with scissors
- adults and children 2 years of age and older: apply to the affected area up to 4 times daily or as directed by a doctor/dentist
- children under 12 years of age: adult supervision should be given in the use of this product
- children under 2 years of age: consult a doctor/dentist
- for denture irritation:
  - apply thin layer to the affected area
  - do not reinsert dental work until irritation/pain is relieved
  - rinse mouth well before reinserting

Anbesol Jr. Gel
- to open tube, cut tip of the tube on score mark with scissors
- adults and children 2 years of age and older: apply to the affected area up to 4 times daily or as directed by a doctor/dentist
- children under 12 years of age: adult supervision should be given in the use of this product
- children under 2 years of age: consult a doctor/dentist

OTHER INFORMATION
Anbesol Regular Strength Liquid and Gel, Anbesol Maximum Strength Liquid, and Anbesol Jr. Gel
Store at 20-25°C (68-77°F)

Anbesol Maximum Strength Gel
Store at 20-25°C (68-77°F). Do not refrigerate.

INACTIVE INGREDIENTS

Anbesol Regular Strength Liquid
benzyl alcohol, D&C red no. 33, D&C yellow no. 10, FD&C blue no. 1, FD&C yellow no. 6, flavor, methylparaben, polyethylene glycol, propylene glycol, saccharin

Anbesol Regular Strength Gel
benzyl alcohol, carbomer 934P, D&C red no. 33, D&C yellow no. 10, FD&C blue no. 1, FD&C yellow no. 6, flavor, glycerin, methylparaben, polyethylene glycol, propylene glycol, saccharin

Anbesol Jr. Gel
artificial flavor, benzyl alcohol, carbomer 934P, D&C red no. 33, glycerin, methylparaben, polyethylene glycol, potassium acesulfame

Anbesol Maximum Strength Liquid
benzyl alcohol, D&C yellow no. 10, FD&C blue no. 1, FD&C red no. 40, flavor, methylparaben, polyethylene glycol, propylene glycol, saccharin

Anbesol Maximum Strength Gel
benzyl alcohol, carbomer 934P, D&C yellow no. 10, FD&C blue no. 1, FD&C red no. 40, flavor, glycerin, methylparaben, polyethylene glycol, propylene glycol, saccharin

---

AQUAPHOR HEALING (petrolatum)

Beiersdorf Inc

Petrolatum 41%
Skin Protectant Ointment
Treatment or Prevention of Diaper Rash

USES
- temporarily protects minor: • cuts • scrapes • burns
- temporarily protects and helps relieve chapped or cracked skin and lips
- helps protect from the drying effects of wind and cold weather
- helps treat and prevent diaper rash
- protects chafed skin associated with diaper rash and helps protect from wetness

DIRECTIONS
- apply as needed
- for diaper rash, change wet and soiled diapers promptly, cleanse the diaper area, and allow to dry. Apply ointment liberally as often as necessary, with each diaper change, especially at bedtime or anytime when exposure to wet diapers may be prolonged.

WHEN USING THIS PRODUCT
- do not get into eyes

DO NOT USE ON
- deep or puncture wounds • animal bites
- serious burns

STOP USE AND ASK A DOCTOR IF
• condition worsens
• symptoms last more than 7 days or clear up and occur again within a few days
Keep out of reach of children. If swallowed, get medical help or contact a Poison Control Center right away.
Mineral Oil, Ceresin, Lanolin Alcohol, Panthenol, Glycerin, Bisabolol

QUESTIONS OR COMMENTS?
1-800-227-4703

ASPERCREME PAIN RELIEVING LOTION
ASPERCREME HEAT PAIN RELIEVING GEL
(trolamine)(menthol)

Chattem, Inc.

DRUG FACTS

Lotion

Active Ingredient(s)	Purpose(s)
Trolamine salicylate 10%	Topical analgesic

Gel

Active Ingredient(s)	Purpose(s)
Menthol 10%	Topical analgesic

USES
• temporarily relieves minor pain associated with:
• arthritis
• simple backache
• muscle strains
• muscle sprains
• bruises
• cramps

WARNINGS
• **For external use only**

Allergy alert: if prone to allergic reaction from aspirin or salicylate, consult a doctor before use.

WHEN USING THIS PRODUCT
Lotion:
• use only as directed
• do not bandage tightly or use with a heating pad
• avoid contact with eyes and mucous membranes
• do not apply to wounds or damaged, broken or irritated skin

Gel:
• use only as directed
• do not bandage tightly or use with a heating pad
• avoid contact with eyes and mucous membranes
• do not apply to wounds or damaged, broken or irritated skin
• a transient burning sensation may occur upon application but generally disappears in several days
• if severe burning sensation occurs, discontinue use immediately
• do not expose the area treated with product to heat or direct sunlight

STOP USE AND ASK A DOCTOR IF
• condition worsens
• symptoms persist for more than 7 days or clear up and occur again within a few days
• redness is present
• irritation develops

If pregnant or breast-feeding, ask a health professional before use.
Keep out of reach of children. In case of accidental ingestion, get medical help or contact a Poison Control Center right away.

DIRECTIONS
Lotion:
• shake well before using

adults and children over 12 years	Apply generously to affected area. Massage into painful area until thoroughly absorbed into skin. Repeat as necessary, but no more than 4 times a daily.
children under 10 years	Do not use

Gel:

adults and children over 18 years	Apply to affected area Squeeze desired amount of Aspercreme Heat Pain Relieving Gel onto affected area Using the sponge-top applicator, massage dispensed gel into painful area until thoroughly absorbed Repeat as necessary, but no more than 3 to 4 times daily IF MEDICINE COMES IN CONTACT WITH HANDS, WASH WITH SOAP AND WATER
children 18 years or younger	Ask a doctor

INACTIVE INGREDIENTS
Lotion: aloe vera gel, cetyl alcohol, glyceryl stearate, isopropyl palmitate, lanolin, methylparaben, potassium phosphate, propylene glycol, propylparaben, sodium lauryl sulfate, stearic acid, water
Gel: acrylates/C10-30, alkyl crosspolymer, allantoin, aloe barbadensis leaf juice, capsaicin, DMDM hydantoin, fragrance, glycerin, methylparaben, phenoxyethanol, propylene glycol, propylparaben, SD alcohol 40-2 (15%), steareth-2, steareth-21, triethanolamine, water

ASPERCREME MAX NO MESS ROLL ON
(menthol)

Chattem, Inc.

ASPERCREME® MAX NO MESS ROLL-ON

Active Ingredient(s)
Menthol 16%

Purpose(s)
Topical analgesic

USES
• temporarily relieves minor pain associated with:
  • arthritis
  • simple backache
  • muscle strains
  • sprains
  • bruises
  • cramps

WARNINGS
For external use only.

WHEN USING THIS PRODUCT
- use only as directed
- do not bandage tightly or use with a heating pad
- avoid contact with eyes and mucous membranes
- do not apply to wounds or damaged, broken or irritated skin
- a transient burning sensation or redness may occur upon application but generally disappears in several days
- if severe burning sensation occurs, discontinue use immediately
- do not expose the area treated with product to heat or direct sunlight

STOP USE AND ASK A DOCTOR IF
- condition worsens
- redness is present
- irritation develops
- symptoms persist for more than 7 days or clear up and occur again within a few days

Flammable
- Keep away from fire or flame.

If pregnant or breast-feeding
ask a health professional before use.

Keep out of reach of children.
If swallowed, get medical help or contact a Poison Control Center right away.

DIRECTIONS
adults and children over 12 years:
- apply generously to affected area
- massage into painful area until thoroughly absorbed into skin
- repeat as necessary, but no more than 3 to 4 times daily
- **IF MEDICINE COMES IN CONTACT WITH HANDS, WASH WITH SOAP AND WATER**

children 12 years or younger: ask a doctor

INACTIVE INGREDIENTS
acrylates/C10-30 alkyl acrylate crosspolymer, capsaicin, glycerin, isopropyl myristate, propylene glycol, SD alcohol 40 (30%), triethanolamine, water (245-256)
Close cap tightly after use. Keep carton as it contains important information.
Distributed by: Chattem, Inc.
P.O. Box 2219
Chattanooga, TN 37409-0219
0043104-01 U.S.A. ©2009 www.chattem.com Recyclable Carton

AVEENO ANTI ITCH CONCENTRATED LOTION (calamine and pramoxine)

Johnson & Johnson Consumer Products Company Division of Johnson & Johnson Consumer Companies, Inc.

DRUG FACTS

Active Ingredient(s)	Purpose(s)
Calamine 3%	Skin protectant
Pramoxine HCl 1%	External analgesic

USES
- For temporary relief of pain and itching associated with minor burns, sunburns, minor cuts, scrapes, insect bites, minor skin irritations, rashes due to poison ivy, poison oak or poison sumac.
- Dries the oozing and weeping of poison ivy/oak/sumac

WARNINGS
For external use only.

WHEN USING THIS PRODUCT
- Do not get into eyes

STOP USE AND ASK A DOCTOR IF
- Condition worsens
- Symptoms last more than 7 days or clear up and occur again within a few days discontinue use and consult a doctor.
- Do not apply to wounds or damaged skin.
- Do not bandage tightly.

Keep out of reach of children. If swallowed, get medical help or contact a Poison Control Center immediately.

DIRECTIONS
- Adults and children 2 years of age and older: Apply to affected area not more than 3 to 4 times daily. Children under 2 years of age: consult a doctor.

OTHER INFORMATION
- Store at room temperature

INACTIVE INGREDIENTS
avena sativa (oat) kernel extract, avena sativa (oat) kernel flour, avena sativa (oat) kernel oil, camphor, cetyl alcohol, dimethicone, distearyldimonium chloride, glycerin, isopropyl palmitate, methylparaben, petrolatum, sodium chloride, water

QUESTIONS OR COMMENTS?
1-866-428-3366

AVEENO BABY ECZEMA THERAPY (colloidal oatmeal)

Johnson & Johnson Consumer Products Company, Division of Johnson & Johnson Consumer Companies, Inc.

DRUG FACTS

Active Ingredient(s)	Purpose(s)
Colloidal oatmeal 1%	Skin protectant

USES
Temporary protects and helps relieve minor skin irritation and itching due to:
- Rashes
- Eczema

WARNINGS
For external use only

WHEN USING THIS PRODUCT DO NOT GET INTO EYES

STOP USE AND ASK A DOCTOR IF
- Condition worsens
- Symptoms last more than 7 days or clear up and occur again within a few days

Keep out of reach of children. If swallowed, get medical help or contact a Poison Control Center immediately.

DIRECTIONS
- Apply as needed

OTHER INFORMATION
- For use on mild to moderate eczema or as directed by a physician.
- Store at room temperature.

INACTIVE INGREDIENTS
water, glycerin, distearyldimonium chloride, panthenol, petrolatum, isopropyl palmitate, cetyl alcohol, dimethicone, avena sativa (Oat) kernel oil, steareth-20, avena sativa (Oat) kernel extract, benzalkonium chloride, ceramide NP, sodium chloride

QUESTIONS OR COMMENTS?
Call **1-866-428-3366** or visit 222.Aveeno.com

AVEENO BABY SOOTHING RELIEF DIAPER RASH FRAGRANCE FREE (zinc oxide)

Johnson & Johnson Consumer Products Company, Division of Johnson & Johnson Consumer Companies, Inc.

DRUG FACTS

Active Ingredient(s)
Zinc Oxide 13%

Purpose(s)
Skin Protectant

USES
- helps treat and prevent diaper rash
- protects chafed skin due to diaper rash
- helps seal out wetness

WARNINGS
For external use only.

WHEN USING THIS PRODUCT
- avoid contact with eyes

STOP USE AND ASK A DOCTOR IF
- condition worsens or does not improve within 7 days.

Keep out of reach of children. If swallowed, get medical help or contact a Poison Control Center immediately.

DIRECTIONS
- Change wet or soiled diapers promptly. Clean the diaper area and allow to dry. Apply cream liberally as often as necessary, with each diaper change, especially at bedtime or any time exposure to wet diapers may be prolonged.

OTHER INFORMATION
- Do not use if quality seal is broken.

INACTIVE INGREDIENTS
Avena sativa (oat) kernel extract, beeswax, benzoic acid, dimethicone, *Epilobium angustifolium* flower/leaf/stem extract (willowherb), glycerin, methylparaben, microcrystalline wax, mineral oil, *Oenothera biennis* (evening primrose) seed extract, potassium hydroxide, propylparaben, sorbitan sesquioleate, synthetic beeswax, water

QUESTIONS OR COMMENTS?
Call 1-866-428-3366 or visit www.aveeno.com

Distributed by:
Johnson & Johnson
CONSUMER PRODUCTS COMPANY
Division of
Johnson &Johnson Consumer Companies, Inc.
Skillman, NJ 08558-9418

AYR ALLERGY & SINUS HYPERTONIC SALINE NASAL MIST

B.F. Ascher & Company, inc.

INGREDIENTS
Ayr Allergy & Sinus is a hypertonic solution of deionized water, sodium chloride (2.65%), potassium phosphate/sodium hydroxide buffer (to minimize nasal irritation), disodium EDTA, and benzalkonium chloride.

DIRECTIONS
Hold head upright and squeeze twice in each nostril. If desired, sniff deeply while squeezing bottle. Use 2 or 3 times daily as needed, or as recommended by your doctor.

USES
Ayr Allergy & Sinus is designed to help dry nasal congestion, help reduce nasal swelling, and is useful as a wash to flush allergens and dust from nasal passages.

WARNINGS
May cause a mild, temporary stinging sensation
Use only as directed.
Keep out of reach of children
The use of this dispenser by more than one person may spread infection.
PRECAUTIONS
Take care not to aspirate nasal contents back into the bottle. If spray tip touches nose, rinse with hot water before replacing cap. Use of he dispenser by more than one person may spread infection.

BABY AYR SALINE NOSE SPRAY/DROPS

B.F. Ascher & Company, inc.

INGREDIENTS
Sodium chloride 0.65% with monobasic potassium phosphate/sodium hydroxide buffer to prevent nasal irritation. Also contains the non-irritating antibacterial and antifungal preservatives disodium EDTA and benzalkonium chloride and is formulated with deionized water.

DIRECTIONS
For Infants: Put child on his/her back with head between your knees. Gently remove excess mucus with warm, moist cloth or cotton swab. With one hand, hold the baby's hands. With your other hand, put 2 to 6 drops in each nostril, taking care not to touch the dropper tip to hands, nose or nasal secretions. Have child remain on back for 1 to 2 minutes. Gently wipe the nose with a tissue or use a nasal aspirator or bulb syringe. The AYR dropper tip should be rinsed with hot water and wiped with a clean towel. Do not use the same bottle for other children.
For older children: Hold bottle upright. Give short, firm squeezes into each nostril. Take care not to aspirate nasal contents back into bottle.
PRECAUTIONS
The use of this dispenser by more than one person may spread infection.

AVAILABILITY

Baby Ayr Saline Nasal Spray/Drops is available in 30 mL bottles.

- Non-medicated formula is safe and gentle on baby's delicate membranes
- Special bottle design eases application
- No burning or stinging
- Loosens and thins mucus secretions to aid aspiration and removal of mucus from nose and sinuses
- Gluten free

Help relieve your baby's delicate nose with non-medicated Baby Ayr Saline Nose Spray/Drops. Baby Ayr restores moisture to dry, crusted and inflamed nasal membranes caused by colds. For babies with congested noses, Baby Ayr loosens and thins secretions to aid in the removal of mucus from the nose and sinuses. Parents will appreciate the unique bottle design which eases application by allowing either drops or spray. The special formula soothes baby's nose while avoiding the unpleasant side effects of decongestant drops or sprays.

AYR SALINE NASAL DROPS (sodium chloride)

B.F. Ascher & Company, inc.

INGREDIENTS

Active Ingredients: A buffered isotonic solution of 0.65% sodium chloride.

DIRECTIONS

Tilt head back, apply 2 to 6 drops in each nostril as often as needed, or as directed by your doctor.

USES

Ayr Drops moisturizes nasal passages relieving dry, crusty and inflamed nasal membranes useful as a nasal wash for sinuses, allergies and colds. Safe and gentle enough for babies. Doctor recommended.

WARNINGS

This bottle is not designed to spray. If tip touches nose, rinse with hot water before replacing cap. Use of bottle by more than one person may spread infection.

AVAILABILITY

Available for purchase in 50 mL bottles.

- Loosens and thins congestion caused by colds or allergies
- Restores moisture to dry nasal membranes
- Safe for babies and pregnant women
- Can be used as often as needed

Ayr Drops restores moisture to dry nasal membranes affected by climate, respiratory infections, travel, oxygen therapy, overuse of nasal decongestants, and hormonal changes brought on by pregnancy. Ayr Drops is specially formulated so there is no burning or stinging, which may be experienced with other saline drops and sprays. Ayr Drops is non-medicated and alcohol free.

AYR SALINE NASAL GEL

B.F. Ascher & Company, inc.

INGREDIENTS

Water, methyl gluceth-10, propylene glycol, glycerin, glyceryl polymethacrylate, triethanolamine, aloe barbadensis leaf juice (aloe vera gel), PEG/PPG-18/18 dimethicone, carbomer, poloxamer 184, sodium chloride, xanthan gum, diazolidinyl urea, methylparaben, propylparaben, glycine soja (soybean) oil, geranium maculatum oil, tocopheryl acetate, blue 1.

DIRECTIONS

Apply Ayr Gel around nostrils and under nose. Ayr Gel may be placed in nostrils to help relieve discomfort. Use during the day and at bedtime to prevent drying and crusting. Use as often as needed. Store at room temperature (59°-86°F).

WARNINGS

For external use only except as directed. Avoid contact with the eyes. Keep out of reach of children.

AVAILABILITY

Ayr Saline Nasal Gel is available in 0.5 oz tubes.

- Restores moisture to dry, irritated nasal membranes
- Formulated to be compatible with nasal tissue
- Gentle enough for babies, and year-round use
- Gives longer moisturization
- Recommended for day and night-time use
- Gluten free

Dry irritated nasal passages can find relief with soothing Ayr Saline Nasal Gel. Created with ingredients chosen by ear, nose, and throat doctors, Ayr Gel is gentle and formulated to be compatible with nasal membranes. Gentle enough for babies, Ayr Gel provides year-round relief. Ayr Gel is recommended for those suffering from dryness due to travel, allergies, mouth breathing, climate, pregnancy, nosebleeds, oxygen therapy, CPAP, and respiratory infections

AYR SALINE NASAL GEL NO-DRIP SINUS SPRAY

B.F. Ascher & Company, inc.

INGREDIENTS

Water, sodium carbomethyl starch, propylene glycol, glycerin, aloe barbadensis leaf juice (aloe vera), sodium chloride, cetylpyridinium chloride, citric acid, disodium EDTA, glycine soja (soybean) oil, tocopheryl acetate, benzyl alcohol, benzalkonium chloride, geranium maculatum oil

DIRECTIONS

Remove cap and safety clip. Spray once into each nostril. Wipe nozzle clean after use.

USES

Helps relieve dry sinus passages due to low humidity, colds, allergies and irritants.

WARNINGS

DO NOT USE

this product if you are allergic to any of the listed ingredients.

USE ONLY AS DIRECTED

KEEP OUT OF REACH OF CHILDREN

AVOID CONTACT with the eyes

PRECAUTIONS

Store at 59°-86° F (15°-30° C)

Mfd. in U.S.A. for B.F. Ascher & Co., Inc.

AVAILABILITY

Ayr Saline Nasal Gel No-Drip Sinus Spray is available in 0.75 fl oz (22 mL) bottles.

- Colds, allergies, sinusitis

AYR SALINE NASAL MIST

B.F. Ascher & Company, inc.

INGREDIENTS

Ayr Saline Nasal Mist is a specially formulated, buffered, isotonic saline solution containing sodium chloride 0.65% adjusted to the proper tonicity and pH with monobasic potassium phosphate/sodium hydroxide buffer to prevent nasal irritation. Ayr also contains the non-irritating antibacterial and antifungal preservatives disodium EDTA and benzalkonium chloride and is formulated with deionized water.

DIRECTIONS
To spray, hold bottle upright and give short, firm squeezes in each nostril as often as needed. For nose drops, hold bottle upside down.

USES
Ayr Mist is a soothing, non-irritating saline solution physiologically compatible with nasal membranes. Ayr Mist restores important moisture to provide relief for dry, crusty and inflamed nasal membranes due to central heating, low humidity environments, or colds and the overuse of nasal decongestant drops or sprays (rebound congestion). Ayr Mist avoids the side effects of decongestant drops or sprays.

PRECAUTIONS
Take care not to aspirate nasal contents back into bottle. If spray tip touches nose, rinse with hot water before replacing cap. Use of bottle by more than one person may spread infection.

AVAILABILITY
Ayr Saline Nasal Mist is available in 50 mL bottles.
- Loosens and thins congestion caused by colds or allergies
- Restores moisture to dry nasal membranes
- Safe for babies and pregnant women
- Can be used as often as needed
- Gluten free

Breathe easier with soothing, non-irritating Ayr Saline Nasal Mist. Ayr Mist effectively washes away mucus and allergens which can lead to nasal congestion. Dry noses will also appreciate the relief of this soothing solution.

Ayr Mist restores moisture to nasal membranes affected by dryness due to climate, respiratory infections, travel, oxygen therapy, overuse of nasal decongestants, and hormonal changes caused by pregnancy. Because Ayr Mist is specially formulated to be compatible with nasal membranes, there is no burning or stinging which may be experienced with other drops and sprays.

BACTINE ORIGINAL FIRST AID LIQUID
(benzalkonium chloride and lidocaine hydrochloride)

Bayer HealthCare LLC.

Active Ingredient(s)
- Benzalkonium Cl 0.13% w/w (First aid antiseptic)
- Lidocaine HCl 2.5% w/w (Pain relieving liquid)

USES
first aid to help prevent skin infection, and for temporary relief of pain and itching associated with minor:
- cuts
- scrapes
- burns
- sunburn
- skin irritations

WARNINGS
- **For external use only**

ASK A DOCTOR BEFORE USE IF YOU HAVE
- deep or puncture wounds
- animal bites
- serious burns

WHEN USING THIS PRODUCT
- do not use in or near the eyes
- do not apply over large areas of the body or in large quantities
- do not apply over raw surfaces or blistered areas

STOP USE AND ASK A DOCTOR IF
- condition worsens
- symptoms persist for more than 7 days, or clear up and occur again within a few days.
- **Keep out of reach of children.** If swallowed, get medical help or contact a Poison Control Center right away.

DIRECTIONS
- adults and children 2 years and older:
  - clean the affected area
  - apply a small amount on the area 1 to 3 times daily
  - may be covered with a sterile bandage
  - if bandaged, let dry first
- children under 2 years: ask a doctor

OTHER INFORMATION
- avoid excessive heat

INACTIVE INGREDIENTS
- edetate disodium
- fragrances
- nonoxynol 9
- propylene glycol
- purified water

QUESTIONS OR COMMENTS?
1-800-986-0369 (Mon - Fri 9AM - 5PM EST) or www.bactine.com

BACTINE PAIN RELIEVING CLEANSING SPRAY (benzalkonium chloride and lidocaine hydrochloride)

Bayer HealthCare LLC.

Active Ingredient(s)
- Benzalkonium CL 0.13% w/w (First aid antiseptic)
- Lidocaine HCL 2.5% w/w (Pain relieving spray)

USES
first aid to help prevent bacterial contamination or skin infection, and temporary relief of pain and itching associated with minor:
- cuts
- scrapes
- burns
- sunburn
- skin irritations
- insect bites

WARNINGS
- **For external use only**

ASK A DOCTOR BEFORE USE IF YOU HAVE
- deep or puncture wounds
- animal bites
- serious burns

WHEN USING THIS PRODUCT
- do not use in or near the eyes
- do not apply over large areas of the body or in large quantities
- do not apply over raw surfaces or blistered areas

STOP USE AND ASK A DOCTOR IF
- condition worsens
- symptoms persist for more than 7 days, or clear up and occur again within a few days.
- **Keep out of reach of children.** If swallowed, get medical help or contact a Poison Control Center right away

DIRECTIONS
- adults and children 2 years and older
  - clean the affected area
  - apply a small amount on the area 1 to 3 times daily
  - may be covered with a sterile bandage (let dry first)
- children under 2 years, ask a doctor

OTHER INFORMATION
- avoid excessive heat

INACTIVE INGREDIENTS
- edetate disodium
- fragrances
- nonoxynol 9
- propylene glycol
- purified water

QUESTIONS OR COMMENTS?
1-800-986-0369 (Mon - Fri 9AM - 5PM EST) or
www.bactine.com

BALMEX DIAPER RASH CREAM (zinc oxide)

Chattem, Inc.

Balmex Diaper Rash Cream

Active Ingredient(s)
Zinc oxide 11.3%

Purpose(s)
Skin protectant

USES
- helps treat and prevent diaper rash
- protects chafed skin due to diaper rash and helps seal out wetness

WARNINGS
For external use only

WHEN USING THIS PRODUCT
avoid contact with eyes

STOP USE AND ASK A DOCTOR IF
condition worsens or lasts more than 7 days

Keep out of reach of children.
If swallowed, get medical help or contact a Poison Control Center immediately.

DIRECTIONS
- change wet or soiled diapers promptly
- cleanse the diaper area and allow to dry
- apply cream liberally as often as necessary, with each diaper change, especially at bedtime or anytime when exposure to wet diapers may be prolonged

OTHER INFORMATION
- do not use if quality seal is broken

INACTIVE INGREDIENTS
beeswax, benzoic acid, dimethicone, fragrance, glycine soja (soybean) oil, magnesium aspartate, methylparaben, microcrystalline wax, mineral oil, oenothera biennis (evening primrose) seed extract, olea europaea (olive) leaf extract, panthenol potassium aspartate, potassium hydroxide, propylene glycol, propylparaben, sarcosine, sodium cocoyl amino acids, sorbitan sesquioleate, synthetic beeswax, tocopherol, water (245-230)

BALMEX DIAPER RASH CREAM STICK (zinc oxide)

Chattem, Inc.

Balmex Diaper Rash Cream Stick

Active Ingredient(s)
Zinc oxide 11.3%

Purpose(s)
Skin protectant

USES
- helps treat and prevent diaper rash
- protects chafed skin due to diaper rash and helps seal out wetness

WARNINGS
For external use only

WHEN USING THIS PRODUCT
avoid contact with eyes

STOP USE AND ASK A DOCTOR IF
condition worsens or lasts more than 7 days

Keep out of reach of children.
If swallowed, get medical help or contact a Poison Control Center immediately.

DIRECTIONS
- change wet or soiled diapers promptly
- cleanse the diaper area and allow to dry
- apply cream liberally as often as necessary, with each diaper change, especially at bedtime or anytime when exposure to wet diapers may be prolonged

INACTIVE INGREDIENTS
beeswax, benzoic acid, dimethicone, fragrance, glycine soja (soybean) oil, magnesium aspartate, methylparaben, microcrystalline wax, mineral oil, oenothera biennis (evening primrose) seed extract, olea europaea (olive) leaf extract, panthenol potassium aspartate, potassium hydroxide, propylene glycol, propylparaben, sarcosine, sodium cocoyl amino acids, sorbitan sesquioleate, synthetic beeswax, tocopherol, water (245-230)
Dist. by Chattem, Inc.
P.O. Box 2219,
Chattanooga, TN 37409-0219
©2009 Chattem, Inc.
*patent pending
0071602-01

BALMEX MULTI-PURPOSE HEALING OINTMENT (petrolatum)

Chattem, Inc.

DRUG FACTS

Active Ingredient(s)
Petrolatum 51.1%

Purpose(s)
Skin protectant

USES
- temporarily protects minor
  - cuts
  - scrapes
  - burns

- temporarily protects and helps relieve chapped or cracked skin
helps treat and prevent diaper rash. Protects chafed skin or
minor skin irritation due to diaper rash and helps seal out
wetness

WARNINGS
For external use only

WHEN USING THIS PRODUCT
- do not get into eyes

STOP USE AND ASK A DOCTOR IF
- condition worsens
- symptoms last more than 7 days or clear up and occur again
within a few days

DO NOT USE ON
- deep puncture wounds
- animal bites
- serious burns

Keep out of reach of children.
If swallowed, get medical help or contact a Poison Control
Center immediately.

DIRECTIONS
- apply as needed for diaper rash:
- change wet or soiled diapers promptly
- cleanse the diaper area and allow to dry
- apply ointment liberally as often as necessary, with each
diaper change, especially at bedtime or any time when
exposure to wet diapers may be prolonged

OTHER INFORMATION
- do not use if quality seal is broken
- see tube for lot number and expiration date

INACTIVE INGREDIENTS
acacia farnesiana flower extract, allantoin, aloe barbadenis leaf
extract, chamomilla recutita (matricaria) flower extract,
cholecalciferol, cyclomethicone, dimethicone, fragrance, isopropyl
myristate, isopropyl palmitate, lavandula angustifolia (lavender)
extract, mineral oil, polyethylene, retinyl palmitate, rosmarinus
officinalis (rosemary) extract, silica, tocopheryl acetate, zea
mays (corn) oil

BALNEOL SOOTHING RELIEF FOR "DOWN THERE"

Meda Consumer Healthcare Inc.

DIRECTIONS FOR USE
To cleanse after a bowel movement:
Squeeze Balneol lotion onto toilet paper and wipe the area.
Balneol is safe to use between bowel movements and at bedtime
for additional comfort.
For feminine cleansing:
Apply Balneol lotion to a clean tissue and gently wipe and pat
the external vaginal area. Excess lotion will help to moisturize
the area. Repeat as frequently as necessary.
For external use only.
Caution: In all cases of rectal bleeding, consult a physician
promptly. If irritation persists or increases, discontinue use and
consult a physician. Keep this and all medications out of the
reach of children. Use as often as necessary.

INGREDIENTS
Below are the ingredients in **Balneol®** hygienic cleansing lotion
and their functions. This gentle, multipurpose lotion for vaginal
or perianal soothing has been recommended for more than 30
years by doctors, surgeons and nurses!

Water	Moisturizer
Mineral oil	A clear odorless oil that does not spoil. It is a common ingredient in lotions, soaps, and cosmetics.
Propylene glycol	Usually an odorless, clear oily liquid that absorbs water. It is used as a moisturizer in medicines and cosmetics.
glyceryl stearate/PEG-100 stearate	Blend of emulsifiers (enable water and oil to mix) that provides excellent appearance and feel. It also has thickening properties and stabilizes essential oils.
PEG-40 stearate	PEG (polyethylene glycol) compounds are mixed with fatty acids and fatty alcohols to create agents that help blend cosmetic ingredients.
Laureth-4	Surfactant (surface active agent) used in cleansers and considered gentle and effective for most skin types.
PEG-4 dilaurate	PEG compound. (See above)
Lanolin oil	Derived from the sebaceous glands of sheep that closely resembles the oil from human oil glands.
Sodium acetate	A buffer which maintains a constant pH even when small amounts of acid or base are added.
Carbomer-934	Used for thickening, suspending, and stabilizing.
Triethanolamine	Used in cosmetics as a pH balancer.
Methylparaben	Preservative used in cosmetics. It is estimated that more than 90% of all cosmetic products contain some form of paraben.
Dioctyl sodium sulfosuccinate	Used as an adjuvant, emulsifier, humectant and stabilizer.
Fragrance	Improves product scent.
Acetic acid	Acid found in vinegar, some fruits, and human sweat. It can be a skin irritant and drying to skin, though it also has disinfecting properties.

BAUSCH & LOMB ALAWAY ANTIHISTAMINE EYE DROPS (ketotifen)

Bausch & Lomb

DRUG FACTS

Active Ingredient(s)	Purpose(s)
Ketotifen 0.025%	Antihistamine

USES
- For the temporary relief of itchy eyes due to ragweed, pollen, grass, animal hair and dander

DO NOT USE
- if you are sensitive to any ingredient in this product
- if the solution changes color or becomes cloudy
- to treat contact lens related irritation

WHEN USING THIS PRODUCT
- remove contact lenses before use

- wait at least 10 minutes before re-inserting contact lenses after use
- do not touch the tip of the container to any surface to avoid contamination
- replace cap after each use

STOP USE AND ASK A DOCTOR IF
you experience any of the following:
- eye pain
- changes in vision
- redness of the eyes
- itching that worsens or lasts for more than 72 hours

Keep out of reach of children. If swallowed, get medical help or contact a Poison Control Center right away.

DIRECTIONS

Adults and children 3 years and older	put 1 drop in the affected eye(s) twice daily, every 8-12 hours, no more than twice per day
Children under 3 years of age	Consult a doctor

OTHER INFORMATION
- Store at 4°- 25°C (39°- 77°F)

INACTIVE INGREDIENTS
benzalkonium chloride (0.01%), glycerin, sodium hydroxide and / or hydrochloric acid and water for injection

---

COLLYRIUM FRESH FOR FRESH EYES (purified water)
Bausch & Lomb

Ingredients
Active Ingredient(s)
Purified water - eyewash

INACTIVE INGREDIENTS
boric acid, sodium borate and sodium chloride. PRESERVATIVE ADDED: benzalkonium chloride (0.01%).

USES
Washes the eye to help relieve:
- irritation
- discomfort
- itching
- stinging

By removing:
- loose foreign material
- air pollutants (smog or pollen)
- chlorinated water

WARNINGS

DO NOT USE
- if you have open wounds in or near the eyes, and get medical help right away
- if solution changes color or becomes cloudy

WHEN USING THIS PRODUCT
- do not touch tip of container to any surface to avoid contamination
- remove contact lenses before using
- replace cap after use

STOP USING AND ASK A DOCTOR IF
- you experience eye pain, changes in vision, continued redness or irritation of the eye
- condition worsens or persists

Keep out of reach of children. If swallowed, get medical help or contact a Poison Control Center right away.

DIRECTIONS
Bottle tip permits use with or without cup.
- flush the affected eye(s) as needed
- control the rate of flow of solution by pressure on the bottle

When using an eye cup
- rinse the eye cup with Collyrium Eye Wash immediately before each use
- avoid contamination of the rim and inside surfaces of cup
- fill the eye cup half full with Collyrium Eye Wash and apply the eye cup to the affected eye(s), pressing tightly to prevent spillage
- tilt the head backward. Open eyelids wide and rotate eyeball to thoroughly wash the eye.
- rinse eye cup with clean water or with Eye Wash after each use
- replace cap after use

OTHER INFORMATION
- store at 15°-30°C (59°-86°F)
- keep tightly closed
- does not contain thimerosal
- enclosed eyecup is sterile if packaging is intact
- use before expiration date marked on the carton or bottle

BAUSCH & LOMB SOOTHE HYDRATION LUBRICANT EYE DROPS (povidone)
Bausch & Lomb

DRUG FACTS

Active Ingredient(s)	Purpose(s)
Povidone 1.25%	Lubricant

USES
- relieves dryness of the eye
- prevents further irritation

WARNINGS
For external use only.

DO NOT USE
- if solution changes color or becomes cloudy

WHEN USING THIS PRODUCT
- do not touch the tip of container to any surface to avoid contamination
- replace cap after using

STOP USE AND ASK A DOCTOR IF
- eye pain
- changes in vision
- continued redness or irritation of the eye
- or if condition worsens or persists more than 72 hours

If pregnant or breastfeeding, ask a health professional before use.
Keep out of reach of children: If swallowed, get medical help or contact a Poison Control Center right away.

DIRECTIONS
Put 1 to 2 drop(s) in the affected eye(s) as needed or directed by your doctor

INACTIVE INGREDIENTS
boric acid, potassium chloride, sodium borate and sodium chloride; preserved with edetate disodium 0.1% and sorbic acid 0.1%

BAUSCH & LOMB SOOTHE NIGHT TIME LUBRICANT EYE OINTMENT (mineral oil and white petrolatum)
Bausch & Lomb

DRUG FACTS

Active Ingredient(s)	Purpose(s)
Mineral oil 20%	Lubricant
White petrolatum 80%	Lubricant

USES
- overnight relief of dry eye
- prevents further irritation

WHEN USING THIS PRODUCT
- do not touch tip of container to any surface to avoid contamination
- do not use with contact lenses
- replace cap after use

STOP USE AND ASK A DOCTOR IF
- you experience eye pain, changes in vision, continued redness or irritation of the eye
- condition worsens or persists for more than 72 hours

Keep out of reach of children. If swallowed, get medical help or contact a Poison Control Center right away.

DIRECTIONS
- pull down the lower lid of the affected eye(s)
- apply a small amount (¼ inch) of ointment to the inside of eyelid
- apply one or more times daily

BAUSCH & LOMB SOOTHE PRESERVATIVE FREE LUBRICANT EYE DROPS (glycerin and propylene glycol)
Bausch & Lomb

DRUG FACTS

Active Ingredient(s)	Purpose(s)
Glycerin 0.6%	Lubricant
Propylene glycol 0.6%	Lubricant

USES
- relieves dryness of the eye
- prevents further irritation

DO NOT USE
- if solution changes color or becomes cloudy
- if single-unit dispenser is not intact

WHEN USING THIS PRODUCT
- do not touch the tip of container to any surface to avoid contamination
- once opened, discard
- do not reuse

STOP USE AND ASK A DOCTOR IF
- you experience eye pain, changes in vision, continued redness or irritation of the eye
- condition worsens or persists more than 72 hours

Keep out of reach of children: If swallowed, get medical help or contact a Poison Control Center right away.

DIRECTIONS
Easy to use sterile dispenser
- to open, completely twist off tab
- instill 1 to 2 drops in the affected eye(s) as needed, or as directed by your doctor
- discard dispenser immediately after use

INACTIVE INGREDIENTS BORIC ACID, HYDROXYALKYL-PHOSPHONATE, PURIFIED WATER, SODIUM ALGINATE, SODIUM BORATE

BAUSCH & LOMB SOOTHE TIRED EYES LUBRICANT EYE DROPS (glycerin)
Bausch & Lomb

DRUG FACTS

Active Ingredient(s)	Purpose(s)
Glycerin 1.0%	Lubricant

USES
- relieves dryness of the eye
- prevents further irritation

WARNINGS
For external use only.

DO NOT USE
- if solution changes color or becomes cloudy

WHEN USING THIS PRODUCT
- do not touch the tip of container to any surface to avoid contamination.
- replace cap after use

STOP USE AND ASK A DOCTOR IF
- eye pain
- changes in vision
- continued redness or irritation of the eye
- or if condition worsens or persists more than 72 hours

Keep out of reach of children: If swallowed, get medical help or contact a Poison Control Center right away.

DIRECTIONS
Put 1 to 2 drop(s) in the affected eye(s) as needed or directed by your doctor

INACTIVE INGREDIENTS
benzalkonium chloride (0.01%), boric acid, edetate disodium, potassium chloride, purified water, sodium borate, sodium chloride. Hydrochloric acid and/or sodium hydroxide may be used to adjust pH

BEANO MELTAWAYS (alpha-galactosidase)
GlaxoSmithKline Consumer Healthcare, L.P.

Beano Meltaways prevent gas, bloating and discomfort caused by many healthful foods.*

How Beano Meltaways works:
Beano Meltaways is a Vegetarian Friendly formula that contains a natural enzyme that breaks down the complex carbohydrates found in many foods, making them easier to digest so they don't cause gas.

How to use Beano Meltaways:
- **Use for the right problem:** Use Beano Meltaways if you experience the symptoms of stomach gas caused by many healthful foods.
- **Use with the right food:** Beano Meltaways prevents gas from a variety of foods*, including:

Beans	Cauliflower	Onions	Seeds
Broccoli	Corn	Peas	Soy
Cabbage	Lettuce	Peanuts	Whole grains
Carrots	Oat Bran	Peppers	And more...

For a complete listing of foods visit www.beanogas.com
- **Use at the right time:** Take right before your first bite of problem food.
- **Use the right amount:** At mealtime, place one Meltaway tablet on your tongue and let it dissolve.

Too much heat can inactivate the enzyme, so don't cook with Beano.

When to use Beano Meltaways:
Use it every day right before every meal with problem food.
Allergy Note: If a rare sensitivity occurs after taking Beano Meltaways, discontinue use. Galactosemics consult your doctor.

	SUPPLEMENT FACTS
	Serving size 1 tablet
	Servings per container 15
Amount Per Serving	%DV
Alpha-galactosidase	300 GAL U†
(derived from Aspergillus niger)	
†Daily Value not established	

OTHER INGREDIENTS
mannitol, povidone, corn starch, water, sodium stearyl fumarate, polyvinyl acetate, **less than 1% of:** maltodextrin, silicon dioxide, calcium gluconate, triacetin, natural & artificial flavor, red 40 lake, acetic acid, sodium lauryl sulfate. **Contains:** wheat
Storage: Store below 25°C (77°F). Avoid heat.

QUESTIONS OR COMMENTS?
call toll-free **1-800-257-8650** (English/Spanish) weekdays or visit www.beanogas.com
If you are pregnant or nursing a baby, ask a doctor before use.
U.S. Patent No. 5,989,544
BEANO® and MELTAWAYS™ are trademarks of the GlaxoSmithKline group of companies.
*This statement has not been evaluated by the Food and Drug Administration. This product is not intended to diagnose, treat, cure or prevent any disease.

BEANO (alpha-galactosidase enzyme)
GlaxoSmithKline Consumer Healthcare, L.P.

Beano prevents gas, and bloating and discomfort caused by many healthful foods.*)

How Beano works:
Beano contains a natural food enzyme that breaks down the complex carbohydrates found in many foods, making them easier to digest so they don't cause gas.

How to use Beano tablets:
- **Use for the right problem:** Use Beano if you experience the symptoms of stomach gas caused by many healthful foods.
- **Use with the right food:** Beano prevents gas from a variety of foods,* including:

Beans	Cauliflower	Onions	Seeds
Broccoli	Corn	Peas	Soy
Cabbage	Lettuce	Peanuts	Whole grains
Carrots	Oat Bran	Peppers	And more . . .

For a complete listing of foods visit www.beanogas.com

- **Use at the right time:** Take right before your first bite of problem food.
- **Use the right amount:** Swallow or chew 2-3 tablets for a typical meal.

Too much heat can inactivate the enzyme, so don't cook with Beano.
When to use Beano:
Use it every day right before every meal with problem food.
Allergy Note: If a rare sensitivity occurs after taking Beano, discontinue use. Galactosemics consult your doctor.

	SUPPLEMENT FACTS
	Serving Size 2 Tablets
	Servings Per Container 15
Amount Per Serving	%DV
Alpha-galactosidase enzyme	300 GAL U†
(derived from Aspergillus niger)	
† Daily Value not established	

OTHER INGREDIENTS
cellulose gel, mannitol, invertase, potato starch, magnesium stearate, colloidal silica, gelatin.
Contains: cod, flounder, redfish, wheat
Storage: Store below 25°C (77°F). Avoid heat.

QUESTIONS OR COMMENTS?
call toll-free **1-800-257-8650** (English/Spanish) weekdays or visit www.beanogas.com
* This statement has not been evaluated by the Food and Drug Administration. This product is not intended to diagnose, treat, cure or prevent any disease.

CHILDRENS BENADRYL ALLERGY
(diphenhydramine hydrochloride)
McNeil Consumer Healthcare Div. McNeil-PPC, Inc

DRUG FACTS

Active Ingredient(s) (in each 5 mL = 1 teaspoonful)
Diphenhydramine HCl 12.5 mg

Purpose(s)
Antihistamine

USES
- temporarily relieves these symptoms due to hay fever or other upper respiratory allergies:
  - runny nose
  - sneezing
  - itchy, watery eyes
  - itching of the nose or throat

WARNINGS

DO NOT USE
- to make a child sleepy
- with any other product containing diphenhydramine, even one used on skin

ASK A DOCTOR BEFORE USE IF THE CHILD HAS
- a breathing problem such as chronic bronchitis
- glaucoma
- a sodium-restricted diet

ASK A DOCTOR OR PHARMACIST BEFORE USE IF THE CHILD IS
taking sedatives or tranquilizers

WHEN USING THIS PRODUCT
- marked drowsiness may occur
- sedatives and tranquilizers may increase drowsiness
- excitability may occur, especially in children

Keep out of reach of children. In case of overdose, get medical help or contact a Poison Control Center right away. (1-800-222-1222)

DIRECTIONS
- find right dose on chart below
- mL = milliliter; tsp = teaspoonful
- take every 4 to 6 hours, as directed by a doctor
- do not take more than 6 doses in 24 hours

children under 2 years	do not use
children 2 to 5 years	do not use unless directed by a doctor
children 6 to 11 years	5 mL (1 tsp) to 10 mL (2 tsp)

Attention: use only enclosed dosing cup specifically designed for use with this product. Do not use any other dosing device.

OTHER INFORMATION
- each 5mL (1 tsp) contains: **sodium 14 mg**
- store between 20-25°C (68-77°F). Protect from light. Store in outer carton until contents used.
- **do not use if bottle wrap, or foil inner seal imprinted "SAFETY SEAL®" is broken or missing**
- see bottom panel for lot number and expiration date

INACTIVE INGREDIENTS
anhydrous citric acid, D&C red #33, FD&C red #40, flavors, glycerin, monoammonium glycyrrhizinate, poloxamer 407, purified water, sodium benzoate, sodium chloride, sodium citrate, sucrose

QUESTIONS OR COMMENTS?
call **1-877-717-2824**

CHILDRENS BENADRYL-D ALLERGY AND SINUS (diphenhydramine hydrochloride and phenylephrine hydrochloride)
McNeil Consumer Healthcare Div. McNeil-PPC, Inc

DRUG FACTS

Active Ingredient(s) (in each 5 mL = 1 teaspoonful)	Purpose(s)
Diphenhydramine HCl 12.5 mg	Antihistamine
Phenylephrine HCl 5 mg	Nasal decongestant

USES
- temporarily relieves these symptoms due to hay fever or other upper respiratory allergies:
  - runny nose
  - sneezing
  - itchy, watery eyes
  - itching of the nose or throat
  - nasal congestion
  - stuffy nose
- temporarily relieves these symptoms due to the common cold:
  - runny nose
  - sneezing
  - nasal congestion
  - stuffy nose
- temporarily relieves sinus congestion and pressure

WARNINGS

DO NOT USE
- to make a child sleepy
- with any other product containing diphenhydramine, even one used on skin
- if you are now taking a prescription monoamine oxidase inhibitor (MAOI) (certain drugs for depression, psychiatric or emotional conditions, or Parkinson's disease), or for 2 weeks after stopping the MAOI drug. If you do not know if your prescription drug contains an MAOI, ask a doctor or pharmacist before taking this product.

ASK A DOCTOR BEFORE USE IF YOU HAVE
- heart disease
- high blood pressure
- thyroid disease
- diabetes
- trouble urinating due to an enlarged prostate gland
- a breathing problem such as emphysema or chronic bronchitis
- glaucoma

ASK A DOCTOR OR PHARMACIST BEFORE USE IF YOU ARE
taking sedatives or tranquilizers

WHEN USING THIS PRODUCT
- **do not exceed recommended dose**
- marked drowsiness may occur
- avoid alcoholic drinks
- alcohol, sedatives, and tranquilizers may increase drowsiness
- be careful when driving a motor vehicle or operating machinery
- excitability may occur, especially in children

STOP USE AND ASK A DOCTOR IF
- nervousness, dizziness, or sleeplessness occur
- symptoms do not improve within 7 days or occur with a fever

If pregnant or breast-feeding, ask a health professional before use.

Keep out of reach of children. In case of overdose, get medical help or contact a Poison Control Center right away. (1-800-222-1222)

DIRECTIONS
- find right dose on chart below
- mL = milliliter; tsp = teaspoonful
- take every 4 hours
- do not take more than 6 doses in 24 hours

Age (yr)	Dose (mL or tsp)
children under 4 years	do not use
children 4 to 5 years	do not use unless directed by a doctor
children 6 to 11 years	5 mL (1 tsp)
adults and children 12 years and over	10 mL (2 tsp)

Attention: use only enclosed dosing cup specifically designed for use with this product. Do not use any other dosing device.

OTHER INFORMATION
- **each 5 mL (1 tsp) contains**: sodium 10 mg
- store between 20-25°C (68-77°F). Protect from light. Store in outer carton until contents are used.
- **do not use if bottle wrap or foil inner seal imprinted with "SAFETY SEAL®" is broken or missing**
- see bottom panel for lot number and expiration date

INACTIVE INGREDIENTS
anhydrous citric acid, carboxymethylcellulose sodium, edetate disodium, FD&C blue no. 1, FD&C red no. 40, flavors, glycerin, purified water, sodium benzoate, sodium citrate, sorbitol solution, sucralose

QUESTIONS OR COMMENTS?
call **1-877-717-2824**

BENADRYL ALLERGY DYE-FREE LIQUI-GELS
(diphenhydramine hydrochloride)

McNeil Consumer Healthcare

PRODUCT DESCRIPTION
- Dye-Free
- Liquid-filled capsules
- Provides relief from allergies

Available In:
- 24 count

Ingredients
Active Ingredient(s) (in each capsule)
- Diphenhydramine HCl 25 mg

Purpose(s)
- Antihistamine

USES
Temporarily relieves these symptoms due to hay fever or other upper respiratory allergies:
- runny nose
- sneezing
- itchy, watery eyes
- itching of the nose or throat

Temporarily relieves these symptoms due to the common cold:
- runny nose
- sneezing

WARNINGS

DO NOT USE
- to make a child sleepy
- with any other product containing diphenhydramine, even one used on skin

ASK A DOCTOR BEFORE USE IF YOU HAVE
- a breathing problem such as emphysema or chronic bronchitis
- glaucoma
- trouble urinating due to an enlarged prostate gland

ASK A DOCTOR OR PHARMACIST BEFORE USE IF YOU ARE
taking sedatives or tranquilizers

WHEN USING THIS PRODUCT
- marked drowsiness may occur
- avoid alcoholic drinks
- alcohol, sedatives, and tranquilizers may increase drowsiness
- be careful when driving a motor vehicle or operating machinery
- excitability may occur, especially in children

If pregnant or breast-feeding, ask a health professional before use.
Keep out of reach of children. In case of overdose, get medical help or contact a Poison Control Center right away. (1-800-222-1222)

DIRECTIONS
- take every 4 to 6 hours
- do not take more than 6 doses in 24 hours
- adults and children 12 years and over:
  - 1 to 2 capsules
    children 6 to under 12 years:
  - 1 capsule
    children under 6 years
  - do not use this product in children under 6 years of age

OTHER INFORMATION
store at 59° to 77° F in a dry place. Protect from heat, humidity, and light.

INACTIVE INGREDIENTS
gelatin, glycerin, polyethylene glycol, purified water, and sorbitol. Capsules are imprinted with edible dye-free ink.

QUESTIONS OR COMMENTS?
Call **1-877-717-2824**
Liqui-Gels® is a registered trademark of R.P. Scherer Technologies, Inc.

BENADRYL ALLERGY ULTRATAB TABLETS
(diphenhydramine hydrochloride)

McNeil Consumer Healthcare

PRODUCT DESCRIPTION
- Small tablet size
- Provides relief from allergies

Available In:
- 24 count
- 48 count
- 100 count

Ingredients
Active Ingredient(s) (in each tablet)
- Diphenhydramine HCl 25 mg

Purpose(s)
- Antihistamine

USES

Temporarily relieves these symptoms due to hay fever or other upper respiratory allergies:
- runny nose
- sneezing
- itchy, watery eyes
- itching of the nose or throat

Temporarily relieves these symptoms due to the common cold:
- runny nose
- sneezing

WARNINGS

DO NOT USE
- to make a child sleepy
- with any other product containing diphenhydramine, even one used on skin

ASK A DOCTOR BEFORE USE IF YOU HAVE
- a breathing problem such as emphysema or chronic bronchitis
- glaucoma
- trouble urinating due to an enlarged prostate gland

ASK A DOCTOR OR PHARMACIST BEFORE USE IF YOU ARE
taking sedatives or tranquilizers

WHEN USING THIS PRODUCT
- marked drowsiness may occur
- avoid alcoholic drinks
- alcohol, sedatives, and tranquilizers may increase drowsiness
- be careful when driving a motor vehicle or operating machinery
- excitability may occur, especially in children

If pregnant or breast-feeding, ask a health professional before use.

Keep out of reach of children. In case of overdose, get medical help or contact a Poison Control Center right away. (1-800-222-1222)

DIRECTIONS

take every 4 to 6 hours, or as directed by a doctor
do not take more than 6 times in 24 hours

adults and children 12 years and over	1 to 2 tablets
children 6 to under 12 years	1 tablet
children under 6 years	do not use

OTHER INFORMATION

each tablet contains: calcium 15 or 20 mg
store between 20-25° C (68-77° F). Avoid high humidity. Protect from light.

INACTIVE INGREDIENTS

carnauba wax, crospovidone, D&C red #27 aluminum lake, dibasic calcium phosphate dihydrate, hypromellose, magnesium stearate, microcrystalline cellulose, polyethylene glycol, polysorbate 80, pregelatinized starch, stearic acid, titanium dioxide
or
carnauba wax, croscarmellose sodium, D&C red no. 27 aluminum lake, dibasic calcium phosphate, hypromellose, magnesium stearate, microcrystalline cellulose, polyethylene glycol, polysorbate 80, titanium dioxide

QUESTIONS OR COMMENTS?

Call **1-877-717-2824** (toll free) or **215-273-8755** (collect) or visit www.benadryl.com

BENADRYL ANTI-ITCH GEL FOR KIDS
(camphor)

McNeil Consumer Healthcare

PRODUCT DESCRIPTION
- Children's Anti-Itch Gel
- External analgesic
- Immediate cooling, soothing itch relief
- Stops the urge to scratch
- For kids ages 2 and up

Available In:
- Gel tube

Ingredients
Active Ingredient(s):
- Camphor 0.45%

Purpose(s):
- External analgesic

USES
Temporarily relieves pain and itching associated with:
- minor burns
  sunburn
  minor cuts
  scrapes
  insect bites
  minor skin irritations
  rashes due to poison ivy, poison oak, and poison sumac

WARNINGS
For external use only.
Flammable. Keep away from fire or flame.

WHEN USING THIS PRODUCT
- avoid contact with eyes.

STOP USE AND ASK A DOCTOR IF
- condition worsens
- symptoms persist for more than 7 days or clear up and occur again within a few days

Keep out of reach of children. If swallowed, get medical help or contact a Poison Control Center right away. (1-800-222-1222)

DIRECTIONS
adults and children 2 years of age and older:
- apply to affected area not more than 3 to 4 times daily

under 2 years of age:
- ask a doctor

OTHER INFORMATION
store at 20° to 25° C (68° to 77° F).

INACTIVE INGREDIENTS
benzyl alcohol, carbomer, EDTA, menthol, SD alcohol 40-B, trolamine, water

QUESTIONS OR COMMENTS?
Call **1-800-524-2624**

BENADRYL EXTRA STRENGTH ITCH RELIEF STICK (diphenhydramine hydrochloride and zinc acetate)

McNeil Consumer Healthcare

PRODUCT DESCRIPTION
- Topical analgesic/skin protectant.
- Diphenhydramine hydrochloride will stop the itch at its source by blocking the histamine that causes itch.
- Skin protectant (Zinc acetate).
- Topical analgesic (Diphenhydramine HCl)
- Portable

Ingredients

Active Ingredient(s)	Purpose(s)
Diphenhydramine HCl 2%	Topical analgesic
Zinc acetate 0.1%	Skin protectant

USES
Temporarily relieves pain and itching associated with:
- insect bites
- minor burns
- sunburn
- minor skin irritations
- minor cuts
- scrapes
- rashes due to poison ivy, poison oak, and poison sumac

Dries the oozing and weeping of poison ivy, poison oak, and poison sumac.

WARNINGS
For external use only.
Flammable. Keep away from fire or flame.

DO NOT USE
- on large areas of the body
- with any other product containing diphenhydramine, even one taken by mouth

ASK A DOCTOR BEFORE USE
- on chicken pox
- measles

WHEN USING THIS PRODUCT
- avoid contact with eyes

STOP USE AND ASK A DOCTOR IF
- condition worsens or does not improve within 7 days
- symptoms persist for more than 7 days or clear up and occur again within a few days

Keep out of reach of children. If swallowed, get medical help or contact a Poison Control Center right away. (1-800-222-1222)

DIRECTIONS
- do not use more than directed
- hold stick straight down over affected skin area
- press tip of stick repeatedly on affected skin area until liquid flows, then dab sparingly
- adults and children 2 years of age and older:
- apply to affected area not more than 3 to 4 times daily
- children under 2 years of age:
- ask a doctor

OTHER INFORMATION
- store at 20° to 25°C (68° to 77°F)

INACTIVE INGREDIENTS
alcohol, glycerin, povidone, purified water, and tromethamine

QUESTIONS OR COMMENTS?
Call 1-800-524-2624

EXTRA STRENGTH BENADRYL ITCH STOPPING CREAM (diphenhydramine hydrochloride and zinc acetate)

McNeil Consumer Healthcare

PRODUCT DESCRIPTION
- Topical analgesic/skin protectant
- Histamine Blocking Itch Relief
- BENADRYL® Extra Strength topical cream stops your itch at the source by blocking the histamine that causes itch
- Topical analgesic (Diphenhydramine HCl)
- Skin protectant (Zinc acetate)

Ingredients

Active Ingredient(s)	Purpose(s)
Diphenhydramine hydrochloride 2%	Topical analgesic
Zinc acetate 0.1%	Skin protectant

USES
Temporarily relieves pain and itching associated with:
- insect bites
- minor burns
- sunburn
- minor skin irritations
- minor cuts
- scrapes
- rashes due to poison ivy, poison oak, and poison sumac

Dries the oozing and weeping of poison ivy, poison oak, and poison sumac

WARNINGS
For external use only.

DO NOT USE
- on large areas of the body
- with any other product containing diphenhydramine, even one taken by mouth

ASK A DOCTOR BEFORE USE
- on chicken pox
- on measles

WHEN USING THIS PRODUCT
- avoid contact with eyes

STOP USE AND ASK A DOCTOR IF
- condition worsens or does not improve within 7 days
- symptoms persist for more than 7 days or clear up and occur again within a few days

Keep out of reach of children. If swallowed, get medical help or contact a Poison Control Center right away. (1-800-222-1222)

DIRECTIONS
- do not use more than directed
- adults and children 2 years of age and older:
- apply to affected area not more than 3 to 4 times daily
- children under 2 years of age:
- ask a doctor

OTHER INFORMATION
- store at 20° to 25°C (68° to 77°F)

INACTIVE INGREDIENTS
cetyl alcohol, diazolidinyl urea, methylparaben, polyethylene glycol monostearate 1000, propylene glycol, propylparaben, and purified water

QUESTIONS OR COMMENTS?
call **1-800-524-2624**

BENADRYL EXTRA STRENGTH SPRAY
(diphenhydramine hydrochloride and zinc acetate)

McNeil Consumer Healthcare

PRODUCT DESCRIPTION
- Topical analgesic/skin protectant
- Histamine Blocking Itch Relief
- BENADRYL® Spray stops your itch at the source by blocking the histamine that causes itch
- Available in Extra Strength (2% Diphenhydramine HCl and 0.1% Zinc acetate)

Ingredients

Active Ingredient(s)	Purpose(s)
Diphenhydramine HCl 2%	Topical analgesic
Zinc acetate 0.1%	Skin protectant

USES
Temporarily relieves pain and itching associated with:
- insect bites
- minor burns
- sunburn
- minor skin irritations
- minor cuts
- scrapes
- rashes due to poison ivy, poison oak, and poison sumac

Dries the oozing and weeping of poison ivy, poison oak, and poison sumac.

WARNINGS
For external use only.
Flammable. Keep away from fire or flame.

DO NOT USE
- on large areas of your body
- with any other product containing diphenhydramine, even one taken by mouth

ASK A DOCTOR BEFORE USE
- on chicken pox
- on measles

WHEN USING THIS PRODUCT
- avoid contact with eyes

STOP USE AND ASK A DOCTOR IF
- condition worsens or does not improve within 7 days
- symptoms persist for more than 7 days or clear up and occur again within a few days

Keep out of reach of children. If swallowed, get medical help or contact a Poison Control Center right away. (1-800-222-1222)

DIRECTIONS
- Do not use more than directed
- adults and children 2 years of age and older:
- spray on affected area not more than 3 to 4 times daily
- children under 2 years of age:
- ask a doctor

OTHER INFORMATION
- store at 20° to 25°C (68° to 77°F)

INACTIVE INGREDIENTS
alcohol, glycerin, povidone, purified water, and tromethamine

QUESTIONS OR COMMENTS?
call **1-800-524-2624**

BENADRYL ITCH STOPPING GEL EXTRA STRENGTH (diphenhydramine hydrochloride)

McNeil Consumer Healthcare

PRODUCT DESCRIPTION
- Topical analgesic
- Histamine Blocking Itch Relief
- BENADRYL® Topical Gel stops your itch at the source by blocking the histamine that causes itch
- Topical pain relief
- Available in Extra Strength (2% Diphenhydramine HCl)

Ingredients
Active Ingredient(s)
- Diphenhydramine hydrochloride 2%

Purpose(s)
- Topical analgesic

USES
Temporarily relieves pain and itching associated with:
- insect bites
- minor burns
- sunburn
- minor skin irritations
- minor cuts
- rashes due to poison ivy, poison oak, and poison sumac

WARNINGS
For external use only.

DO NOT USE
- on large areas of the body
- with any other product containing diphenhydramine, even one taken by mouth

ASK A DOCTOR BEFORE USE
- on chicken pox
- on measles

WHEN USING THIS PRODUCT
- avoid contact with eyes

STOP USE AND ASK A DOCTOR IF
- condition worsens
- symptoms persist for more than 7 days or clear up and occur again within a few days

Keep out of reach of children. If swallowed, get medical help or contact a Poison Control Center right away. (1-800-222-1222)

DIRECTIONS
- do not use more than directed
- adults and children 2 years of age and older:
- apply to affected area not more than 3 to 4 times daily
- children under 2 years of age:
- ask a doctor

OTHER INFORMATION
- store at 20° to 25°C (68° to 77°F)

INACTIVE INGREDIENTS
SD alcohol 38-B, camphor, citric acid, diazolidinyl urea, glycerin, hypromellose, methylparaben, propylene glycol, propylparaben, purified water, and sodium citrate

QUESTIONS OR COMMENTS?
Call 1-800-524-2624

ORIGINAL STRENGTH BENADRYL ITCH STOPPING CREAM (diphenhydramine hydrochloride and zinc acetate)
McNeil Consumer Healthcare

PRODUCT DESCRIPTION
- Topical analgesic/skin protectant
- Histamine Blocking Itch Relief
- BENADRYL® topical cream stops your itch at the source by blocking the histamine that causes itch.
- Topical analgesic (Diphenhydramine HCl)
- Skin protectant (Zinc acetate)

Ingredients

Active Ingredient(s)	Purpose(s)
Diphenhydramine hydrochloride 1%	Topical analgesic
Zinc acetate 0.1%	Skin protectant

USES
Temporarily relieves pain and itching associated with:
- insect bites
- minor burns
- sunburn
- minor skin irritations
- minor cuts
- scrapes
- rashes due to poison ivy, poison oak, and poison sumac

Dries the oozing and weeping of poison ivy, poison oak, and poison sumac

WARNINGS
For external use only.

DO NOT USE
- on large areas of the body
- with any other product containing diphenhydramine, even one taken by mouth

ASK A DOCTOR BEFORE USE
- on chicken pox
- on measles

WHEN USING THIS PRODUCT
- avoid contact with eyes

STOP USE AND ASK A DOCTOR IF
- condition worsens or does not improve within 7 days
- symptoms persist for more than 7 days or clear up and occur again within a few days

Keep out of reach of children. If swallowed, get medical help or contact a Poison Control Center right away.

DIRECTIONS
- do not use more than directed
- adults and children 2 years of age and older:
- apply to affected area not more than 3 to 4 times daily
- children under 2 years of age:
- ask a doctor

OTHER INFORMATION
- store at 20° to 25°C (68° to 77°F)

INACTIVE INGREDIENTS
cetyl alcohol, diazolidinyl urea, methylparaben, polyethylene glycol monostearate 1000, propylene glycol, propylparaben, and purified water

QUESTIONS OR COMMENTS?
call 1-800-524-2624

BENADRYL READYMIST ITCH STOPPING SPRAY (diphenhydramine hydrochloride and zinc acetate)
McNeil Consumer Healthcare

PRODUCT DESCRIPTION
- On-the-go Itch Stopping Spray
- Topical analgesic/skin protectant
- Histamine Blocking Itch Relief
- BENADRYL® Spray stops your itch at the source by blocking the histamines that cause itch

Available In:
- Spray package

Ingredients

Active Ingredient(s)	Purpose(s)
Diphenhydramine hydrochloride 2%	Topical analgesic
Zinc acetate 0.1%	Skin protectant

USES
Temporarily relieves pain and itching associated with:
- insect bites
- minor burns
- sunburn
- minor skin irritations
- minor cuts
- scrapes
- rashes due to poison ivy, poison oak, and poison sumac

Dries the oozing and weeping of poison ivy, poison oak, and poison sumac.

WARNINGS
For external use only.
Flammable. Keep away from fire or flame.

DO NOT USE
- on large areas of the body
- with any other product containing diphenhydramine, even one taken by mouth

ASK A DOCTOR BEFORE USE
- on chicken pox
- on measles

WHEN USING THIS PRODUCT
- avoid contact with eyes

STOP USE AND ASK A DOCTOR IF
- condition worsens or does not improve within 7 days
- symptoms persist for more than 7 days or clear up and occur again within a few days

Keep out of reach of children. If swallowed, get medical help or contact a Poison Control Center right away. (1-800-222-1222)

DIRECTIONS
- do not use more than directed
- adults and children 2 years of age and older:
- spray on affected area not more than 3 to 4 times daily
- under 2 years of age:
- ask a doctor

OTHER INFORMATION
- store at 20° to 25°C (68° to 77°F)

INACTIVE INGREDIENTS
alcohol, glycerin, povidone, purified water, tromethamine

QUESTIONS OR COMMENTS?
call **1-800-524-2624**

BENEFIBER CAPLETS (wheat dextrin, microcrystalline cellulose, magnesium stearate, and colloidal silicon dioxide)

Novartis Consumer Health, Inc.

Ingredients
Wheat dextrin, microcrystalline cellulose, magnesium stearate, colloidal silicon dioxide
Gluten-free (less than 20 ppm gluten)

SUPPLEMENT FACTS		
Serving Size: 3 Tablets		
	Amount Per Serving	**%DV***
Calories	15	
Sodium	0mg	0%
Total Carbohydrates	4g	1%
Dietary Fiber	3g	12%
Soluble Fiber	3g	†
Sugar	0g	†
*Percent Daily Values (DV) are based on a 2,000 calorie diet.		
†Daily Value not established.		

DIRECTIONS
Adults: Take 3 caplets up to 3 times daily to supplement the fiber content of your diet. Swallow with liquid. Do not exceed 9 caplets per day.
Keep out of reach of children.
If you are pregnant or nursing a baby, ask a health professional before use.

BENEFIBER PLUS HEART HEALTH CAPLETS
(wheat dextrin, microcrystalline cellulose, magnesium stearate, colloidal silicon dioxide, modified food starch, pyridoxine hydrochloride, [vitamin b_6], sodium citrate, citric acid, folic acid, sodium benzoate, sorbic acid, cyanocobalamin [vitamin b_{12}])

INGREDIENTS
Wheat dextrin, microcrystalline cellulose, magnesium stearate, colloidal silicon dioxide, modified food starch, pyridoxine hydrochloride, (vitamin B_6), sodium citrate, citric acid, folic acid, sodium benzoate, sorbic acid, cyanocobalamin (vitamin B_{12})
Gluten-free (less than 20 ppm gluten)

SUPPLEMENT FACTS		
Serving Size: 3 Tablets		
	Amount Per Serving	**%DV***
Calories	15	
Sodium	0mg	0%
Total Carbohydrate	4g	1%
Dietary Fiber	3g	12%
Soluble Fiber	3g	†
Sugar	0g	†
B_6	0.7mg	35%
Folic Acid	134mcg	34%
B_{12}	2mcg	33%
*Percent Daily Values (DV) are based on a 2,000 calorie diet.		
†Daily Value not established.		

DIRECTIONS
Adults: Take 3 caplets up to 3 times daily to supplement the fiber content of your diet. Swallow with liquid.
Do not exceed 9 caplets per day.
Keep out of reach of children.
If you are pregnant or nursing a baby, ask a health professional before use.

BENGAY ARTHRITIS PAIN RELIEVING
(menthol and methyl salicylate)

Johnson & Johnson Consumer Products Company, Division of Johnson & Johnson Consumer Companies, Inc.

DRUG FACTS

Active Ingredient(s)	Purpose(s)
Menthol 8%	Topical analgesic
Methyl salicylate 30%	Topical analgesic

USES
temporarily relieves the minor aches and pains of muscles and joints associated with:
- simple backache
- arthritis
- strains
- bruises
- sprains

WARNINGS
For external use only.

DO NOT USE
- on wounds or damaged skin
- with a heating pad
- on a child under 12 years of age with arthritis-like conditions

ASK A DOCTOR BEFORE USE IF YOU HAVE
redness over the affected area.

WHEN USING THIS PRODUCT
- avoid contact with eyes or mucous membranes
- do not bandage tightly

STOP USE AND ASK A DOCTOR IF
• condition worsens or symptoms persist for more than 7 days
• symptoms clear up and occur again within a few days
• excessive skin irritation occurs

Keep out of reach of children to avoid accidental ingestion. If swallowed, get medical help or contact a Poison Control Center immediately.

DIRECTIONS
• use only as directed
• adults and children 12 years of age and older: apply to affected area not more than 3 to 4 times daily
• children under 12 years of age: ask a doctor

OTHER INFORMATION
• store at 20° to 25°C (68° to 77°F)

INACTIVE INGREDIENTS
glyceryl stearate se, lanolin, methylparaben, potassium cetyl phosphate, potassium hydroxide, propylparaben, stearic acid, water

QUESTIONS OR COMMENTS?
call 1-800-223-0182
Dist: **Johnson & Johnson Consumer Products Company**
Division of Johnson & Johnson Consumer Companies Inc.
Skillman, NJ 08558 USA

BENGAY COLD THERAPY WITH PRO-COOL TECHNOLOGY (menthol)

Johnson & Johnson Consumer Products company, Division of Johnson & Johnson Consumer Companies, Inc.

DRUG FACTS

Active Ingredient(s)
Menthol 5%

Purpose(s)
Topical analgesic

USES
temporarily relieves the minor aches and pains of muscles and joints associated with:
• simple backache
• bruises
• arthritis
• sprains
• strains

WARNINGS
For external use only.
Flammable: Keep away from fire or flame.

DO NOT USE
• on wounds or damaged skin
• with a heating pad
• on a child under 12 years of age with arthritis-like conditions

ASK A DOCTOR BEFORE USE IF YOU HAVE
redness over the affected area.

WHEN USING THIS PRODUCT
• avoid contact with eyes or mucous membranes
• do not bandage tightly

STOP USE AND ASK A DOCTOR IF
• condition worsens or symptoms persist for more than 7 days
• symptoms clear up and occur again within a few days
• excessive skin irritation occurs

Keep out of reach of children. If swallowed, get medical help or contact a Poison Control Center immediately.

DIRECTIONS
• adults and children 12 years of age and older: apply to affected area not more than 3 to 4 times daily
• children under 12 years of age: ask a doctor

OTHER INFORMATION
• store at 20° to 25°C (68° to 77°F)

INACTIVE INGREDIENTS
alcohol, aminomethyl propanol, camphor, carbomer, disteareth-75 IPDI, ethylhexyl isononanoate, FD&C blue no. 1, glycerin, isopropyl alcohol, PEG-7 caprylic/capric glycerides, polysorbate 60, water

QUESTIONS OR COMMENTS?
call 1-800-223-0182

BENGAY PAIN RELIEF AND MASSAGE (menthol)

Johnson & Johnson Consumer Products Company, Division of Johnson Consumer Companies, Inc.

DRUG FACTS

Active Ingredient(s)
Menthol 2.5%

Purpose(s)
Topical analgesic

USES
temporarily relieves the minor aches and pains of muscles and joints associated with:
• simple backache
• bruises
• arthritis
• sprains
• strains

WARNINGS
For external use only.

DO NOT USE
• on wounds or damaged skin
• with a heating pad
• on a child under 12 years of age with arthritis-like conditions

ASK A DOCTOR BEFORE USE IF YOU HAVE
redness over the affected area.

WHEN USING THIS PRODUCT
• avoid contact with eyes or mucous membranes
• do not bandage tightly

STOP USE AND ASK A DOCTOR IF
• condition worsens or symptoms persist for more than 7 days
• symptoms clear up and occur again within a few days
• excessive skin irritation occurs

Keep out of reach of children. If swallowed, get medical help or contact a Poison Control Center immediately.

DIRECTIONS
- **adults and children 12 years of age and older:**
  - apply to affected area not more than 3 to 4 times daily
  - remove protective cap
  - to open: twist applicator counter-clockwise until it stops
  - squeeze tube to dispense gel
  - to close: twist applicator clockwise until it stops
  - after closing, use applicator to massage in gel
  - after use, clean applicator with damp cloth or paper towel - do not rinse under or immerse in water
  - replace protective cap
- **children under 12 years of age:** ask a doctor

OTHER INFORMATION
- store at 20° to 25°C (68° to 77°F)

INACTIVE INGREDIENTS
camphor, carbomer, DMDM hydantoin, isoceteth-20, isopropyl alcohol, PEG-40 hydrogenated castor oil, sodium hydroxide, water

QUESTIONS OR COMMENTS?
call **1-800-223-0182**

BENGAY ZERO DEGREES MENTHOL PAIN RELIEVING (menthol)

Johnson & Johnson Consumer Products Company, Division of Johnson & Johnson Consumer Companies, Inc.

DRUG FACTS

Active Ingredient(s)
Menthol 5%

Purpose(s)
Topical analgesic

USES
temporarily relieves the minor aches and pains of muscles and joints associated with:
- simple backache
- arthritis
- strains
- bruises
- sprains

WARNINGS
For external use only.
Flammable: Keep away from fire or flame.

DO NOT USE
- on wounds or damaged skin
- with a heating pad
- on a child under 12 years of age with arthritis-like Conditions

ASK A DOCTOR BEFORE USE IF YOU HAVE
redness over the affected area

WHEN USING THIS PRODUCT
- avoid contact with eyes or mucous membranes
- do not bandage tightly

STOP USE AND ASK A DOCTOR IF
- condition worsens or symptoms persist for more than 7 days
- symptoms clear up and occur again within a few days
- excessive skin irritation occurs

Keep out of reach of children. If swallowed, get medical help or contact a Poison Control Center immediately.

DIRECTIONS
- **adults and children 12 years of age and older:**
  - apply to affected area not more than 3 to 4 times daily
  - for first use: remove and discard foil on applicator head
  - after use, wipe off applicator head, turn dial back slightly, and replace protective cap
  - clean outside with damp cloth or paper towel. Do not rinse under or immerse in water.
  - return product to storage
- **children under 12 years of age:** ask a doctor

OTHER INFORMATION
- product may be stored in freezer out of reach of children. Place product in freezer a minimum of 2 hours before use, or
- product may be stored at 20° to 25°C (68° to 77°F) and applied at room temperature, but will not feel as refreshing as when stored in freezer

INACTIVE INGREDIENTS
alcohol, aminomethyl propanol, camphor, carbomer, disteareth-75 IPDI, ethylhexyl isononanoate, FD&C blue no. 1, glycerin, isopropyl alcohol, PEG-7 caprylic/capric glycerides, polysorbate 60, propylene glycol, water

QUESTIONS OR COMMENTS?
call toll-free **800-223-0182** or **215-273-8755** (collect)
DIST: JOHNSON & JOHNSON CONSUMER PRODUCTS COMPANY
Division of Johnson & Johnson Consumer Companies Inc.
Skillman, NJ 08558-9418 USA

BENGAY PAIN RELIEVING GREASELESS
(menthol and methyl salicylate)

Johnson & Johnson Consumer Products Company, Division of Johnson & Johnson Consumer Companies, Inc.

DRUG FACTS

Active Ingredient(s)	Purpose(s)
Menthol 10%	Topical analgesic
Methyl salicylate 15%	Topical analgesic

USES
temporarily relieves the minor aches and pains of muscles and joints associated with:
- simple backache
- arthritis
- strains
- bruises
- sprains

WARNINGS
For external use only.

DO NOT USE
- on wounds or damaged skin
- with a heating pad
- on a child under 12 years of age with arthritis-like conditions

ASK A DOCTOR BEFORE USE IF YOU HAVE
redness over the affected area.

WHEN USING THIS PRODUCT
- avoid contact with eyes or mucous membranes
- do not bandage tightly

STOP USE AND ASK A DOCTOR IF
• condition worsens or symptoms persist for more than 7 days
• symptoms clear up and occur again within a few days
• excessive skin irritation occurs

Keep out of reach of children to avoid accidental ingestion. If swallowed, get medical help or contact a Poison Control Center immediately.

DIRECTIONS
• use only as directed
• adults and children 12 years of age and older: apply to affected area not more than 3 to 4 times daily
• children under 12 years of age: ask a doctor

OTHER INFORMATION
• store at 20° to 25°C (68° to 77°F)

INACTIVE INGREDIENTS
carbomer, cetyl alcohol, glycerin, glyceryl stearate se, isopropyl palmitate, methylparaben, potassium cetyl phosphate, propylparaben, stearic acid, stearyl alcohol, trolamine, water

QUESTIONS OR COMMENTS?
call 1-800-223-0182
Dist: **Johnson & Johnson Consumer Products Company**
Division of Johnson & Johnson Consumer Companies Inc.
Skillman, NJ 08558 USA

ULTRA STRENGTH BENGAY (camphor, menthol, and methyl salicylate)

Johnson & Johnson Consumer Products Company, Division of Johnson & Johnson Consumer Companies, Inc.

DRUG FACTS

Active Ingredient(s)
Camphor 4%
Menthol 10%
Methyl Salicylate 30%

Purpose(s)
Topical analgesic
Topical analgesic
Topical analgesic

USES
Temporarily relieves the minor aches and pains of muscles and joints associated with:
• simple backache
• arthritis
• strains
• bruises
• sprains

WARNINGS
For external use only.

DO NOT USE
• on wounds or damaged skin
• with a heating pad
• on a child under 12 years of age with arthritis-like conditions

ASK A DOCTOR BEFORE USE IF YOU HAVE
redness over the affected area.

DIRECTIONS

WHEN USING THIS PRODUCT
• avoid contact with eyes or mucous membranes
• do not bandage tightly

STOP USE AND ASK A DOCTOR IF
• condition worsens or symptoms persist for more than 7 days
• symptoms clear up and occur again within a few days
• excessive skin irritation occurs

Keep out of reach of children to avoid accidental ingestion. If swallowed, get medical help or contact a Poison Control Center immediately.
• use only as directed
• adults and children 12 years of age and older: apply to affected area not more than 3 to 4 times daily
• children under 12 years of age: ask a doctor

OTHER INFORMATION
• Store between 20° to 25° C (68° to 77°F).

INACTIVE INGREDIENTS
carbomer, edetate disodium, glyceryl sterate se, lanolin, polysorbate 80, potassium hydroxide, purified water, stearic acid, trolamine.

QUESTIONS OR COMMENTS?
call 1-800-223-0182.

BENGAY ULTRA STRENGTH PAIN RELIEVING REGULAR SIZE (menthol)

Johnson & Johnson Consumer Products Company, Division of Johnson & Johnson Consumer Companies, Inc.

DRUG FACTS

Active Ingredient(s)
Menthol 5%

Purpose(s)
Topical analgesic

USES
• temporarily relieves minor aches and pains of muscles and joints associated with:
  • simple backache
  • arthritis
  • strains
  • bruises
  • sprains

WARNINGS
For external use only.

DO NOT USE
• on wounds or damaged skin
• with a heating pad
• on a child under 12 years of age with arthritis-like conditions

ASK A DOCTOR BEFORE USE IF YOU HAVE
• redness over the affected area

WHEN USING THIS PRODUCT
• avoid contact with eyes or mucous membranes
• do not bandage tightly

STOP USE AND ASK A DOCTOR IF
• condition worsens or symptoms persist for more than 7 days
• symptoms clear up and occur again within a few days
• excessive skin irritation occurs

Keep out of reach of children. If swallowed, get medical help or contact a Poison Control Center immediately.

DIRECTIONS
• open pouch and remove patch
• if desired, cut patch to size
• peel off protective backing and apply sticky side to affected area
• adults and children 12 years of age and older: apply to affected area not more than 3 to 4 times daily
• children under 12 years of age: consult a doctor

OTHER INFORMATION
• store at 20° to 25°C (68° to 77°F)

INACTIVE INGREDIENTS
carboxymethylcellulose sodium, glycerin, kaolin, methyl acrylate/2-ethylhexyl acrylate copolymer, polyacrylic acid, polysorbate 80, sodium polyacrylate, tartaric acid, titanium dioxide, and water

QUESTIONS OR COMMENTS?
call 1-800-223-0182
Dist: **Johnson & Johnson Consumer Products Company**
Division of Johnson & Johnson Consumer Companies Inc.
Skillman, NJ 08558 USA

BENGAY VANISHING SCENT (menthol)

Johnson & Johnson Consumer Products Company,
Division of Johnson & Johnson Consumer Companies,
Inc.

DRUG FACTS

Active Ingredient(s)
Menthol 2.5%

Purpose(s)
Topical analgesic

USES
temporarily relieves the minor aches and pains of muscles and joints associated with:
• simple backache
• arthritis
• strains
• bruises
• sprains

WARNINGS
For external use only.

DO NOT USE
• on wounds or damaged skin
• with a heating pad
• on a child under 12 years of age with arthritis-like conditions

ASK A DOCTOR BEFORE USE IF YOU HAVE
redness over the affected area.

WHEN USING THIS PRODUCT
• avoid contact with eyes or mucous membranes
• do not bandage tightly

STOP USE AND ASK A DOCTOR IF
• condition worsens or symptoms persist for more than 7 days
• symptoms clear up and occur again within a few days
• excessive skin irritation occurs

Keep out of reach of children. If swallowed, get medical help or contact a Poison Control Center immediately.

DIRECTIONS
• adults and children 12 years of age and older: apply to affected area not more than 3 to 4 times daily
• children under 12 years of age: ask a doctor

OTHER INFORMATION
• store at 20° to 25°C (68° to 77°F)

INACTIVE INGREDIENTS
camphor, carbomer, DMDM hydantoin, isoceteth-20, isopropyl alcohol, PEG-40 hydrogenated castor oil, sodium hydroxide, water

QUESTIONS OR COMMENTS?
call **1-800-223-0182**

BLINK TEARS LUBRICATING EYE DROPS
(polyethylene glycol)
Abbott

DRUG FACTS

Active Ingredient(s)	Purpose(s)
Polyethylene glycol 0.25%	Lubricant

USES
• For the temporary relief of burning, irritation and discomfort due to dryness of the eye or exposure to wind or sun.
• May be used as a protectant against further irritation.

WARNINGS
• For external use only.
• To avoid contamination, do not touch tip of container to any surface. Replace cap after using.
• Do not use if solution changes color or becomes cloudy.

KEEP OUT OF REACH OF CHILDREN SECTION. If swallowed, get medical help of contact a Poison Control Center right away.

STOP USE AND ASK A DOCTOR IF
• You experience eye pain, changes in vision, continued redness or irritation of the eye, or if the condition worsens or persists for more than 72 hours

DIRECTIONS
• Instill 1 or 2 drops in the affected eye(s) as needed.

OTHER INFORMATION
• Use only if tape seals on top and bottom flaps are intact.
• RETAIN THIS CARTON FOR FUTURE REFERENCE.

INACTIVE INGREDIENTS
boric acid, calcium chloride, magnesium chloride, potassium chloride, purified water, sodium borate, sodium chloride, sodium chlorite (OcuPure® Brand) as a preservative; sodium hyaluronate

QUESTIONS OR COMMENTS?
call **1-800-347-5005**
www.yourhealthyeyes.com

BLISTEX COLD AND ALLERGY LIP SOOTHER (dimethicone and pramoxine hydrochloride)
Blistex Inc.

DRUG FACTS

Active Ingredient(s)	Purpose(s)
Dimethicone 2.0%(w/w)	Skin protectant
Pramoxine HCL 1.0%(w/w)	External analgesic

USES
- for the temporary relief of pain and itching associated with minor lip irritations
- temporarily protects and helps relieve chapped or cracked lips

WARNINGS
For external use only

WHEN USING THIS PRODUCT
- Do not get into eyes

STOP USE AND ASK A DOCTOR IF
- condition worsens, or if symptoms persist for more than 7 days or clear up and occur again within a few days

Keep out of reach of children.
If swallowed, get medical help or contact a Poison Control Center right away.

DIRECTIONS
- adults and children 2 years of age and older: apply liberally to affected area not more than 3 to 4 times daily. Children under 2 years of age: consult a doctor.

INACTIVE INGREDIENTS
C20-40 pareth-3, camellia sinensis leaf extract, castor oil bis-hydroxypropyl dimethicone esters, chamomilla recutita (matricaria) flower extract, ethyl menthane carboxamide, flavor, glycerin, glyceryl stearate, helianthus annuus (sunflower) seed oil, honey, lanolin, lecithin, microcrystalline wax, myristyl myristate, ozokerite, paraffin, phenoxyethanol, polybutene, purified water, sambucus nigra fruit extract, sodium ascorbyl phosphate, sodium hyaluronate, sodium saccharin, tocopheryl acetate, tridecyl neopentanoate, triethanolamine, triisononanoin

BLISTEX COMPLETE MOISTURE (dimethicone, octinoxate, and oxybenzone)
Blistex Inc.

DRUG FACTS

Active Ingredient(s)	Purpose(s)
Dimethicone 2.0%(w/w)	Lip protectant
Octinoxate 7.5%(w/w)	Sunscreen
Oxybenzone 2.5%(w/w)	Sunscreen

USES
- temporarily protects and helps relieve chapped or cracked lips
- helps prevent sunburn

WARNINGS
Skin Cancer/Skin Aging Alert
Spending time in the sun increases your risk of skin cancer and early skin aging. This product has been shown only to help prevent sunburn, **not** skin cancer or early skin aging.

For external use only

DO NOT USE
on damaged or broken skin

WHEN USING THIS PRODUCT
keep out of eyes. Rinse with water to remove.

STOP USE AND ASK A DOCTOR IF
rash occurs
Keep out of reach of children. If swallowed, get medical help or contact a Poison Control Center right away.

DIRECTIONS
- apply liberally 15 minutes before sun exposure
- reapply at least every 2 hours
- use a water resistant sunscreen if swimming or sweating
- children under 6 months of age: Ask a doctor

INACTIVE INGREDIENTS
behenoyl stearic acid, butylparaben, caprylic/capric triglyceride, cholesteryl/behenyl/octyldodecyl lauroyl glutamate, diethylhexyl adipate, ethylhexyl palmitate, ethylhexyl stearate, ethylparaben, flavor, glycerin, jojoba esters, lecithin, methylparaben, microcrystalline wax, ozokerite, panthenol, petrolatum, propylparaben, purified water, sodium borate, sodium saccharin, squalane

OTHER INFORMATION
- protect the product in this container from excessive heat and direct sun

BLISTEX FIVE STAR (homosalate, octinoxate, octisalate, oxybenzone, and petrolatum)
Blistex Inc.

DRUG FACTS

Active Ingredient(s)	Purpose(s)
Homosalate 9.6%(w/w)	Sunscreen
Octinoxate 7.5%(w/w)	Sunscreen
Octisalate 5.0%(w/w)	Sunscreen
Oxybenzone 5.0%(w/w)	Sunscreen
Petrolatum 30.1%(w/w)	Skin Protectant

USES
- temporarily protects and helps relieve chapped or cracked lips
- helps protect lips from the drying effects of wind and cold weather
- helps prevent sunburn

WARNINGS
- Do not use on
- deep or puncture wounds
- animal bites
- serious burns
- Stop use if skin rash occurs

DIRECTIONS
- apply liberally before sun exposure and as needed
- children under six months of age: ask a doctor

INACTIVE INGREDIENTS
alumina, calendula officinalis flower extract, carthamus tinctorius (safflower) oil, citric acid, euphorbia cerifera (candelilla) wax, flavor, glycerin, glyceryl laurate, helianthus annuus (sunflower) seed oil, hydrogenated coconut oil, isopropyl

myristate, jojoba esters, lanolin, lecithin, microcrystalline wax, phenoxyethanol, polyhydroxystearic acid, purified water, saccharin, silica, theobroma cacao (cocoa) seed butter, titanium dioxide, tocopheryl acetate, triticum vulgare (wheat) germ oil, vanillin

BLISTEX HERBAL ANSWER (oxtinoxate, oxybenzone, and petrolatum)
Blistex Inc.

DRUG FACTS

Active Ingredient(s)	Purpose(s)
Oxtinoxate 7.5%	Sunscreen
Oxybenzone 2.5%	Sunscreen
Petrolatum 43%	Lip protectant

USES
• Temporarily protects and helps relieve chapped or cracked lips
• Helps prevent sunburn

WARNINGS
Skin Cancer/Skin Aging Alert: Spending time in the sun increases your risk of skin cancer and early skin aging. This product has been shown to help prevent sunburn, **not** skin cancer or early skin aging.
For external use only.

DO NOT USE
• On damaged or broken skin

WHEN USING THIS PRODUCT
• Keep out of eyes. Rinse with warm water to remove.

STOP USE AND ASK A DOCTOR IF
• Rash occurs

Keep out of reach of children. If swallowed, get medical help or contact a Poison Control Center right away.

DIRECTIONS
• apply liberally 15 minutes before sun exposure
• Reapply at least every 2 hours
• Use a water resistant sunscreen if swimming or sweating
• Children under 6 months of age: ask a doctor

OTHER INFORMATION
• protect this product in this container from excessive heat and direct sun

INACTIVE INGREDIENTS
aloe barbadensis leaf extract beeswax, butyrospermum parkii (shea butter), cetyl alcohol, chamomilla recutita (matricaria) flower extract, flavor, helianthus annus (sunflower) seed oil, isopropyl lanolate, lanolin, methylparaben, microcrystalline wax, ozokenite, paraffin, persea gratissima (avocado) oil, phenyl trimethicone, propylparaben, simmondsia chinensis (jojoba) seed oil

BLISTEX LIP MEDEX (camphor, menthol, petrolatum, and phenol)
Blistex Inc.

DRUG FACTS

Active Ingredient(s)	Purpose(s)
Camphor 1.0%	External analgesic
Menthol 1.0%	External analgesic
Petrolatum 59%	Lip protectant
Phenol 0.54%	External analgesic

USES
• for the temporary relief of pain and itching associated with minor lip irritation
• temporarily protects and helps relieve chapped or cracked lips
• helps protect lips from the drying effects of wind and cold weather

WARNINGS
For external use only.

DO NOT USE
• deep or puncture wounds
• animal bites
• serious burns

WHEN USING THIS PRODUCT
• do not get into eyes
• do not apply over large areas of the body or bandage

STOP USE AND ASK A DOCTOR IF
• condition worsens
• symptoms last more than 7 days or clear up and occur again within a few days

Keep out of reach of children. If swallowed, get medical help or contact a Poison Control Center right away.

DIRECTIONS
• adults and children 2 years of age and older: Apply to affected area not more than 3 to 4 times daily
• children under 2 years of age: Consult a doctor

INACTIVE INGREDIENTS
beeswax, benzyl alcohol, diisopropyl adipate, flavors, fragrances, lanolin, menthoxypropanediol, microcrystalline wax, myristyl myristate, ricinus communis (castor) seed oil, saccharin, theobroma cacao (cocoa) seed butter

BLISTEX MEDICATED LIP BALM (dimethicone, oxybenzone, and padimate O)
Blistex Inc.

DRUG FACTS

Active Ingredient(s)	Purpose(s)
Dimethicone 2.0%(w/w)	Lip protectant
Oxybenzone 2.5%(w/w)	Sunscreen
Padimate O 6.6%(w/w)	Sunscreen

USES
• temporarily protects and helps relieve chapped or cracked lips
• helps prevent sunburn

WARNINGS
Skin Cancer/Skin Aging Alert
Spending time in the sun increases your risk of skin cancer and early skin aging. This product has been shown only to help prevent sunburn, **not** skin cancer or early skin aging.
For external use only

DO NOT USE
on damaged or broken skin

WHEN USING THIS PRODUCT
keep out of eyes. Rinse with water to remove.

STOP USE AND ASK A DOCTOR IF
rash occurs
Keep out of reach of children. If swallowed, get medical help or contact a Poison Control Center right away.

DIRECTIONS
- apply liberally 15 minutes before sun exposure
- reapply at least every 2 hours
- use a water resistant sunscreen if swimming or sweating
- children under 6 months of age: Ask a doctor

INACTIVE INGREDIENTS
beeswax, camphor, cetyl alcohol, cetyl palmitate, euphorbia cerifera (candelilla) wax, flavor, isopropyl myristate, isopropyl palmitate, isopropyl stearate, lanolin, lanolin oil, menthol, methylparaben, mineral oil, ozokerite, paraffin, petrolatum, polybutene, propylparaben, red 6 lake, theobroma cacao (cocoa) seed butter, titanium dioxide

OTHER INFORMATION
- protect the product in this container from excessive heat and direct sun

---

BLISTEX MEDICATED LIP OINTMENT
(dimethicone, camphor, menthol, and phenol)

Blistex Inc.

DRUG FACTS

Active Ingredient(s)	Purpose(s)
Dimethicone 1.1%(w/w)	Lip protectant
Camphor 0.5%(w/w)	External analgesic
Menthol 0.6%(w/w)	External analgesic
Phenol 0.5%(w/w)	External analgesic

USES
- for the temporary relief of pain and itching associated with minor lip irritations and cold sores
- temporarily protects and helps relieve chapped or cracked lips

WARNINGS
For external use only

DO NOT USE ON
deep or puncture wounds
animal bites
serious burns

WHEN USING THIS PRODUCT
- Do not get into eyes
- Do not apply over large areas of the body or bandage

STOP USE AND ASK A DOCTOR IF
- condition worsens
- symptoms last more than 7 days or clear up and occur again within a few days

Keep out of reach of children.
If swallowed, get medical help or contact a Poison Control Center right away.

DIRECTIONS
- adults and children 2 years of age and older: apply to affected area not more than 3 to 4 times daily. Children under 2 years of age: consult a doctor.

INACTIVE INGREDIENTS
allantoin, ammonium hydroxide, beeswax, calcium disodium EDTA, calcium hydroxide, cetyl alcohol, flavors, glycerin, hydrated silica, lanolin, lauric acid, mineral oil, myristic acid, oleic acid, palmitic acid, paraffin, petrolatum, polyglyceryl-3 diisostearate, potassium hydroxide, purified water, SD alcohol 36, sodium hydroxide, sodium saccharin, stearyl alcohol

---

BLISTEX REVIVE & RESTORE (dimethicone, octinoxate, oxybenzone, and lanolin)

Blistex Inc.

DRUG FACTS – REVIVE

Active Ingredient(s)	Purpose(s)
Dimethicone 1.0% (w/w)	Skin protectant
Octinoxate 7.5%% (w/w)	Sunscreen
Oxybenzone 2.5% (w.w)	Sunscreen

USES
- temporarily protects and helps relieve chapped or cracked lips
- helps protect lips from the drying effects of wind and cold weather
- helps prevent sunburn

WARNINGS
- Stop use if skin rash occurs

DIRECTIONS
- apply liberally before sun exposure and as needed
- children under 6 months of age: Ask a doctor

INACTIVE INGREDIENTS
acer saccharum (sugar maple) extract, aloe barbadensis leaf extract, beeswax, bis-diglyceryl polyacyladipate-2, butyrospermum parkii (shea butter), C10-30 cholesterol/lanosterol esters, caprylic/capric triglyceride, cholesteryl/behenyl/octyldodecyl lauroyl glutamate, citrus aurantium dulcis (orange) fruit extract, citrus medica limonum (lemon) extract, flavors, menthol, microcrystalline wax, myristyl myristate, octyldodecanol, phenoxyethanol, polybutene, purified water, ricinus communis (castor) seed oil, saccharin, saccharum officinarum (sugar cane) extract, vaccinium myrtillus (bilberry) extract

DRUG FACTS – RESTORE

Active Ingredient(s)	Purpose(s)
Lanolin 15.0% (w/w)	Skin protectant

USES
- temporarily protects and helps relieve chapped or cracked lips
- helps protect lips from the drying effects of wind and cold weather

DIRECTIONS
• apply as needed

INACTIVE INGREDIENTS
beeswax, bis-diglyceryl polyacyladipate-2, brassica campestris/aleurites fordi oil copolymer, C10-30 cholesterol/lanosterol esters, flavors, hydrogenated polyisobutene, jojoba esters, microcrystalline wax, myristyl myristate, octyldodecanol, phenoxyethanol, polybutene, saccharin, simmondsia chinensis (jojoba) seed oil, squalane, theobroma cacao (cocoa) seed butter, tocopheryl acetate

BONINE (meclizine hydrochloride)
Insight Pharmaceuticals

DRUG FACTS

Active Ingredient(s) (in each tablet)
Meclizine HCl 25 mg

Purpose(s)
Antiemetic

USES
prevents and treats nausea, vomiting or dizziness associated with motion sickness

WARNINGS

DO NOT USE
for children under 12 years of age unless directed by a doctor
Do not take unless directed by a doctor if you have
• glaucoma
• trouble urinating due to an enlarged prostate gland
• a breathing problem such as emphysema or chronic bronchitis

Do not take if you are taking sedatives or tranquilizers, without first consulting your doctor.

WHEN USING THIS PRODUCT
• do not exceed recommended dosage
• drowsiness may occur
• alcohol, sedatives, and tranquilizers may increase drowsiness
• avoid alcoholic drinks
• be careful when driving a motor vehicle or operating machinery

If pregnant or breast-feeding, ask a health professional before use.
Keep out of reach of children. In case of overdose, get medical help or contact a Poison Control Center right away.

DIRECTIONS
• dosage should be taken one hour before travel starts
• adults and children 12 years of age and over: take 1 to 2 tablets once daily or as directed by a doctor

OTHER INFORMATION
store at room temperature 20°- 25°C (68°-77°F)

INACTIVE INGREDIENTS
croscarmellose sodium, crospovidone, FD&C red #40 lake, lactose, magnesium stearate, raspberry flavor, silica, sodium saccharin, stearic acid, vanilla flavor.

QUESTIONS OR COMMENTS?
call 1-800-344-7239 or visit us on the web at www.insightpharma.com
Dist. by: INSIGHT Pharmaceuticals Corp.
Langhorne, PA 19047-1749

BOUDREAUX'S BUTT PASTE ALL NATURAL
(zinc oxide)
C B Fleet

Instructions & Usage
Active Ingredient(s)
Zinc Oxide, 16%
Purpose(s)
Skin Protectant

USES
• Helps treat and prevent diaper rash
• Protects chafed skin due to diaper rash and helps seal out wetness

WARNINGS
• For external use only.
• When using this product avoid contact with the eyes
• Stop use and ask a doctor if condition worsens or does not improve after 7 days
• Keep out of the reach of children
• If swallowed, seek medical help or call Poison Control Center immediately

DIRECTIONS FOR USE
• Change wet and soiled diaper immediately
• Cleanse the diaper area and allow to dry
• Apply ointment liberally and as often as necessary with each diaper change and especially when exposed to wet diapers for a prolonged period of time, such as bedtime

OTHER INFORMATION
• Store at room temperature, 15°C to 30°C (59°F to 86°F)

INACTIVE INGREDIENTS
aloe vera, beeswax, carnauba wax, castor oil, citric acid, hydrogenated castor oil, peruvian balsam oil
855-785-2888
buttpaste@cbfleet.com

BOUDREAUX'S BUTT PASTE MAXIMUM STRENGTH (zinc oxide)
C B Fleet

Instructions & Usage
Active Ingredient(s)
Zinc Oxide, 40%
Purpose(s)
Skin Protectant

USES
• Helps treat and prevent diaper rash
• Protects chafed skin due to diaper rash and helps seal out wetness

WARNINGS
• **For external use only**
• **When using this product** avoid contact with the eyes
• **Stop use and ask a doctor if** condition worsens or does not improve after 7 days
• **Keep out of the reach of children**
• If swallowed seek medical help or call Poison Control Center immediately

DIRECTIONS FOR USE
• Change wet and soiled diaper immediately
• Cleanse the diaper area and allow to dry

- Apply ointment liberally and often as necessary with each diaper change and especially when exposed to wet diapers for a prolonged period of time, such as bedtime.

OTHER INFORMATION
- Store at room temperature, 20°-27° (68°-80°F)
- Use with infants, children, and adults
- Will stain clothing and fabric

INACTIVE INGREDIENTS
castor oil, mineral oil, paraffin, peruvian balsam, petrolatum.
855-785-2888

BOUDREAUX'S BUTT PASTE (zinc oxide)

C B Fleet

Instructions & Usage
Active Ingredient(s)
Zinc Oxide, 16%
Purpose(s)
Skin Protectant

USES
- Helps treat and prevent diaper rash
- Protects chafed skin due to diaper rash and helps seal out wetness

WARNINGS
- For external use only
- Avoid contact with the eyes
- Stop use and ask a doctor if condition worsens or does not improve after 7 days
- Keep out of the reach of children
- If swallowed seek medical help or call Poison Control Center immediately

DIRECTIONS FOR USE
- Change wet and soiled diaper immediately
- Cleanse the diaper area and allow to dry
- Apply ointment liberally and often as necessary with each diaper change and especially when exposed to wet diapers for a prolonged period of time, such as bedtime.

OTHER INFORMATION
- Store at room temperature, 20-27°C (68-80°F)
- Use with infants, children and adults
- Will stain clothing and fabric

INACTIVE INGREDIENTS
castor oil, mineral oil, paraffin, peruvian balsam, petrolatum
855-785-2888
buttpaste@cbfleet.com

BOUDREAUX'S RASH PROTECTOR

(dimethicone)

C B Fleet

Instructions & Usage
Active Ingredient(s)
Dimethicone 10%

Purpose(s)
Skin Protectant

USES
- Temporarily protects and helps relieve chapped or cracked skin

- Helps protect from minor skin irritations associated with diaper rash

WARNINGS
For external use only.

WHEN USING THIS PRODUCT:
- do not get into eyes

STOP USE AND ASK A DOCTOR IF:
- condition worsens
- symptoms last more than 7 days or clear up and occur again within a few days

DO NOT USE ON
- deep or puncture wounds
- animal bites
- serious burns

Keep out of the reach of children. If swallowed, get medical help or contact a Poison Control Center right away.

DIRECTIONS
- Change wet and soiled diaper promptly
- Cleanse the diaper area and allow to dry
- Remove nozzle cap
- Apply 1-2 sprays to affected area as often as needed
- Apply during each diaper change, especially at bedtime or anytime when exposure to wet diaper may be prolonged.

OTHER INFORMATION
- Do not use if safety seal is missing or broken
- Store at room temperature 15-30°C (59-86°F)

Do not store near saline nasal spray. In case of accidental inhalation, seek medical attention immediately.

INACTIVE INGREDIENTS
aloe oil extract, caprylic/capric triglyceride, mineral oil, peruvian balsam oil, shea liquid, tocopheryl acetate (vitamin E)
855-785-2888
buttpaste@cbfleet.com

BUFFERIN LOW DOSE BUFFERED ASPIRIN

(aspirin)

Novartis Consumer Health, Inc.

DRUG FACTS

Active Ingredient(s) (in each tablet)	Purpose(s)
Buffered aspirin equal to 81 mg aspirin	Pain reliever

USES
- temporarily relieves minor aches and pains or as recommended by your doctor
- ask your doctor about other uses of buffered aspirin 81 mg

WARNINGS
Reye's syndrome: Children and teenagers who have or are recovering from chicken pox or flu-like symptoms should not use this product. When using this product, if changes in behavior with nausea and vomiting occur, consult a doctor because these symptoms could be an early sign of Reye's syndrome, a rare but serious illness.

Allergy Alert

Aspirin may cause a severe allergic reaction which may include:
- hives
- facial swelling
- asthma (wheezing)
- shock

Stomach bleeding warning: This product contains an NSAID, which may cause severe stomach bleeding. The chance is higher if you:
- are age 60 or older
- have had stomach ulcers or bleeding problems
- take a blood thinning (anticoagulant) or steroid drug
- take other drugs containing prescription or nonprescription NSAIDs (aspirin, ibuprofen, naproxen, or others)
- have 3 or more alcoholic drinks every day while using this product
- take more or for a longer time than directed

DO NOT USE
- if you have ever had an allergic reaction to aspirin or any other pain reliever/fever reducer

ASK A DOCTOR BEFORE USE IF YOU HAVE
- stomach bleeding warning applies to you
- you have a history of stomach problems, such as heartburn
- you have high blood pressure, heart disease, liver cirrhosis, or kidney disease
- you are taking a diuretic
- you are on a magnesium-restricted diet
- you have asthma

ASK A DOCTOR OR PHARMACIST BEFORE IF YOU ARE TAKING
- any other drug containing an NSAID (prescription or nonprescription)
- a blood thinning (anticoagulant) or steroid drug
- a prescription drug for diabetes, gout, or arthritis
- any other drug, or are under a doctor's care for any serious condition

STOP USE AND ASK A DOCTOR IF
- an allergic reaction occurs. Seek medical help right away.
- you experience any of the following signs of stomach bleeding:
  - feel faint
  - vomit blood
  - have bloody or black stools
  - have stomach pain that does not get better
- ringing in the ears or loss of hearing occurs
- painful area is red or swollen
- pain gets worse or lasts for more than 10 days
- fever gets worse or lasts for more than 3 days
- any new symptoms appear

If pregnant or breast feeding; ask a health professional before use. It is especially important not to use aspirin during the last 3 months of pregnancy unless definitely directed to do so by a doctor because it may cause problems in the unborn child or complications during delivery.
Keep out of reach of children

OVERDOSE WARNING
- In case of overdose, get medical help or contact a Poison Control Center right away.

DIRECTIONS
- **do not use more than directed**
- drink a full glass of water with each dose
- adults and children 12 years and over: take 4 to 8 tablets every 4 hours; not more than 48 tablets in 24 hours or as directed by a doctor
- children under 12 years: ask a doctor

OTHER INFORMATION
- **each tablet contains:** calcium 18 mg, and magnesium 15 mg
- store at controlled room temperature 200 - 250 C (680 - 770 F)
- protect from freezing
- read all product information before using. Keep this box for important information.

INACTIVE INGREDIENTS
benzoic acid, carnauba wax, corn starch, FD&C blue #1, hypromellose, light mineral oil, magnesium stearate, microcrystalline cellulose, polysorbate 20, polysorbate 80, povidone, pregelatinized starch, propylene glycol, simethicone emulsion, sorbitan monolaurate, talc, titanium dioxide

QUESTIONS OR COMMENTS?
1-800-468-7746

CALADRYL (calamine and pramoxine hydrochloride)

Johnson & Johnson Consumer Products Company, and Division of Johnson & Johnson Consumer Companies Inc.

DRUG FACTS

Active Ingredient(s)	Purpose(s)
Calamine 8%	Skin protectant
Pramoxine HCl 1%	Topical analgesic

USES
- temporarily relieves pain and itching associated with:
  - rashes due to poison ivy, poison oak or poison sumac
  - insect bites
  - minor skin irritation
  - minor cuts
- dries the oozing and weeping of poison ivy, poison oak and poison sumac

WARNINGS
For external use only.

WHEN USING THIS PRODUCT
do not get into eyes

STOP USE AND ASK A DOCTOR IF
- condition worsens or does not improve within 7 days
- symptoms persist for more than 7 days or clear up and occur again within a few days

Keep out of reach of children. If swallowed, get medical help or contact a Poison Control Center right away.

DIRECTIONS
- shake well before use
- adults and children 2 years of age and older: apply to affected area not more than 3 to 4 times daily
- children under 2 years of age: ask a doctor

OTHER INFORMATION
- store at 20° to 25°C (68° to 77°F)

INACTIVE INGREDIENTS
SD alcohol 38-B, camphor, diazolidinyl urea, fragrance, hypromellose, methylparaben, polysorbate 80, propylene glycol, propylparaben, purified water, xanthan gum

QUESTIONS OR COMMENTS?
call **1-800-223-0182**

Dist: **Johnson & Johnson Consumer Products Company**
Division of Johnson & Johnson Consumer Companies Inc.
Skillman, NJ 08558 USA·

CALADRYL CLEAR (pramoxine hydrochloride and zinc acetate)

Johnson & Johnson Consumer Products Company,
Division of Johnson & Johnson Consumer Companies,
Inc.

DRUG FACTS

Active Ingredient(s)	Purpose(s)
Pramoxine HCl 1%	Topical analgesic
Zinc acetate 0.1%	Skin protectant

USES
- temporarily relieves pain and itching associated with:
  - rashes due to poison ivy, poison oak or poison sumac
  - insect bites
  - minor skin irritation
  - minor cuts
- dries the oozing and weeping of poison ivy, poison oak and poison sumac

WARNINGS
For external use only.

WHEN USING THIS PRODUCT
do not get into eyes

STOP USE AND ASK A DOCTOR IF
- condition worsens or does not improve within 7 days
- symptoms persist for more than 7 days or clear up and occur again within a few days

Keep out of reach of children. If swallowed, get medical help or contact a Poison Control Center right away.

DIRECTIONS
- shake well before use
- adults and children 2 years of age and older: apply to affected area not more than 3 to 4 times daily
- children under 2 years of age: ask a doctor

OTHER INFORMATION
- store at 20° to 25°C (68° to 77°F)

INACTIVE INGREDIENTS
SD alcohol 38-B, camphor, citric acid, diazolidinyl urea, fragrance, glycerin, hypromellose, methylparaben, polysorbate 40, propylene glycol, propylparaben, purified water, sodium citrate

QUESTIONS OR COMMENTS?
call **1-800-223-0182**
Dist: **Johnson & Johnson Consumer Products Company**
Division of Johnson & Johnson Consumer Companies Inc.
Skillman, NJ 08558 USA

CALTRATE 600 + D$_3$ (vitamin D$_3$ and calcium)
Pfizer

Suggested Use
Adults: Take one (1) tablet up to two times daily with food or as directed by your physician. Take with a full glass of water. Not formulated for use in children.

SUPPLEMENT FACTS

Serving Size 1 Tablet

Amount Per Tablet	% Daily Value
Vitamin D$_3$ 800 IU	200%
Calcium 600 mg	60%

INGREDIENTS
Calcium Carbonate, Maltodextrin. **Contains < 2% of:** Blue 2 Lake, Cholecalciferol (Vit. D$_3$), Croscarmellose Sodium, Magnesium Stearate, Polyethylene Glycol, Polyvinyl Alcohol, Red 40 Lake, Talc, Titanium Dioxide, Tocopherols (to preserve freshness), Yellow 6 Lake.
As with any supplement, if you are pregnant, nursing, or taking medication, consult your doctor before use. Do not exceed suggested use.
Keep out of reach of children.
Store at room temperature. Keep bottle tightly closed.
Bottle sealed with printed foil under cap. Do Not Use if foil is torn.
Marketed by: Pfizer, Madison, NJ 07940 USA

QUESTIONS OR COMMENTS?
Call 1-800-282-8805

CALTRATE 600 + D$_3$ PLUS MINERALS
Pfizer

Suggested Use
Adults: Take one (1) tablet up to two times daily with food or as directed by your physician. Take with a full glass of water. Not formulated for use in children.

SUPPLEMENT FACTS

Serving Size 1 Tablet

Amount Per Tablet	% Daily Value
Vitamin D$_3$ 800 IU	200%
Calcium 600 mg	60%
Magnesium 50 mg	13%
Zinc 7.5 mg	50%
Copper 1 mg	50%
Manganese 1.8 mg	90%
Boron 250 mcg	*
*Daily Value not established.	

Ingredients
Calcium Carbonate, Pregelatinized Corn Starch, Magnesium Oxide, Maltodextrin, Microcrystalline Cellulose. **Contains < 2% of:** Blue 2 Lake, Cholecalciferol (Vit. D$_3$), Croscarmellose Sodium, Cupric Sulfate, Magnesium Stearate, Manganese Sulfate, Polyethylene Glycol, Polyvinyl Alcohol, Red 40 Lake, Sodium Borate, Talc, Titanium Dioxide, Tocopherols (to preserve freshness), Yellow 6 Lake, Zinc Oxide.
As with any supplement, if you are pregnant, nursing, or taking medication, consult your doctor before use. Do not exceed suggested use.
Keep out of reach of children.

Store at room temperature. Keep bottle tightly closed.
Bottle sealed with printed foil under cap. Do Not Use if foil is torn.
Marketed by: Pfizer, Madison, NJ 07940 USA

QUESTIONS OR COMMENTS?
Call 1-800-282-8805

CALTRATE GUMMY BITES
Pfizer

SUPPLEMENT FACTS

Serving Size 2 Gummy Bites

Each Serving Contains	Amount Per Serving	%DV
Calories	35	
Total Carbohydrate	9g	3%†
Sugars	7g	*
Vitamin D₃	800 IU	200%
Calcium	500 mg	50%
Phosphorus	230 mg	23%
Sodium	20 mg	<1%
†Percent Daily Value based on a 2,000 calorie diet.		
*Daily Value not established.		

ASK A DOCTOR BEFORE USE IF YOU HAVE
As with any supplement, if you are pregnant, nursing, or taking medication, consult your doctor before use.
Keep out of reach of children.

WHEN USING THIS PRODUCT
• Do not exceed suggested use.

DIRECTIONS
• Take two (2) gummy bites up to two times daily with or without food, or as directed by your physician.
• Not formulated for use in children under 13.

OTHER INFORMATION
Store at room temperature. Keep bottle tightly closed.
Bottle sealed with printed foil under cap. Do Not Use if foil is torn.

OTHER INGREDIENTS
corn syrup, sucrose, tribasic calcium phosphate, water. Contains <2% of: acacia, annatto (color), black carrot juice concentrate (color), cholecalciferol (Vit. D₃), citric acid, corn starch, ethyl alcohol, glycerin, invert sugar, medium-chain triglycerides, modified corn starch, natural flavors, pectin, polysorbate 80, potassium hydroxide, propylene glycol, silicon dioxide, sodium ascorbate (to preserve freshness), sodium citrate, tocopherols (to preserve freshness).

QUESTIONS OR COMMENTS?
Call **1-800-282-8805**

CAPZASIN NO MESS APPLICATOR (capsaicin)
Chattem, Inc.

Capzasin No Mess Applicator

Active Ingredient(s)
Capsaicin 0.15%

Purpose(s)
Topical analgesic

USES
temporarily relieves minor pain associated with:
• arthritis
• simple backache
• muscle strains
• sprains
• bruises
• cramps

WARNINGS
For external use only

WHEN USING THIS PRODUCT
• read inside of carton before using
• use only as directed
• do not bandage
• do not use with a heating pad
• avoid contact with eyes and mucous membranes
• do not apply to wounds, damaged, broken or irritated skin
• a transient burning sensation may occur upon application but generally disappears in several days
• if severe burning sensation occurs, discontinue use immediately and read information printed inside carton
• do not expose the area treated with product to heat or direct sunlight

STOP USE AND ASK A DOCTOR IF
• condition worsens
• redness is present
• irritation develops
• symptoms persist for more than 7 days or clear up and occur again within a few days

Flammable
keep away from fire or flame

If pregnant or breast-feeding
ask a health professional before use.

Keep out of reach of children.
If swallowed, get medical help or contact a Poison Control Center right away.

DIRECTIONS
adults and children over 18 years:
• apply to affected area
• place applicator on skin, press firmly and hold to activate the dispensing of liquid
• massage into painful area until thoroughly absorbed
• repeat as necessary, but no more than 3 to 4 times daily
• IF MEDICINE COMES IN CONTACT WITH HANDS, WASH WITH SOAP AND WATER

children 18 years or younger: ask a doctor

INACTIVE INGREDIENTS
carbomer, glycerin, propylene glycol, SD alcohol 40-2 (35%), triethanolamine, water (245-130)
KEEP CARTON AS IT CONTAINS IMPORTANT INFORMATION.
Close cap tightly after use. 0042763-04
Dist. by Chattem, Inc., P.O. Box 2219
Chattanooga, TN 37409-0219
U.S.A. © 2009 www.chattem.com Recyclable Carton

CAPZASIN QUICK RELIEF (capsaicin and menthol)

Chattem, Inc.

Capzasin Quick Relief Gel

Active Ingredient(s)
Capsaicin 0.025%

Purpose(s)
Topical analgesic

Active Ingredient(s)
Menthol 10%

Purpose(s)
Topical analgesic

USES
temporarily relieves minor pain associated with:
- arthritis
- simple backache
- muscle strains
- sprains
- bruises
- cramps

WARNINGS
For external use only

WHEN USING THIS PRODUCT
- read inside of carton before using
- use only as directed
- do not bandage tightly or use with a heating pad
- avoid contact with eyes and mucous membranes
- do not apply to wounds or damaged, broken or irritated skin
- a transient burning sensation may occur upon application but generally disappears in several days
- if severe burning sensation occurs, discontinue use immediately and read inside carton for important information
- do not expose the area treated with product to heat or direct sunlight

STOP USE AND ASK A DOCTOR IF
- condition worsens
- redness is present
- irritation develops
- symptoms persist for more than 7 days or clear up and occur again within a few days

If pregnant or breast-feeding
ask a health professional before use.

Keep out of reach of children.
If swallowed, get medical help or contact a Poison Control Center right away.

DIRECTIONS
adults and children over 18 years:
- squeeze desired amount of Capzasin Quick Relief Gel onto affected area
- using the sponge-top applicator, massage dispensed gel into painful area until thoroughly absorbed
- repeat as necessary, but no more than 3 to 4 times daily
- **IF MEDICINE COMES IN CONTACT WITH HANDS, WASH WITH SOAP AND WATER**

children 18 years or younger: ask a doctor

INACTIVE INGREDIENTS
acrylates/C10-30 alkyl acrylate crosspolymer, allantoin, aloe barbadensis leaf juice, DMDM hydantoin, fragrance, glycerin, methylparaben, phenoxyethanol, propylene glycol, propylparaben, SD alcohol 40-2 (15%), steareth-2, steareth-21, triethanolamine, water (245-285)
KEEP CARTON AS IT CONTAINS IMPORTANT INFORMATION.

Distributed by: Chattem, Inc.
P.O. Box 2219
Chattanooga, TN 37409-0219
0049618-03 U.S.A. ©2010 www.chattem.com Recyclable Carton

CAPZASIN HP ARTHRITIS PAIN RELIEF
(capsaicin)

Chattem, Inc.

Capzasin HP Arthritis Pain Relief

Active Ingredient(s)
Capsaicin 0.1%

Purpose(s)
Topical analgesic

USES
temporarily relieves minor pain of muscles and joints associated with:
- arthritis
- simple backache
- strains
- sprains
- bruises

WARNINGS
For external use only

WHEN USING THIS PRODUCT
- use only as directed
- do not bandage tightly or use with a heating pad
- avoid contact with eyes and mucous membranes
- do not apply to wounds, damaged, broken or irritated skin
- a transient burning sensation may occur upon application but generally disappears in several days
- if severe burning sensation occurs, discontinue use immediately and read important information printed inside carton
- do not expose the area treated with product to heat or direct sunlight

STOP USE AND ASK A DOCTOR IF
- condition worsens
- symptoms persist for more than 7 days or clear up and occur again within a few days
- redness is present
- irritation develops

If pregnant or breast-feeding
ask a health professional before use.

Keep out of reach of children.
If swallowed, get medical help or contact a Poison Control Center right away.

DIRECTIONS
adults and children over 18 years:
- apply to affected area
- massage into painful area until thoroughly absorbed
- repeat as necessary, but no more than 3 to 4 times daily
- **WASH HANDS WITH SOAP AND WATER AFTER APPLYING**

children 18 years or younger: ask a doctor

INACTIVE INGREDIENTS
benzyl alcohol, cetyl alcohol, glyceryl stearate, isopropyl myristate, PEG-40 stearate, petrolatum, sorbitol, water (238-10)

READ INFORMATION PRINTED INSIDE CARTON BEFORE USING.
KEEP CARTON AS IT CONTAINS IMPORTANT INFORMATION. Recyclable Carton

Dist. by Chattem, Inc., P.O. Box 2219
Chattanooga, TN 37409-0219 U.S.A.
© 2009 www.chattem.com

CAPZASIN P ARTHRITIS PAIN RELIEF
(capsaicin)

Chattem, Inc.

Capzasin P Arthritis Pain Relief

Active Ingredient(s)
Capsaicin 0.035%

Purpose(s)
Topical analgesic

USES
temporarily relieves minor pain associated with:
• arthritis
• simple backache
• strains
• sprains
• bruises

WARNINGS
For external use only

WHEN USING THIS PRODUCT
• use only as directed
• do not bandage
• do not use with a heating pad
• avoid contact with eyes and mucous membranes
• do not apply to wounds or damaged skin

STOP USE AND ASK A DOCTOR IF
• condition worsens
• symptoms persist for more than 7 days or clear up and occur
  again within a few days
• redness is present
• irritation develops

If pregnant or breast-feeding
ask a health professional before use.

Keep out of reach of children.
In case of accidental ingestion, get medical help or contact a
Poison Control Center right away.

DIRECTIONS
adults and children over 18 years:
• apply to affected area
• massage into painful area until thoroughly absorbed
• repeat as necessary, but no more than 4 times daily
• **WASH HANDS WITH SOAP AND WATER AFTER
  APPLYING**

children 18 years or younger: ask a doctor

INACTIVE INGREDIENTS
benzyl alcohol, cetyl alcohol, glyceryl stearate, isopropyl
myristate, PEG-40 stearate, petrolatum, sorbitol, water (238-9)

**READ PACKAGE INSERT BEFORE USING. KEEP
CARTON AND INSERT AS THEY CONTAIN IMPORTANT
INFORMATION.**

Dist. by Chattem, Inc., P.O. Box 2219
Chattanooga, TN 37409-0219 U.S.A.
© 2006 www.chattem.com

CENTRUM ADULTS UNDER 50

Pfizer

SUPPLEMENT FACTS

Serving Size 1 Tablet

Each Tablet Contains	% Daily Value
Vitamin A 3,500 IU (29% as Beta-Carotene)	70%
Vitamin C 60 mg	100%
Vitamin D 400 IU	100%
Vitamin E 30 IU	100%
Vitamin K 25 mcg	31%
Thiamin 1.5 mg	100%
Riboflavin 1.7 mg	100%
Niacin 20 mg	100%
Vitamin B_6 2 mg	100%
Folic Acid 400 mcg	100%
Vitamin B_{12} 6 mcg	100%
Biotin 30 mcg	10%
Pantothenic Acid 10 mg	100%
Calcium 200 mg	20%
Iron 18 mg	100%
Phosphorus 20 mg	2%
Iodine 150 mcg	100%
Magnesium 50 mg	13%
Zinc 11 mg	73%
Selenium 55 mcg	79%
Copper 0.5 mg	25%
Manganese 2.3 mg	115%
Chromium 35 mcg	29%
Molybdenum 45 mcg	60%
Chloride 72 mg	2%
Potassium 80 mg	2%
Boron 75 mcg	*
Nickel 5 mcg	*
Silicon 2 mg	*
Tin 10 mcg	*
Vanadium 10 mcg	*

*Daily Value not established.

INGREDIENTS
Calcium Carbonate, Potassium Chloride, Dibasic Calcium
Phosphate, Magnesium Oxide, Microcrystalline Cellulose,
Ascorbic Acid (Vit. C), Ferrous Fumarate, Pregelatinized Corn
Starch, dl-Alpha Tocopheryl Acetate (Vit. E). **Contains < 2% of:**
Acacia, Beta-Carotene, BHT, Biotin, Boric Acid, Calcium
Pantothenate, Calcium Stearate, Cholecalciferol (Vit. D_3),
Chromium Picolinate, Citric Acid, Corn Starch, Crospovidone,
Cupric Sulfate, Cyanocobalamin (Vit. B_{12}), FD&C Yellow No. 6
Aluminum Lake, Folic Acid, Gelatin, Hydrogenated Palm Oil,
Hypromellose, Manganese Sulfate, Medium-Chain Triglycerides,
Modified Food Starch, Niacinamide, Nickelous Sulfate,
Phytonadione (Vit. K), Polyethylene Glycol, Polyvinyl Alcohol,
Potassium Iodide, Pyridoxine Hydrochloride (Vit. B_6), Riboflavin
(Vit. B_2), Silicon Dioxide, Sodium Ascorbate, Sodium Benzoate,
Sodium Citrate, Sodium Metavanadate, Sodium Molybdate,
Sodium Selenate, Sorbic Acid, Stannous Chloride, Sucrose, Talc,
Thiamine Mononitrate (Vit. B_1), Titanium Dioxide, Tocopherols,
Tribasic Calcium Phosphate, Vitamin A Acetate (Vit. A), Zinc
Oxide. **May also contain < 2% of:** Ascorbyl Palmitate,
Maltodextrin, Sodium Aluminosilicate, Sunflower Oil.

SUGGESTED USE

Adults - Take one tablet daily with food. Not formulated for use in children. Do not exceed suggested use.

As with any supplement, if you are pregnant, nursing, or taking medication, consult your doctor before use.

> **WARNING:** Accidental overdose of iron-containing products is a leading cause of fatal poisoning in children under 6. Keep this product out of reach of children. In case of accidental overdose, call a doctor or poison control center immediately.

IMPORTANT INFORMATION

Long-term intake of high levels of vitamin A (excluding that sourced from beta-carotene) may increase the risk of osteoporosis in adults. Do not take this product if taking other vitamin A supplements.

Store at room temperature. Keep bottle tightly closed.

Bottle sealed with printed foil under cap. Do Not Use if foil is torn.

Marketed by: Pfizer, Madison, NJ 07940 USA

QUESTIONS OR COMMENTS?

Call 1-877-CENTRUM

CENTRUM FLAVOR BURST MIXED FRUIT
CENTRUM FLAVOR BURST TROPICAL FRUIT
CENTRUM FLAVOR BURST WILD GRAPE
CENTRUM FLAVOR BURST RASPBERRY LEMONADE DRINK MIX

Pfizer

SUPPLEMENT FACTS

Mixed Fruit, Tropical Fruit, Wild Grape: Serving Size 4 Chews

Each Serving Contains	Amount Per Serving	%DV
Calories	25	
Total Carbohydrate	6 g	2%†
Sugar	4 g	*
Vitamin A	2,000 IU	40%
Vitamin C	60 mg	100%
Vitamin D	800 mg	200%
Vitamin E	40 IU	133%
Vitamin B_6	2 mg	100%
Folic Acid	400 mcg	100%
Vitamin B_{12}	10 mcg	167%
Biotin	150 mcg	50%
Pantothenic Acid	10 mg	100%
Iodine	80 mcg	53%
Zinc	5 mg	33%
Choline	76 mg	*
Inositol	40 mcg	*
† Percent Daily Values are based on a 2,000 calorie diet.		
* Daily Value not established.		

Raspberry Lemonade Drink Mix: Serving Size 1 Packet

Each Serving Contains	Amount Per Serving	%DV
Calories 30	30	
Total Carbohydrate 8 g	8 g	3%†
Sugars 6 g	6 g	*
Vitamin A 2,000 IU	2,000 IU	40%
Vitamin C 60 mg	60 mg	100%
Vitamin D 800 IU	800 IU	200%
Vitamin E 40 IU	40 IU	133%
Thiamine 0.38 mg	0.38 mg	25%
Riboflavin 0.43 mg	0.43 mg	25%
Niacin 4 mg	4 mg	20%
Vitamin B_6 10 mg	10 mg	500%
Folic Acid 400 mcg	400 mcg	100%
Vitamin B_{12} 25 mcg	25 mcg	417%
Biotin 30 mcg	30 mcg	10%
Pantothenic Acid 10 mg	10 mg	100%
Calcium 65 mg	65 mg	7%
Phosphorous 38 mg	38 mg	4%
Magnesium 60 mg	60 mg	15%
Zinc 2 mg	2 mg	13%
Manganese 0.5 mg	0.5 mg	25%
Chromium 10 mcg	10 mcg	8%
Sodium 30 mg	30 mg	<2%
Potassium 200 mg	200 mg	6%
† Percent Daily Values are based on a 2,000 calorie diet.		
* Daily Value not established.		

WARNINGS

Long-term intake of high levels of vitamin A (excluding that sourced from beta-carotene) may increase the risk of osteoporosis in adults. Do not take this product if taking other vitamin A supplements.

This product must not be taken with products containing high levels of vitamins A, D, folic acid, or zinc.

Keep out of reach of children.

ASK A DOCTOR BEFORE USE IF YOU

• are pregnant, nursing, or taking medication

WHEN USING THIS PRODUCT

• Do not exceed suggested use.

DIRECTIONS

Chews:

• Adults &8211; Take 4 chews daily with or without food.
• Not formulated for use in children.

Drink Mix:

• Adults ages 18 and older: One (1) packet daily with or without food. Empty contents into a glass, add 4-6 oz of water, stir.
• Not formulated for use in children.

OTHER INFORMATION

• Store at room temperature.
• Keep bottle tightly closed.
• Bottle sealed with printed foil under cap. Do Not Use if foil is torn.

OTHER INGREDIENTS

Mixed Fruit: sucrose, corn syrup, water, hydrogenated coconut oil, choline bitartrate, maltodextrin, acacia. **Contains < 2% of:**

ascorbic acid (vit. C), beeswax, biotin, blue 1 lake, blue 2 lake, calcium pantothenate, carmine (color), carnauba wax, cholecalciferol (vit. D3), cyanocobalamin (vit. B_{12}), dl-alpha tocopheryl acetate (vit. E), folic acid, inositol, lac-resin, lecithin (soy), modified corn starch, natural and artificial flavors, potassium iodide, pregelatinized corn starch, pyridoxine hydrochloride (vit. B_6), titanium dioxide, vitamin a palmitate, zinc sulfate. **Contains:** soy.

Tropical Fruit: sucrose, corn syrup, water, hydrogenated coconut oil, choline bitartrate, acacia, modified corn starch, maltodextrin. **Contains < 2% of:** annatto seed extract (color), ascorbic acid (vit. C), beeswax, beet juice concentrate (color), beta-carotene (color), biotin, calcium pantothenate, carnauba wax, cholecalciferol (vit. D_3), cyanocobalamin (vit. B_{12}), dl-alpha tocopheryl acetate (vit. E), folic acid, inositol, lac-resin, lecithin (soy), natural & artificial flavor, potassium iodide, pregelatinized corn starch, pyridoxine hydrochloride (vit. B_6), titanium dioxide, tumeric oleoresin (color), vitamin a palmitate, zinc sulfate. **Contains:** soy.

Wild Grape: sucrose, corn syrup, water, hydrogenated coconut oil, choline bitartrate, maltodextrin, acacia. **Contains < 2% of:** ascorbic acid (vit. C), beeswax, biotin, blue 2 lake, calcium pantothenate, carmine (color), carnauba wax, cholecalciferol (vit. D_3), cyanocobalamin (vit. B_{12}), dl-alpha tocopheryl acetate (vit. E), folic acid, inositol, lac-resin, lecithin (soy), modified corn starch, natural and artificial flavors, potassium iodide, pregelatinized corn starch, pyridoxine hydrochloride (vit. B_6), titanium dioxide, vitamin a palmitate, zinc sulfate. **Contains:** soy.

Raspberry Lemonade Drink Mix: fructose, citric acid, maltodextrin, potassium bicarbonate, sucrose. **Contains < 2% of:** ascorbic acid (vit. C), beta-carotene, biotin, calcium carbonate, calcium pantothenate, cholecalciferol (vit. D_3), chromium picolinate, cyanocobalamin (vit. B_{12}), d-alpha tocopheryl acetate (vit. E) (soy), dibasic calcium phosphate, dried fruit and vegetable juice concentrates (beet, raspberry, cherry) (color and/or flavor), folic acid, glycine, l-aspartic acid, lemon juice solids, magnesium carbonate, magnesium hydroxide, manganese gluconate, monobasic calcium phosphate, monobasic potassium phosphate, monobasic sodium phosphate, natural flavors, niacin, potassium carbonate, pyridoxine hydrochloride (vit. B_6), riboflavin-5'-phosphate (vit. B_2), silicon dioxide, sodium bicarbonate, sucralose, tartaric acid, thiamine hydrochloride (vit. B_1), tocopherols (to preserve freshness), tribasic calcium phosphate, vitamin a acetate, zinc ascorbate. **Contains:** soy.

CENTRUM KIDS
Pfizer

SUPPLEMENT FACTS

Serving Size	½ Tablet	1 Tablet
	%DV for Children 2 and 3 years	%DV for Children 4 years and older
Amount Per Tablet	(½ Tablet)	(1 Tablet)
Calories 5		
Total Carbohydrate 1 g	*	<1%†
Sugars <1 g	*	*
Vitamin A 3,500 IU (29% as Beta-Carotene)	70%	70%
Vitamin C 60 mg	75%	100%
Vitamin D 400 IU	50%	100%
Vitamin E 30 IU	150%	100%
Vitamin K 10 mcg	*	13%
Thiamin 1.5 mg	107%	100%
Riboflavin 1.7 mg	106%	100%
Niacin 20 mg	111%	100%
Vitamin B_6 2 mg	143%	100%
Folic Acid 400 mcg	100%	100%
Vitamin B_{12} 6 mcg	100%	100%
Biotin 45 mcg	15%	15%
Pantothenic Acid 10 mg	100%	100%
Calcium 108 mg	7%	11%
Iron 18 mg	90%	100%
Phosphorus 50 mg	3%	5%
Iodine 150 mcg	107%	100%
Magnesium 40 mg	10%	10%
Zinc 15 mg	94%	100%
Copper 2 mg	100%	100%
Manganese 1 mg	*	50%
Chromium 20 mcg	*	17%
Molybdenum 20 mcg	*	27%

*Daily Value (DV) not established.

†Percent Daily Values are based on a 2,000 calorie diet.

INGREDIENTS
Sucrose, Dibasic Calcium Phosphate, Microcrystalline Cellulose, Mannitol (wheat), Calcium Carbonate, Ascorbic Acid (Vit. C), Magnesium Oxide, Pregelatinized Corn Starch, Mono- and Di-glycerides, Stearic Acid (soybean), Maltodextrin. **Contains < 2% of:** Aspartame,** Beta-Carotene, BHT (to retard oxidation), Biotin, Blue 2 Lake, Calcium Pantothenate, Carbonyl Iron, Carrageenan, Cholecalciferol (Vit. D_3), Chromic Chloride, Citric Acid, Cupric Oxide, Cyanocobalamin (Vit. B_{12}), Dextrose, dl-Alpha Tocopheryl Acetate (Vit. E), Folic Acid, Gelatin, Guar Gum, Lactose (milk), Magnesium Stearate, Malic Acid, Manganese Sulfate, Modified Corn Starch, Natural and Artificial Flavors, Niacinamide, Phytonadione (Vit. K), Potassium Iodide, Pyridoxine Hydrochloride (Vit. B_6), Red 40 Lake, Riboflavin (Vit. B_2), Silicon Dioxide, Sodium Molybdate, Thiamine Mononitrate (Vit. B_1), Tocopherols (to retard oxidation), Vanillin, Vitamin A Acetate, Yellow 6 Lake, Zinc Oxide. **Contains:** Milk, Soybean, Wheat.

SUGGESTED USE

Children 2 and 3 years of age, chew approximately ½ tablet daily with food. Children 4 years of age and older, chew 1 tablet daily with food. Not formulated for use in children less than 2 years of age. Do not exceed suggested use.

As with any supplement, if your child is taking medication, consult your pediatrician before use.

> **WARNING:** Accidental overdose of iron-containing products is a leading cause of fatal poisoning in children under 6. Keep this product out of reach of children. In case of accidental overdose, call a doctor or poison control center immediately.

**PHENYLKETONURICS: CONTAINS PHENYLALANINE.

IMPORTANT INFORMATION

Long-term intake of high levels of vitamin A (excluding that sourced from beta-carotene) may increase the risk of osteoporosis in adults. Do not take this product if taking other vitamin A supplements.

Store at room temperature. Keep bottle tightly closed. Protect from moisture.

Bottle sealed with printed foil under cap. Do Not Use if foil is torn.

Marketed by: Pfizer, Madison, NJ 07940 USA

Made in Canada

QUESTIONS OR COMMENTS?

Call 1-877-CENTRUM

CENTRUM MEN

Pfizer

SUPPLEMENT FACTS

Serving Size 1 Tablet

Amount Per Serving	% Daily Value
Vitamin A 3,500 IU (29% as Beta-Carotene)	70%
Vitamin C 90 mg	150%
Vitamin D 600 IU	150%
Vitamin E 45 IU	150%
Vitamin K 60 mcg	75%
Thiamin 1.2 mg	80%
Riboflavin 1.3 mg	76%
Niacin 16 mg	80%
Vitamin B_6 2 mg	100%
Folic Acid 200 mcg	50%
Vitamin B_{12} 6 mcg	100%
Biotin 40 mcg	13%
Pantothenic Acid 15 mg	150%
Calcium 210 mg	21%
Iron 8 mg	44%
Phosphorus 20 mg	2%
Iodine 150 mcg	100%
Magnesium 100 mg	25%
Zinc 11 mg	73%
Selenium 100 mcg	143%
Copper 0.9 mg	45%
Manganese 2.3 mg	115%
Chromium 35 mcg	29%
Molybdenum 50 mcg	67%
Chloride 72 mg	2%
Potassium 80 mg	2%
Boron 150 mcg	*
Nickel 5 mcg	*
Silicon 2 mg	*
Tin 10 mcg	*
Vanadium 10 mcg	*
Lycopene 600 mcg	*

*Daily Value not established.

INGREDIENTS

Calcium Carbonate, Magnesium Oxide, Potassium Chloride, Ascorbic Acid (Vit. C), Dibasic Calcium Phosphate, Microcrystalline Cellulose, dl-Alpha Tocopheryl Acetate (Vit. E), Corn Starch. **Contains < 2% of:** Beta-Carotene, BHT (to retard oxidation), Biotin, Calcium Pantothenate, Cholecalciferol (Vit. D_3), Chromium Picolinate, Crospovidone, Cupric Sulfate, Cyanocobalamin (Vit. B_{12}), Ferrous Fumarate, Folic Acid, Gelatin, Hydrogenated Palm Oil, Lecithin (Soy), Lycopene, Magnesium Borate, Magnesium Stearate, Maltodextrin, Manganese Sulfate, Modified Corn Starch, Niacinamide, Nickelous Sulfate, Phytonadione (Vit. K), Polyethylene Glycol, Polyvinyl Alcohol, Potassium Iodide, Pregelatinized Corn Starch, Pyridoxine Hydrochloride (Vit. B_6), Red 40 Lake, Riboflavin (Vit. B_2), Silicon Dioxide, Sodium Ascorbate (to retard oxidation), Sodium Metavanadate, Sodium Molybdate, Sodium Selenate, Stannous Chloride, Talc, Thiamine Mononitrate (Vit. B_1), Titanium Dioxide, Tocopherols (to retard oxidation), Vitamin A Acetate, Yellow 6 Lake, Zinc Oxide. **Contains:** Soy.

SUGGESTED USE

Adults - Take one tablet daily with food. Not formulated for use in children. Do not exceed suggested use.
As with any supplement, if you are taking medication, consult your doctor before use.

WARNING: Accidental overdose of iron-containing products is a leading cause of fatal poisoning in children under 6. Keep this product out of reach of children. In case of accidental overdose, call a doctor or poison control center immediately.

IMPORTANT INFORMATION

Long-term intake of high levels of vitamin A (excluding that sourced from beta-carotene) may increase the risk of osteoporosis in adults. Do not take this product if taking other vitamin A supplements.
Store at room temperature. Keep bottle tightly closed.
Bottle sealed with printed foil under cap. Do Not Use if foil is torn.
Marketed by: Pfizer, Madison, NJ 07940 USA
Made in Canada

QUESTIONS OR COMMENTS?

Call 1-877-CENTRUM

CENTRUM SILVER ADULTS 50+

Pfizer

SUPPLEMENT FACTS

Serving Size 1 Tablet

Each Tablet Contains	% Daily Value
Vitamin A 2,500 IU (40% as Beta-Carotene)	50%
Vitamin C 60 mg	100%
Vitamin D 500 IU	125%
Vitamin E 50 IU	167%
Vitamin K 30 mcg	38%
Thiamin 1.5 mg	100%
Riboflavin 1.7 mg	100%
Niacin 20 mg	100%
Vitamin B_6 3 mg	150%
Folic Acid 400 mcg	100%
Vitamin B_{12} 25 mcg	417%
Biotin 30 mcg	10%
Pantothenic Acid 10 mg	100%
Calcium 220 mg	22%
Phosphorus 20 mg	2%
Iodine 150 mcg	100%
Magnesium 50 mg	13%
Zinc 11 mg	73%
Selenium 55 mcg	79%
Copper 0.5 mg	25%
Manganese 2.3 mg	115%
Chromium 45 mcg	38%
Molybdenum 45 mcg	60%
Chloride 72 mg	2%
Potassium 80 mg	2%
Boron 150 mcg	*
Nickel 5 mcg	*
Silicon 2 mg	*
Vanadium 10 mcg	*
Lutein 250 mcg	*
Lycopene 300 mcg	*

*Daily Value not established.

INGREDIENTS

Calcium Carbonate, Potassium Chloride, Dibasic Calcium Phosphate, Magnesium Oxide, Ascorbic Acid (Vit. C), Microcrystalline Cellulose, dl-Alpha Tocopheryl Acetate (Vit. E), Pregelatinized Corn Starch, Modified Food Starch. **Contains < 2% of:** Acacia, Ascorbyl Palmitate, Beta-Carotene, BHT, Biotin, Boric Acid, Calcium Pantothenate, Calcium Stearate, Cholecalciferol (Vit. D_3), Chromium Picolinate, Citric Acid, Corn Starch, Crospovidone, Cupric Sulfate, Cyanocobalamin (Vit. B_{12}), FD&C Blue No. 2 Aluminum Lake, FD&C Red No. 40 Aluminum Lake, FD&C Yellow No. 6 Aluminum Lake, Folic Acid, Gelatin, Hydrogenated Palm Oil, Hypromellose, Lutein, Lycopene, Manganese Sulfate, Medium-Chain Triglycerides, Niacinamide, Nickelous Sulfate, Phytonadione (Vit. K), Polyethylene Glycol, Polyvinyl Alcohol, Potassium Iodide, Pyridoxine Hydrochloride (Vit. B_6), Riboflavin (Vit. B_2), Silicon Dioxide, Sodium Ascorbate, Sodium Benzoate, Sodium Borate, Sodium Citrate, Sodium Metavanadate, Sodium Molybdate, Sodium Selenate, Sorbic Acid, Sucrose, Talc, Thiamine Mononitrate (Vit. B_1), Titanium Dioxide, Tocopherols, Tribasic Calcium Phosphate, Vitamin A Acetate (Vit. A), Zinc Oxide. **May**

also contain < 2% of: Maltodextrin, Sodium Aluminosilicate, Sunflower Oil.

SUGGESTED USE

Adults - Take one tablet daily with food. Not formulated for use in children. Do not exceed suggested use.

As with any supplement, if you are pregnant, nursing, or taking medication, consult your doctor before use.

IMPORTANT INFORMATION

Long-term intake of high levels of vitamin A (excluding that sourced from beta-carotene) may increase the risk of osteoporosis in adults. Do not take this product if taking other vitamin A supplements.

Keep out of reach of children.

Store at room temperature. Keep bottle tightly closed.

Bottle sealed with printed foil under cap. Do Not Use if foil is torn.

Marketed by: Pfizer, Madison, NJ 07940 USA

QUESTIONS OR COMMENTS?

Call 1-877-CENTRUM

CENTRUM SILVER MEN

Pfizer

SUPPLEMENT FACTS

Serving Size 1 Tablet

Amount Per Serving	% Daily Value
Vitamin A 3,500 IU (29% as Beta-Carotene)	70%
Vitamin C 120 mg	200%
Vitamin D 600 IU	150%
Vitamin E 60 IU	200%
Vitamin K 60 mcg	75%
Thiamin 1.5 mg	100%
Riboflavin 1.7 mg	100%
Niacin 20 mg	100%
Vitamin B_6 6 mg	300%
Folic Acid 300 mcg	75%
Vitamin B_{12} 100 mcg	1667%
Biotin 30 mcg	10%
Pantothenic Acid 10 mg	100%
Calcium 250 mg	25%
Phosphorus 20 mg	2%
Iodine 150 mcg	100%
Magnesium 50 mg	13%
Zinc 15 mg	100%
Selenium 100 mcg	143%
Copper 0.7 mg	35%
Manganese 4 mg	200%
Chromium 60 mcg	50%
Molybdenum 50 mcg	67%
Chloride 72 mg	2%
Potassium 80 mg	2%
Boron 150 mcg	*
Nickel 5 mcg	*
Silicon 2 mg	*
Vanadium 10 mcg	*
Lutein 300 mcg	*
Lycopene 600 mcg	*

*Daily Value not established.

INGREDIENTS

Calcium Carbonate, Potassium Chloride, Ascorbic Acid (Vit. C), Dibasic Calcium Phosphate, Magnesium Oxide, dl-Alpha Tocopheryl Acetate (Vit. E), Microcrystalline Cellulose, Modified Corn Starch, Corn Starch, Crospovidone, Maltodextrin, Pregelatinized Corn Starch. **Contains < 2% of:** Beta-Carotene, BHT (to retard oxidation), Biotin, Blue 2 Lake, Calcium Pantothenate, Cholecalciferol (Vit. D_3), Chromium Picolinate, Cupric Sulfate, Cyanocobalamin (Vit. B_{12}), Folic Acid, Gelatin, Hydrogenated Palm Oil, Lecithin (Soy), Lutein, Lycopene, Magnesium Borate, Magnesium Stearate, Manganese Sulfate, Niacinamide, Nickelous Sulfate, Phytonadione (Vit. K), Polyethylene Glycol, Polyvinyl Alcohol, Potassium Iodide, Pyridoxine Hydrochloride (Vit. B_6),Red 40 Lake, Riboflavin (Vit. B_2), Silicon Dioxide, Sodium Ascorbate (to retard oxidation), Sodium Borate, Sodium Metavanadate, Sodium Molybdate, Sodium Selenate, Talc, Thiamine Mononitrate (Vit. B_1), Titanium Dioxide, Tocopherols (to retard oxidation), Vitamin A Acetate, Yellow 6 Lake, Zinc Oxide. **Contains:** Soy.

SUGGESTED USE

Adults - Take one tablet daily with food. Not formulated for use in children. Do not exceed suggested use.

As with any supplement, if you are taking medication, consult your doctor before use.

IMPORTANT INFORMATION

Long-term intake of high levels of vitamin A (excluding that sourced from beta-carotene) may increase the risk of osteoporosis in adults. Do not take this product if taking other vitamin A supplements.

Keep out of reach of children.

Store at room temperature. Keep bottle tightly closed.

Bottle sealed with printed foil under cap. Do Not Use if foil is torn.

Marketed by: Pfizer, Madison, NJ 07940 USA

Made in Canada

QUESTIONS OR COMMENTS?

Call 1-877-CENTRUM

CENTRUM SILVER WOMEN

Pfizer

SUPPLEMENT FACTS

Serving Size 1 Tablet

Amount Per Serving	% Daily Value
Vitamin A 3,500 IU (43% as Beta-Carotene)	70%
Vitamin C 100 mg	167%
Vitamin D 800 IU	200%
Vitamin E 35 IU	117%
Vitamin K 50 mcg	63%
Thiamin 1.1 mg	73%
Riboflavin 1.1 mg	65%
Niacin 14 mg	70%
Vitamin B$_6$ 5 mg	250%
Folic Acid 400 mcg	100%
Vitamin B$_{12}$ 50 mcg	833%
Biotin 30 mcg	10%
Pantothenic Acid 5 mg	50%
Calcium 500 mg	50%
Iron 8 mg	44%
Phosphorus 20 mg	2%
Iodine 150 mcg	100%
Magnesium 50 mg	13%
Zinc 15 mg	100%
Selenium 55 mcg	79%
Copper 0.5 mg	25%
Manganese 2.3 mg	115%
Chromium 50 mcg	42%
Molybdenum 50 mcg	67%
Chloride 72 mg	2%
Potassium 80 mg	2%
Boron 150 mcg	*
Nickel 5 mcg	*
Silicon 2 mg	*
Vanadium 10 mcg	*
Lutein 300 mcg	*
*Daily Value not established.	

INGREDIENTS

Calcium Carbonate, Potassium Chloride, Ascorbic Acid (Vit. C), Dibasic Calcium Phosphate, Magnesium Oxide, Microcrystalline Cellulose, Pregelatinized Corn Starch, Maltodextrin, dl-Alpha Tocopheryl Acetate (Vit. E), Crospovidone. **Contains < 2% of:** Beta-Carotene, BHT (to preserve freshness), Biotin, Blue 2 Lake, Calcium Pantothenate, Cholecalciferol (Vit. D$_3$), Chromium Picolinate, Corn Starch, Cupric Sulfate, Cyanocobalamin (Vit. B$_{12}$), Ferrous Fumarate, Folic Acid, Gelatin, Hydrogenated Palm Oil, Lecithin (Soy), Lutein, Magnesium Borate, Magnesium Stearate, Manganese Sulfate, Niacinamide, Nickelous Sulfate, Phytonadione (Vit. K), Polyethylene Glycol, Polyvinyl Alcohol, Potassium Iodide, Pyridoxine Hydrochloride (Vit. B$_6$), Riboflavin (Vit. B$_2$), Silicon Dioxide, Sodium Ascorbate (To Preserve Freshness), Sodium Borate, Sodium Metavanadate, Sodium Molybdate, Sodium Selenate, Talc, Thiamine Mononitrate (Vit. B$_1$), Titanium Dioxide, Tocopherols (To Preserve Freshness), Vitamin A Acetate, Zinc Oxide. **Contains:** Soy.

SUGGESTED USE

Adults - Take one tablet daily with food. Not formulated for use in children. Do not exceed suggested use.

As with any supplement, if you are pregnant, nursing, or taking medication, consult your doctor before use.

WARNING: Accidental overdose of iron-containing products is a leading cause of fatal poisoning in children under 6. Keep this product out of reach of children. In case of accidental overdose, call a doctor or poison control center immediately.

IMPORTANT INFORMATION

Long-term intake of high levels of vitamin A (excluding that sourced from beta-carotene) may increase the risk of osteoporosis in adults. Do not take this product if taking other vitamin A supplements.

Store at room temperature. Keep bottle tightly closed.

Bottle sealed with printed foil under cap. Do Not Use if foil is torn.

Marketed by: Pfizer, Madison, NJ 07940 USA

QUESTIONS OR COMMENTS?

Call 1-877-CENTRUM

CENTRUM SPECIALIST ENERGY
Pfizer

SUPPLEMENT FACTS

Serving Size 1 Tablet

Each Tablet Contains	% Daily Value
Vitamin A 3,500 IU (29% as Beta-Carotene)	70%
Vitamin C 120 mg	200%
Vitamin D 400 IU	100%
Vitamin E 60 IU	200%
Vitamin K 25 mcg	31%
Thiamin 4.5 mg	300%
Riboflavin 5.1 mg	300%
Niacin 40 mg	200%
Vitamin B_6 6 mg	300%
Folic Acid 400 mcg	100%
Vitamin B_{12} 18 mcg	300%
Biotin 50 mcg	17%
Pantothenic Acid 12 mg	120%
Calcium 100 mg	10%
Iron 18 mg	100%
Phosphorus 48 mg	5%
Iodine 150 mcg	100%
Magnesium 40 mg	10%
Zinc 11 mg	73%
Selenium 70 mcg	100%
Copper 0.9 mg	45%
Manganese 4 mg	200%
Chromium 120 mcg	100%
Molybdenum 75 mcg	100%
Chloride 72 mg	2%
Potassium 80 mg	2%
Ginseng Root (Panax ginseng) 50 mg Standardized Extract	*
Boron 60 mcg	*
Nickel 5 mcg	*
Tin 10 mcg	*
Vanadium 10 mcg	*
*Daily Value not established.	

INGREDIENTS
Dibasic Calcium Phosphate, Potassium Chloride, Ascorbic Acid (Vit. C), Microcrystalline Cellulose, Calcium Carbonate, Magnesium Oxide, dl-Alpha Tocopheryl Acetate (Vit. E), Ginseng Root (*Panax ginseng*) Standardized Extract, Ferrous Fumarate, Niacinamide, Modified Corn Starch, Crospovidone. **Contains < 2% of:** Acacia, Beta-Carotene, BHT, Biotin, Calcium Pantothenate, Calcium Stearate, Cholecalciferol (Vit. D_3), Chromium Picolinate, Citric Acid, Corn Starch, Cupric Sulfate, Cyanocobalamin (Vit. B_{12}), Folic Acid, Gelatin, Hydrogenated Palm Oil, Hypromellose, Magnesium Borate, Magnesium Stearate, Maltodextrin, Manganese Sulfate, Medium-Chain Triglycerides, Nickelous Sulfate, Phytonadione (Vit. K), Polyethylene Glycol, Polyvinyl Alcohol, Potassium Iodide, Pregelatinized Corn Starch, Pyridoxine Hydrochloride (Vit. B_6), Riboflavin (Vit. B_2), Silicon Dioxide, Sodium Ascorbate (to retard oxidation), Sodium Benzoate, Sodium Citrate, Sodium Metavanadate, Sodium Molybdate, Sodium Selenate, Sorbic Acid, Stannous Chloride, Sucrose, Talc, Thiamine Mononitrate (Vit. B_1), Titanium Dioxide, Tocopherols (to retard oxidation), Vitamin A Acetate, Yellow 6 Lake, Zinc Oxide. **May also contain < 2% of:** Ascorbyl Palmitate, Corn Syrup Solids, Sodium Aluminosilicate, Sunflower Oil, Tribasic Calcium Phosphate.

SUGGESTED USE
Adults - Take one tablet daily with food. Not formulated for use in children. Do not exceed suggested use.
As with any supplement, if you are pregnant, nursing, or taking medication, consult your doctor before use.

> **WARNING:** Accidental overdose of iron-containing products is a leading cause of fatal poisoning in children under 6. Keep this product out of reach of children. In case of accidental overdose, call a doctor or poison control center immediately.

IMPORTANT INFORMATION
Long-term intake of high levels of vitamin A (excluding that sourced from beta-carotene) may increase the risk of osteoporosis in adults. Do not take this product if taking other vitamin A supplements.
Store at room temperature. Keep bottle tightly closed.
Bottle sealed with printed foil under cap. Do Not Use if foil is torn.
Marketed by: Pfizer, Madison, NJ 07940 USA
Made in Canada

QUESTIONS OR COMMENTS?
Call 1-877-CENTRUM

CENTRUM SPECIALIST PRENATAL
Pfizer

SUPPLEMENT FACTS

Serving Size 1 Tablet and 1 DHA Softgel

Each Serving Contains	% Daily Value for Pregnant and Lactating Women
Calories 5	
Calories from fat 5	
Total Fat 0.5 g	*
Vitamin A 2,500 IU (60% as Beta-Carotene)	31%
Vitamin C 90 mg	150%
Vitamin D 400 IU	100%
Vitamin E 35 IU	116%
Vitamin K 30 mcg	*
Thiamin 1.4 mg	82%
Riboflavin 1.4 mg	70%
Niacin 18 mg	90%
Vitamin B_6 1.9 mg	76%
Folic Acid 800 mcg	100%
Vitamin B_{12} 2.6 mcg	32%
Biotin 30 mcg	10%
Pantothenic Acid 6 mg	60%
Calcium 250 mg	19%
Iron 27 mg	150%
Phosphorus 20 mg	2%
Iodine 220 mcg	147%
Magnesium 50 mg	11%
Zinc 11 mg	73%
Selenium 30 mcg	*
Copper 0.9 mg	45%
Manganese 2 mg	*
Chromium 30 mcg	*
Molybdenum 50 mcg	*
Chloride 72 mg	*
Potassium 80 mg	*
DHA (Docosahexaenoic acid) 200 mg	*
EPA (Eicosapentaenoic acid) 15 mg	*

*Daily Value not established.

INGREDIENTS (TABLET)
Calcium Carbonate, Potassium Chloride, Dibasic Calcium Phosphate, Ascorbic Acid (Vit. C), Ferrous Fumarate, Magnesium Oxide, Microcrystalline Cellulose, Pregelatinized Corn Starch, dl-Alpha-Tocopheryl Acetate (Vit. E). **Contains < 2% of:** Acacia, Beta-Carotene, BHT (to retard oxidation), Biotin, Calcium Pantothenate, Calcium Stearate, Carmine (Color), Cholecalciferol (Vit. D_3), Chromic Chloride, Citric Acid, Corn Starch, Corn Syrup Solids, Crospovidone, Cupric Sulfate, Cyanocobalamin (Vit. B_{12}), Folic Acid, Gelatin, Hypromellose, Lecithin (Soy), Magnesium Stearate, Maltodextrin, Manganese Sulfate, Medium-Chain Triglycerides, Modified Corn Starch, Niacinamide, Phytonadione (Vit. K), Polyethylene Glycol, Polyvinyl Alcohol, Potassium Iodide, Pyridoxine Hydrochloride (Vit. B_6), Riboflavin (Vit. B_2), Silicon Dioxide, Sodium Ascorbate (to retard oxidation), Sodium Benzoate (preservative), Sodium Citrate, Sodium Molybdate, Sodium Selenate, Sorbic Acid (preservative), Sucrose, Talc, Thiamine Mononitrate (Vit. B_1), Titanium Dioxide, Tocopherols (to retard oxidation), Vitamin A Acetate, Zinc Oxide. **May also contain < 2% of:** Sodium Aluminosilicate. **Contains:** Soy.

INGREDIENTS (SOFTGEL)
Fish Oil Concentrate, Gelatin, Glycerin, Purified Water. **Contains < 2% of:** Medium-Chain Triglycerides, Sunflower Oil, Tocopherols (to retard oxidation).

SUGGESTED USE
Adults - Take one tablet and one DHA softgel daily with food. Not formulated for use in children. Do not exceed suggested use. As with any supplement, if you are pregnant, nursing, or taking medication, consult your doctor before use.
The safe upper limit for daily intake of folic acid is 1000 mcg (1 mg).
Do not take Centrum Specialist Prenatal with other multivitamin formulas unless recommended by your doctor.

WARNING: Accidental overdose of iron-containing products is a leading cause of fatal poisoning in children under 6. Keep this product out of reach of children. In case of accidental overdose, call a doctor or poison control center immediately.

IMPORTANT INFORMATION
Long-term intake of high levels of vitamin A (excluding that sourced from beta-carotene) may increase the risk of osteoporosis in adults. Do not take this product if taking other vitamin A supplements.
Store at room temperature. Avoid excessive heat above 40°C (104°F.)
Product inside sealed in plastic blister with foil backing. Do Not Use if plastic blister or foil barrier is broken.
Marketed by: Pfizer, Madison, NJ 07940 USA
Made in Canada

QUESTIONS OR COMMENTS?
Call 1-877-CENTRUM

CENTRUM SPECIALIST VISION
Pfizer

SUPPLEMENT FACTS

Serving Size 2 Tablets

Amount Per Serving	% Daily Value
Total Carbohydrate <1 g	<1%*
Vitamin A 3,500 IU (29% as Beta-Carotene)	70%
Vitamin C 90 mg	150%
Vitamin D 400 IU	100%
Vitamin E 60 IU	200%
Vitamin K 25 mcg	31%
Thiamin 1.5 mg	100%
Riboflavin 1.7 mg	100%
Niacin 20 mg	100%
Vitamin B_6 3 mg	150%
Folic Acid 200 mcg	50%
Vitamin B_{12} 25 mcg	417%
Biotin 30 mcg	10%
Pantothenic Acid 5 mg	50%
Calcium 200 mg	20%
Phosphorus 50 mg	5%
Iodine 150 mcg	100%
Magnesium 100 mg	25%
Zinc 15 mg	100%
Selenium 55 mcg	79%
Copper 0.5 mg	25%
Manganese 2.3 mg	115%
Chromium 35 mcg	29%
Molybdenum 45 mcg	60%
Chloride 72 mg	2%
Potassium 80 mg	2%
Lutein 10 mg	†
Zeaxanthin 2 mg	†

*Percent Daily Value based on a 2,000 calorie diet.

†Daily Value not established.

INGREDIENTS

Calcium Carbonate, Dibasic Calcium Phosphate, Modified Corn Starch, Microcrystalline Cellulose, Magnesium Oxide, Potassium Chloride, Corn Starch, Ascorbic Acid (Vit. C), dl-Alpha Tocopheryl Acetate (Vit. E), Corn Syrup Solids. **Contains < 2% of:** Beta-Carotene, BHT (to retard oxidation), Biotin, Blue 2 Lake, Calcium Pantothenate, Cholecalciferol (Vit. D_3), Chromium Picolinate, Crospovidone, Cupric Sulfate, Cyanocobalamin (Vit. B_{12}), Folic Acid, Gelatin, Hypromellose, Lutein, Magnesium Stearate, Maltodextrin, Manganese Sulfate, Niacinamide, Phytonadione (Vit. K), Polysorbate 80, Potassium Iodide, Pyridoxine Hydrochloride (Vit. B_6), Riboflavin (Vit. B_2), Silicon Dioxide, Sodium Ascorbate (to retard oxidation), Sodium Molybdate, Sodium Selenate, Thiamine Mononitrate (Vit. B_1), Titanium Dioxide, Tocopherols (to retard oxidation), Triethyl Citrate, Vitamin A Acetate, Zeaxanthin, Zinc Oxide.

SUGGESTED USE

Adults - Take two tablets daily with food. Not formulated for use in children. Do not exceed suggested use.

As with any supplement, if you are pregnant, nursing, or taking medication, consult your doctor before use.

Keep out of reach of children.

IMPORTANT INFORMATION

Long-term intake of high levels of vitamin A (excluding that sourced from beta-carotene) may increase the risk of osteoporosis in adults. Do not take this product if taking other vitamin A supplements.

Store at room temperature. Keep bottle tightly closed.

Bottle sealed with printed foil under cap. Do Not Use if foil is torn.

Marketed by: Pfizer, Madison, NJ 07940 USA

Made in Canada

QUESTIONS OR COMMENTS?
Call 1-877-CENTRUM

CENTRUM WOMEN UNDER 50
Pfizer

SUPPLEMENT FACTS

Serving Size 1 Tablet

Each Tablet Contains	% Daily Value
Vitamin A 3,500 IU (29% as Beta-Carotene)	70%
Vitamin C 75 mg	125%
Vitamin D 800 IU	200%
Vitamin E 35 IU	117%
Vitamin K 50 mcg	63%
Thiamin 1.1 mg	73%
Riboflavin 1.1 mg	65%
Niacin 14 mg	70%
Vitamin B_6 2 mg	100%
Folic Acid 400 mcg	100%
Vitamin B_{12} 6 mcg	100%
Biotin 40 mcg	13%
Pantothenic Acid 15 mg	150%
Calcium 500 mg	50%
Iron 18 mg	100%
Phosphorus 20 mg	2%
Iodine 150 mcg	100%
Magnesium 100 mg	25%
Zinc 8 mg	53%
Selenium 55 mcg	79%
Copper 0.9 mg	45%
Manganese 1.8 mg	90%
Chromium 25 mcg	21%
Molybdenum 50 mcg	67%
Chloride 72 mg	2%
Potassium 80 mg	2%
Boron 150 mcg	*
Nickel 5 mcg	*
Silicon 2 mg	*
Tin 10 mcg	*
Vanadium 10 mcg	*

*Daily Value not established.

INGREDIENTS

Calcium Carbonate, Magnesium Oxide, Potassium Chloride, Pregelatinized Corn Starch, Dibasic Calcium Phosphate, Ascorbic Acid (Vit. C), Microcrystalline Cellulose, Ferrous Fumarate. **Contains < 2% of:** Acacia, Beta Carotene, BHT,

Biotin, Calcium Pantothenate, Calcium Stearate, Cholecalciferol (Vit. D_3), Chromium Picolinate, Citric Acid, Corn Starch, Crospovidone, Cupric Sulfate, Cyanocobalamin (Vit. B_{12}), dl-Alpha Tocopheryl Acetate (Vit. E), FD&C Blue No. 2 Aluminum Lake, FD&C Red No. 40 Aluminum Lake, FD&C Yellow No. 6 Aluminum Lake, Folic Acid, Gelatin, Hydrogenated Palm Oil, Hypromellose, Lecithin (Soy), Magnesium Borate, Magnesium Stearate, Manganese Sulfate, Medium-Chain Triglycerides, Modified Corn Starch, Niacinamide, Nickelous Sulfate, Phytonadione (Vit. K), Polyethylene Glycol, Polyvinyl Alcohol, Potassium Iodide, Pyridoxine Hydrochloride (Vit. B_6), Riboflavin (Vit. B_2), Silicon Dioxide, Sodium Ascorbate, Sodium Benzoate, Sodium Citrate, Sodium Metavanadate, Sodium Molybdate, Sodium Selenate, Sorbic Acid, Stannous Chloride, Sucrose, Talc, Thiamine Mononitrate (Vit. B_1), Titanium Dioxide, Tocopherols, Vitamin A Acetate (Vit. A), Zinc Oxide. **May also contain < 2% of:** Ascorbyl Palmitate, Maltodextrin, Sodium Aluminosilicate, Sunflower Oil, Tribasic Calcium Phosphate. **Contains:** Soy.

SUGGESTED USE
Adults - Take one tablet daily with food. Not formulated for use in children. Do not exceed suggested use.
As with any supplement, if you are pregnant, nursing, or taking medication, consult your doctor before use.

> **WARNING:** Accidental overdose of iron-containing products is a leading cause of fatal poisoning in children under 6. Keep this product out of reach of children. In case of accidental overdose, call a doctor or poison control center immediately.

IMPORTANT INFORMATION
Long-term intake of high levels of vitamin A (excluding that sourced from beta-carotene) may increase the risk of osteoporosis in adults. Do not take this product if taking other vitamin A supplements.
Store at room temperature. Keep bottle tightly closed.
Bottle sealed with printed foil under cap. Do Not Use if foil is torn.
Marketed by: Pfizer, Madison, NJ 07940 USA

QUESTIONS OR COMMENTS?
Call 1-877-CENTRUM

CHAPSTICK CLASSIC STRAWBERRY
(petrolatum)

Pfizer Consumer Healthcare

DRUG FACTS

Active Ingredient(s)
White petrolatum 45%

Purpose(s)
Skin protectant

USES
• helps prevent and temporarily protects chafed, chapped or cracked lips
• helps prevent and protects from the drying effects of wind and cold weather

WARNINGS
For external use only

Keep out of reach of children.
If swallowed, get medical help or contact a Poison Control Center right away.

DIRECTIONS
• apply as needed

OTHER INFORMATION
store at 20-25°C (68-77°F)

INACTIVE INGREDIENTS
arachidyl propionate, camphor, carnauba wax, cetyl alcohol, fragrance, isopropyl lanolate, isopropyl myristate, lanolin, lemon oil, light mineral oil, maltol, methylparaben, octyldodecanol, paraffin, phenyl trimethicone, propylparaben, red 6 lake, saccharin, white wax

QUESTIONS OR COMMENTS?
Call weekdays from 9 AM to 5 PM EST at **1-877-227-3421**
For most recent product information, visit www.chapstick.com

CHILDREN'S TRIAMINIC CHEST AND NASAL CONGESTION (guaifenesin and phenylephrine HCl)

Novartis Consumer Health, Inc.

DRUG FACTS

Active Ingredient(s) (in each 5 mL, and 1 teaspoonful)
Guaifenesin 50 mg
Phenylephrine HCl 2.5 mg

Purpose(s)
Expectorant
Nasal decongestant

USES
• helps loosen phlegm (mucus) and thins bronchial secretions to make coughs more productive
• temporarily relieves nasal and sinus congestion as may occur with a cold

WARNINGS

DO NOT USE
• in a child under 4 years of age
• in a child who is taking a prescription monoamine oxidase inhibitor (MAOI) (certain drugs for depression, psychiatric or emotional conditions, or Parkinson's disease), or for 2 weeks after stopping the MAOI drug. If you do not know if the child's prescription drug contains an MAOI, ask a doctor or pharmacist before giving this product.

ASK A DOCTOR BEFORE USE IF YOUR CHILD HAS
• heart disease
• high blood pressure
• thyroid disease
• diabetes
• cough that occurs with too much phlegm (mucus)
• chronic cough that lasts, or as occurs with asthma

WHEN USING THIS PRODUCT
• **do not exceed recommended dosage**

STOP USE AND ASK A DOCTOR IF
• nervousness, dizziness or sleeplessness occurs
• symptoms do not improve within 7 days or occur with a fever
• cough persists for more than 7 days, comes back or occurs with a fever, rash or persistent headache. These could be signs of a serious condition.

Keep Out of Reach of Children
In case of overdose, get medical help or contact a Poison Control Center right away.

DIRECTIONS
• may be given every 4 hours. Do not give more than 6 doses in 24 hours unless directed by a doctor

Age	Dose
children 4 years of age	**do not use**
children 4 to under 6 years of age	1 teaspoonful (5 mL)
children 6 to under 12 years of age	2 teaspoonfuls (10 mL)

OTHER INFORMATION
- **each teaspoonful contains:** sodium 3 mg
- store at controlled room temperature 20-25°C (68-77°F).

INACTIVE INGREDIENTS
acesulfame K, benzoic acid, citric acid, D&C yellow #10, edetate disodium, FD&C yellow #6, flavors, maltitol solution, propylene glycol, purified water, sodium citrate

QUESTIONS OR COMMENTS?
Call **1-800-452-0051** 24 hours a day, 7 days a week

CHILDREN'S TRIAMINIC FEVER REDUCER
(acetaminophen)

Novartis Consumer Health, Inc.

DRUG FACTS

Active Ingredient(s) (in each 5 mL, and 1 teaspoonful)
Acetaminophen 160 mg

Purpose(s)
Pain reliever/fever reducer

USES
- temporarily relieves minor aches and pains due to:
  - the common cold
  - flu
  - headache
  - minor sore throat pain
  - toothache
- temporarily reduces fever

WARNINGS
Liver warning
This product contains acetaminophen. Severe liver damage may occur if your child take
- more than 5 doses in 24 hours, which is the maximum daily amount
- with other drugs containing acetaminophen

Sore throat warning
If sore throat is severe, persists for more than 2 days, is accompanied or followed by fever, headache, rash, nausea, or vomiting consult a doctor promptly.

DO NOT USE
- if your child is allergic to acetaminophen
- with any other drug containing acetaminophen (prescription or nonprescription). If you are not sure whether a drug contains acetaminophen, ask a doctor or pharmacist.

ASK A DOCTOR BEFORE USE IF YOUR CHILD HAS
- liver disease

ASK A DOCTOR OR PHARMACIST BEFORE USE IF YOUR CHILD IS
- taking the blood thinning drug warfarin

WHEN USING THIS PRODUCT
- **do not exceed recommended dosage**

STOP USE AND ASK A DOCTOR IF
- pain gets worse or lasts more than 5 days
- fever gets worse or lasts more than 3 days
- redness or swelling is present
- new symptoms occur

Keep Out of Reach of Children
In case of overdose, get medical help or contact a Poison Control Center right away. Prompt medical attention is critical for adults as well as for children even if you do not notice any signs or symptoms.

DIRECTIONS
- **this product does not contain directions or complete warnings for adult use**
- **do not give more than directed**
- may be given every 4 hours. Do not give more than 5 doses in 24 hours unless directed by a doctor

Age	Weight	Dose
under 2 years of age	**Under 24 lbs**	**ask a doctor**
2 to 3 years of age	24-35 lbs	1 teaspoon (5 mL)
4 to 5 years of age	36-47 lbs	1 ½ teaspoons (7.5 mL)
6 to 8 years of age	48-59 lbs	2 teaspoons (10 mL)
9 to 10 years of age	60-71 lbs	2 ½ teaspoons (12.5 mL)
11 years of age	72-95 lbs	3 teaspoons (15 mL)

OTHER INFORMATION
- **each teaspoonful contains:** sodium 5 mg [for grape flavor], sodium 6 mg [for bubblegum flavor]
- contains no aspirin
- store at controlled room temperature 20-25°C (68-77°F).

INACTIVE INGREDIENTS
[for grape flavor]
citric acid, edetate disodium, FD&C blue #1, FD&C red #40, flavor, glycerin, polyethylene glycol, purified water, sodium benzoate, sodium citrate, sorbitol, sucrose
[for bubblegum flavor]
benzoic acid, citric acid, dibasic sodium phosphate, edetate disodium, FD&C red #40, flavor, glycerin, polyethylene glycol, purified water, sorbitol, sucrose

QUESTIONS OR COMMENTS?
Call **1-800-452-0051**
For more information plus helpful tips visit www.triaminic.com

CITRACAL CALCIUM GUMMIES
CITRACAL SUGAR FREE CALCIUM SOFT CHEWS

Bayer HealthCare LLC

SUPPLEMENT FACTS

Gummies: Serving Size 2 Gummies

Each Serving Contains	Amount Per Serving	%DV
Calories	30	
Total Carbohydrate	7 g	2%†
Sugars	7 g	*
Vitamin D (as cholecalciferol)	500 IU	125%
Calcium (elemental)	500 mg	50%
Phosphorous	230 mg	23%
Sodium	60 mg	3%
† Percent Daily Values are based on a 2,000 calorie diet.		
* Daily Value not established.		

Soft Chews: Serving Size 1 Chew

Each Serving Contains	Amount Per Serving	%DV
Calories	15	
Total Carbohydrate	3 g	1%†
Sugar	0 g	*
Sugar Alcohol	2 g	*
Vitamin C	2.3 mg	4%
Vitamin D (as cholecalciferol)	1000 IU	250%
Vitamin K	40 mcg	50%
Calcium (elemental)	500 mg	50%
Iron	1 mg	6%
Sodium	10 mg	<1%
† Percent Daily Values are based on a 2,000 calorie diet.		
* Daily Value not established.		

WARNINGS
Accidental overdose of iron-containing products is a leading cause of fatal poisoning in children under 6. Keep this product out of reach of children. In case of accidental overdose, call a doctor or poison control center immediately.
Not for children under 2 years of age due to risk of choking
KEEP OUT OF REACH OF CHILDREN.

ASK A DOCTOR OR A PHARMACIST BEFORE USE IF YOU ARE
pregnant, nursing, or have a medical condition ask a health care professional before use.

DIRECTIONS
Gummies: Adults: Chew 1 serving (2 gummies) twice daily with food or as recommended by your physician, pharmacist or health care professional.
Soft Chews: Adults: Chew 1 serving (1 Soft Chew) twice daily with food or as recommended by your physician, pharmacist or health care professional.

OTHER INGREDIENTS
Gummies: corn syrup, sucrose, tricalcium phosphate, water, sodium citrate, citric acid, pectin, maqui berry juice concentrate (color), artificial flavoring, fd&c yellow #6, fd&c red #40, vitamin D_3 (cholecalciferol). Soft Chews: maltitol syrup, calcium carbonate, isomalt, hydrogenated coconut oil, water, cocoa processed with alkali, nonfat dry milk; less than 2% of: acesulfame potassium, natural and artificial flavor, sodium ascorbate, sodium chloride, soy lecithin, sucralose, vitamin D_3 (cholecalciferol), vitamin K_1. Contains: milk, soy, tree nuts (coconut).

QUESTIONS OR COMMENTS?
Please call 1-866-511-9328
Visit our website at www.citracal.com

CITRACAL SLOW RELEASE 1200

Bayer HealthCare LLC

SUPPLEMENT FACTS

Serving Size 2 Tablets

Each Serving Contains	Amount Per Serving	%DV
Vitamin D	1000 IU	250%
Calcium (elemental)	1200mg	120%
Phosphorous	80 mg	20%
Sodium	5 mg	<1%

WARNINGS
KEEP OUT OF REACH OF CHILDREN

ASK A DOCTOR OR A PHARMACIST BEFORE USE
Due to the sustained release nature of this product, you should seek advice from your pharmacist about use with certain prescription medications

STOP USE AND ASK A DOCTOR IF
pregnant or breast-feeding, ask a health professional before use.

DIRECTIONS
Adults: Take 1 serving (2 tablets) once daily in the morning with food or as recommended by your physician, pharmacist or health care professional.

OTHER INGREDIENTS
calcium carbonate, calcium citrate, magnesium hydroxide, acacia, hydroxypropyl methylcellulose, croscarmellose sodium, magnesium silicate, titanium dioxide (color), propylene glycol dicaprylate/dicaprate, magnesium stearate, inulin (oligofructose enriched), vitamin D3 (cholecalciferol)

QUESTIONS OR COMMENTS?
Please call 1-866-511-9328
Visit our website at www.citracal.com

CITRACAL REGULAR

Bayer HealthCare LLC.

DIRECTIONS
Adults: Take 1 serving (2 tablets) twice daily with or without food or as recommended by your physician, pharmacist or healthcare professional.

SUPPLEMENT FACTS

Serving Size: 2 tablets

	Amount Per Serving	% Daily Value
Vitamin D	400 IU	100%
Calcium (elemental)	500 mg	50%
Sodium	5 mg	< 1%

INGREDIENTS
Calcium Citrate, Polyethylene Glycol, Croscarmellose Sodium, Hydroxypropyl Methylcellulose, Magnesium Silicate, Titanium Dioxide (color), Propylene Glycol Dicaprylate/Dicaprate, Oligofructose Enriched Inulin, Magnesium Stearate, Vitamin D_3 (Cholecalciferol).

WARNINGS
KEEP OUT OF REACH OF CHILDREN

QUESTIONS OR COMMENTS?
Please call 1-866-511-9328
Visit our website at www.citracal.com

CITRUCEL (methylcellulose)
GlaxoSmithKline Consumer Healthcare LP

Active Ingredient(s) CITRUCEL® Orange (in each heaping tablespoon)
Methylcellulose (a non-allergenic fiber) 2g

Active Ingredient(s) CITRUCEL® Sugar Free (in each rounded tablespoon)
Methylcellulose (a non-allergenic fiber) 2g

Purpose(s)
Bulk-forming fiber laxative

USES
- relieves constipation (irregularity)
- helps to restore and maintain regularity
- for constipation associated with other bowel disorders like IBS when recommended by a doctor
- generally produces a bowel movement in 12-72 hours

WARNINGS
Choking: taking this product without adequate fluid may cause it to swell and block your throat or esophagus and may cause choking. Do not take this product if you have difficulty in swallowing. If you experience chest pain, vomiting, or difficulty in swallowing or breathing after taking this product, seek immediate medical attention.

ASK A DOCTOR BEFORE USE IF YOU HAVE
- a sudden change in bowel habits that persists for two weeks
- abdominal pain, nausea or vomiting

STOP USE AND ASK A DOCTOR IF
- constipation lasts more than 7 days
- you have rectal bleeding

These could be signs of a serious condition.

Keep out of reach of children.
In case of overdose, get medical help or contact a Poison Control Center right away.

DIRECTIONS
- **MIX THIS PRODUCT (CHILD OR ADULT DOSE) WITH AT LEAST 8 OUNCES (A FULL GLASS) OF WATER OR OTHER FLUID. TAKING THIS PRODUCT WITHOUT ENOUGH LIQUID MAY CAUSE CHOKING. SEE CHOKING WARNING**
- use product at the first sign of constipation or irregularity
- put one dose in a full glass of cold water
- stir briskly and drink promptly
- drinking another glass of water is helpful

CITRUCEL® Orange

Age	Dose
adults & children 12 years of age and over	start with 1 heaping *tablespoon*. Increase as needed, 1 heaping *tablespoon* at a time, up to 3 times per day.
children 6 - 11 years of age	start with 2.5 level *teaspoons*. Increase as needed, 2.5 level *teaspoons* at a time, up to 3 times per day.
children under 6 years of age	consult a physician

CITRUCEL® Sugar Free

Age	Dose
adults & children 12 years of age and over	start with 1 rounded *tablespoon*. Increase as needed, 1 rounded *tablespoon* at a time, up to 3 times per day.
children 6 - 11 years of age	start with 2 level *teaspoons*. Increase as needed, 2 level *teaspoons* at a time, up to 3 times per day.
children under 6 years of age	consult a physician

OTHER INFORMATION (Citrucel® Orange)
- **each heaping tablespoon contains:** calcium 80mg and potassium 110mg
- each heaping tablespoon contributes 60 calories from sucrose and maltodextrin
- store below 77°F (25°C)
- protect contents from humidity
- keep tightly closed

OTHER INFORMATION (Citrucel® Sugar Free)
- **each rounded tablespoon contains:** calcium 85mg and potassium 125mg
- each rounded tablespoon contributes 24 calories from maltodextrin
- store below 77°F (25°C)
- protect contents from humidity
- keep tightly closed
- **Phenylketonurics: CONTAINS PHENYLALANINE** 52mg per adult dose

INACTIVE INGREDIENTS (Citrucel® Orange)
citric acid, dibasic calcium phosphate, FD&C yellow #6 lake, maltodextrin, orange flavors (natural and artificial), potassium citrate, riboflavin, sucrose, titanium dioxide, tricalcium phosphate

INACTIVE INGREDIENTS (Citrucel® Sugar Free)
aspartame, dibasic calcium phosphate, FD&C yellow #6 lake, malic acid, maltodextrin, orange flavors (natural and artificial), potassium citrate, riboflavin

QUESTIONS OR COMMENTS?
call toll-free 1-800-897-6081 (English/Spanish) weekdays

Citrucel® is a registered trademark of the Sanofi group of companies and licensed by the GlaxoSmithKline group of companies.
For more information on Citrucel®, visit citrucel.com.

CITRUCEL® Orange
DIRECTIONS FOR USE (NO SCOOP DOSING):**
1. Fill glass with at least 8 oz. of cold water.
2. Measure heaping tablespoon of product (one dose) and stir product into water. Stir briskly and drink promptly.
**We are as concerned about the environment as you are so we have removed the scoop from our Citrucel powder products. Doing so helps save energy, reduce the amount of plastic produced and improve environmental footprints.

CITRUCEL® Sugar Free
DIRECTIONS FOR USE (NO SCOOP DOSING):**
1. Fill glass with at least 8 oz. of cold water.
2. Measure rounded tablespoon of product (one dose) and stir product into water. Stir briskly and drink promptly.
**We are as concerned about the environment as you are so we have removed the scoop from our Citrucel powder products. Doing so helps save energy, reduce the amount of plastic produced and improve environmental footprints.

CHILDRENS CLARITIN GRAPE CHEWABLE TABLETS (loratadine)

MSD Consumer Care, Inc.

Active Ingredient(s) (in each tablet)
Loratadine 5 mg

Purpose(s)
Antihistamine

USES
temporarily relieves these symptoms due to hay fever or other upper respiratory allergies:
• runny nose
• sneezing
• itchy, watery eyes
• itching of the nose or throat

WARNINGS

DO NOT USE
if you have ever had an allergic reaction to this product or any of its ingredients.

ASK A DOCTOR BEFORE USE IF YOU HAVE
liver or kidney disease. Your doctor should determine if you need a different dose.

WHEN USING THIS PRODUCT
do not take more than directed. Taking more than directed may cause drowsiness.

STOP USE AND ASK A DOCTOR IF
an allergic reaction to this product occurs. Seek medical help right away.
If pregnant or breast-feeding, ask a health professional before use.
Keep out of reach of children. In case of overdose, get medical help or contact a Poison Control Center right away.

DIRECTIONS

adults and children 6 years and over	chew 2 tablets daily; not more than 2 tablets in 24 hours
children 2 to under 6 years of age	chew 1 tablet daily; not more than 1 tablet in 24 hours
children under 2 years of age	ask a doctor
consumers with liver or kidney disease	ask a doctor

OTHER INFORMATION
• phenylketonurics: contains phenylalanine 1.4 mg per tablet
• safety sealed: do not use if the individual blister unit imprinted with Children's Claritin® is open or torn
• store between 20° to 25°C (68° to 77°F)

INACTIVE INGREDIENTS
aspartame, citric acid anhydrous, colloidal silicon dioxide, D&C red no. 27 aluminum lake, FD&C blue no. 2 aluminum lake, flavor, magnesium stearate, mannitol, microcrystalline cellulose, sodium starch glycolate, stearic acid

QUESTIONS OR COMMENTS?
1-800-CLARITIN (1-800-252-7484) or www.claritin.com

CHILDRENS CLARITIN ORAL SOLUTION (loratadine)

MSD Consumer Care, Inc.

Active Ingredient(s) (in each 5 mL teaspoonful)
Loratadine 5 mg

Purpose(s)
Antihistamine

USES
temporarily relieves these symptoms due to hay fever or other upper respiratory allergies:
• runny nose
• sneezing
• itchy, watery eyes
• itching of the nose or throat

WARNINGS

DO NOT USE
if you have ever had an allergic reaction to this product or any of its ingredients.

ASK A DOCTOR BEFORE USE IF YOU HAVE
liver or kidney disease. Your doctor should determine if you need a different dose.

WHEN USING THIS PRODUCT
do not take more than directed. Taking more than directed may cause drowsiness.

STOP USE AND ASK A DOCTOR IF
an allergic reaction to this product occurs. Seek medical help right away.
If pregnant or breast-feeding, ask a health professional before use.
Keep out of reach of children. In case of overdose, get medical help or contact a Poison Control Center right away.

DIRECTIONS
Use only with enclosed dosing cup
• adults and children 6 years and over: 2 teaspoonfuls (TSP) daily; do not take more than 2 teaspoonfuls (TSP) in 24 hours

- children 2 to under 6 years of age: 1 teaspoonful (TSP) daily; do not take more than 1 teaspoonful (TSP) in 24 hours
- children under 2 years of age: ask a doctor
- consumers with liver or kidney disease: ask a doctor

OTHER INFORMATION
- each teaspoonful contains: sodium 5 mg
- do not use if tape imprinted with "SEALED FOR YOUR PROTECTION" on top and bottom flaps of carton is not intact.
- store between 20° and 25°C (68° and 77°F)

INACTIVE INGREDIENTS
edetate disodium, flavor, glycerin, maltitol, monobasic sodium phosphate, phosphoric acid, propylene glycol, sodium benzoate, sorbitol, sucralose, purified water

QUESTIONS OR COMMENTS?
1-800-CLARITIN (1-800-252-7484) or www.claritin.com

CLARITIN LIQUI-GELS (loratadine)

MSD Consumer Care, Inc.

DRUG FACTS

Active Ingredient(s) (in each capsule)
Loratadine 10 mg

Purpose(s)
Antihistamine

USES
temporarily relieves these symptoms due to hay fever or other upper respiratory allergies:
- runny nose
- itchy, watery eyes
- sneezing
- itching of the nose or throat

WARNINGS

DO NOT USE
if you have ever had an allergic reaction to this product or any of its ingredients.

ASK A DOCTOR BEFORE USE IF YOU HAVE
liver or kidney disease. Your doctor should determine if you need a different dose.

WHEN USING THIS PRODUCT
do not take more than directed. Taking more than directed may cause drowsiness.

STOP USE AND ASK A DOCTOR IF
an allergic reaction to this product occurs. Seek medical help right away.
If pregnant or breast-feeding, ask a health professional before use.
Keep out of reach of children. In case of overdose, get medical help or contact a Poison Control Center right away.

DIRECTIONS

adults and children 6 years and over	1 capsule daily; not more than 1 capsule in 24 hours
children under 6 years of age	ask a doctor
consumers with liver or kidney disease	ask a doctor

OTHER INFORMATION
- safety sealed: do not use if the individual blister unit imprinted with Claritin® Liqui-Gels® is open or torn
- store between 20° to 25°C (68° to 77°F)
- protect from freezing

INACTIVE INGREDIENTS
caprylic/capric glycerides, FD&C blue no.1, gelatin, glycerin, pharmaceutical ink, polysorbate 80, povidone, purified water, sorbitol

QUESTIONS OR COMMENTS?
1-800-CLARITIN (1-800-252-7484) or www.claritin.com
© Copyright & Distributed by MSD Consumer Care, Inc., PO Box 377, Memphis, TN 38151 USA, a subsidiary of Merck & Co., Inc., Whitehouse Station, NJ USA.

CLARITIN REDITABS 12 HOUR (loratadine)

MSD Consumer Care, Inc.

DRUG FACTS

Active Ingredient(s) (in each tablet)
Loratadine 5 mg

Purpose(s)
Antihistamine

USES
temporarily relieves these symptoms due to hay fever or other upper respiratory allergies:
- runny nose
- itchy, watery eyes
- sneezing
- itching of the nose or throat

WARNINGS

DO NOT USE
if you have ever had an allergic reaction to this product or any of its ingredients.

ASK A DOCTOR BEFORE USE IF YOU HAVE
liver or kidney disease. Your doctor should determine if you need a different dose.

WHEN USING THIS PRODUCT
do not take more than directed. Taking more than directed may cause drowsiness.

STOP USE AND ASK A DOCTOR IF
an allergic reaction to this product occurs. Seek medical help right away.
If pregnant or breast-feeding, ask a health professional before use.
Keep out of reach of children. In case of overdose, get medical help or contact a Poison Control Center right away.

DIRECTIONS
- place 1 tablet on tongue; tablet disintegrates, with or without water

adults and children 6 years and over	1 tablet every 12 hours; not more than 2 tablets in 24 hours
children under 6 years of age	ask a doctor
consumers with liver or kidney disease	ask a doctor

OTHER INFORMATION
- safety sealed: do not use if the individual blister unit imprinted with Claritin® RediTabs® is open or torn
- store between 20° to 25°C (68° to 77°F)
- use tablet immediately after opening individual blister

INACTIVE INGREDIENTS
anhydrous citric acid, gelatin, mannitol, mint flavor

QUESTIONS OR COMMENTS?
1-800-CLARITIN (1-800-252-7484) or www.claritin.com
Distributed by MSD Consumer Care, Inc.,
PO Box 377, Memphis, TN 38151 USA,
a subsidiary of Merck & Co., Inc., Whitehouse Station, NJ USA.

CLARITIN REDITABS 24 HOUR (loratadine)

MSD Consumer Care, Inc.

DRUG FACTS

Active Ingredient(s) (in each tablet)
Loratadine 10 mg

Purpose(s)
Antihistamine

USES
temporarily relieves these symptoms due to hay fever or other upper respiratory allergies:
- runny nose
- itchy, watery eyes
- sneezing
- itching of the nose or throat

WARNINGS

DO NOT USE
if you have ever had an allergic reaction to this product or any of its ingredients.

ASK A DOCTOR BEFORE USE IF YOU HAVE
liver or kidney disease. Your doctor should determine if you need a different dose.

WHEN USING THIS PRODUCT
do not take more than directed. Taking more than directed may cause drowsiness.

STOP USE AND ASK A DOCTOR IF
an allergic reaction to this product occurs. Seek medical help right away.
If pregnant or breast-feeding, ask a health professional before use.
Keep out of reach of children. In case of overdose, get medical help or contact a Poison Control Center right away.

DIRECTIONS
- place 1 tablet on tongue; tablet disintegrates, with or without water

adults and children 6 years and over	1 tablet daily; not more than 1 tablet in 24 hours
children under 6 years of age	ask a doctor
consumers with liver or kidney disease	ask a doctor

OTHER INFORMATION
- safety sealed: do not use if the individual blister unit imprinted with Claritin® RediTabs® is open or torn

- store between 20° to 25°C (68° to 77°F)
- use tablet immediately after opening individual blister

INACTIVE INGREDIENTS
anhydrous citric acid, gelatin, mannitol, mint flavor

QUESTIONS OR COMMENTS?
1-800-CLARITIN (1-800-252-7484) or www.claritin.com
Distributed by MSD Consumer Care, Inc.,
PO Box 377, Memphis, TN 38151 USA,
a subsidiary of Merck & Co., Inc., Whitehouse Station, NJ USA.

CLARITIN (loratadine)

MSD Consumer Care, Inc.

DRUG FACTS

Active Ingredient(s) (in each tablet)
Loratadine 10 mg

Purpose(s)
Antihistamine

USES
temporarily relieves these symptoms due to hay fever or other upper respiratory allergies:
- runny nose
- itchy, watery eyes
- sneezing
- itching of the nose or throat

WARNINGS

DO NOT USE
if you have ever had an allergic reaction to this product or any of its ingredients.

ASK A DOCTOR BEFORE USE IF YOU HAVE
liver or kidney disease. Your doctor should determine if you need a different dose.

WHEN USING THIS PRODUCT
do not take more than directed. Taking more than directed may cause drowsiness.

STOP USE AND ASK A DOCTOR IF
an allergic reaction to this product occurs. Seek medical help right away.
If pregnant or breast-feeding, ask a health professional before use.
Keep out of reach of children. In case of overdose, get medical help or contact a Poison Control Center right away.

DIRECTIONS
adults and children 6 years and over: 1 tablet daily; not more than 1 tablet in 24 hours; children under 6 years of age: ask a doctor; consumers with liver or kidney disease: ask a doctor

OTHER INFORMATION (BOTTLES)
- Tamper-evident: do not use if foil seal under cap, printed with "SEALED for YOUR PROTECTION" is missing, open or broken
- store between 20° to 25°C (68° to 77°F)

OTHER INFORMATION (BLISTER FOIL UNITS)
- safety sealed: do not use if the individual blister unit imprinted with Claritin (R) is open or torn
- store between 20° to 25° C (68° to 77°F)
- protect from excessive moisture

INACTIVE INGREDIENTS
corn starch, lactose monohydrate, magnesium stearate

QUESTIONS OR COMMENTS?
1-800-CLARITIN (1-800-252-7484) or www.claritin.com

CLARITIN-D 12 HOUR (loratadine and pseudoephedrine sulfate)
MSD Consumer Care, Inc.

DRUG FACTS

Active Ingredient(s) (in each tablet)	Purpose(s)
Loratadine 5 mg	Antihistamine
Pseudoephedrine sulfate 120 mg	Nasal decongestant

USES
- temporarily relieves these symptoms due to hay fever or other upper respiratory allergies:
  - sneezing
  - itchy, watery eyes
  - runny nose
  - itching of the nose or throat
- temporarily relieves nasal congestion due to the common cold, hay fever or other upper respiratory allergies
- reduces swelling of nasal passages
- temporarily relieves sinus congestion and pressure
- temporarily restores freer breathing through the nose

WARNINGS

DO NOT USE
- if you have ever had an allergic reaction to this product or any of its ingredients
- if you are now taking a prescription monoamine oxidase inhibitor (MAOI) (certain drugs for depression, psychiatric, or emotional conditions, or Parkinson's disease), or for 2 weeks after stopping the MAOI drug. If you do not know if your prescription drug contains an MAOI, ask a doctor or pharmacist before taking this product.

ASK A DOCTOR BEFORE USE IF YOU HAVE
- heart disease
- thyroid disease
- high blood pressure
- diabetes
- trouble urinating due to an enlarged prostate gland
- liver or kidney disease. Your doctor should determine if you need a different dose.

WHEN USING THIS PRODUCT
do not take more than directed.
Taking more than directed may cause drowsiness.

STOP USE AND ASK A DOCTOR IF
- an allergic reaction to this product occurs. Seek medical help right away.
- symptoms do not improve within 7 days or are accompanied by a fever
- nervousness, dizziness or sleeplessness occurs

If pregnant or breast-feeding, ask a health professional before use.
Keep out of reach of children. In case of overdose, get medical help or contact a Poison Control Center right away.

DIRECTIONS
- do not divide, crush, chew or dissolve the tablet

adults and children 12 years and over	1 tablet every 12 hours; not more than 2 tablets in 24 hours
children under 12 years of age	ask a doctor
consumers with liver or kidney disease	ask a doctor

OTHER INFORMATION
- **each tablet contains:** calcium 30 mg
- safety sealed: do not use if the individual blister unit imprinted with Claritin-D® 12 Hour is open or torn
- store between 20° to 25°C (68° to 77°F)
- keep in a dry place

INACTIVE INGREDIENTS
croscarmellose sodium, dibasic calcium phosphate, hypromellose, lactose monohydrate, magnesium sterararate, pharmaceutical ink, povidone, titanium dioxide

QUESTIONS OR COMMENTS?
1-800-CLARITIN (1-800-252-7484) or www.claritin.com
© Copyright & Distributed by MSD Consumer Care, Inc., PO Box 377,
Memphis, TN 38151 USA, a subsidiary of Merck & Co., Inc., Whitehouse Station, NJ USA.

CLARITIN-D 24 HOUR (loratadine and pseudoephedrine sulfate)
MSD Consumer Care, Inc.

DRUG FACTS

Active Ingredient(s) (in each tablet)	Purpose(s)
Loratadine 10 mg	Antihistamine
Pseudoephedrine sulfate 240 mg	Nasal decongestant

USES
- temporarily relieves these symptoms due to hay fever or other upper respiratory allergies:
  - sneezing
  - itchy, watery eyes
  - runny nose
  - itching of the nose or throat
- temporarily relieves nasal congestion due to the common cold, hay fever or other upper respiratory allergies
- reduces swelling of nasal passages
- temporarily relieves sinus congestion and pressure
- temporarily restores freer breathing through the nose

WARNINGS

DO NOT USE
- if you have ever had an allergic reaction to this product or any of its ingredients
- if you are now taking a prescription monoamine oxidase inhibitor (MAOI) (certain drugs for depression, psychiatric, or emotional conditions, or Parkinson's disease), or for 2 weeks after stopping the MAOI drug. If you do not know if your prescription drug contains an MAOI, ask a doctor or pharmacist before taking this product.

ASK A DOCTOR BEFORE USE IF YOU HAVE
- heart disease
- thyroid disease
- high blood pressure
- diabetes
- trouble urinating due to an enlarged prostate gland
- liver or kidney disease. Your doctor should determine if you need a different dose.

WHEN USING THIS PRODUCT
do not take more than directed.
Taking more than directed may cause drowsiness.

STOP USE AND ASK A DOCTOR IF
- an allergic reaction to this product occurs. Seek medical help right away.
- symptoms do not improve within 7 days or are accompanied by a fever
- nervousness, dizziness or sleeplessness occurs

If pregnant or breast-feeding, ask a health professional before use.
Keep out of reach of children. In case of overdose, get medical help or contact a Poison Control Center right away.

DIRECTIONS
- do not divide, crush, chew or dissolve the tablet

adults and children 12 years and over	1 tablet daily with a full glass of water; not more than 1 tablet in 24 hours
children under 12 years of age	ask a doctor
consumers with liver or kidney disease	ask a doctor

OTHER INFORMATION
- **each tablet contains:** calcium 25 mg
- safety sealed: do not use if the individual blister unit imprinted with Claritin-D® 24 hour is open or torn
- store between 20° to 25°C (68° to 77°F)
- protect from light and store in a dry place

INACTIVE INGREDIENTS
carnauba wax, dibasic calcium phosphate dihydrate, ethylcellulose, hydroxypropyl cellulose, hypromellose, magnesium stearate, pharmaceutical ink, polyethylene glycol, povidone, silicon dioxide, sucrose, titanium dioxide, white wax

QUESTIONS OR COMMENTS?
1-800-CLARITIN (1-800-252-7484) or www.claritin.com
Distributed by MSD Consumer Care, Inc., PO Box 377, Memphis, TN 38151 USA, a subsidiary of Merck & Co., Inc., Whitehouse Station, NJ USA.

CLEAR EYES COOLING ITCHY EYE RELIEF
(naphazoline hydrochloride, glycerin, and zinc sulfate)
Prestige Brands Holdings, Inc.

DRUG FACTS

Active Ingredient(s)
Glycerin 0.25%

Purpose(s)
Lubricant

Active Ingredient(s)
Naphazoline hydrochloride 0.012%

Purpose(s)
Redness Reliever

Active Ingredient(s)
Zinc sulfate 0.25%

Purpose(s)
Astringent

USES
- For use as a protectant against further irritation or to relieve dryness of the eye.
- For the temporary relief of burning & irritation due to the dryness of the eye.
- Relieves redness of the eye due to minor eye irritations.

WARNINGS
For external use only.

DO NOT USE
if solution changes color or becomes cloudy.

ASK A DOCTOR BEFORE USE IF
you have narrow angle glaucoma.

WHEN USING THIS PRODUCT
- To avoid contamination, do not touch tip of container to any surface.
- Replace cap after using.
- Overuse may produce increased redness of the eye.
- Pupils may become enlarged temporarily.

STOP USE & ASK A DOCTOR IF
- you experience eye pain
- you experience changes in vision
- you experience continued redness or irritation of the eye
- the condition worsens or persists for more than 72 hours.

Keep out of reach of children.
If swallowed, get medical help or contact a Poison Control Center (1-800-222-1222) right away.

DIRECTIONS
Instill 1 to 2 drops in the affected eye(s) up to four times daily.

OTHER INFORMATION
- Store at room temperature.
- Remove contact lenses before using.
- **Tamper Evident:** Do not use if neckband on bottle is broken or missing.

INACTIVE INGREDIENTS
benzalkonium chloride, boric acid, cyclodextrin, edetate disodium, menthol, purified water, sodium chloride, sodium citrate

QUESTIONS OR COMMENTS?
1-877-274-1787 www.cleareyes.com

CLEAR EYES COOLING REDNESS RELIEF
(glycerin and naphazoline hydrochloride)
Prestige Brands Holdings, Inc.

DRUG FACTS

Active Ingredient(s)
Glycerin 0.5%

Purpose(s)
Lubricant

Active Ingredient(s)
Naphazoline hydrochloride 0.03%

Purpose(s)
Redness Reliever

USES
- For the relief of redness of the eye due to minor eye irritations.
- For the temporary relief of burning and irritation due to dryness of the eye.
- For use as a protectant against further irritation or dryness of the eye.

WARNINGS
For external use only.

DO NOT USE IF
solution changes color or becomes cloudy.

ASK A DOCTOR BEFORE USE IF
you have narrow angle glaucoma.

WHEN USING THIS PRODUCT
- To avoid contamination, do not touch tip of container to any surface.
- Replace cap after using.
- Overuse may produce increased redness of the eye.
- Pupils may become enlarged temporarily.

STOP USE & ASK A DOCTOR IF
- you experience eye pain
- you experience changes in vision
- you experience continued redness or irritation of the eye
- the condition worsens or persists for more than 72 hours

Keep out of reach of children.
If swallowed, get medical help or contact a Poison Control Center (1-800-222-1222) right away.

DIRECTIONS
Instill 1 to 2 drops in the affected eye(s) up to four times daily.

OTHER INFORMATION
- Store at room temperature.
- Remove contact lenses before using.
- **Tamper Evident:** Do not use if neckband on bottle is broken or missing.

INACTIVE INGREDIENTS
benzalkonium chloride, boric acid, cyclodextrin, edetate disodium, menthol, purified water, sodium borate

QUESTIONS OR COMMENTS?
1-877-274-1787 www.cleareyes.com

CLEAR EYES MAXIMUM ITCHY EYE RELIEF
(glycerin, naphazoline hydrochloride, and zinc sulfate)

Prestige Brands Holdings, Inc.

DRUG FACTS

Active Ingredient(s)
Glycerin 0.25%

Purpose(s)
Lubricant

Active Ingredient(s)
Naphazoline hydrochloride 0.012%

Purpose(s)
Redness Reliever

Active Ingredient(s)
Zinc Sulfate 0.25%

Purpose(s)
Astringent

USES
- For use as a protectant against further irritation or to relieve dryness of the eye.
- For the temporary relief of burning & irritation due to dryness of the eye.
- Relieves redness of the eye due to minor eye irritations.

WARNINGS
For external use only.

DO NOT USE
if solution changes color or becomes cloudy.

ASK A DOCTOR BEFORE USE IF YOU HAVE
narrow angle glaucoma.

WHEN USING THIS PRODUCT
- To avoid contamination, do not touch tip to any surface.
- Replace cap after using.
- Overuse may produce increased redness of the eye.
- Pupils may become enlarged temporarily.

STOP USE & ASK A DOCTOR IF
- you experience eye pain
- you experience changes in vision
- you experience continued redness or irritation of the eye
- the condition worsens
- symptoms last for more than 72 hours

Keep out of reach of children.
If swallowed, get medical help or contact a Poison Control Center right away.

DIRECTIONS
Instill 1 to 2 drops in the affected eye(s) up to four times daily.

OTHER INFORMATION
- Store at room temperature.
- Remove contact lenses before using.
- **Tamper Evident.** Do not use if neckband on bottle is broken or missing.

INACTIVE INGREDIENTS
benzalkonium chloride, boric acid, edetate disodium, purified water, sodium chloride, sodium citrate

QUESTIONS OR COMMENTS?
1-877-274-1787 www.cleareyes.com

CLEAR EYES MAXIMUM REDNESS RELIEF
(naphazoline hydrochloride and glycerin)

Prestige Brands Holdings, Inc.

DRUG FACTS

Active Ingredient(s)
Glycerin 0.5%

Purpose(s)
Lubricant

Active Ingredient(s)
Naphazoline hydrochloride 0.03%

Purpose(s)
Redness Reliever

USES
- for the relief of redness of the eye due to minor eye irritations.
- for the temporary relief of burning and irritation due to the dryness of the eye.
- for the use as a protectant against further irritation or dryness of the eye.

WARNINGS
For external use only.

DO NOT USE
if solution changes color or becomes cloudy.

ASK A DOCTOR BEFORE USE IF
you have narrow angle glaucoma.

WHEN USING THIS PRODUCT
- To avoid contamination, do not touch tip of container to any surface.
- Replace cap after using.
- Overuse may produce increased redness of the eye.
- Pupils may become enlarged temporarily.

STOP USE & ASK A DOCTOR IF
- you experience eye pain
- you experience changes in vision
- you experience continued redness or irritation of the eye
- the condition worsens or persists for more than 72 hours

Keep out of reach of children.
If swallowed, get medical help or contact a Poison Control Center right away.

DIRECTIONS
Instill 1 to 2 drops in the affected eye(s) up to four times daily

OTHER INFORMATION
- Store at room temperature.
- Remove contact lenses before using.
- **Tamper Evident**: Do not use if neckband on bottle is broken or missing.

INACTIVE INGREDIENTS
benzalkonium chloride, boric acid, edetate disodium, purified water, sodium borate

QUESTIONS OR COMMENTS?
1-877-274-1787 www.cleareyes.com

CLEAR EYES NATURAL TEARS LUBRICANT
(polyvinyl alcohol and povidone)
Prestige Brands Holdings, Inc.

Active Ingredient(s)

Ingredient		Purpose
Polyvinyl alcohol	0.5%	Lubricant
Povidone	0.6%	Lubricant

USES
- For the temporary relief of burning and irritation due to dryness of the eye.
- For use as a protectant against further irritation or to relieve dryness of the eye.

WARNINGS
For external use only. Do not use if solution changes color or becomes cloudy.

WHEN USING THIS PRODUCT
- To avoid contamination, do not touch tip of container to any surface.
- Replace cap after using.

STOP USE AND ASK A DOCTOR IF
- you experience eye pain
- you experience changes in vision
- you experience continued redness or irritation of the eye
- the condition worsens
- symptoms last for more than 72 hours

Keep out of reach of children. If swallowed, get medical help or contact a Poison Control Center right away.

DIRECTIONS
Instill 1 or 2 drops in the affected eye(s) as needed.

OTHER INFORMATION
- Store at room temperature.
- Remove contact lenses before using.
- Tamper evident: Do not use if neckband on bottle is broken or missing.

INACTIVE INGREDIENTS
benzalkonium chloride, dextrose, edetate disodium, potassium chloride, purified water, sodium bicarbonate, sodium chloride, sodium citrate, sodium phosphate (mono- and dibasic)

QUESTIONS?
1-877-274-1787 www.cleareyes.com

COLACE (docusate sodium)
Cardinal Health

DRUG FACTS

Colace® (docusate sodium) Capsules 50 mg

Stool Softener
Gentle, Effective, Stimulant-Free for Comfortable Relief

Active Ingredient(s) (in each capsule)
Docusate sodium 50 mg

Purpose(s)
Stool softener

USES
- relieves occasional constipation (irregularity)
- generally produces a bowel movement in 12 to 72 hours

WARNINGS

DO NOT USE
- if you are presently taking mineral oil, unless told to do so by a doctor

ASK A DOCTOR BEFORE USE IF YOU HAVE
- stomach pain
- nausea
- vomiting
- noticed a sudden change in bowel habits that lasts over 2 weeks

STOP USE AND ASK A DOCTOR IF
- you have rectal bleeding or fail to have a bowel movement after use of a laxative.
  These could be signs of a serious condition.
- you need to use a stool softener laxative for more than 1 week

If pregnant or breast-feeding, ask a health professional before use.

KEEP OUT OF REACH OF CHILDREN
Keep out of reach of children. In case of overdose, get medical help or contact a Poison Control Center right away. This package is intended for institutional use only. This package is not child resistant.

DIRECTIONS
Take only by mouth. Doses may be taken as a single daily dose or in divided doses.

adults and children 12 years and over	take 1-6 capsules daily
children 2 to under 12 years of age	take 1-3 capsules daily
children under 2 years	ask a doctor

OTHER INFORMATION
- each capsule contains: **sodium 3 mg**
  VERY LOW SODIUM
- store at 25°C (77°F); excursions permitted between 15°-30°C (59°-86°F)
- #1 Doctor Recommended Stool-Softener Brand
- see window for lot number and expiration date

QUESTIONS OR COMMENTS?
1-888-726-7535 (8am-5pm, EST, Mon.-Fri.). www.colacecapsules.com

INACTIVE INGREDIENTS
D&C red no. 33, FD&C red no. 40, gelatin, glycerin, PEG 400, propylene glycol, sorbitol
Dist. by: **Purdue Products L.P.**
Stamford, CT 06901-3431
Made in USA Packaged in Canada
Repackaged by: Cardinal Health Zanesville, OH 43701

COLACE STOOL SOFTENER SYRUP (docusate sodium)

Purdue Products L.P.

How Supplied
Each 15 mL of syrup (1 tablespoonful) contains 60 mg of docusate sodium. One pint (473 mL).
Mechanism of action
The active ingredient in Colace Syrup is docusate sodium. Docusate sodium allows water and fats to get into the stool. This helps soften fecal material and makes defecation easier. Docusate sodium is not a stimulant laxative.
Recommended Doses
Each 15 mL of syrup (1 tablespoonful) contains 60 mg of docusate sodium.
- Doses must be given in a 6-8 oz glass of milk or fruit juice, to prevent throat irritation.
- Take only by mouth. Doses may be taken as a single daily dose or in divided doses.
- Adults and children 12 years of age and older: 1 to 6 tablespoonfuls daily, or as directed by a doctor.
- Children 2 to under 12 years of age: 1 to 2 ½ tablespoonfuls daily or as directed by a doctor.
- Children under 2 years of age: Consult a doctor.

WARNINGS
- Do not use laxative products for longer than 1 week unless told to do so by a doctor.
- Do not use if you are presently taking mineral oil unless told to do so by a doctor.
- Ask a doctor before use if you have:
  - Stomach pain
  - Nausea
  - Vomiting

- Noticed a sudden change in bowel habits that lasts over two weeks
- Stop use and ask a doctor if you have rectal bleeding or fail to have a bowel movement after use of a laxative. These could be signs of a serious condition.
- If pregnant or breast-feeding, ask a health professional before use.
- Keep out of reach of children. In case of overdose, get medical help or contact a Poison Control Center right away.

COLD-EEZE (zinc gluconate)

ProPhase Labs, Inc.

DRUG FACTS

Active Ingredient(s) (per lozenge)
Zincum Gluconicum 2x (13.3mg)

Purpose(s)
Cold Remedy

USES
- to reduce the duration of the common cold
- reduces the severity of cold symptoms: cough, sore throat, stuffy nose, sneezing, post nasal drip and/or hoarseness

WARNINGS

ASK A DOCTOR BEFORE USE IF YOU
- are taking minocycline, doxycycline, tetracycline or are on coumadin therapy,
  zinc treatment may inhibit the absorption of these medicines

STOP USE AND ASK YOUR HEALTHCARE PRACTITIONER
if symptoms persist beyond 7 days.
COLD-EEZE® Lozenges are formulated to reduce the duration of common cold symptoms and may be insufficient treatment for Influenza or Allergies.
Diabetic Warning: sugar replacements may affect blood sugar levels.
If pregnant or breast-feeding, ask a health professional before use.

Keep out of reach of children.

DIRECTIONS
- adults and children 12 years and over
- for best results, begin treatment at start of symptoms (within 24-48 hours of onset)
- repeat every 2 - 4 hours as needed until all symptoms subside
- completely dissolve a COLD-EEZE® lozenge in mouth (do not chew)
- recommended daily dosage is 6 lozenges for adults and 4 lozenges for ages 12-17
- children under 12 years of age should consult a health professional prior to use

OTHER INFORMATION
- avoid minor stomach upset - Do not dissolve COLD-EEZE® lozenges on an empty stomach
- avoid citrus fruits or juices and products containing citric acid 1/2 hour before or after taking COLD-EEZE® lozenges as they may diminish product effectiveness, otherwise, drink plenty of fluids
- store in a cool dry place after opening
- gluten-free
- product may produce a laxative effect

INACTIVE INGREDIENTS
acesulfame-K, glycine, isomalt, natural flavors. No artificial colors or preservatives.

QUESTIONS OR COMMENTS?
Call 1-800-505-COLD
(9AM-5PM EST)

CORICIDIN HBP (acetaminophen and chlorpheniramine maleate)
Schering-Plough HealthCare Products, Inc.

DRUG FACTS

Active Ingredient(s) (in each tablet)	Purpose(s)
Acetaminophen 325 mg	Pain reliever/fever reducer
Chlorpheniramine maleate 2 mg	Antihistamine

USES
- temporarily relieves
  - minor aches and pains
  - sneezing
  - headache
  - runny nose
- temporarily reduces fever

LIVER WARNING
This product contains acetaminophen. Sever liver damage may occur if
- adult takes more than 12 tablets in 24 hours
- child takes more than 5 tablets in 24 hours
- taken with other drugs containing acetaminophen
- adult has 3 or more alcoholic drinks everyday while using this product.

DO NOT USE
with any other drug containing acetaminophen (prescription or non prescription). If you are not sure whether a drug contains acetaminophen, ask a doctor or pharmacist.

ASK A DOCTOR BEFORE USE IF
the user has
- liver disease
- a breathing problem such as emphysema or chronic bronchitis
- glaucoma
- trouble urinating due to an enlarged prostate gland

ASK A DOCTOR OR PHARMACIST BEFORE USE IF
the user is
- taking the blood thinning drug warfarin
- taking sedatives or tranquilizers

WHEN USING THIS PRODUCT
- excitability may occur, expecially in children
- drowsiness may occur
- avoid alcoholic beverages alcohol, sedatives and tranquilizers may increase drowsiness
- use caution when driving a motor vehicle or operating machinery

STOP USE AND ASK A DOCTOR IF
- pain gets worse or lasts more than 5 days (children 6 to under 12 years) or 10 days (adults)
- fever gets worse or lasts more than 3 days
- redness or swelling is present
- new symptoms occur

If pregnant or breast-feeding, ask a health professional before use.
Keep out of reach of children.

OVERDOSE WARNING
Taking more than the recommended dose may cause liver damage. In case of overdose, get medical help or contact a Poison Control Center right away. Quick medical attention is critical for adults as well as children even if you do not notice any signs or symptoms.

DIRECTIONS
- do not use more than directed (see overdose warning)

Adults and children 12 years and over	2 tablets every 4 to 6 hours, not more than 12 tablets in 24 hours
Children 6 to under 12 years of age	1 tablet every 4 to 6 hours, not more than 5 tablets in 24 hours

OTHER INFORMATION
- **each tablet contains:** magnesium 10 mg
- store between 20° to 25°C (68° to 77°F)
- protect from excessive moisture

INACTIVE INGREDIENTS
acacia, calcium sulfate, carnauba wax, corn starch, FD&C red no. 40 aluminum lake, FD&C yellow no. 6 aluminum lake, lactose, magnesium stearate, microcrystalline cellulose, pharmaceutical ink, povidone, sugar, talc, titanium dioxide, white wax
© Copyright & Distributed by
Schering-Plough HealthCare Products, Inc.,
P.O. Box 377
Memphis, TN 38151 USA.
All rights reserved. Made in Canada.
For more information, visit www.coricidin hbp.com

CORTAID 12-HOUR ADVANCED ANTI-ITCH CREAM (hydrocortisone)
Valeant Consumer

Active Ingredient(s)
Hydrocortisone 1%

Purpose(s)
Anti-Itch

USES
- Temporarily relieves itching associated with minor skin irritations, inflammation and rashes due to:
  - eczema
  - insect bites
  - poison ivy, oak, or sumac
  - soaps
  - detergents
  - cosmetics
  - jewelry
  - seborrheic dermatitis
  - psoriasis
- Other uses of this product should only be under advice and supervision of a doctor

WARNINGS
For external use only

DO NOT USE
for the treatment of diaper rash. Ask a doctor

WHEN USING THIS PRODUCT
avoid contact with eyes **Stop use and ask a doctor if** condition worsens, symptoms persist for more than 7 days or clear up and occur again within a few days, and do not begin

use of any other hydrocortisone product unless you have asked a doctor **Keep out of reach of children.** If swallowed, get medical help or contact a Poison Control Center right away

DIRECTIONS
- Adults and children 2 years of age and older: apply to affected area not more than 3 to 4 times daily
- Children under 2 years of age: ask a doctor

OTHER INFORMATION
- Store at 20° to 25°C (68° to 77°F)

INACTIVE INGREDIENTS
aloe barbadensis leaf juice, benzyl alcohol, ceteareth-20, cetearyl alcohol, cetyl palmitate, citric acid, cyclopentasiloxane, dimethicone/vinyltrimethylsiloxysilicate crosspolymer, dimethyl MEA, feverfew extract, glycerin, isopropyl myristate, isostearyl neopentanoate, methylparaben, oat kernel extract, PEG-40 stearate, potassium lactate, *sodium hydroxide, water *may contain this ingredient

CORTAID MAXIMUM STRENGTH
(hydrocortisone)

Valeant Consumer

DRUG FACTS

Active Ingredient(s)
Hydrocortisone 1%

Purpose(s)
Anti-itch

USES
- temporarily relieves itching associated with minor skin irritations, inflammation, and rashes due to:
  - eczema
  - insect bites
  - poison ivy, oak, or sumac
  - soaps
  - detergents
  - cosmetics
  - jewelry
  - seborrheic dermatitis
  - psoriasis
- temporarily relieves external anal and genital itching
- other uses of this product should only be under the advice and supervision of a doctor

WARNINGS
For external use only

DO NOT USE
- in the genital area if you have a vaginal discharge. Consult a doctor.
- for the treatment of diaper rash. Ask a doctor.

WHEN USING THIS PRODUCT
- avoid contact with eyes
- do not use more than directed unless told to do so by a doctor
- do not put directly into the rectum by using fingers or any mechanical device or applicator

STOP USE AND ASK A DOCTOR IF
- condition worsens, symptoms persist for more than 7 days or clear up and occur again within a few days, and do not begin use of any other hydrocortisone product unless you have asked a doctor
- rectal bleeding occurs

Keep out of reach of children. If swallowed, get medical help or contact a Poison Control Center right away.

DIRECTIONS
- **for itching of skin irritation, inflammation, and rashes:**
  - adults and children 2 years of age and older: apply to affected area not more than 3 to 4 times daily
  - children under 2 years: Ask a doctor
- **for external anal and genital itching, adults:**
  - when practical, clean the affected area with mild soap and water and rinse thoroughly
  - gently dry by patting or blotting with toilet tissue or a soft cloth before applying
  - apply to affected area not more than 3 to 4 times daily
  - children under 12 years of age: Ask a doctor

OTHER INFORMATION
- store at 20° to 25°C (68° to 77°F)
- see end of carton or tube crimp for lot number and expiration date

INACTIVE INGREDIENTS
water, petrolatum, glycerin, mineral oil, ceteareth-6, dimethicone, VP/eicosene copolymer, phenoxyethanol, stearyl alcohol, ammonium acryloyldimethyltaurate/VP copolymer, cetyl alcohol, carbomer, edetate disodium, methylparaben, sodium citrate, ethylparaben, citric acid, propylparaben, [1]sodium hydroxide
[1]may contain this ingredient

QUESTIONS OR COMMENTS?
call **1-800-321-4576**

CORTAID INTENSIVE THERAPY COOLING SPRAY (hydrocortisone)

Valeant Consumer

Relieves your worst itches due to:
Eczema
Psoriasis
Dry, itchy skin
Seborrheic dermatitis
Rashes
Also relieves itching due to:
Insect bites
Poison ivy, oak, sumac
Active ingredient & Uses
Active Ingredient(s):
Hydrocortisone 1%
Purpose(s):
Anti-Itch

USES
- Temporarily relieves itching associated with minor skin irritations, inflammation and rashes due to:
  - eczema
  - insect bites
  - poison ivy, oak, or sumac
  - soaps
  - detergents
  - cosmetics
  - jewelry
  - seborrheic dermatitis
  - psoriasis
- Other uses of this product should only be under advice and supervision of a doctor.

WARNINGS
For external use only
Flammable: Keep away from fire or flame

DO NOT USE
- For the treatment of diaper rash. Consult a doctor.
- For external anal, genital or vaginal itching.
- In or near the eyes.

WHEN USING THIS PRODUCT
avoid contact with eyes. If contact with eyes occurs, flush liberally with water. **Stop use and ask a doctor** If condition worsens, symptoms persist for more than 7 days or clear up and occur again within a few days, and do not begin use of any other hydrocortisone product unless you have asked a doctor **Keep out of reach of children.** If swallowed, get medical help or contact a Poison Control Center right away.

DIRECTIONS
- Adults and children 2 years of age and older: apply to affected area not more than 3 to 4 times daily.
- Children under 2 years of age: ask a doctor

OTHER INFORMATION
- Store at 20° to 25°C (68° to 77°F).
- Protect from freezing.
- See end of carton or tube crimp for lot number and expiration date.

INACTIVE INGREDIENTS
citric acid, disodium EDTA, glycerin, poloxamer 188, polysorbate 20, SD alcohol 40-B, water

---

CORTIZONE-10® CREME (hydrocortisone)
Chattem, Inc.

Active Ingredient(s)
Hydrocortisone 1%

Purpose(s)
Anti-itch

USES
- temporarily relieves itching associated with minor skin irritations, inflammation, and rashes due to:
  - eczema
  - psoriasis
  - poison ivy, oak, sumac
  - insect bites
  - detergents
  - jewelry
  - cosmetics
  - soaps
  - seborrheic dermatitis
  - temporarily relieves external anal and genital itching
  - other uses of this product should only be under the advice and supervision of a doctor

WARNINGS
For external use only

DO NOT USE
- in the genital area if you have a vaginal discharge. Consult a doctor.
- for the treatment of diaper rash. Consult a doctor.

WHEN USING THIS PRODUCT
- avoid contact with eyes
- do not use more than directed unless told to do so by a doctor.
- do not put directly into the rectum by using fingers or any mechanical device or applicator

STOP USE AND ASK A DOCTOR IF
- condition worsens, symptoms persist for more than 7 days or clear up and occur again within a few days, and do not begin use of any other hydrocortisone product unless you have asked a doctor
- rectal bleeding occurs

Keep out of reach of children.
If swallowed, get medical help or contact a Poison Control Center right away.

DIRECTIONS
- **for itching of skin irritation, inflammation, and rashes:**
  - adults and children 2 years of age and older: apply to affected area not more than 3 to 4 times daily
  - children under 2 years of age: ask a doctor
- **for external anal and genital itching, adults:**
  - when practical, clean the affected area with mild soap and warm water and rinse thoroughly
  - gently dry by patting or blotting with toilet tissue or a soft cloth before applying
  - apply to affected area not more than 3 to 4 times daily
  - children under 12 years of age: ask a doctor

OTHER INFORMATION
- contents filled by weight, not volume

INACTIVE INGREDIENTS
aloe barbadensis leaf juice, aluminum sulfate, beeswax, calcium acetate, cetearyl alcohol, glycerin, maltodextrin, methylparaben, mineral oil, petrolatum, propylparaben, sodium cetearyl sulfate, sodium lauryl sulfate, water
*Refers to the ingredient hydrocortisone

CORTIZONE-10® PLUS CREME (hydrocortisone)
Chattem, Inc.

Active Ingredient(s)
Hydrocortisone 1%

Purpose(s)
Anti-itch

USES
- temporarily relieves itching associated with minor skin irritations, inflammation, and rashes due to:
  - eczema
  - psoriasis
  - poison ivy, oak, sumac
  - insect bites
  - detergents
  - jewelry
  - cosmetics
  - soaps
  - seborrheic dermatitis
  - temporarily relieves external anal and genital itching
  - other uses of this product should only be under the advice and supervision of a doctor

WARNINGS
For external use only

DO NOT USE
- in the genital area if you have a vaginal discharge. Consult a doctor.
- for the treatment of diaper rash. Consult a doctor.

WHEN USING THIS PRODUCT
- avoid contact with eyes
- do not use more than directed unless told to do so by a doctor.

- do not put directly into the rectum by using fingers or any mechanical device or applicator

STOP USE AND ASK A DOCTOR IF
- condition worsens, symptoms persist for more than 7 days or clear up and occur again within a few days, and do not begin use of any other hydrocortisone product unless you have asked a doctor
- rectal bleeding occurs

Keep out of reach of children.
If swallowed, get medical help or contact a Poison Control Center right away.

DIRECTIONS
- **for itching of skin irritation, inflammation, and rashes:**
  - adults and children 2 years of age and older: apply to affected area not more than 3 to 4 times daily
  - children under 2 years of age: ask a doctor
- **for external anal and genital itching, adults:**
  - when practical, clean the affected area with mild soap and warm water and rinse thoroughly
  - gently dry by patting or blotting with toilet tissue or a soft cloth before applying
  - apply to affected area not more than 3 to 4 times daily
  - children under 12 years of age: ask a doctor

OTHER INFORMATION
- contents filled by weight, not volume

INACTIVE INGREDIENTS
aloe barbadensis leaf juice, aluminum sulfate, beeswax, calcium acetate, cetearyl alcohol, cetyl alcohol, cholecalciferol, dextrin, glycerin, isopropyl palmitate, maltodextrin, methylparaben, mineral oil, petrolatum, propylene glycol, propylparaben, retinyl palmitate, sodium cetearyl sulfate, sodium lauryl sulfate, tocopheryl acetate, water, zea mays (corn) oil
*Refers to the ingredient hydrocortisone

CORTIZONE-10® OINTMENT (hydrocortisone)

Chattem, Inc.

Active Ingredient(s)
Hydrocortisone 1%

Purpose(s)
Anti-itch

USES
- temporarily relieves itching associated with minor skin irritations, inflammation, and rashes due to:
  - eczema
  - psoriasis
  - poison ivy, oak, sumac
  - insect bites
  - detergents
  - jewelry
  - cosmetics
  - soaps
  - seborrheic dermatitis
  - temporarily relieves external anal and genital itching
  - other uses of this product should only be under the advice and supervision of a doctor

WARNINGS
For external use only

DO NOT USE
- in the genital area if you have a vaginal discharge. Consult a doctor.
- for the treatment of diaper rash. Consult a doctor.

WHEN USING THIS PRODUCT
- avoid contact with eyes
- do not use more than directed unless told to do so by a doctor
- do not put directly into the rectum by using fingers or any mechanical device or applicator

STOP USE AND ASK A DOCTOR IF
- condition worsens, symptoms persist for more than 7 days or clear up and occur again within a few days, and do not begin use of any other hydrocortisone product unless you have asked a doctor
- rectal bleeding occurs

Keep out of reach of children.
If swallowed, get medical help or contact a Poison Control Center right away.

DIRECTIONS
- **for itching of skin irritation, inflammation, and rashes:**
  - adults and children 2 years of age and older: apply to affected area not more than 3 to 4 times daily
  - children under 2 years of age: ask a doctor
- **for external anal and genital itching, adults:**
  - when practical, clean the affected area with mild soap and warm water and rinse thoroughly
  - gently dry by patting or blotting with toilet tissue or a soft cloth before applying
  - apply to affected area not more than 3 to 4 times daily
  - children under 12 years of age: ask a doctor

OTHER INFORMATION
- contents filled by weight, not volume

INACTIVE INGREDIENTS
petrolatum
*Refers to the ingredient hydrocortisone

CULTURELLE DIGESTIVE HEALTH CAPSULES (*Lactobacillus* GG and inulin)

i-Health, Inc.

INGREDIENTS
Lactobacillus GG (10 Billion Cells), Inulin
Contains none of the following: synthetic colors, preservatives, dairy, yeast, wheat, gluten or lactose.

SUGGESTED USE
As a dietary supplement, take one (1) capsule per day to support digestive and immune health. Continued daily use is suggested. If experiencing digestive upset, two (2) capsules daily are recommended until discomfort subsides.
When Traveling, take two (2) capsules twice daily throughout the trip. Best results if started two to three days prior to travel.
For children 1 year or older, take one (1) capsule daily. Capsule may be opened and mixed into cool drink or food. Do not add to warm or hot foods or beverages. Consult your medical professionals for more information.

WARNING
This product is intended for use under adult supervision only. Keep out of reach of children. Not intended for children under 1 year of age. This product should not be used by those with immune problems unless directed by a physician.

STORAGE INSTRUCTIONS
Keep Culturelle in a cool, dry place away from direct sunlight. Keep Culturelle at room temperature or below.

INACTIVE INGREDIENTS
gelatin (capsule), vegetable magnesium stearate, silica, titanium dioxide (color)

QUESTIONS OR COMMENTS?
For questions, concerns, or to report an adverse event, please call **1-800-722-3476** www.Culturelle.com

---

VICKS ALCOHOL FREE NYQUIL COLD AND FLU NIGHTTIME RELIEF (acetaminophen, chlorpheniramine maleate, and dextromethorphan hydrobromide)

Procter & Gamble

DRUG FACTS

Active Ingredient(s) (in each 30 mL dose cup)	Purpose(s)
Acetaminophen 650 mg	Pain reliever/fever reducer
Chlorpheniramine maleate 4 mg	Antihistamine
Dextromethorphan HBr 30 mg	Cough suppressant

USES
temporarily relieves common cold/flu symptoms:
• cough due to minor throat & bronchial irritation
• sore throat
• headache
• minor aches & pains
• fever
• runny nose & sneezing

WARNINGS
Liver warning
This product contains acetaminophen. Severe liver damage may occur if you take
• more than 4 doses in 24 hours, which is the maximum daily amount for this product
• with other drugs containing acetaminophen
• 3 or more alcoholic drinks daily while using this product

Sore throat warning
If sore throat is severe, lasts for more than 2 days, occurs with or is followed by fever, headache, rash, nausea, or vomiting, see a doctor promptly.

DO NOT USE
• with any other drug containing acetaminophen (prescription or nonprescription). If you are not sure whether a drug contains acetaminophen, ask a doctor or pharmacist
• if you are now taking a prescription monoamine oxidase inhibitor (MAOI) (certain drugs for depression, psychiatric or emotional conditions, or Parkinson's disease), or for 2 weeks after stopping the MAOI drug. If you do not know if your prescription drug contains an MAOI, ask a doctor or pharmacist before taking this product.
• to make a child sleep

ASK A DOCTOR BEFORE USE IF YOU HAVE
• liver disease
• glaucoma
• cough that occurs with too much phlegm (mucus)
• a breathing problem or chronic cough that lasts or as occurs with smoking, asthma, chronic bronchitis or emphysema
• trouble urinating due to enlarged prostate gland
• a sodium-restricted diet

ASK A DOCTOR OR PHARMACIST BEFORE USE IF YOU ARE
• taking sedatives or tranquilizers
• taking the blood thinning drug warfarin

WHEN USING THIS PRODUCT
• **do not use more than directed**
• excitability may occur, especially in children
• marked drowsiness may occur
• avoid alcoholic drinks
• be careful when driving a motor vehicle or operating machinery
• alcohol, sedatives, & tranquilizers may increase drowsiness

STOP USE AND ASK A DOCTOR IF
• pain or cough gets worse or lasts more than 7 days
• fever gets worse or lasts more than 3 days
• redness or swelling is present
• new symptoms occur
• cough comes back or occurs with rash or headache that lasts. These could be signs of a serious condition.
If pregnant or breast-feeding, ask a health professional before use.
Keep out of reach of children.

OVERDOSE WARNING
Taking more than directed can cause serious health problems. In case of overdose, get medical help or contact a Poison Control Center right away. Quick medical attention is critical for adults & for children even if you do not notice any signs or symptoms.

DIRECTIONS
• take only as directed-see Overdose warning
• use dose cup or tablespoon (TBSP)
• do not exceed 4 doses per 24 hrs

adults & children 12 yrs & over	30 ml (2 TBSP) every 6 hrs
children 4 to under 12 yrs	ask a doctor
children under 4 yrs	do not use

• **when using other DayQuil® or NyQuil products, carefully read each label to insure correct dosing**

OTHER INFORMATION
• **each 30 mL dose cup contains:** potassium 7 mg, sodium 47 mg
• store at room temperature

INACTIVE INGREDIENTS
acesulfame potassium, carboxymethylcellulose sodium, citric acid, FD&C red no. 40, flavor, high fructose corn syrup, polyethylene glycol, propylene glycol, purified water, saccharin sodium, sodium benzoate, sodium citrate

QUESTIONS OR COMMENTS?
1-800-362-1683
Dist. by Procter & Gamble, Cincinnati OH 45202.
www.vicks.com

VICKS DAYQUIL COLD & FLU (acetaminophen, dextromethorphan HBr, and phenylephrine HCl)

Procter & Gamble

DRUG FACTS

Active Ingredient(s) (in each 15 mL tablespoon)	Purpose(s)
Acetaminophen 325 mg	Pain reliever/fever reducer
Dextromethorphan HBr 10 mg	Cough suppressant
Phenylephrine HCl 5 mg	Nasal decongestant

USES TEMPORARILY RELIEVES COMMON COLD/FLU SYMPTOMS:
- nasal congestion
- cough due to minor throat & bronchial irritation
- sore throat
- headache
- minor aches & pains
- fever

WARNINGS

LIVER WARNING THIS PRODUCT CONTAINS ACETAMINO-PHEN. SEVERE LIVER DAMAGE MAY OCCUR IF ADULT/CHILD TAKES
- more than 4 doses in 24 hours, which is the maximum daily amount for this product
- with other drugs containing acetaminophen
- adult has 3 or more alcoholic drinks every day while using this product

SORE THROAT WARNING
If sore throat is severe, lasts for more than 2 days, occurs with or is followed by fever, headache, rash, nausea, or vomiting, see a doctor promptly.

DO NOT USE
- with any other drug containing acetaminophen (prescription or nonprescription). If you are not sure whether a drug contains acetaminophen, ask a doctor or pharmacist.
- if you are now taking a prescription monoamine oxidase inhibitor (MAOI) (certain drugs for depression, psychiatric or emotional conditions, or Parkinson's disease), or for 2 weeks after stopping the MAOI drug. If you do not know if your prescription drug contains an MAOI, ask a doctor or pharmacist before taking this product.

ASK A DOCTOR BEFORE USE IF YOU HAVE
- liver disease
- heart disease
- thyroid disease
- diabetes
- high blood pressure
- trouble urinating due to enlarged prostate gland
- cough that occurs with too much phlegm (mucus)
- persistent or chronic cough as occurs with smoking, asthma, or emphysema
- a sodium-restricted diet

ASK A DOCTOR OR PHARMACIST BEFORE USE IF YOU ARE
- taking the blood thinning drug warfarin.

WHEN USING THIS PRODUCT
- do not use more than directed.

STOP USE AND ASK A DOCTOR IF
- you get nervous, dizzy or sleepless

- symptoms get worse or last more than 5 days (children) or 7 days (adults)
- fever gets worse or lasts more than 3 days
- redness or swelling is present
- new symptoms occur
- cough comes back, or occurs with rash or headache that lasts.

These could be signs of a serious condition.
If pregnant or breast-feeding, ask a health professional before use.
Keep out of reach of children.

OVERDOSE WARNING TAKING MORE THAN DIRECTED CAN CAUSE SERIOUS HEALTH PROBLEMS. IN CASE OF OVERDOSE, GET MEDICAL HELP OR CONTACT A POISON CONTROL CENTER RIGHT AWAY. QUICK MEDICAL ATTENTION IS CRITICAL FOR ADULTS & FOR CHILDREN EVEN IF YOU DO NOT NOTICE ANY SIGNS OR SYMPTOMS.

DIRECTIONS
- take only as directed - see **OVERDOSE WARNING**
- use dose cup or tablespoon (TBSP)
- do not exceed 4 doses per 24 hrs

adults & children 12 yrs & over	30 mL (2 TBSP) every 4 hrs
children 6 to under 12 yrs	15 mL (1 TBSP) every 4 hrs
children 4 to under 6 yrs	ask a doctor
children under 4 yrs	do not use

- **when using other DayQuil or NyQuil products, carefully read each label to insure correct dosing**

OTHER INFORMATION
- **each tablespoon contains:** sodium 50 mg
- store at room temperature

INACTIVE INGREDIENTS
carboxymethylcellulose sodium, citric acid, disodium EDTA, FD&C Yellow No. 6, flavor, glycerin, propylene glycol, purified water, saccharin sodium, sodium benzoate, sodium chloride, sodium citrate, sorbitol, sucralose

QUESTIONS OR COMMENTS?
1-800-251-3374
www.vicks.com

VICKS DAYQUIL COLD & FLU MULTI-SYMPTOM RELIEF (acetaminophen, dextromethorphan HBr, and phenylephrine HCl)

Procter & Gamble

DRUGS FACTS

Active Ingredient(s) (in each LiquiCap)	Purpose(s)
Acetaminophen 325 mg	Pain reliever/fever reducer
Dextromethorphan HBr 10 mg	Cough suppressant
Phenylephrine HCl 5 mg	Nasal decongestant

USES
temporarily relieves common cold/flu symptoms:
- nasal congestion
- cough due to minor throat & bronchial irritation
- sore throat
- headache
- minor aches & pains
- fever

WARNINGS
Liver warning
This product contains acetaminophen. Severe liver damage may occur if you take
- more than 4 doses in 24 hrs, which is the maximum daily amount for this product
- with other drugs containing acetaminophen
- 3 or more alcoholic drinks daily while using this product

Sore throat warning
If sore throat is severe, lasts for more than 2 days, occurs with or is followed by fever, headache, rash, nausea, or vomiting, see a doctor promptly.

DO NOT USE
- with any other drug containing acetaminophen (prescription or nonprescription). If you are not sure whether a drug contains acetaminophen, ask a doctor or pharmacist.
- if you are now taking a prescription monoamine oxidase inhibitor (MAOI) (certain drugs for depression, psychiatric or emotional conditions, or Parkinson's disease), or for 2 weeks after stopping the MAOI drug. If you do not know if your prescription drug contains an MAOI, ask a doctor or pharmacist before taking this product.

ASK A DOCTOR BEFORE USE IF YOU HAVE
- liver disease
- heart disease
- thyroid disease
- diabetes
- high blood pressure
- trouble urinating due to enlarged prostate gland
- cough that occurs with too much phlegm (mucus)
- persistent or chronic cough as occurs with smoking, asthma, or emphysema

ASK A DOCTOR OR PHARMACIST BEFORE USE IF YOU ARE
- taking the blood thinning drug warfarin.

WHEN USING THIS PRODUCT
- do not use more than directed.

STOP USE AND ASK A DOCTOR IF
- you get nervous, dizzy or sleepless
- symptoms get worse or last more than 5 days (children) or 7 days (adults)
- fever gets worse or lasts more than 3 days
- redness or swelling is present
- new symptoms occur
- cough comes back, or occurs with rash or headache that lasts. These could be signs of a serious condition.

If pregnant or breast-feeding, ask a health professional before use.
Keep out of reach of children.

OVERDOSE WARNING
Taking more than directed can cause serious health problems. In case of overdose, get medical help or contact a Poison Control Center right away. Quick medical attention is critical for adults & for children even if you do not notice any signs or symptoms.

DIRECTIONS
- take only as directed - see **OVERDOSE WARNING**
- do not exceed 4 doses per 24 hrs

adults & children 12 yrs & over	2 LiquiCaps with water every 4 hrs
children 4 to under 12 yrs	ask a doctor
children under 4 yrs	do not use

- when using other DayQuil or NyQuil products, carefully read each label to insure correct dosing

OTHER INFORMATION
- store at room temperature

INACTIVE INGREDIENTS
FD&C Red No. 40, FD&C Yellow No. 6, gelatin, glycerin, polyethylene glycol, povidone, propylene glycol, purified water, sorbitol special, titanium dioxide

QUESTIONS OR COMMENTS?
Call 1-800-251-3374

VICKS DAYQUIL COUGH (dextromethorphan hydrobromide)
Procter & Gamble

DRUG FACTS

Active Ingredient(s) (in each 15 mL tablespoon)
Dextromethorphan HBr 15 mg

Purpose(s)
Cough suppressant

USE
temporarily relieves cough due to minor throat and bronchial irritation

WARNINGS

DO NOT USE
if you are now taking a prescription monoamine oxidase inhibitor (MAOI) (certain drugs for depression, psychiatric or emotional conditions, or Parkinson's disease), or for 2 weeks after stopping the MAOI drug. If you do not know if your prescription drug contains an MAOI, ask a doctor or pharmacist before taking this product.

ASK A DOCTOR BEFORE USE IF YOU HAVE
- cough that occurs with too much phlegm (mucus)
- persistent or chronic cough such as occurs with smoking, asthma, or emphysema

WHEN USING THIS PRODUCT
do not use more than directed.

STOP USE AND ASK A DOCTOR IF
cough lasts more than 7 days, comes back, or occurs with fever, rash, or headache that lasts. These could be signs of a serious condition.
If pregnant or breast-feeding, ask a health professional before use.
Keep out of reach of children. In case of overdose, get medical help or contact a Poison Control Center right away.

DIRECTIONS
- take only as recommended
- use dose cup or tablespoon (TBSP)
- do not exceed 4 doses per 24 hours

adults and children 12 years and over	30 mL (2 TBSP) every 6-8 hours
children 6 to under 12 years	15 mL (1 TBSP) every 6-8 hours
children 4 to under 6 years	ask a doctor
children under 4 years	do not use

- when using other DayQuil or NyQuil® products, carefully read each label to insure correct dosing

OTHER INFORMATION
- **each tablespoon contains:** sodium 15 mg
- store at room temperature

INACTIVE INGREDIENTS
citric acid, D&C yellow no. 10, FD&C yellow no. 6, flavor, high fructose corn syrup, polyethylene glycol, propylene glycol, purified water, saccharin sodium, sodium citrate

QUESTIONS OR COMMENTS?
1-800-251-3374

VICKS DAYQUIL MUCUS CONTROL DM
(dextromethorphan hydrobromide and guaifenesin)

Procter & Gamble

DRUG FACTS

Active Ingredient(s) (in each 15 mL tablespoon)	Purpose(s)
Dextromethorphan HBr 10 mg	Cough suppressant
Guaifenesin 200 mg	Expectorant

USES
- temporarily relieves cough associated with the common cold
- helps loosen phlegm and thin bronchial secretions to rid the bronchial passageways of bothersome mucus

WARNINGS

DO NOT USE
if you are now taking a prescription monoamine oxidase inhibitor (MAOI) (certain drugs for depression, psychiatric or emotional conditions, or Parkinson's disease), or for 2 weeks after stopping the MAOI drug. If you do not know if your prescription drug contains an MAOI, ask a doctor or pharmacist before taking this product.

ASK A DOCTOR BEFORE USE IF YOU HAVE
- persistent or chronic cough such as occurs with smoking, asthma, chronic bronchitis, or emphysema
- cough that occurs with too much phlegm (mucus)
- a sodium-restricted diet

STOP USE AND ASK A DOCTOR IF
- cough lasts more than 7 days, comes back, or occurs with fever, rash, or headache that lasts.
  These could be signs of a serious condition.

If pregnant or breast-feeding, ask a health professional before use.
Keep out of reach of children. In case of overdose, get medical help or contact a Poison Control Center right away.

DIRECTIONS
- use dose cup or tablespoon (TBSP)
- do not exceed 6 doses per 24 hours

adults and children 12 years and over	30 mL (2 TBSP) every 4 hours
children 6 to under 12 years	15 mL (1 TBSP) every 4 hours
children 4 to under 6 years	ask a doctor
children under 4 years	do not use

- when using other DayQuil or NyQuil® products, carefully read each label to insure correct dosing

OTHER INFORMATION
- **each tablespoon contains:** sodium 25 mg
- store at room temperature

INACTIVE INGREDIENTS
carboxymethylcellulose sodium, citric acid, D&C yellow no. 10, FD&C yellow no. 6, flavor, high fructose corn syrup, propylene glycol, purified water, saccharin sodium, sodium benzoate, sodium citrate

QUESTIONS OR COMMENTS?
1-800-251-3374
www.vicks.com
Dist. by Procter & Gamble,
Cincinnati OH 45202.

VICKS NYQUIL COLD & FLU RELIEF LIQUICAPS (acetaminophen, dextromethorphan hydrobromide, and doxylamine succinate)

Procter & Gamble

RELIEVES
Temporarily relieves common cold and flu symptoms: cough due to minor throat and bronchial irritation, sore throat, headache, minor aches and pains, fever, runny nose and sneezing
- Cough
- Runny Nose/Sneezing
- Fever
- Sore Throat
- Aches and Pain

DIRECTIONS
- Take only as recommended—see Overdose warning.
- Do not exceed 4 doses per 24 hours

Adults and children 12 years and over	2 LiquiCaps® with water every 6 hours
Children 4 to under 12 years	Ask a doctor.
Children under 4 years	Do not use.

When using other DayQuil® or NyQuil products, carefully read each label to ensure correct dosing.

INGREDIENTS
Active Ingredient(s) (in each LiquiCap®) (Purpose(s))
Acetaminophen 325 mg (Pain reliever/fever reducer)
Dextromethorphan HBr 15 mg (Cough suppressant)
Doxylamine succinate 6.25 mg (Antihistamine)

INACTIVE INGREDIENTS
D&C yellow no. 10, FD&C blue no. 1, gelatin, glycerin, polyethylene glycol, povidone, propylene glycol, purified water, sorbitol special, titanium dioxide

OTHER INFORMATION
- Store at room temperature.

WARNINGS
Liver warning: This product contains acetaminophen. Severe liver damage may occur if you take:
- More than 4 doses in 24 hours, which is the maximum daily amount for this product
- With other drugs containing acetaminophen
- 3 or more alcoholic drinks daily while using this product

Sore throat warning: If sore throat is severe, lasts for more than 2 days, or occurs with or is followed by fever, headache, rash, nausea, or vomiting, see a doctor promptly.

DO NOT USE
- With any other drug containing acetaminophen (prescription or nonprescription). If you are not sure whether a drug contains acetaminophen, ask a doctor or pharmacist.
- If you are now taking a prescription monoamine oxidase inhibitor (MAOI) (certain drugs for depression, psychiatric or emotional conditions, or Parkinson's disease), or for 2 weeks after stopping the MAOI drug. If you do not know if your prescription drug contains an MAOI, ask a doctor or pharmacist before taking this product.
- To make a child sleep

ASK A DOCTOR BEFORE USE IF YOU HAVE
- Liver disease
- Glaucoma
- Cough that occurs with too much phlegm (mucus)
- A breathing problem or chronic cough that lasts or as occurs with smoking, asthma, chronic bronchitis, or emphysema
- Trouble urinating due to enlarged prostate gland

ASK A DOCTOR OR PHARMACIST BEFORE USE IF YOU ARE
- Taking sedatives or tranquilizers
- Taking the blood-thinning drug Warfarin

WHEN USING THIS PRODUCT
- **Do not use more than directed.**
- Excitability may occur, especially in children.
- Marked drowsiness may occur.
- Avoid alcoholic drinks.
- Be careful when driving a motor vehicle or operating machinery.
- Alcohol, sedatives, and tranquilizers may increase drowsiness.

STOP USE AND ASK A DOCTOR IF
- Pain or cough gets worse or lasts more than 7 days
- Fever gets worse or lasts more than 3 days
- Redness or swelling is present
- New symptoms occur
- Cough comes back or occurs with rash or headache that lasts

These could be signs of a serious condition.
If pregnant or breast-feeding, ask a health professional before use.
Keep out of reach of children.

OVERDOSE WARNING
Taking more than directed can cause serious health problems. In case of overdose, get medical help or contact a Poison Control Center right away. Quick medical attention is critical for adults as well as for children, even if you do not notice any signs or symptoms.
Tamper evident:
- 16-, 24-, 48-, and 72-count packages: This package is safety sealed and child resistant. Use only if blisters are intact. If difficult to open, use scissors.
- 2-count pouch is **Safety Sealed:** Use only if foil is intact. TO OPEN, FOLD, AND TEAR

QUESTIONS OR COMMENTS?
Call 1-800-362-1683.

VICKS NYQUIL COLD & FLU RELIEF LIQUID
(acetaminophen, dextromethorphan hydrobromide, and doxylamine succinate)

Procter & Gamble
RELIEVES
Temporarily relieves common cold and flu symptoms: cough due to minor throat and bronchial irritation, sore throat, headache, minor aches and pains, fever, runny nose and sneezing
- Cough
- Runny Nose/Sneezing
- Fever
- Sore Throat
- Aches and Pain

DIRECTIONS
- Take only as recommended—see Overdose warning.
- Use dose cup or tablespoon (TBSP).
- Do not exceed 4 doses per 24 hours

Adults and children 12 years and over	30 mL (2 TBSP) every 6 hours
Children 4 to under 12 years	Ask a doctor.
Children under 4 years	Do not use.

When using other DayQuil® or NyQuil products, carefully read each label to ensure correct dosing.

INGREDIENTS
Active Ingredient(s) (in each 30 mL dose cup) (Purpose(s))
Acetaminophen 650 mg (Pain reliever/fever reducer)
Dextromethorphan HBr 30 mg (Cough suppressant)
Doxylamine succinate 12.5 mg (Antihistamine)

INACTIVE INGREDIENTS
Original: acesulfame potassium, alcohol, citric acid, D&C yellow no. 10, FD&C green no. 3, FD&C yellow no. 6, flavor, high fructose corn syrup, polyethylene glycol, propylene glycol, purified water, saccharin sodium, sodium citrate
Cherry: acesulfame potassium, alcohol, citric acid, FD&C blue no. 1, FD&C red no. 40, flavor, high fructose corn syrup, polyethylene glycol, propylene glycol, purified water, saccharin sodium, sodium citrate

OTHER INFORMATION
- Each 30 mL dose cup contains 5 mg potassium and 37 mg sodium (Original) or 5 mg potassium and 38 mg sodium (Cherry).
- Store at room temperature.

WARNINGS
Liver warning: This product contains acetaminophen. Severe liver damage may occur if you take:
- More than 4 doses in 24 hours, which is the maximum daily amount for this product
- With other drugs containing acetaminophen
- 3 or more alcoholic drinks daily while using this product

Sore throat warning: If sore throat is severe, lasts for more than 2 days, or occurs with or is followed by fever, headache, rash, nausea, or vomiting, see a doctor promptly.

DO NOT USE
- With any other drug containing acetaminophen (prescription or nonprescription). If you are not sure whether a drug contains acetaminophen, ask a doctor or pharmacist.
- If you are now taking a prescription monoamine oxidase inhibitor (MAOI) (certain drugs for depression, psychiatric or emotional conditions, or Parkinson's disease), or for 2 weeks after stopping the MAOI drug. If you do not know if your

prescription drug contains an MAOI, ask a doctor or pharmacist before taking this product.
- To make a child sleep

ASK A DOCTOR BEFORE USE IF YOU HAVE
- Liver disease
- Glaucoma
- Cough that occurs with too much phlegm (mucus)
- A breathing problem or chronic cough that lasts or as occurs with smoking, asthma, chronic bronchitis, or emphysema
- Trouble urinating due to enlarged prostate gland
- A sodium-restricted diet

ASK A DOCTOR OR PHARMACIST BEFORE USE IF YOU ARE
- Taking sedatives or tranquilizers
- Taking the blood-thinning drug Warfarin

WHEN USING THIS PRODUCT
- **Do not use more than directed.**
- Excitability may occur, especially in children.
- Marked drowsiness may occur.
- Avoid alcoholic drinks.
- Be careful when driving a motor vehicle or operating machinery.
- Alcohol, sedatives, and tranquilizers may increase drowsiness.

STOP USE AND ASK A DOCTOR IF
- Pain or cough gets worse or lasts more than 7 days
- Fever gets worse or lasts more than 3 days
- Redness or swelling is present
- New symptoms occur
- Cough comes back or occurs with rash or headache that lasts

These could be signs of a serious condition.
If pregnant or breast-feeding, ask a health professional before use
Keep out of reach of children.

OVERDOSE WARNING
Taking more than directed can cause serious health problems. In case of overdose, get medical help or contact a Poison Control Center right away. Quick medical attention is critical for adults as well as for children, even if you do not notice any signs or symptoms.
Tamper evident: Do not use if printed shrinkband is missing or broken.

QUESTIONS OR COMMENTS?
Call 1-800-362-1683.

VICKS NYQUIL COUGH (dextromethorphan hydrobromide and doxylamine succinate)
Procter & Gamble

DRUG FACTS

Active Ingredient(s) (in each 30 mL dose cup)	Purpose(s)
Dextromethorphan HBr 30 mg	Cough suppressant
Doxylamine succinate 12.5 mg	Antihistamine

USES
temporarily relieves cold symptoms:
- cough
- runny nose and sneezing

WARNINGS
DO NOT USE
- if you are now taking a prescription monoamine oxidase inhibitor (MAOI) (certain drugs for depression, psychiatric or emotional conditions, or Parkinson's disease), or for 2 weeks after stopping the MAOI drug. If you do not know if your prescription drug contains an MAOI, ask a doctor or pharmacist before taking this product.
- to make a child sleep

ASK A DOCTOR BEFORE USE IF YOU HAVE
- glaucoma
- excessive phlegm (mucus)
- a breathing problem or chronic cough that lasts or as occurs with smoking, asthma, chronic bronchitis or emphysema
- trouble urinating due to enlarged prostate gland
- a sodium-restricted diet

ASK A DOCTOR OR PHARMACIST BEFORE USE IF YOU ARE
taking sedatives or tranquilizers.

WHEN USING THIS PRODUCT
- **do not use more than directed**
- excitability may occur, especially in children
- marked drowsiness may occur
- avoid alcoholic drinks
- be careful when driving a motor vehicle or operating machinery
- alcohol, sedatives, and tranquilizers may increase drowsiness

STOP USE AND ASK A DOCTOR IF
- cough lasts more than 7 days, comes back, or occurs with fever, rash, or headache that lasts.
  These could be signs of a serious condition.

If pregnant or breast-feeding, ask a health professional before use.
Keep out of reach of children. In case of overdose, get medical help or contact a Poison Control Center right away.

DIRECTIONS
- use dose cup or tablespoon (TBSP)
- do not exceed 4 doses per 24 hrs

adults & children 12 yrs & over	30 mL (2 TBSP) every 6 hrs
children 4 to under 12 yrs	ask a doctor
children under 4 yrs	do not use

- **when using other DayQuil® or NyQuil products, carefully read each label to insure correct dosing**

OTHER INFORMATION
- **each 30 mL dose cup contains:** sodium 36 mg
- store at room temperature

INACTIVE INGREDIENTS
alcohol, citric acid, FD&C blue no. 1, FD&C red no. 40, flavor, high fructose corn syrup, polyethylene glycol, propylene glycol, purified water, saccharin sodium, sodium citrate

QUESTIONS OR COMMENTS?
1-800-362-1683
Dist. by
Procter & Gamble,
Cincinnati OH 45202.

DELSYM NIGHT TIME COUGH AND COLD

(acetaminophen, dextromethorphan hydrobromide, and doxylamine succinate)

Reckitt Benckiser Inc.

DRUG FACTS

Active Ingredient(s) (in each 15 mL)	Purpose(s)
Acetaminophen 500 mg	Pain reliever/Fever reducer
Dextromethorphan HBr 15 mg	Cough suppressant
Doxylamine Succinate 6.25 mg	Antihistamine

USES

temporarily relieves these common cold and flu symptoms:
- cough due to minor throat and bronchial irritation
- runny nose and sneezing
- minor aches and pains
- sore throat
- headache
- fever
- the impulse to cough to help you get to sleep

WARNINGS

Liver warning

This product contains acetaminophen. Severe liver damage may occur if you take:
- more than 4 doses in 24 hours, which is the maximum daily amount
- with other drugs containing acetaminophen
- 3 or more alcoholic drinks daily while using this product

Sore throat warning

If sore throat is severe, persists for more than 2 days, is accompanied or followed by fever, headache, rash, nausea or vomiting, consult a doctor promptly.

DO NOT USE

- **with any other drug containing acetaminophen** (prescription or nonprescription). If you are not sure whether a drug contains acetaminophen, ask a doctor or pharmacist.
- if you are now taking a prescription monoamine oxidase inhibitor (MAOI) (certain drugs for depression, psychiatric, or emotional conditions, or Parkinson's disease), or for 2 weeks after stopping the MAOI drug. If you do not know if your prescription drug contains an MAOI, ask a doctor or pharmacist before taking this product.

ASK A DOCTOR BEFORE USE IF YOU HAVE

- liver disease
- glaucoma
- trouble urinating due to an enlarged prostate gland
- a breathing problem such as emphysema or chronic bronchitis
- persistent or chronic cough such as occurs with smoking, asthma or emphysema
- cough that occurs with too much phlegm (mucus)
- a sodium restricted diet

ASK A DOCTOR OR PHARMACIST BEFORE USE IF

- you are taking the blood thinning drug warfarin.
- you are taking sedatives or tranquilizers.

WHEN USING THIS PRODUCT

- **do not use more than directed**
- excitability may occur, especially in children
- marked drowsiness may occur
- alcohol, sedatives and tranquilizers may increase drowsiness
- avoid alcoholic drinks
- be careful when driving a motor vehicle or operating machinery

STOP USE AND ASK A DOCTOR IF

- pain or cough gets worse or lasts more than 7 days
- fever gets worse or lasts more than 3 days
- redness or swelling is present
- new symptoms occur
- cough comes back or occurs with rash or persistent headache. These could be signs of a serious condition.

If pregnant or breast feeding, ask a health professional before use.

Keep out of reach of children.

OVERDOSE WARNING

Taking more than the recommended dose (overdose) may cause liver damage. In case of overdose, get medical help or contact a Poison Control Center right away. Quick medical attention is critical for adults as well as for children even if you do not notice any signs or symptoms.

DIRECTIONS

- **do not take more than directed (see OVERDOSE WARNING)**
- do not take more than 4 doses in any 24-hour period
- measure only with dosing cup provided
- do not use dosing cup with other products
- dose as follows or as directed by a doctor
- mL = milliliter

| Adults and Children 12 years and older | 30 mL in dosing cup provided every 6 hours |
| Children under 12 years of age | Do not use. |

OTHER INFORMATION

- each 15 mL contains: **sodium 23 mg**
- tamper evident: do not use if seal under bottle cap printed "SEALED for YOUR PROTECTION" is torn or missing
- dosing cup provided
- store between 15-30°C (59-86°F)
- **Keep carton for full directions for use**

INACTIVE INGREDIENTS

anhydrous citric acid, anhydrous trisodium citrate, FD&C blue #1, FD&C Red #40, flavors, glycerin, polyethylene glycol, propylene glycol, purified water, saccharin sodium, sodium benzoate, sugar

QUESTIONS OR COMMENTS?

1-888-963-3382
You may also report side effects to this phone number.

DELSYM ADULT 12 HOUR COUGH LIQUID (ORANGE FLAVOR) (dextromethorphan polistirex)

Reckitt Benckiser LLC

DRUG FACTS

Active Ingredient(s) (in each 5 mL)	Purpose(s)
Dextromethorphan polistirex equivalent to 30 mg dextromethorphan hydrobromide	Cough suppressant

USES

temporarily relieves
- cough due to minor throat and bronchial irritation as may occur with the common cold or inhaled irritants
- the impulse to cough to help you get to sleep

WARNINGS

DO NOT USE

if you are now taking a prescription monoamine oxidase inhibitor (MAOI) (certain drugs for depression, psychiatric or emotional conditions, or Parkinson's disease), or for 2 weeks after stopping the MAOI drug. If you do not know if your prescription drug contains an MAOI, ask a doctor or pharmacist before taking this product.

ASK A DOCTOR BEFORE USE IF YOU HAVE
- chronic cough that lasts as occurs with smoking, asthma or emphysema
- cough that occurs with too much phlegm (mucus)

STOP USE AND ASK A DOCTOR IF

cough lasts more than 7 days, cough comes back, or occurs with fever, rash or headache that lasts. These could be signs of a serious condition.
If pregnant or breast-feeding, ask a health professional before use.
Keep out of reach of children. In case of overdose, get medical help or contact a Poison Control Center right away.

DIRECTIONS
- **shake bottle well before use**
- measure only with dosing cup provided. Do not use dosing cup with other products.
- dose as follows or as directed by a doctor
- mL = milliliter

adults and children 12 years of age and over	10 mL every 12 hours, not to exceed 20 mL in 24 hours
children 6 to under 12 years of age	5 mL every 12 hours, not to exceed 10 mL in 24 hours
children 4 to under 6 years of age	2.5 mL every 12 hours, not to exceed 5 mL in 24 hours
children under 4 years of age	do not use

OTHER INFORMATION
- store at 20-25°C (68-77°F)
- each 5 mL contains: **sodium 7 mg**
- dosing cup provided

INACTIVE INGREDIENTS
citric acid, edetate disodium, ethylcellulose, FD&C yellow no. 6, flavor, high fructose corn syrup, methylparaben, polyethylene glycol 3350, polysorbate 80, propylene glycol, propylparaben, purified water, sucrose, tragacanth, vegetable oil, xanthan gum

QUESTIONS OR COMMENTS?
1-888-963-3382
You may also report side effects to this phone number.

DELSYM COUGH RELIEF PLUS SOOTHING ACTION (dextromethorphan hydrobromide and menthol)

Reckitt Benckiser LLC

DRUG FACTS

Active Ingredient(s) (in each lozenge)	Purpose(s)
Dextromethorphan HBr 5 mg	Cough suppressant
Menthol 5 mg	Oral pain reliever

USES
temporarily relieves
- sore throat
- sore mouth
- minor mouth irritation
- cough due to minor throat and bronchial irritation as may occur with the common cold

WARNINGS
Sore throat warning
- If sore throat is severe, persists for more than 2 days, is accompanied or followed by fever, headache, rash, nausea or vomiting consult a doctor promptly.

DO NOT USE
in a child under 6 years of age.

DO NOT USE
if you are now taking a prescription monoamine oxidase inhibitor (MAOI) (certain drugs for depression, psychiatric, or emotional conditions, or Parkinson's disease), or for 2 weeks after stopping the MAOI drug. If you do not know if your prescription drug contains an MAOI, ask a doctor or pharmacist before taking this product.

ASK A DOCTOR BEFORE USE IF YOU HAVE
- persistent or chronic cough such as occurs with smoking, asthma, or emphysema
- cough that is accompanied by excessive phlegm (mucus)

STOP USE AND ASK A DOCTOR OR DENTIST IF
- sore mouth symptoms do not improve in 7 days
- irritation, pain or redness persists or worsens
- swelling develops
- cough lasts more than 7 days, comes back, or occurs with fever, rash, or persistent headache. These could be signs of a serious illness

If pregnant or breast-feeding, ask a health professional before use.
Keep this and all drugs out of the reach of children. In case of overdose, get medical help or contact a Poison Control Center right away.

DIRECTIONS
- adults and children 12 years and older: take 2 lozenges (one immediately after the other) and allow each lozenge to dissolve slowly in the mouth; may be repeated every 4 hours, not to exceed 12 lozenges in any 24-hour period, or as directed by a doctor
- children 6 to under 12 years of age: take 1 lozenge and allow to dissolve slowly in the mouth; may be repeated every 4 hours, not to exceed 6 lozenges in 24 hours, or as directed by a doctor
- children under 6 years of age: do not use

OTHER INFORMATION
- tamper evident: product is sealed in blister package for your protection. Do not use if carton is damaged or if printed seal on blister is broken or missing.
- store at room temperature 20-25°C (68-77°F)

INACTIVE INGREDIENTS
D&C red #33, FD&C red #40, flavors, isomalt, maltitol syrup, propylene glycol, sorbitol, sucralose, water

QUESTIONS OR COMMENTS?
Call 1-888-963-3382
You may also report side effects to this phone number.
Dist. by: Reckitt Benckiser
Parsippany, NJ 07054-0224

DELSYM NIGHT TIME MULTI-SYMPTOM
(acetaminophen, dextromethorphan hydrobromide, and doxylamine succinate)

Reckitt Benckiser LLC

DRUGS FACTS

Active Ingredient(s) (in each: 15 mL)	Purpose(s)
Acetaminophen 325 mg	Pain reliever/Fever reducer
Dextromethorphan HBr 10 mg	Cough suppressant
Doxylamine Succinate 6.25 mg	Antihistamine
Phenylephrine HCl 5 mg	Nasal decongestant

USES
temporarily relieves these common cold and flu symptoms:
- nasal congestion
- cough due to minor throat and bronchial irritation
- runny nose and sneezing
- minor aches and pains
- sore throat
- headache
- fever
- the impulse to cough to help you get to sleep

WARNINGS
Liver warning
This product contains acetaminophen. Severe liver damage may occur if you take:
- more than 6 doses in 24 hours, which is the maximum daily amount
- with other drugs containing acetaminophen
- 3 or more alcoholic drinks daily while using this product

Sore throat warning
If sore throat is severe, persists for more than 2 days, is accompanied or followed by fever, headache, rash, nausea or vomiting, consult a doctor promptly.

DO NOT USE
- **with any other drug containing acetaminophen** (prescription or nonprescription). If you are not sure whether a drug contains acetaminophen, ask a doctor or pharmacist.
- if you are now taking a prescription monoamine oxidase inhibitor (MAOI) (certain drugs for depression, psychiatric, or emotional conditions, or Parkinson's disease), or for 2 weeks after stopping the MAOI drug. If you do not know if your prescription drug contains an MAOI, ask a doctor or pharmacist before taking this product.

ASK A DOCTOR BEFORE USE IF YOU HAVE
- liver disease
- heart disease
- diabetes
- high blood pressure
- thyroid disease
- glaucoma
- trouble urinating due to an enlarged prostate gland
- a breathing problem such as emphysema or chronic bronchitis
- persistent or chronic cough such as occurs with smoking, asthma or emphysema
- cough that occurs with too much phlegm (mucus)

ASK A DOCTOR OR PHARMACIST BEFORE USE IF YOU ARE
- taking the blood thinning drug warfarin.
- taking sedatives or tranquilizers.

WHEN USING THIS PRODUCT
- **do not use more than directed**
- excitability may occur, especially in children
- marked drowsiness may occur
- alcohol, sedatives and tranquilizers may increase drowsiness
- avoid alcoholic drinks
- be careful when driving a motor vehicle or operating machinery

STOP USE AND ASK A DOCTOR IF
- nervousness, dizziness, or sleeplessness occurs
- pain, nasal congestion or cough gets worse or lasts more than 7 days
- fever gets worse or lasts more than 3 days
- redness or swelling is present
- new symptoms occur
- cough comes back, or occurs with rash or persistent headache. These could be signs of a serious condition.

If pregnant or breast feeding, ask a health professional before use.
Keep out of reach of children.

OVERDOSE WARNING
Taking more than the recommended dose (overdose) may cause liver damage. In case of overdose, get medical help or contact a Poison Control Center right away. Quick medical attention is critical for adults as well as for children even if you do not notice any signs or symptoms.

DIRECTIONS
- **do not take more than directed (see OVERDOSE WARNING)**
- do not take more than 6 doses in any 24-hour period
- measure only with dosing cup provided
- do not use dosing cup with other products
- dose as follows or as directed by a doctor
- mL = milliliter
- **Adults and Children 12 years and older:** 30 mL in dosing cup provided every 4 hours.
- **Children under 12 years of age:** Do not use.

OTHER INFORMATION
- each 15 mL contains: **sodium 5 mg**
- tamper evident: do not use if seal under bottle cap printed "SEALED for YOUR PROTECTION" is torn or missing
- dosing cup provided
- store between 15-30 °C (59-86 °F)
- **Keep carton for full directions for use**

INACTIVE INGREDIENTS
anhydrous citric acid, FD&C blue #1, FD&C red #40, FD&C yellow #6, flavors, glycerin, propylene glycol, purified water, sodium benzoate, sorbitol, sucralose

QUESTIONS OR COMMENTS?
1-888-963-3382
You may also report side effects to this phone number.

DESITIN MAXIMUM STRENGTH ORIGINAL
(zinc oxide)

Johnson & Johnson Consumer Products Company, Division of Johnson & Johnson Consumer Companies, Inc.

DRUG FACTS

Active Ingredient(s)
Zinc Oxide 40%

Purpose(s)
Skin Protectant

USES
- Helps treat and prevent diaper rash
- Protects chafed skin due to diaper rash
- Helps seal out wetness

WARNINGS
For external use only.

WHEN USING THIS PRODUCT
- Do not get into eyes

STOP USE AND ASK A DOCTOR IF
- Condition worsens
- Symptoms last more than 7 days or clear up and occur within a few days.

Keep out of reach of children. If swallowed, get medical help or contact a Poison Control Center right away.

DIRECTIONS
- Change wet or soiled diapers promptly
- Clean the diaper area
- Allow to dry
- Apply cream liberally as often as necessary, with each diaper change, especially at bedtime or any time prolonged exposure to wet diapers may be prolonged.

OTHER INFORMATION
Store at 20° to 25°C (68°F to 77°F)

INACTIVE INGREDIENTS
BHA, cod liver oil, fragrance, lanolin, methylparaben, petrolatum, talc, water

QUESTIONS OR COMMENTS?
Call 1-800-720-3843 weekdays 9AM - 5PM EST
Distributed in the U.S. by:
JOHNSON & JOHNSON CONSUMER PRODUCTS COMPANY
Division of Johnson & Johnson Consumer Companies, Inc.
Skillman, NJ 08558-9418

DESITIN MULTI-PURPOSE FRAGRANCE FREE (petrolatum)

Johnson & Johnson Consumer Products Company, Division of Johnson & Johnson Consumer Companies, Inc.

DRUG FACTS

Active Ingredient(s)
Petrolatum 70.3%

Purpose(s)
Skin Protectant

USES
- helps treat and prevent diaper rash
- protects chafed skin due to diaper rash and helps seal out wetness
- temporarily protects and helps relieve chapped, or cracked skin
- helps prevent and protect from the drying effects of wind and cold weather
- temporarily protects minor:
  - cuts
  - scrapes
  - burns

WARNINGS
For external use only.

WHEN USING THIS PRODUCT
- Do not get into eyes

STOP USE AND ASK A DOCTOR IF
- condition worsens
- symptoms last more than 7 days or clear up and occur again within a few days.

DO NOT USE ON
- deep or puncture wounds
- animal bites
- serious burns

Keep out of reach of children. If swallowed, get medical help or contact a Poison Control Center right away.

DIRECTIONS
For diaper rash:
- Change wet or soiled diapers promptly
- Cleanse the diaper area and allow to dry
- Apply ointment liberally as often as necessary, with each diaper change, especially at bedtime or any time when exposure to wet diapers may be prolonged

For skin irritation:
- apply as needed.

OTHER INFORMATION
- store between 20° - 25°C (68° -77°F)
- twist off cap, remove quality seal. Do not use if quality seal is broken.

INACTIVE INGREDIENTS
mineral oil, paraffin, theobroma cacao (cocoa) seed butter, tocopheryl acetate, sodium pyruvate, retinyl palmitate, cholecalciferol

QUESTIONS OR COMMENTS?
Call 1-800-720-3843, weekdays, 9AM - 5PM EST

DESITIN SOOTHING RASH BATH TREATMENT (oatmeal)

Johnson & Johnson Consumer Products Company, Division of Johnson & Johnson Consumer Companies, Inc.

DRUG FACTS

Active Ingredient(s)
Colloidal Oatmeal (43%)

Purpose(s)
Skin Protectant

USES
Temporary protects and helps relieve minor skin irritation and itching due to:
- Rashes

WARNINGS
For external use only.

WHEN USING THIS PRODUCT
- Do not get into eyes
- To avoid slipping use mat in tub or shower
- In some skin conditions, soaking too long may overdry

STOP USE AND ASK A DOCTOR IF
• Condition worsens
• Symptoms last more than 7 days or clear up and occur again within a few days.

Keep out of reach of children. If swallowed, get medical help or contact a Poison Control Center right away.

DIRECTIONS
For dispersal in water:
• Turn warm water faucet on to full force
• Slowly sprinkle packette of colloidal oatmeal directly under faucet into the tub or container
• Stir any colloidal oatmeal settled on the bottom

For use as a soak in a bath:
• Slowly sprinkle one packette in an infant tub filled with warm water. Stir any colloidal oatmeal that may have settled on the bottom.
• Soak affected area for 15 to 30 minutes as needed, or as directed by a doctor
• Pat dry (do not rub) to keep a thin layer on the skin.

INACTIVE INGREDIENTS
mineral oil, calcium silicate, laureth-4, tocopheryl acetate, aloe barbadensis leaf extract

QUESTIONS OR COMMENTS?
Call 1-800-720-3843 Weekdays, 8AM - 8PM EST

CHILDRENS DIMETAPP COLD AND ALLERGY LIQUID (brompheniramine maleate and phenylephrine HCl)

Richmond Division of Wyeth LLC

DRUG FACTS

Active Ingredient(s) (in each 5 mL tsp)
Brompheniramine maleate, USP 1 mg
Phenylephrine HCl, USP 2.5 mg

Purpose(s)
Antihistamine
Nasal decongestant

USES
• temporarily relieves nasal congestion due to the common cold, hay fever or other upper respiratory allergies
• temporarily relieves these symptoms due to hay fever (allergic rhinitis):
  • runny nose
  • sneezing
  • itchy, watery eyes
  • itching of the nose or throat
• temporarily restores freer breathing through the nose

WARNINGS

DO NOT USE
• to sedate a child or to make a child sleepy
• if you are now taking a prescription monoamine oxidase inhibitor (MAOI) (certain drugs for depression, psychiatric, or emotional conditions, or Parkinson's disease), or for 2 weeks after stopping the MAOI drug. If you do not know if your prescription drug contains an MAOI, ask a doctor or pharmacist before taking this product.

ASK A DOCTOR BEFORE USE IF YOU HAVE
• heart disease
• high blood pressure
• thyroid disease
• diabetes
• trouble urinating due to an enlarged prostate gland
• glaucoma
• a breathing problem such as emphysema, asthma, or chronic bronchitis

ASK A DOCTOR OR PHARMACIST BEFORE USE IF YOU ARE
• taking any other oral nasal decongestant or stimulant
• taking sedatives or tranquilizers

WHEN USING THIS PRODUCT
• **do not use more than directed**
• drowsiness may occur
• avoid alcoholic beverages
• alcohol, sedatives, and tranquilizers may increase drowsiness
• be careful when driving a motor vehicle or operating machinery
• excitability may occur, especially in children

STOP USE AND ASK A DOCTOR IF
• you get nervous, dizzy, or sleepless
• symptoms do not get better within 7 days or are accompanied by fever

If pregnant or breast-feeding,
ask a health professional before use.

Keep out of reach of children.
In case of overdose, get medical help or contact a Poison Control Center right away.

DIRECTIONS
• do not take more than 6 doses in any 24-hour period

age	dose
adults and children 12 years and over	4 tsp every 4 hours
children 6 to under 12 years	2 tsp every 4 hours
children under 6 years	do not use

OTHER INFORMATION
• **each teaspoon contains:** sodium 3 mg
• store at 20-25°C (68-77°F)
• dosage cup provided

INACTIVE INGREDIENTS
anhydrous citric acid, artificial flavor, FD&C blue no. 1, FD&C red no. 40, glycerin, propylene glycol, purified water, sodium benzoate, sodium citrate, sorbitol solution, sucralose

QUESTIONS OR COMMENTS?
Call weekdays from 9 AM to 5 PM EST at **1-800-762-4675**

CHILDRENS DIMETAPP COLD AND ALLERGY CHEWABLE TABLETS
(brompheniramine maleate and phenylephrine HCl)

Richmond Division of Wyeth LLC

DRUG FACTS

Active Ingredient(s) (in each tablet)
Brompheniramine maleate, USP 1 mg
Phenylephrine HCl, USP 2.5 mg

Purpose(s)
Antihistamine
Nasal decongestant

USES
- temporarily relieves nasal congestion due to the common cold, hay fever or other upper respiratory allergies
- temporarily relieves these symptoms due to hay fever (allergic rhinitis) or other upper respiratory allergies:
  - runny nose
  - sneezing
  - itchy, watery eyes
  - itching of the nose or throat
- temporarily restores freer breathing through the nose

WARNINGS

DO NOT USE
- to sedate a child or to make a child sleepy
- if you are now taking a prescription monoamine oxidase inhibitor (MAOI) (certain drugs for depression, psychiatric, or emotional conditions, or Parkinson's disease), or for 2 weeks after stopping the MAOI drug. If you do not know if your prescription drug contains an MAOI, ask a doctor or pharmacist before taking this product.

ASK A DOCTOR BEFORE USE IF YOU HAVE
- heart disease
- high blood pressure
- thyroid disease
- diabetes
- trouble urinating due to an enlarged prostate gland
- glaucoma
- a breathing problem such as emphysema, asthma or chronic bronchitis

ASK A DOCTOR OR PHARMACIST BEFORE USE IF YOU ARE
- taking any other oral nasal decongestant or stimulant
- taking sedatives or tranquilizers

WHEN USING THIS PRODUCT
- **do not use more than directed**
- drowsiness may occur
- avoid alcoholic beverages
- alcohol, sedatives and tranquilizers may increase drowsiness
- be careful when driving a motor vehicle or operating machinery
- excitability may occur, especially in children

STOP USE AND ASK A DOCTOR IF
- you get nervous, dizzy, or sleepless
- symptoms do not get better within 7 days or are accompanied by fever

If pregnant or breast feeding,
ask a health professional before use.

Keep out of reach of children.
In case of overdose, get medical help or contact a Poison Control Center right away.

DIRECTIONS
- do not take more than 6 doses in any 24-hour period

age	dose
adults and children 12 years and over	4 tablets every 4 hours
children 6 to under 12 years	2 tablets every 4 hours
children under 6 years	do not use

OTHER INFORMATION
- store at 20-25°C (68-77°F)

INACTIVE INGREDIENTS
carmine, carrageenan, croscarmellose sodium, fructose, fumaric acid, glycine, magnesium stearate, maltodextrin, mannitol, microcrystalline cellulose, modified starch, natural and artificial flavor, polyethylene oxide, silicon dioxide, sorbitol, sucralose, tribasic calcium phosphate

QUESTIONS OR COMMENTS?
call weekdays from 9 AM to 5 PM EST at **1-800-762-4675**

CHILDRENS DIMETAPP COLD AND COUGH
(brompheniramine maleate, dextromethorphan HBr, and phenylephrine HCl)
Richmond Division of Wyeth LLC

DRUG FACTS

Active Ingredient(s) (in each 5 mL tsp)
Brompheniramine maleate, USP 1 mg
Dextromethorphan HBr, USP 5 mg
Phenylephrine HCl, USP 2.5 mg

Purpose(s)
Antihistamine
Cough suppressant
Nasal decongestant

USES
- temporarily relieves cough due to minor throat and bronchial irritation occurring with a cold, and nasal congestion due to the common cold, hay fever or other upper respiratory allergies
- temporarily relieves these symptoms due to hay fever (allergic rhinitis):
  - runny nose
  - sneezing
  - itchy, watery eyes
  - itching of the nose or throat
- temporarily restores freer breathing through the nose

WARNINGS

DO NOT USE
- to sedate a child or to make a child sleepy
- if you are now taking a prescription monoamine oxidase inhibitor (MAOI) (certain drugs for depression, psychiatric, or emotional conditions, or Parkinson's disease), or for 2 weeks after stopping the MAOI drug. If you do not know if your prescription drug contains an MAOI, ask a doctor or pharmacist before taking this product.

ASK A DOCTOR BEFORE USE IF YOU HAVE
- heart disease
- high blood pressure
- thyroid disease
- diabetes
- trouble urinating due to an enlarged prostate gland
- glaucoma
- cough that occurs with too much phlegm (mucus)
- a breathing problem or persistent or chronic cough that lasts such as occurs with smoking, asthma, chronic bronchitis, or emphysema

ASK A DOCTOR OR PHARMACIST BEFORE USE IF YOU ARE
- taking any other oral nasal decongestant or stimulant
- taking sedatives or tranquilizers

WHEN USING THIS PRODUCT
- **do not use more than directed**
- may cause marked drowsiness
- avoid alcoholic beverages
- alcohol, sedatives, and tranquilizers may increase drowsiness

- be careful when driving a motor vehicle or operating machinery
- excitability may occur, especially in children

STOP USE AND ASK A DOCTOR IF
- you get nervous, dizzy, or sleepless
- symptoms do not get better within 7 days or are accompanied by fever
- cough lasts more than 7 days, comes back, or is accompanied by fever, rash, or persistent headache. These could be signs of a serious condition.

If pregnant or breast-feeding,
ask a health professional before use.

Keep out of reach of children.
In case of overdose, get medical help or contact a Poison Control Center right away.

DIRECTIONS
- do not take more than 6 doses in any 24-hour period

age	dose
adults and children 12 years and over	4 tsp every 4 hours
children 6 to under 12 years	2 tsp every 4 hours
children under 6 years	do not use

OTHER INFORMATION
- **each teaspoon contains:** sodium 3 mg
- store at 20-25°C (68-77°F)
- dosage cup provided

INACTIVE INGREDIENTS
anhydrous citric acid, artificial flavor, FD&C blue no. 1, FD&C red no. 40, glycerin, propylene glycol, purified water, sodium benzoate, sodium citrate, sorbitol solution, sucralose

QUESTIONS OR COMMENTS?
Call weekdays from 9 AM to 5 PM EST at **1-800-762-4675**

CHILDRENS DIMETAPP LONG ACTING COUGH PLUS COLD (chlorpheniramine maleate and dextromethorphan HBr)

Richmond Division of Wyeth

DRUG FACTS

Active Ingredient(s) (in each 5 mL teaspoon)
Chlorpheniramine maleate, USP 1.0 mg
Dextromethorphan HBr, USP 7.5 mg

Purpose(s)
Antihistamine
Cough suppressant

USES
- temporarily relieves cough due to minor throat and bronchial irritation as may occur with a cold
- temporarily relieves these symptoms due to hay fever or other upper respiratory allergies:
  - runny nose
  - sneezing
  - itchy, watery eyes
  - itching of the nose or throat

WARNINGS

DO NOT USE
- to sedate a child or to make a child sleepy
- if you are now taking a prescription monoamine oxidase inhibitor (MAOI) (certain drugs for depression, psychiatric, or emotional conditions, or Parkinson's disease), or for 2 weeks after stopping the MAOI drug. If you do not know if your prescription drug contains an MAOI, ask a doctor or pharmacist before taking this product.

ASK A DOCTOR BEFORE USE IF YOU HAVE
- trouble urinating due to an enlarged prostate gland
- glaucoma
- a cough that occurs with too much phlegm (mucus)
- a breathing problem or chronic cough that lasts or as occurs with smoking, asthma, chronic bronchitis or emphysema

ASK A DOCTOR OR PHARMACIST BEFORE USE IF YOU ARE
taking sedatives or tranquilizers

WHEN USING THIS PRODUCT
- **do not use more than directed**
- marked drowsiness may occur
- avoid alcoholic drinks
- alcohol, sedatives, and tranquilizers may increase drowsiness
- be careful when driving a motor vehicle or operating machinery
- excitability may occur, especially in children

STOP USE AND ASK A DOCTOR IF
cough lasts more than 7 days, comes back, or is accompanied by fever, rash, or persistent headache. These could be signs of a serious condition.

If pregnant or breast-feeding,
ask a health professional before use.

Keep out of reach of children.
In case of overdose, get medical help or contact a Poison Control Center right away.

DIRECTIONS
- do not take more than 4 doses in any 24-hour period

age	dose
12 years and over	4 tsp every 6 hours
6 to under 12 years	2 tsp every 6 hours
under 6 years	do not use

OTHER INFORMATION
- **each teaspoon contains:** sodium 3 mg
- store at 20-25°C (68-77°F)
- dosage cup provided

INACTIVE INGREDIENTS
anhydrous citric acid, artificial flavor, FD&C blue no. 1, FD&C red no. 40, glycerin, propylene glycol, purified water, sodium benzoate, sodium citrate, sorbitol solution, sucralose

QUESTIONS OR COMMENTS?
Call weekdays from 9 AM to 5 PM EST at **1-800-762-4675**

CHILDRENS DIMETAPP MULTISYMPTOM COLD AND FLU (acetaminophen, chlorpheniramine maleate, dextromethorphan HBr, and phenylephrine HCl)

Richmond Division of Wyeth

DRUG FACTS

Active Ingredient(s) (in each 5 mL tsp)
Acetaminophen, USP 160 mg
Chlorpheniramine maleate, USP 1 mg
Dextromethorphan HBr, USP 5 mg
Phenylephrine HCl, USP 2.5 mg

Purpose(s)
Pain reliever/Fever reducer
Antihistamine
Cough suppressant
Nasal decongestant

USES
- temporarily relieves these symptoms associated with a cold, or flu:
  - headache
  - sore throat
  - fever
  - minor aches and pains
- temporarily relieves nasal congestion, and cough due to minor throat and bronchial irritation occurring with a cold
- temporarily relieves these symptoms due to hay fever or other upper respiratory allergies:
  - sneezing
  - itching of the nose or throat
  - itchy, watery eyes
  - runny nose
- temporarily restores freer breathing through the nose

WARNINGS
Liver warning:
This product contains acetaminophen. Severe liver damage may occur if user takes
- more than 5 doses in any 24-hour period, which is the maximum daily amount
- with other drugs containing acetaminophen
- 3 or more alcoholic drinks every day while using this product

Sore throat warning:
If sore throat is severe, persists for more than 2 days, is accompanied or followed by fever, headache, rash, nausea, or vomiting, consult a doctor promptly.

DO NOT USE
- to sedate a child or to make a child sleepy
- in a child under 6 years of age
- if user is now taking a prescription monoamine oxidase inhibitor (MAOI) (certain drugs for depression, psychiatric, or emotional conditions, or Parkinson's disease), or for 2 weeks after stopping the MAOI drug. If you do not know if your prescription drug contains an MAOI, ask a doctor or pharmacist before taking this product.
- with any other drug containing acetaminophen (prescription or nonprescription). If you are not sure whether a drug contains acetaminophen ask a doctor or pharmacist.

ASK A DOCTOR BEFORE USE IF USER HAS
- liver disease
- heart disease
- high blood pressure
- thyroid disease
- diabetes
- trouble urinating due to an enlarged prostate gland
- glaucoma
- cough that occurs with too much phlegm (mucus)
- a breathing problem or chronic cough that lasts or as occurs with smoking, asthma, chronic bronchitis, or emphysema

ASK A DOCTOR OR PHARMACIST BEFORE USE IF USER IS
- taking the blood thinning drug warfarin
- taking any other oral nasal decongestant or stimulant
- taking any other pain reliever/fever reducer
- taking sedatives or tranquilizers

WHEN USING THIS PRODUCT
- **do not use more than directed**
- marked drowsiness may occur
- avoid alcoholic drinks
- alcohol, sedatives, and tranquilizers may increase drowsiness

- be careful when driving a motor vehicle or operating machinery
- excitability may occur, especially in children

STOP USE AND ASK A DOCTOR IF
- user gets nervous, dizzy, or sleepless
- pain, cough, or nasal congestion gets worse or lasts more than 5 days (children) or 7 days (adults)
- fever gets worse or lasts more than 3 days
- redness or swelling is present
- cough comes back or occurs with rash or headache that lasts. These could be signs of a serious condition.
- new symptoms occur

If pregnant or breast-feeding,
ask a health professional before use.

Keep out of reach of children.
In case of overdose, get medical help or contact a Poison Control Center right away. Prompt medical attention is critical for adults as well as for children, even if you do not notice any signs or symptoms.

DIRECTIONS
- do not take more than 5 doses in any 24-hour period
- do not exceed recommended dosage. Taking more than the recommended dose (overdose) may cause serious liver damage.

age	dose
adults and children 12 years and over	4 teaspoons every 4 hours
children 6 to 12 years	2 teaspoons every 4 hours
children under 6 years	do not use

OTHER INFORMATION
- **each teaspoon contains:** sodium 2 mg
- store at 20-25°C (68-77°F)
- dosage cup provided

INACTIVE INGREDIENTS
anhydrous citric acid, artificial flavor, FD&C red no. 40, glycerin, menthol, polyethylene glycol, propyl gallate, propylene glycol, purified water, sodium benzoate, sodium citrate, sorbitol solution, sucralose

QUESTIONS OR COMMENTS?
Call weekdays from 9 AM to 5 PM EST at **1-800-762-4675**

CHILDRENS DIMETAPP NIGHTTIME COLD AND CONGESTION (diphenhydramine HCl and phenylephrine HCl)

Richmond Division of Wyeth LLC, and a subsidiary of Pfizer Inc.

DRUG FACTS

Active Ingredient(s) (in each 5 mL tsp)
Diphenhydramine HCl, USP 6.25 mg
Phenylephrine HCl, USP 2.5 mg

Purpose(s)
Antihistamine/Cough suppressant
Nasal decongestant

USES
- temporarily relieves these symptoms occurring with a cold, hay fever, or other upper respiratory allergies:
  - nasal congestion
  - cough
  - runny nose
  - sneezing

- itchy, watery eyes
- itching of the nose or throat

WARNINGS

DO NOT USE
- to sedate a child or to make a child sleepy
- If you are now taking a prescription monoamine oxidase inhibitor (MAOI) (certain drugs for depression, psychiatric, or emotional conditions, or Parkinson's disease), or for 2 weeks after stopping the MAOI drug. If you do not know if your prescription drug contains an MAOI, ask a doctor or pharmacist before taking this product.
- with any other product containing diphenhydramine, even one used on skin

ASK A DOCTOR BEFORE USE IF YOU HAVE
- heart disease
- high blood pressure
- thyroid disease
- diabetes
- trouble urinating due to an enlarged prostate gland
- glaucoma
- cough that occurs with too much phlegm (mucus)
- a breathing problem or chronic cough that lasts or as occurs with smoking, asthma, chronic bronchitis, or emphysema

ASK A DOCTOR OR PHARMACIST BEFORE USE IF YOU ARE
- taking any other oral nasal decongestant or stimulant
- taking sedatives or tranquilizers

WHEN USING THIS PRODUCT
- **do not use more than directed**
- marked drowsiness may occur
- avoid alcoholic drinks
- alcohol, sedatives, and tranquilizers may increase drowsiness
- be careful when driving a motor vehicle or operating machinery
- excitability may occur, especially in children

STOP USE AND ASK A DOCTOR IF
- you get nervous, dizzy, or sleepless
- symptoms do not get better within 7 days or are accompanied by fever
- cough lasts more than 7 days, comes back, or is accompanied by fever, rash or persistent headache. These could be signs of a serious condition.

If pregnant or breast-feeding,
ask a health professional before use.

Keep out of reach of children.
In case of overdose, get medical help or contact a Poison Control Center right away.

DIRECTIONS
- do not take more than 6 doses in any 24-hour period
- do not exceed recommended dosage

age	dose
adults and children 12 years and over	4 tsp every 4 hours
children 6 to under 12 years	2 tsp every 4 hours
children under 6 years	do not use

OTHER INFORMATION
- **each teaspoon contains:** sodium 4 mg
- store at 20 -25°C (68 -77°F)
- dosage cup provided

INACTIVE INGREDIENTS
anhydrous citric acid, artificial flavor, FD&C blue no.1, FD&C red no. 40, glycerin, propyl gallate, propylene glycol, purified water, sodium benzoate, sodium citrate, sorbitol solution, sucralose

QUESTIONS OR COMMENTS?
Call weekdays from 9 AM to 5 PM EST at **1-800-762-4675**

DRAMAMINE CHEWABLE FORMULA
(dimenhydrinate)

McNeil Consumer Healthcare Div McNeil-PPC, Inc

DRUG FACTS

Active Ingredient(s) (in each tablet)
Dimenhydrinate 50 mg

Purpose(s)
Antiemetic

USE
for prevention and treatment of these symptoms associated with motion sickness:
- nausea
- vomiting
- dizziness

WARNINGS

DO NOT USE
for children under 2 years of age unless directed by a doctor

ASK A DOCTOR BEFORE USE IF YOU HAVE
- a breathing problem such as emphysema or chronic bronchitis
- glaucoma
- trouble urinating due to an enlarged prostate gland

ASK A DOCTOR OR PHARMACIST BEFORE USE IF YOU ARE
taking sedatives or tranquilizers

WHEN USING THIS PRODUCT
- marked drowsiness may occur
- avoid alcoholic drinks
- alcohol, sedatives, and tranquilizers may increase drowsiness
- be careful when driving a motor vehicle or operating machinery

If pregnant or breast-feeding, ask a health professional before use.
Keep out of reach of children. In case of overdose, get medical help or contact a Poison Control Center right away. (1-800-222-1222)

DIRECTIONS
- to prevent motion sickness, the first dose should be taken ½ to 1 hour before starting activity
- to prevent or treat motion sickness, see below:

adults and children 12 years and over	take 1 to 2 chewable tablets every 4-6 hours do not take more than 8 chewable tablets in 24 hours, or as directed by a doctor
children 6 to under 12 years	give ½ to 1 chewable tablet every 6-8 hours do not give more than 3 chewable tablets in 24 hours, or as directed by a doctor
children 2 to under 6 years	give ½ chewable tablet every 6-8 hours do not give more than 1-1/2 chewable tablets in 24 hours, or as directed by a doctor

OTHER INFORMATION
- Phenylketonurics: contains phenylalanine 0.84 mg per tablet
- store between 20-25°C (68-77°F)
- **do not use if carton is opened or if blister unit is broken or torn**
- see side panel for lot number and expiration date

INACTIVE INGREDIENTS
anhydrous citric acid, aspartame, FD&C yellow #6 aluminum lake, flavors, magnesium stearate, maltodextrin, methacrylic acid copolymer, modified starch, sorbitol

QUESTIONS OR COMMENTS?
call **1-800-382-7219**

DRAMAMINE FOR KIDS (dimenhydrinate)
Medtech Products Inc.

DRUG FACTS

Active Ingredient(s)
(in each tablet)
Dimenhydrinate 25 mg

Purpose(s)
Antiemetic

USE
for prevention and treatment of these symptoms associated with motion sickness:
- nausea
- vomiting
- dizziness

WARNINGS

DO NOT USE
for children under 2 years of age unless directed by a doctor

ASK A DOCTOR BEFORE USE IF THE CHILD HAS
- a breathing problem such as emphysema or chronic bronchitis
- glaucoma

ASK A DOCTOR OR PHARMACIST BEFORE USE IF THE CHILD IS
taking sedatives or tranquilizers

WHEN USING THIS PRODUCT
- marked drowsiness may occur
- avoid alcoholic drinks
- alcohol, sedatives, and tranquilizers may increase drowsiness

- be careful when driving a motor vehicle or operating machinery

If pregnant or breast-feeding,
ask a doctor before use.

Keep out of reach of children.
In case of accidental overdose, get medical help or contact a Poison Control Center (1-800-222-1222) right away.

DIRECTIONS
- to prevent motion sickness, the first dose should be taken ½ to 1 hour before starting activity
- to prevent or treat motion sickness, see below:

Children 2 to under 6 years	give ½ to 1 chewable tablet every 6-8 hours do not give more than 3 chewable tablets in 24 hours, or as directed by a doctor
Children 6 to under 12 years	give 1 to 2 chewable tablets every 6-8 hours do not give more than 6 chewable tablets in 24 hours, or as directed by a doctor

OTHER INFORMATION
- Phenylketonurics: contains phenylalanine 0.84 mg per tablet
- store at room temperature 68° - 77°F (20° - 25°C)
- **do not use if blister is broken or torn**

INACTIVE INGREDIENTS
aspartame, citric acid, flavor, magnesium stearate, methacrylic acid copolymer, sorbitol

QUESTIONS OR COMMENTS?
1-800-382-7219 Dramamine.com

DRAMAMINE LESS DROWSY (meclizine hydrochloride)
Medtech Products Inc.

DRUG FACTS

Active Ingredient(s)
(in each tablet)
Meclizine HCl 25 mg

Purpose(s)
Antiemetic

USE
for prevention and treatment of these symptoms associated with motion sickness:
- nausea
- vomiting
- dizziness

WARNINGS

DO NOT USE
for children under 12 years of age unless directed by a doctor

ASK A DOCTOR BEFORE USE IF YOU HAVE
- a breathing problem such as emphysema or chronic bronchitis
- glaucoma
- trouble urinating due to an enlarged prostate gland

ASK A DOCTOR OR PHARMACIST BEFORE USE IF YOU ARE
taking sedatives or tranquilizers

WHEN USING THIS PRODUCT
• drowsiness may occur
• avoid alcoholic drinks
• alcohol, sedatives, and tranquilizers may increase drowsiness
• be careful when driving a motor vehicle or operating machinery

If pregnant or breast-feeding,
ask a doctor before use.

Keep out of reach of children.
In case of overdose, get medical help or contact a Poison Control Center (1-800-222-1222) right away.

DIRECTIONS
• take first dose one hour before starting activity
• adults and children 12 years and over: 1 to 2 tablets once daily, or as directed by a doctor

OTHER INFORMATION
• store between 20 - 25°C (68 - 77°F)
• do not use if blister is broken or torn

INACTIVE INGREDIENTS
anhydrous lactose, corn starch, colloidal silicon dioxide, D&C yellow # 10 aluminum lake, magnesium stearate, microcrystalline cellulose

QUESTIONS OR COMMENTS?
call 1-800-382-7219

DRAMAMINE ORIGINAL FORMULA
(dimenhydrinate)

McNeil Consumer Healthcare Div McNeil-PPC, Inc

DRUG FACTS

Active Ingredient(s) (in each tablet)
Dimenhydrinate 50 mg

Purpose(s)
Antiemetic

USE
for prevention and treatment of these symptoms associated with motion sickness:
• nausea
• vomiting
• dizziness

WARNINGS

DO NOT USE
for children under 2 years of age unless directed by a doctor

ASK A DOCTOR BEFORE USE IF YOU HAVE
• a breathing problem such as emphysema or chronic bronchitis
• glaucoma
• trouble urinating due to an enlarged prostate gland

ASK A DOCTOR OR PHARMACIST BEFORE USE IF YOU ARE
taking sedatives or tranquilizers

WHEN USING THIS PRODUCT
• marked drowsiness may occur
• avoid alcoholic drinks

• alcohol, sedatives, and tranquilizers may increase drowsiness
• be careful when driving a motor vehicle or operating machinery

If pregnant or breast-feeding, ask a health professional before use.
Keep out of reach of children. In case of overdose, get medical help or contact a Poison Control Center right away. (1-800-222-1222)

DIRECTIONS
• to prevent motion sickness, the first dose should be taken ½ to 1 hour before starting activity
• to prevent or treat motion sickness, see below:

adults and children 12 years and over	take 1 to 2 tablets every 4-6 hours do not take more than 8 tablets in 24 hours, or as directed by a doctor
children 6 to under 12 years	give ½ to 1 tablet every 6-8 hours do not give more than 3 tablets in 24 hours, or as directed by a doctor
children 2 to under 6 years	give ½ tablet every 6-8 hours do not give more than 1-1/2 tablets in 24 hours, or as directed by a doctor

OTHER INFORMATION
• store between 20-25°C (68-77°F)
• **do not use if carton is opened or if blister unit is broken or torn**
• see side panel for lot number and expiration date

INACTIVE INGREDIENTS
anhydrous lactose, colloidal silicon dioxide, croscarmellose sodium, magnesium stearate, microcrystalline cellulose

QUESTIONS OR COMMENTS?
call **1-800-382-7219**

DULCOLAX BALANCE (polyethylene glycol 3350)

Boehringer Ingelheim Pharmaceuticals Inc

Active Ingredient(s) (in each dose) (Pouches Only)
Polyethylene Glycol 3350, 17 g

Active Ingredient(s) (in each dose) (Bottle Only)
Polyethylene Glycol 3350, 17 g (cap filled to line)

Purpose(s)
Laxative

USES
• relieves occasional constipation (irregularity)
• generally produces a bowel movement in 1 to 3 days

WARNINGS
Allergy alert: Do not use if you are allergic to polyethylene glycol

DO NOT USE
if you have kidney disease, except under the advice and supervision of a doctor

ASK A DOCTOR BEFORE USE IF YOU HAVE

- nausea, vomiting or abdominal pain
- a sudden change in bowel habits that lasts over 2 weeks
- irritable bowel syndrome

ASK A DOCTOR OR PHARMACIST BEFORE USE IF YOU ARE

taking a prescription drug

WHEN USING THIS PRODUCT

you may have loose, watery, more frequent stools

STOP USE AND ASK A DOCTOR IF

- you have rectal bleeding or your nausea, bloating, cramping or abdominal pain gets worse. These may be signs of a serious condition.
- you get diarrhea
- you need to use a laxative for longer than 1 week

If pregnant or breast-feeding,
ask a health professional before use.

Keep out of reach of children.
In case of overdose, get medical help or contact a Poison Control Center right away.

DIRECTIONS (POUCHES ONLY)

- do not take more than directed unless advised by your doctor
- adults and children 17 years of age and older:
- stir and dissolve one packet of powder (17 g) in any 4 to 8 ounces of beverage (cold, hot or room temperature) then drink
- use once a day
- use no more than 7 days
- children 16 years of age or under: ask a doctor

DIRECTIONS (BOTTLE ONLY)

- do not take more than directed unless advised by your doctor
- the bottle top is a measuring cap marked to contain 17 grams of powder when filled to the indicated line (white section in cap)
- adults and children 17 years of age or older:
- fill to top of white section in cap which is marked to indicate the correct dose (17 g)
- stir and dissolve in any 4 to 8 ounces of beverage (cold, hot or room temperature) then drink
- use once a day
- use no more than 7 days
- children 16 years of age or under: ask a doctor

OTHER INFORMATION

- store at 20°-25°C (68°-77°F)
- tamper-evident: do not use if printed foil pouch is open or broken (Pouches Only)
- tamper-evident: do not use if printed foil seal under cap is missing, open or broken (Bottle Only)

INACTIVE INGREDIENTS

QUESTIONS OR COMMENTS?

about DULCOLAX BALANCE? 1-888-285-9159
(English/Spanish) or www.Dulcolax.com

DULCOLAX (bisacodyl)

Boehringer Ingelheim Pharmaceuticals, Inc.

DRUG FACTS

Active Ingredient(s) (in each suppository)	Purpose(s)
Bisacodyl USP 10 mg	Stimulant laxative

USES

- for temporary relief of occasional constipation and irregularity
- this product generally produces bowel movement in 15 minutes to 1 hour

WARNINGS

For rectal use only

ASK A DOCTOR BEFORE USE IF YOU HAVE

- stomach pain, nausea or vomiting
- a sudden change in bowel habits that lasts more than 2 weeks

WHEN USING THIS PRODUCT IT

may cause stomach discomfort, faintness, rectal burning and mild cramps

STOP USE AND ASK A DOCTOR IF

- you have rectal bleeding or no bowel movement after using this product. These could be signs of a serious condition.
- you need to use a laxative for more than 1 week

If pregnant or breast-feeding, ask a health professional before use.
Keep out of reach of children. If swallowed, get medical help or contact a Poison Control Center right away.

DIRECTIONS

adults and children 12 years of age and over	1 suppository in a single daily dose. Peel open plastic. Insert suppository well into rectum, pointed end first. Retain about 15 to 20 minutes.
children 6 to under 12 years of age	1/2 suppository in a single daily dose
children under 2 years of age	ask a doctor

OTHER INFORMATION

- do not store above 30°C (86°F)

INACTIVE INGREDIENT

hydrogenated vegetable oil

ECOTRIN (aspirin)

GlaxoSmithKline Consumer Healthcare LP

Active Ingredient(s) (in each tablet) (Low Strength)
Aspirin (NSAID)* 81mg
*nonsteroidal anti-inflammatory drug

Active Ingredient(s) (in each tablet) (Regular Strength)
Aspirin (NSAID)* 325mg
*nonsteroidal anti-inflammatory drug

Purpose(s)
Pain reliever

USES
- temporarily relieves minor aches and pains due to:
  - headache
  - menstrual pain
  - minor arthritis pain
  - muscle pain
  - toothache
  - colds
- or as recommended by a doctor

WARNINGS
Reye's syndrome: Children and teenagers who have or are recovering from chicken pox or flu-like symptoms should not use this product. When using this product, if changes in behavior with nausea and vomiting occur, consult a doctor because these symptoms could be an early sign of Reye's syndrome, a rare but serious illness.
Allergy alert: Aspirin may cause a severe allergic reaction which may include:
- hives
- facial swelling
- shock
- asthma (wheezing)

Stomach bleeding warning: This product contains an NSAID, which may cause severe stomach bleeding. The chance is higher if you
- are age 60 or older
- have had stomach ulcers or bleeding problems
- take a blood thinning (anticoagulant) or steroid drug
- take other drugs containing prescription or nonprescription NSAIDs (aspirin, ibuprofen, naproxen, or others)
- have 3 or more alcoholic drinks every day while using this product
- take more or for a longer time than directed

DO NOT USE
if you have ever had an allergic reaction to aspirin or any other pain reliever/fever reducer

ASK A DOCTOR BEFORE USE IF
- stomach bleeding warnings applies to you
- you have a history of stomach problems, such as heartburn
- you have high blood pressure, heart disease, liver cirrhosis, or kidney disease
- you are taking a diuretic
- you have asthma

ASK A DOCTOR OR PHARMACIST BEFORE USE IF YOU ARE
taking a prescription drug for diabetes, gout, or arthritis

STOP USE AND ASK A DOCTOR IF
- allergic reaction occurs. Seek medical help right away.
- you experience any of the following signs of stomach bleeding:
  - feel faint
  - vomit blood
  - have bloody or black stools
  - have stomach pain that does not get better
- pain gets worse or lasts more than 10 days
- redness or swelling is present
- any new symptoms appear
- ringing in the ears or a loss of hearing occurs

These could be signs of a serious condition.
If pregnant or breast-feeding, ask a health professional before use. It is especially important not to use aspirin during the last 3 months of pregnancy unless definitely directed to do so by a doctor because it may cause problems in the unborn child or complications during delivery.
Keep out of reach of children. In case of overdose, get medical help or contact a Poison Control Center right away.

DIRECTIONS (LOW STRENGTH)
- adults and children 12 years of age or over: take 4 to 8 tablets every 4 hours, while symptoms persist. Drink a full glass of water with each dose.
- do not take more than 48 tablets in 24 hours unless directed by a doctor
- children under 12 years of age: ask a doctor

DIRECTIONS (REGULAR STRENGTH)
- adults and children 12 years of age or over: take 1 to 2 tablets every 4 hours, while symptoms persist. Drink a full glass of water with each dose.
- do not take more than 12 tablets in 24 hours unless directed by a doctor
- children under 12 years of age: ask a doctor

OTHER INFORMATION
- Tamper Evident Feature: Do not use if printed inner-seal beneath cap is missing or broken.
- store below 25°C (77°F)

INACTIVE INGREDIENTS (LOW STRENGTH)
carnauba wax, colloidal silicon dioxide, EDTA, FD&C yellow#6, glyceryl monostearate, hypromellose, methacrylic acid copolymer, methylparaben, microcrystalline cellulose, polysorbate 80, propylparaben, starch, stearic acid, talc, titanium dioxide, triethyl citrate. Printed with edible black ink.

INACTIVE INGREDIENTS (REGULAR STRENGTH)
carnauba wax, colloidal silicon dioxide, EDTA, FD&C yellow#6, glyceryl monostearate, hypromellose, methacrylic acid copolymer, methylparaben, microcrystalline cellulose, polysorbate 80, pregelatinized starch, propylparaben, sodium starch glycolate, stearic acid, talc, titanium dioxide, triethyl citrate. Printed with edible ink.

QUESTIONS OR COMMENTS?
call toll-free **1-800-245-1040** (English/Spanish) weekdays ECOTRIN is a registered trademark of the GlaxoSmithKline group of companies.
GlaxoSmithKline Consumer Healthcare, L.P. Moon Township, PA 15108, Made in Thailand www.ecotrin.com

ECOTRIN REGULAR STRENGTH (aspirin)
Medtech Products Inc.

DRUG FACTS

Active Ingredient(s)
(in each tablet)
Aspirin (NSAID) *325mg
*nonsteroidal anti-inflammatory drug

Purpose(s)
Pain reliever

USES
- temporarily relieves minor aches and pains due to:
  - headache
  - minor arthritis pain
  - toothache
  - menstrual pain
  - colds
- or as recommended by a doctor

WARNINGS
Reye's syndrome: Children and teenagers who have or are recovering from chicken pox or flu-like symptoms should not use this product. When using this product, if changes in behavior with nausea and vomiting occur, consult a doctor because these

symptoms could be an early sign of Reye's syndrome, a rare but serious illness.

Allergy alert: Aspirin may cause a severe allergic reaction which may include:
- hives
- shock
- facial swelling
- asthma (wheezing)

Stomach bleeding warning: This product contains an NSAID, which may cause severe stomach bleeding. The chance is higher if you
- are age 60 or older
- have had stomach ulcers or bleeding problems
- take a blood thinning (anticoagulant) or steroid drug
- take other drugs containing prescription or nonprescription NSAIDs (aspirin, ibuprofen, naproxen, or others)
- have 3 or more alcoholic drinks every day while using this product
- take more or for a longer time than directed

DO NOT USE
if you have ever had an allergic reaction to aspirin or any other pain reliever/fever reducer

ASK A DOCTOR BEFORE USE IF
- stomach bleeding warning applies to you
- you have a history of stomach problems, such as heartburn
- you have high blood pressure, heart disease, liver cirrhosis, or kidney disease
- you are taking a diuretic
- you have asthma

ASK A DOCTOR OR PHARMACIST BEFORE USE IF YOU ARE
taking a prescription drug for diabetes, gout, or arthritis

STOP USE AND ASK A DOCTOR IF
- allergic reaction occurs. Seek medical help right away.
- you experience any of the following signs of stomach bleeding:
  - feel faint
  - vomit blood
  - have bloody or black stools
  - have stomach pain that does not get better
- pain gets worse or lasts more than 10 days
- redness or swelling is present
- any new symptoms appear
- ringing in the ears or a loss of hearing occurs

These could be signs of a serious condition.

If pregnant or breast-feeding,
ask a health professional before use. It is especially important not to use aspirin during the last 3 months of pregnancy unless definitely directed to do so by a doctor because it may cause problems in the unborn child or complications during delivery.

Keep out of reach of children.
In case of overdose, get medical help or contact a Poison Control Center right away.

DIRECTIONS
- adults and children 12 years of age and over: take 1 to 2 tablets every 4 hours, while symptoms persist. Drink a full glass of water with each dose.
- do not take more than 12 tablets in 24 hours unless directed by a doctor
- children under 12 years of age: ask a doctor

OTHER INFORMATION
- Tamper Evident Feature: Do not use if printed inner-seal beneath cap is missing or broken.
- store below 25°C (77°F)

INACTIVE INGREDIENTS
carnauba wax, colloidal silicon dioxide, EDTA, FD&C yellow#6, glyceryl monostearate, hypromellose, methacrylic acid copolymer, methylparaben, microcrystalline cellulose, polysorbate 80, pregelatinized starch, propylparaben, sodium starch glycolate, stearic acid, talc, titanium dioxide, triethyl citrate. Printed with edible ink.

QUESTIONS OR COMMENTS?
call toll-free **1-866-255-5202** (English/Spanish) weekdays

EMETROL CHERRY (phosphorated carbohydrate)
WellSpring Pharmaceutical Corporation

Active Ingredient(s)
Phosphorated carbohydrate solution*
*each 5 mL contains:
- 3.74 g Total sugar
- 21.5 mg Phosphoric acid

Purpose(s)
Upset Stomach Reliever

USES
For relief of upset stomach associated with nausea due to overindulgence in food and drink.

WARNINGS
- This product contains fructose and should not be taken by persons with hereditary fructose intolerance (HFI).

DO NOT USE IF YOU HAVE
- allergic reactions to any of the ingredients in this product

ASK A DOCTOR BEFORE USE IF YOU HAVE
- diabetes

STOP USE AND ASK A DOCTOR IF
- symptoms persist, return or get worse

If pregnant or breast-feeding,
ask a health professional before use.

Keep out of reach of children.
In case of overdose, get medical help or contact a Poison Control Center right away. (1-800-222-1222)

DIRECTIONS
- For maximum effectiveness never dilute or drink fluids of any kind immediately before or after taking this product
- adults and children 12 years of age and over: one to two tablespoons
- children 2 to under 12: one or two teaspoons
- repeat dose every 15 minutes or until distress subsides
- do not take more than 5 doses in 1 hour without consulting a doctor

OTHER INFORMATION
- Store between 20-25°C (68-77°F) away from heat and direct light; keep from freezing
- **Do not use if printed foil seal under bottle cap is broken or missing**

INACTIVE INGREDIENTS
FD&C red no. 40, flavors, glycerin, methylparaben, and purified water.

QUESTIONS OR COMMENTS?
call 1-866-337-4500

DISTRIBUTED BY
WellSpring Pharmaceutical Corporation
Sarasota, FL 34243 USA
(c) WellSpring 2009

EUCERIN Q10 ANTI-WRINKLE SENSITIVE SKIN LOTION (octinoxate, octisalate, and oxybenzone)

Beiersdorf Inc
Active ingredient(s)
Octinoxate 7.5%
Octisalate 3.0%
Oxybenzone 3.0%
Purpose(s)
Sunscreen

WARNINGS
Skin Cancer/Skin Aging Alert: Spending time in the sun increases your risk of skin cancer and early skin aging. This product has been shown only to help prevent sunburn, not skin cancer or early skin aging.
For external use only
Do not use on damaged or broken skin.
Stop use and ask a doctor if irritation occurs.
When using this product keep out of eyes. Rinse with water to remove.
Keep out of reach of children. If swallowed, get medical help or contact a Poison Control Center right away.

USES
• helps prevent sunburn

DIRECTIONS
For sunscreen use:
• apply liberally 15 minutes before sun exposure
• use a water resistant sunscreen if swimming or sweating
• reapply at least every 2 hours
• Children under 6 months of age: Ask a doctor

INACTIVE INGREDIENTS
water, glycerin, stearic acid, cetyl alcohol, cetearyl isononanoate, cyclopentasiloxane, glyceryl stearate SE, alcohol denat., cyclohexasiloxane, caprylic/capric triglyceride, octyldodecanol, ubiquinone, tocopheryl acetate, panthenol, carbomer, EDTA, sodium hydroxide, phenoxyethanol, methylparaben, ethylparaben, propylparaben, butylparaben, isobutylparaben

QUESTIONS OR COMMENTS?
1-800-227-4703

EUCERIN CALMING ITCH RELIEF TREATMENT (menthol)

Beiersdorf Inc

Your dry skin can become so uncomfortable and itchy that it seems like nothing will provide relief fast enough. The Solution? Eucerin Calming Itch-Relief Treatment with cooling menthol for immediate itch relief. Its soothing oatmeal formula provides relief that lasts for up to 8 hours.
• Preferred by dermatologists
• Provides immediate relief of itchy, dry skin
• Fast absorbing lightweight lotion spreads easily over skin
• Appropriate for use on children and for atopic dermatitis
• Free of fragrances that can irritate sensitive skin

Menthol 0.1%
External analgesic lotion
Use for the temporary relief of itching associated with minor skin irritations.
For external use only.

WHEN USING THIS PRODUCT
avoid contact with eyes.

STOP USE AND ASK A DOCTOR IF
• condition worsens
• symptoms last more than 7 days or clear up and occur again within a few days
• irritation occurs

Keep out of reach of children. If swallowed, get medical help or contact a Poison Control Center right away.

QUESTIONS OR COMMENTS?
1-800-227-4703

INACTIVE INGREDIENTS
water, glycerin, octyldodecanol, caprylic/capric triglyceride, isopropyl stearate, myristyl myristate, cetyl alcohol, colloidal oatmeal, cetearyl alcohol, dimethicone, glyceryl stearate SE, oenothera biennis (evening primrose) oil, benzyl alcohol, phenoxyethanol, DMDM hydantoin, PEG-40 castor oil, caprylyl glycol, acrylates/C10-30 alkyl acrylate crosspolymer, sodium cetearyl sulfate, sodium citrate, polyglyceryl-3 methyl glucose distearate, potassium sorbate, citric acid

EXCEDRIN BACK AND BODY (acetaminophen and aspirin)

Novartis Consumer Health, Inc.
Active Ingredient(s)
Acetaminophen 250
Buffered aspirin equal to 250 mg aspirin (NSAID)*
(buffered with calcium carbonate)
*nonsteroidal anti-inflammatory drug

Purpose(s)
Pain reliever
Pain reliever

USES
• for the temporary relief of minor aches and pains due to:
  • minor pain of arthritis
  • backache
  • muscular aches

WARNINGS
Reye's syndrome: Children and teenagers who have or are recovering from chicken pox or flu-like symptoms should not use this product. When using this product, if changes in behavior with nausea and vomiting occur, consult a doctor because these symptoms could be an early sign of Reye's syndrome, a rare but serious illness.
Allergy alert: Aspirin may cause a severe allergic reaction which may include:
• hives
• facial swelling
• asthma (wheezing)
• shock

Liver warning: This product contains acetaminophen. Severe liver damage may occur if you take
• more than 8 caplets in 24 hours, which is the maximum daily amount
• with other drugs containing acetaminophen
• 3 or more alcoholic drinks every day while using this product

Stomach bleeding warning: This product contains an NSAID, which may cause severe stomach bleeding. The chance is higher if you
- are age 60 or older
- have had stomach ulcers or bleeding problems
- take a blood thinning (anticoagulant) or steroid drug
- take other drugs containing prescription or nonprescription NSAIDs (aspirin, ibuprofen, naproxen, or others)
- have 3 or more alcoholic drinks every day while using this product
- take more or for a longer time than directed

DO NOT USE
- if you have ever had an allergic reaction to acetaminophen, aspirin or any other pain reliever/fever reducer
- with any other drug containing acetaminophen (prescription or nonprescription). If you are not sure whether a drug contains acetaminophen, ask a doctor or pharmacist.

ASK DOCTOR BEFORE USE IF
- you have liver disease
- stomach bleeding warning applies to you
- you have a history of stomach problems, such as heartburn
- you have high blood pressure, heart disease, liver cirrhosis, or kidney disease
- you are taking a diuretic
- you have asthma

ASK THE DOCTOR OR PHARMACIST BEFORE USE IF YOU ARE TAKING
- any other drug containing an NSAID (prescription or nonprescription)
- a blood thinning (anticoagulant) or steroid drug.
- a prescription drug for diabetes, gout, or arthritis
- any other drug, or are under a doctor's care for any serious condition

STOP USE AND ASK A DOCTOR IF
- an allergic reaction occurs. Seek medical help right away
- you experience any of the following signs of stomach bleeding:
  - feel faint
  - vomit blood
  - have bloody or black stools
  - have stomach pain that does not get better
- ringing in the ears or loss of hearing occurs
- painful area is red or swollen
- pain gets worse or lasts for more than 10 days
- fever gets worse or lasts for more than 3 days
- any new symptoms appear

PREGNANCY OR BREAST FEEDING
ask a health professional before use. It is especially important not to use aspirin during the last 3 months of pregnancy unless definitely directed to do so by a doctor because it may cause problems in the unborn child or complications during delivery.

KEEP OUT OF REACH OF CHILDREN
In case of overdose, get medical help or contact a Poison Control Center right away. Quick medical attention is critical for adults as well as for children even if you do not notice any signs or symptoms.

DIRECTIONS
- **do not use more than directed**
- drink a full glass of water with each dose
- adults and children 12 years and over: take 2 caplets every 6 hours; not more than 8 caplets in 24 hours
- children under 12 years: ask a doctor

OTHER INFORMATION
- **each caplet contains:** calcium 80 mg
- store at controlled room temperature 20°-25°C (68°-77°F)

- read all product information before using. Keep this box for important information.

QUESTIONS OR COMMENTS?
1-800-468-7746
Distr. By: **Novartis Consumer Health, Inc.**
Parsippany, NJ 07054-0622 ©20XX
Visit us at www.excedrin.com

EXCEDRIN EXTRA STRENGTH PAIN RELIEVER (acetaminophen, aspirin (NSAID), and caffeine)

Novartis Consumer Health, Inc.

Active Ingredient(s) (in each caplet)
Acetaminophen 250 mg
Aspirin 250 mg (NSAID)*
Caffeine 65 mg
*nonsteroidal anti-inflammatory drug

Purpose(s)
Pain reliever
Pain reliever
Pain reliever aid

USES
- temporarily relieves minor aches and pains due to:
  - headache
  - a cold
  - arthritis
  - muscular aches
  - sinusitis
  - toothache
  - premenstrual & menstrual cramps

WARNINGS
Reye's syndrome:
Children and teenagers who have or are recovering from chicken pox or flu-like symptoms should not use this product. When using this product, if changes in behavior with nausea and vomiting occur, consult a doctor because these symptoms could be an early sign of Reye's syndrome, a rare but serious illness.

Allergy alert:
Aspirin may cause a severe allergic reaction which may include:
- hives
- facial swelling
- asthma (wheezing)
- shock

Liver warning:
This product contains acetaminophen. Severe liver damage may occur if you take
- more than 8 caplets in 24 hours, which is the maximum daily amount
- with other drugs containing acetaminophen
- 3 or more alcoholic drinks every day while using this product

Stomach bleeding warning:
This product contains a nonsteroidal anti-inflammatory drug (NSAID), which may cause stomach bleeding. The chance is higher if you
- are age 60 or older
- have had stomach ulcers or bleeding problems
- take a blood thinning (anticoagulant) or steroid drug
- take other drugs containing an NSAID (aspirin, ibuprofen, naproxen, or others)

- have 3 or more alcoholic drinks every day while using this product
- take more or for a longer time than directed

Caffeine warning:
The recommended dose of this product contains about as much caffeine as a cup of coffee. Limit the use of caffeine-containing medications, foods, or beverages while taking this product because too much caffeine may cause nervousness, irritability, sleeplessness, and, occasionally, rapid heart beat.

DO NOT USE
- if you have ever had an allergic reaction to aspirin or any other pain reliever/fever reducer
- with any other drug containing acetaminophen (prescription or nonprescription). If you are not sure whether a drug contains acetaminophen, ask a doctor or pharmacist.

ASK DOCTOR BEFORE USE IF
- you have liver disease
- stomach bleeding warning applies to you
- you have a history of stomach problems, such as heartburn
- you have high blood pressure, heart disease, liver cirrhosis. or kidney disease
- you are taking a diuretic
- high blood pressure
- you have asthma

ASK A DOCTOR OR PHARMACIST BEFORE USE
- any other drug containing an NSAID (prescription or nonprescription)
- a blood thinning (anticoagulant) or steroid drug
- a prescription drug for diabetes, gout, or arthritis
- any other drug, or are under a doctor's care for any serious condition

STOP USE AND ASK DOCTOR IF
- an allergic reaction occurs. Seek medical help right away.
- you experience any of the following signs os stomach bleeding
  - feel faint
  - vomit blood
  - have bloody or black stools
  - have stomach pain that does not get better
- ringing in the ears or loss of hearing occurs
- painful area is red or swollen
- pain gets worse or lasts for more than 10 days
- fever gets worse or lasts for more than 3 days
- any new symptoms appear

If pregnant or breast-feeding
ask a health professional before use. It is especially important not to use aspirin during the last 3 months of pregnancy unless definitely directed to do so by a doctor because it may cause problems in the unborn child or complications during delivery.

Keep out of reach of children

OVERDOSE WARNING
In case of overdose, get medical help or contact a Poison Control Center right away. Quick medical attention is critical for adults as well as for children even if you do not notice any signs or symptoms.

DIRECTIONS
- do not use more than directed **(see Overdose Warning)**
- drink a full glass of water with each dose
- adults and children 12 years and over: take 2 caplets every 6 hours; not more than 8 caplets in 24 hours
- children under 12 years: ask a doctor

OTHER INFORMATION
- store at controlled room temperature 20^0 - 25^0 C (68^0 - 77^0 F)
- read all product information before using. Keep this box for important information

INACTIVE INGREDIENTS
benzoic acid, carnauba wax, FD&C blue #1, hydroxypropylcellulose, hypromellose, light mineral oil, microcrystalline cellulose, polysorbate 20, povidone, propylene glycol, simethicone emulsion, sorbitan monolaurate, stearic acid, titanium dioxide

EXCEDRIN MENSTRUAL COMPLETE
(acetaminophen, aspirin (NSAID), and caffeine)
Novartis Consumer Health, Inc.

Active Ingredient(s) (in each gelcap)
Acetaminophen 250 mg
Aspirin 250 mg (NSAID)*
Caffeine 65 mg
*nonsteroidal anti-inflammatory drug

Purpose(s)
Pain reliever
Pain reliever
Diuretic

USES
- temporarily relieves minor aches and pains due to:
- muscular aches • headache • backache • premenstrual & menstrual cramps
- temporarily relieves these symptoms associated with menstrual periods:
- water-weight gain • bloating • swelling • full feeling • fatigue

WARNINGS
Reye's syndrome: Children and teenagers who have or are recovering from chicken pox or flu-like symptoms should not use this product. When using this product, if changes in behavior with nausea and vomiting occur, consult a doctor because these symptoms could be an early sign of Reye's syndrome, a rare but serious illness.
Liver warning: This product contains acetaminophen. Severe liver damage may occur if you take
- more than 8 gelcaps in 24 hours, which is the maximum daily amount
- with other drugs containing acetaminophen
- 3 or more alcoholic drinks every day while using this product

Stomach bleeding warning: This product contains an NSAID, which may cause severe stomach bleeding. The chance is higher if you
- are age 60 or older
- have had stomach ulcers or bleeding problems
- take a blood thinning (anticoagulant) or steroid drug
- take other drugs containing prescription or nonprescription NSAIDs (aspirin, ibuprofen, naproxen, or others)
- have 3 or more alcoholic drinks every day while using this product
- take more or for a longer time than directed

Caffeine warning: The recommended dose of this product contains about as much caffeine as a cup of coffee. Limit the use of caffeine-containing medications, foods, or beverages while taking this product because too much caffeine may cause nervousness, irritability, sleeplessness, and, occasionally, rapid heart beat.

ALLERGY ALERT
Allergy alert: Aspirin may cause a severe allergic reaction which may include:
- hives • facial swelling • asthma (wheezing) • shock

DO NOT USE
- if you have ever had an allergic reaction to acetaminophen, aspirin or any other pain reliever/fever reducer

• with any other drug containing acetaminophen (prescription or nonprescription). If you are not sure whether a drug contains acetaminophen, ask a doctor or pharmacist.

ASK A DOCTOR BEFORE USE IF
• you have liver disease
• stomach bleeding warning applies to you
• you have a history of stomach problems, such as heartburn
• you have high blood pressure, heart disease, liver cirrhosis, or kidney disease
• you are taking a diuretic
• you have asthma

ASK A DOCTOR OR PHARMACIST BEFORE USE IF YOU ARE
taking:
• any other drug containing an NSAID (prescription or nonprescription)
• a blood thinning (anticoagulant) or steroid drug
• a prescription drug for diabetes, gout, or arthritis
• any other drug, or are under a doctor's care for any serious condition

STOP USE AND ASK A DOCTOR IF
• an allergic reaction occurs. Seek medical help right away.
• you experience any of the following signs of stomach bleeding
  • feel faint
  • vomit blood
  • have bloody or black stools
  • have stomach pain that does not get better
• ringing in the ears or loss of hearing occurs
• painful area is red or swollen
• pain gets worse or lasts for more than 10 days
• fever gets worse or lasts for more than 3 days
• any new symptoms appear

PREGNANCY OR BREAST FEEDING
If pregnant or breast-feeding, ask a health professional before use. It is especially important not to use aspirin during the last 3 months of pregnancy unless definitely directed to do so by a doctor because it may cause problems in the unborn child or complications during delivery.

KEEP OUT OF REACH OF CHILDREN
Keep out of reach of children.

OVERDOSE
In case of overdose, get medical help or contact a Poison Control Center right away. Quick medical attention is critical for adults as well as for children even if you do not notice any signs or symptoms.

DIRECTIONS
• **do not use more than directed**
• drink a full glass of water with each dose
• adults and children 12 years and over: take 2 gelcaps every 4-6 hours; not more than 8 gelcaps in 24 hours
• children under 12 years: ask a doctor

OTHER INFORMATION
• store at controlled room temperature 20°-25°C (68°-77°F)
• read all product information before using. Keep this box for important information.

INACTIVE INGREDIENTS
benzoic acid, D&C red # 28, D&C yellow #10, FD&C green #3, gelatin, hydroxypropyl cellulose, hypromellose, light mineral oil, microcrystalline cellulose, pepsin, polysorbate 20, povidone, propylene glycol, simethicone emulsion, sorbitan monolaurate, stearic acid, titanium dioxide

QUESTIONS OR COMMENTS?
1-800-468-7746
Distr. By: Novartis Consumer Health, Inc.
Parsippany, NJ 07054-0622 ©2009
Visit us at www.excedrin.com

EXCEDRIN MIGRAINE (acetaminophen, aspirin (NSAID), and caffeine)

Novartis Consumer Health, Inc.

Active Ingredient(s)
Acetaminophen 250 mg
Aspirin 250 mg (NSAID) *
Caffeine 65 mg
* nonsteroidal anti-inflammatory drug

Purpose(s)
Pain reliever
Pain reliever
Pain reliever aid

USES
• treats migraine

WARNINGS
Reye's syndrome: Children and teenagers who have or are recovering from chicken pox or flu-like symptoms should not use this product. When using this product, if changes in behavior with nausea and vomiting occur, consult a doctor because these symptoms could be an early sign of Reye's syndrome, a rare but serious illness.
Allergy alert: Aspirin may cause a severe allergic reaction which may include:
• hives
• facial swelling
• asthma (wheezing)
• shock

Liver warning: This product contains acetaminophen. Severe liver damage may occur if you take
• more than 2 tablets in 24 hours, which is the maximum daily amount
• with other drugs containing acetaminophen
• 3 or more alcoholic drinks every day while using this product

Stomach bleeding warning: This product contains an NSAID, which may cause severe stomach bleeding. The chance is higher if you
• are age 60 or older
• have had stomach ulcers or bleeding problems
• take a blood thinning (anticoagulant) or steroid drug
• take other drugs containing prescription or nonprescription NSAIDs (aspirin, ibuprofen, naproxen, or others)
• have 3 or more alcoholic drinks every day while using this product
• take more or for a longer time than directed

Caffeine warning: The recommended dose of this product contains about as much caffeine as a cup of coffee. Limit the use of caffeine-containing medications, foods, or beverages while taking this product because too much caffeine may cause nervousness, irritability, sleeplessness, and, occasionally, rapid heart beat.

DO NOT USE
• if you have ever had an allergic reaction to acetaminophen, aspirin or any other pain reliever/fever reducer
• with any other drug containing acetaminophen (prescription or nonprescription). If you are not sure whether a drug contains acetaminophen, ask a doctor or pharmacist

ASK DOCTOR BEFORE USE IF
• you have never had migraines diagnosed by a health professional

- you have a headache that is different from your usual migraines
- you have the worst headache of your life
- you have fever and stiff neck
- you have headaches beginning after or caused by head injury, exertion, coughing or bending
- you experienced your first headache after the age of 50
- you have daily headaches
- you have a migraine so severe as to require bed rest
- you have liver disease
- stomach bleeding warning applies to you
- you have a history of stomach problems, such as heartburn
- you have high blood pressure, heart disease, liver cirrhosis, or kidney disease
- you are taking a diuretic
- you have asthma
- you have problems or serious side effects from taking pain relievers or fever reducers
- you have vomiting with your migraine headache

ASK A DOCTOR OR PHARMACIST BEFORE USE IF YOU ARE
- taking a prescription drug for:
  - anticoagulation (thinning of the blood)
  - diabetes
  - gout
  - arthritis
- under a doctor's care for any serious condition
- taking any other drug
- taking any other product that contains aspirin, acetaminophen, or any other pain reliever/fever reducer

STOP USE AND ASK A DOCTOR IF
- an allergic reaction occurs. Seek medical help right away.
- you experience any of the following signs of stomach bleeding
  - feel faint
  - vomit blood
  - have bloody or black stools
  - have stomach pain that does not get better
- your migraine is not relieved or worsens after first dose
- new or unexpected symptoms occur
- ringing in the ears or loss of hearing occurs

IF PREGNANT OR BREAST-FEEDING
ask a health professional before use. It is especially important not to use aspirin during the last 3 months of pregnancy unless definitely directed to do so by a doctor because it may cause problems in the unborn child or complications during delivery.

KEEP OUT OF REACH OF CHILDREN
In case of overdose, get medical help or contact a Poison Control Center right away. Quick medical attention is critical for adults as well as for children even if you do not notice any signs or symptoms.

DIRECTIONS
- **do not use more than directed**
- adults: take 2 tablets with a glass of water
- if symptoms persist or worsen, ask your doctor
- do not take more than 2 tablets in 24 hours, unless directed by a doctor
- under 18 years of age: ask a doctor

OTHER INFORMATION
- store at 20°-25°C (68°-77°F)
- read all product information before using. Keep this box for important information.

INACTIVE INGREDIENTS
carnauba wax, crospovidone, FD&C blue #1 aluminum lake, hypromellose, microcrystalline cellulose, povidone, pregelatinized starch, propylene glycol, saccharin sodium, stearic acid, titanium dioxide

QUESTIONS OR COMMENTS?
1-800-468-7746
Distr. By:
Novartis Consumer Health, Inc.
Parsippany, NJ 07054-0622

EXCEDRIN PM (acetaminophen and diphenhydramine citrate)
Novartis Consumer Health, Inc.

Active Ingredient(s)
Acetaminophen 500 mg
Diphenhydramine citrate 38 mg

Purpose(s)
Pain reliever
Nighttime sleep-aid

USES
for the temporary relief of occasional headaches and minor aches and pains with accompanying sleeplessness.

WARNINGS
Liver warning: This product contains acetaminophen. Severe liver damage may occur if you take
- more than 2 caplets in 24 hours, which is the maximum daily amount
- with other drugs containing acetaminophen
- 3 or more alcoholic drinks every day while using this product

DO NOT USE
- if you are allergic to acetaminophen
- with any other drug containing acetaminophen (prescription or nonprescription). If you are not sure whether a drug contains acetaminophen, ask a doctor or pharmacist.
- with any other product containing diphenhydramine, even one used on skin
- in children under 12 years of age

ASK A DOCTOR BEFORE USE IF YOU HAVE
- liver disease
- glaucoma
- a breathing problem such as emphysema or chronic bronchitis
- trouble urinating due to an enlarged prostate gland

ASK A DOCTOR OR PHARMACIST BEFORE USE IF YOU ARE
- taking the blood thinning drug warfarin
- taking sedatives or tranquilizers

WHEN USING THIS PRODUCT
- avoid alcoholic drinks
- drowsiness may occur
- be careful when driving a motor vehicle or operating machinery

STOP USE AND ASK A DOCTOR IF
- any new symptoms occur
- sleeplessness lasts continuously for more than 2 weeks. Insomnia may be a symptom of serious underlying medical illness.
- pain gets worse or lasts for more than 10 days
- painful area is red or swollen
- fever gets worse or lasts for more than 3 days

IF PREGNANT OR BREAST-FEEDING,
ask a health professional before use.

KEEP OUT OF REACH OF CHILDREN

OVERDOSE
In case of overdose, get medical help or contact a Poison Control Center right away. Quick medical attention is critical for adults as well as for children even if you do not notice any signs or symptoms

DIRECTIONS
- **do not use more than directed**
- do not use in children under 12 years of age
- adults and children 12 years of age and over: take 2 caplets at bedtime, if needed, or as directed by a doctor

OTHER INFORMATION
- store at controlled room temperature 20°-25°C (68°-77°F)
- read all product information before using. Keep this box for important information.

INACTIVE INGREDIENTS
benzoic acid, carnauba wax, croscarmellose sodium, D&C yellow #10 lake, FD&C blue #1 lake, hypromellose, light mineral oil, magnesium stearate, microcrystalline cellulose, polysorbate 20, povidone, pregelatinized starch, propylene glycol, simethicone emulsion, sodium citrate, sorbitan monolaurate, stearic acid, titanium dioxide

QUESTIONS OR COMMENTS?
1-800-468-7746
Distr. By: Novartis Consumer Health, Inc.
Parsippany, NJ 07054-0622 ©2008
Visit us at www.excedrin.com

ADDITIONAL INFORMATION
Country of origin -- USA per NAFTA requirements

Tamper-Evident Feature -

> TAMPER-EVIDENT BOTTLE DO NOT USE IF INNER FOIL SEAL IMPRINTED WITH "SEALED for YOUR PROTECTION" IS BROKEN OR MISSING

Exempt packaging statement --

> THIS PACKAGE FOR HOUSEHOLDS WITHOUT YOUNG CHILDREN

READ ALL PRODUCT INFORMATION BEFORE USING. KEEP BOX FOR IMPORTANT INFORMATION.

EXCEDRIN SINUS HEADACHE CAPLETS
(acetaminophen and phenylephrine hydrochloride)

Novartis Consumer Health, Inc.

DRUG FACTS

Active Ingredient(s) (in each caplet)	Purpose(s)
Acetaminophen 325 mg	Pain reliever
Phenylephrine HCl 5 mg	Nasal decongestant

USES
- temporarily relieves:
  - headache
  - minor aches and pains
  - nasal congestion
  - sinus congestion and pressure
- helps clear nasal passages; shrinks swollen membranes

WARNINGS
Liver warning
This product contains acetaminophen. Sever liver damage may occur if you take
- more than 12 caplets in 24 hours, which is the maximum daily amount
- with other drugs containing acetaminophen
- 3 or more alcoholic drinks every day while using this product

DO NOT USE
- if you are allergic to acetaminophen
- with any other drug containing acetaminophen (presciption or nonprescription). If you are not sure whether a drug contains acetaminophen, ask a doctor or pharmacist.
- if you are now taking a prescription monoamine oxidase inhibitor (MAOI) (certain drugs for depression, psychiatric or emotional conditions, or Parkinson's disease), or for 2 weeks after stopping the MAOI drug. If you do not know if your prescription drug contains an MAOI, ask a doctor or pharmacist before taking this product.

ASK A DOCTOR BEFORE USE IF YOU HAVE
- liver disease
- trouble urinating due to an enlarged prostate gland
- heart disease
- high blood pressure
- thyroid disease
- diabetes

ASK A DOCTOR OR PHARMACIST BEFORE USE IF YOU ARE
- taking the blood thinning drug warfarin

WHEN USING THIS PRODUCT
- do not use more than directed

STOP USE AND ASK A DOCTOR IF
- any new symptoms occur
- you get nervous, dizzy, or sleepless
- painful area is red or swollen
- pain or nasal congestion gets worse or lasts for more than 7 days
- fever gets worse or lasts for more than 3 days

If pregnant or breast-feeding, ask a health professional before use.

Keep out of reach of children.
In case of overdose, get medical help or contact a Poison Control Center right away. Quick medical attention is critical for adults as well as for children even if you do not notice any signs or symptoms.

DIRECTIONS
- **do not use more than directed**
- adults and children 12 years and over: take 2 caplets every 4 hours; not more than 12 caplets in 24 hours
- children under 12 years: ask a doctor

OTHER INFORMATION
- store at controlled room temperature 20°-25°C (68°-77°F)
- read all product information before using.

INACTIVE INGREDIENTS
benzoic acid, carnauba wax, corn starch, FD&C blue #1, hypromellose, light mineral oil, magnesium stearate, microcrystalline cellulose, polysorbate 20, povidone, propylene glycol, simethicone emulsion, sorbitan monolaurate, stearic acid, titanium dioxide

QUESTIONS OR COMMENTS?
1-800-468-7746

EXCEDRIN TENSION HEADACHE
(acetaminophen and caffeine)

Novartis Consumer Health, Inc.

Active Ingredient(s)
Acetaminophen 500 mg
Caffeine 65 mg

Purpose(s)
Pain reliever

USES
• temporarily relieves minor aches and pains due to:
• headache • muscular aches

WARNINGS
Liver warning: This product contains acetaminophen. Severe liver damage may occur if you take
• more than 8 caplets in 24 hours, which is the maximum daily amount
• with other drugs containing acetaminophen
• 3 or more alcoholic drinks every day while using this product
Caffeine warning: The recommended dose of this product contains about as much caffeine as a cup of coffee. Limit the use of caffeine-containing medications, foods, or beverages while taking this product because too much caffeine may cause nervousness, irritability, sleeplessness, and, occasionally, rapid heart beat.

DO NOT USE
• if you are allergic to acetaminophen
• with any other drug containing acetaminophen (prescription or nonprescription). If you are not sure whether a drug contains acetaminophen, ask a doctor or pharmacist.

ASK A DOCTOR BEFORE USE IF YOU HAVE
• liver disease

ASK A DOCTOR OR PHARMACISTS
• taking the blood thinning drug warfarin

STOP USE AND ASK A DOCTOR IF
• any new symptoms occur
• painful area is red or swollen
• pain gets worse or lasts for more than 10 days
• fever gets worse or lasts for more than 3 days

PREGNANCY OR BREAST FEEDING
ask a health professional before use.

KEEP OUT OF REACH OF CHILDREN
In case of overdose, get medical help or contact a Poison Control Center right away. Quick medical attention is critical for adults as well as for children even if you do not notice any signs or symptoms.

DIRECTIONS
• **do not use more than directed**
• adults and children 12 years and over: take 2 caplets every 6 hours; not more than 8 caplets in 24 hours

OTHER INFORMATION
• store at controlled room temperature 20°-25°C (68°-77°F)
• read all product information before using. Keep this box for important information.

INACTIVE INGREDIENTS
benzoic acid, carnauba wax, D&C red # 27 lake, D&C yellow # 10 lake, FD&C blue # 1 lake, FD&C red # 40, hypromellose, light mineral oil, magnesium stearate, microcrystalline cellulose, polysorbate 20, povidone, pregelatinized starch, propylene glycol, simethicone emulsion, sorbitan monolaurate, stearic acid, titanium dioxide

QUESTIONS OR COMMENTS?
1-800-468-7746
Distr. By:
Novartis Consumer Health, Inc.
Parsippany, NJ 07054-0622
Visit us at www.excedrin.com

EX-LAX MAXIMUM STRENGTH (sennosides)

Novartis Consumer Health, Inc.

DRUG FACTS

Active Ingredient(s) (in each pill)	Purpose(s)
Sennosides, USP, 25 mg	Stimulant laxative

USES
• relieves occasional constipation (irregularity)
• generally produces bowel movement in 6 to 12 hours

WARNINGS

DO NOT USE
laxative products when abdominal pain, nausea, or vomiting are present unless directed by a doctor

ASK A DOCTOR BEFORE USE IF YOU HAVE
• noticed a sudden change in bowel habits that persists over a period of 2 weeks

ASK A DOCTOR OR PHARMACIST BEFORE USE IF YOU
• are taking a prescription drug. Laxatives may affect how other drugs work. Take this product 2 or more hours before or after other drugs.

WHEN USING THIS PRODUCT
• do not use for a period longer than 1 week

STOP USE AND ASK A DOCTOR IF
• rectal bleeding or failure to have a bowel movement occur after use of a laxative. These may be signs of a serious condition.

If pregnant or breast-feeding, ask a health professional before use.
Keep out of reach of children. In case of overdose, get medical help or contact a Poison Control Center right away.

DIRECTIONS
• Swallow pill(s) with a glass of water.
• Swallow pill(s) whole, do not crush, break, or chew.

adults and children 12 years of age and older	2 pills once or twice daily
children 6 to under 12 years of age	1 pill once or twice daily
children under 6 years of age	ask a doctor

OTHER INFORMATION
• each piece contains: **calcium 50mg**
• sodium free
• store at controlled room temperature 20-25 °C (68-77°F) Protect from moisture.

INACTIVE INGREDIENTS

acacia, alginic acid, carnauba wax, colloidal silicon dioxide, dibasic calcium phosphate, FD&C blue no.1 aluminum lake, iron oxide black, magnesium stearate, microcrystalline cellulose, potassium hydroxide, povidone, pregelatinized starch, propylene glycol, shellac, sodium benzoate, sodium lauryl sulfate, stearic acid, sucrose, talc, titanium dioxide.

QUESTIONS OR COMMENTS?

call **1-800-452-0051**

EX-LAX REGULAR STRENGTH CHOCOLATE

(sennosides)

Novartis Consumer Health, Inc.

DRUG FACTS

Active Ingredient(s) (in each piece)	Purpose(s)
Sennosides, USP, 15 mg	Stimulant laxative

USES

• relieves occasional constipation (irregularity)
• generally produces bowel movement in 6 to 12 hours

WARNINGS

DO NOT USE

laxative products when abdominal pain, nausea, or vomiting are present unless directed by a doctor

ASK A DOCTOR BEFORE USE IF YOU HAVE

• noticed a sudden change in bowel habits that persists over a period of 2 weeks

ASK A DOCTOR OR PHARMACIST BEFORE USE IF YOU

• are taking a prescription drug. Laxatives may affect how other drugs work. Take this product 2 or more hours before or after other drugs.

WHEN USING THIS PRODUCT

• do not use for a period longer than 1 week.

STOP USE AND ASK A DOCTOR IF

• rectal bleeding or failure to have a bowel movement occur after use of a laxative. These may be signs of a serious condition.

If pregnant or breast-feeding, ask a health professional before use.
Keep out of reach of children. In case of overdose, get medical help or contact a Poison Control Center right away.

DIRECTIONS

adults and children 12 years of age and older	chew 2 chocolated pieces once or twice daily
children 6 to under 12 years of age	chew 1 chocolated piece once or twice daily
children under 6 years of age	ask a doctor

OTHER INFORMATION

• each piece contains: **potassium 10mg**
• sodium free
• store at controlled room temperature 20-25°C (68-77°F)

INACTIVE INGREDIENTS

cocoa, confectioners sugar, hydrogenated palm kernel oil, lecithin, non-fat dry milk, vanillin

QUESTIONS OR COMMENTS?

call **1-800-452-0051**

FEVERALL ADULTS (acetaminophen)

Actavis Mid Atlantic LLC

Active Ingredient(s)
Acetaminophen 650 mg

Purpose(s)
Pain reliever/fever reducer

USES

Temporarily
• reduces fever
• relieves minor aches, pains, and headache

WARNINGS

Liver warning: This product contains acetaminophen. Severe liver damage may occur if
• an adult or child 12 years and older takes more than 6 doses in 24 hours, which is the maximum daily amount
• taken with other drugs containing acetaminophen
• an adult takes 3 or more alcoholic drinks everyday while using this product

For rectal use only

DO NOT USE

• in children under 12 years.
• if you are allergic to acetaminophen.
• with any other drug containing acetaminophen (prescription or nonprescription). If you are not sure whether a drug contains acetaminophen, ask a doctor or pharmacist

ASK A DOCTOR BEFORE USE IF

• you have liver disease.
• you are taking the blood thinning drug warfarin.

STOP USE AND ASK A DOCTOR IF

• fever lasts more than 3 days (72 hours), or recurs.
• pain gets worse or lasts more than 10 days.
• new symptoms occur.
• redness or swelling is present in the painful area.

These may be signs of a serious condition.

OTC - PREGNANCY OR BREAST FEEDING

If pregnant or breast-feeding, ask a health professional before use.

KEEP OUT OF REACH OF CHILDREN

If swallowed or in case of overdose, get medical help or contact a Poison Control Center right away. Quick medical attention is critical in case of overdose for adults and for children even if you do not notice any signs or symptoms.

DIRECTIONS

• **do not use more than directed**
• remove wrapper
• carefully insert suppository well up into the rectum
• adults and children 12 years and older:
  • 1 suppository every 4 to 6 hours while symptoms last
  • do not exceed 6 suppositories in any 24-hour period
• **children under 12 years: ask a doctor**

OTHER INFORMATION
- store at 2°-27°C (35°-80°F)
- do not use if imprinted suppository wrapper is opened or damaged

INACTIVE INGREDIENTS
glycerol monostearate, hydrogenated vegetable oil, polyoxyethylene stearate, polysorbate 80

QUESTIONS OR COMMENTS?
1-800-432-8534 (select option #2) between 9 am and 4 pm EST, Monday - Friday.

FEVERALL CHILDREN (acetaminophen)
Actavis Mid Atlantic LLC

Active Ingredient(s)
Acetaminophen 120 mg

Purpose(s)
Pain reliever/fever reducer

USES
Temporarily
- reduces fever
- relieves minor aches, pains, and headache

WARNINGS
Liver warning: This product contains acetaminophen. Severe liver damage may occur if your child takes
- more than 5 doses in 24 hours, which is the maximum daily amount
- with other drugs containing acetaminophen

For rectal use only

DO NOT USE
- if you are allergic to acetaminophen.
- with any other drug containing acetaminophen (prescription or nonprescription). If you are not sure whether a drug contains acetaminophen, ask a doctor or pharmacist

ASK A DOCTOR BEFORE USE IF
- the child has liver disease.
- the child is taking the blood thinning drug warfarin.

STOP USE AND ASK A DOCTOR IF
- fever lasts more than 3 days (72 hours), or recurs.
- pain lasts more than 5 days or gets worse.
- new symptoms occur.
- redness or swelling is present in the painful area.

These may be signs of a serious condition.

KEEP OUT OF REACH OF CHILDREN
If swallowed or in case of overdose, get medical help or contact a Poison Control Center right away. Quick medical attention is critical in case of overdose for adults and for children even if you do not notice any signs or symptoms.

DIRECTIONS
- **this product does not contain directions or warnings for adult use**
- **do not use more than directed**
- remove wrapper
- carefully insert suppository well up into the rectum

Dosing Chart

Age	Dose
under 3 years	Do not use unless directed by a doctor
3 to 6 years	Use 1 suppository every 4 to 6 hours (maximum of 5 doses in 24 hours)

OTHER INFORMATION
- store at 2°-27°C (35°-80°F)
- do not use if imprinted suppository wrapper is opened or damaged

INACTIVE INGREDIENTS
glycerol monostearate, hydrogenated vegetable oil, polyoxyethylene stearate, polysorbate 80

QUESTIONS OR COMMENTS?
1-800-432-8534 (select option #2) between 9 am and 4 pm EST, Monday - Friday.

FEVERALL INFANTS (acetaminophen)
Actavis Mid Atlantic LLC

Active Ingredient(s)
Acetaminophen 80 mg

Purpose(s)
Pain reliever/fever reducer

USES
Temporarily
- reduces fever
- relieves minor aches, pains, and headache

WARNINGS
Liver warning: This product contains acetaminophen. Severe liver damage may occur if your child takes
- more than 4 doses in 24 hours, which is the maximum daily amount for ages 6 to 11 months
- more than 5 doses in 24 hours, which is the maximum daily amount for ages 12 to 36 months
- with other drugs containing acetaminophen

For rectal use only

DO NOT USE
- if you are allergic to acetaminophen.
- with any other drug containing acetaminophen (prescription or nonprescription). If you are not sure whether a drug contains acetaminophen, ask a doctor or pharmacist

ASK A DOCTOR BEFORE USE IF
- the child has liver disease.
- the child is taking the blood thinning drug warfarin.

STOP USE AND ASK A DOCTOR IF
- fever lasts more than 3 days (72 hours), or recurs.
- pain lasts more than 3 days or gets worse.
- new symptoms occur.
- redness or swelling is present in the painful area.

These may be signs of a serious condition.

KEEP OUT OF REACH OF CHILDREN
If swallowed or in case of overdose, get medical help or contact a Poison Control Center right away. Quick medical attention is critical in case of overdose for adults and for children even if you do not notice any signs or symptoms.

DIRECTIONS
- **this product does not contain directions or warnings for adult use**
- **do not use more than directed**
- remove wrapper
- carefully insert suppository well up into the rectum

Dosing Chart	
Age	Dose
under 6 months	Do not use unless directed by a doctor
6 to 11 months	Use 1 suppository every 6 hours (maximum of 4 doses in 24 hours)
12 to 36 months	Use 1 suppository every 4 to 6 hours (maximum of 5 doses in 24 hours)

OTHER INFORMATION
- store at 2(-27(C (35(-80(F)
- do not use if imprinted suppository wrapper is opened or damaged

INACTIVE INGREDIENTS
glycerol monostearate, hydrogenated vegetable oil, polyoxyethylene stearate, polysorbate 80

QUESTIONS OR COMMENTS?
1-800-432-8534 (select option #2) between 9 am and 4 pm EST, Monday - Friday.

FEVERALL JUNIOR (acetaminophen)
Actavis Mid Atlantic LLC

Active Ingredient(s)
Acetaminophen 325 mg

Purpose(s)
Pain reliever/fever reducer

USES
Temporarily
- reduces fever
- relieves minor aches, pains, and headache

WARNINGS
Liver warning: This product contains acetaminophen. Severe liver damage may occur if
- a child 6 to 12 years takes more than 5 doses in 24 hours
- an adult or child 12 years and older takes more than 6 doses in 24 hours, which is the maximum daily amount
- taken with other drugs containing acetaminophen
- an adult takes 3 or more alcoholic drinks everyday while using this product

For rectal use only

DO NOT USE
- in children under 6 years
- if you are allergic to acetaminophen.
- with any other drug containing acetaminophen (prescription or nonprescription). If you are not sure whether a drug contains acetaminophen, ask a doctor or pharmacist

ASK A DOCTOR BEFORE USE IF
- you have liver disease.
- you are taking the blood thinning drug warfarin.

STOP USE AND ASK A DOCTOR IF
- fever lasts more than 3 days (72 hours), or recurs.
- pain gets worse or lasts more than 10 days.
- new symptoms occur.
- redness or swelling is present in the painful area.

These may be signs of a serious condition.

PREGNANCY OR BREAST FEEDING
If pregnant or breast-feeding, ask a health professional before use.

KEEP OUT OF REACH OF CHILDREN
If swallowed or in case of overdose, get medical help or contact a Poison Control Center right away. Quick medical attention is critical in case of overdose for adults and for children even if you do not notice any signs or symptoms.

DIRECTIONS
- **do not use more than directed**
- remove wrapper
- carefully insert suppository well up into the rectum

Dosing Chart	
Age	Dose
under 6 years	do not use
6 to 12 years	Use 1 suppository every 4 to 6 hours (maximum of 5 doses in 24 hours)
adults and children 12 years and older	Use 2 suppositories every 4 to 6 hours (maximum of 6 doses)

OTHER INFORMATION
- store at 2°-27°C (35°-80°F)
- do not use if imprinted suppository wrapper is opened or damaged

INACTIVE INGREDIENTS
glycerol monostearate, hydrogenated vegetable oil, polyoxyethylene stearate, polysorbate 80

QUESTIONS OR COMMENTS?
1-800-432-8534 (select option #2) between 9 am and 4 pm EST, Monday - Friday.

FIBERCON (calcium polycarbophil)
Wyeth Pharmaceutical Division of Wyeth Holdings Corporation and a subsidiary of Pfizer Inc.

DRUG FACTS

Active Ingredient(s) (in each caplet)
Calcium polycarbophil 625 mg equivalent to 500 mg polycarbophil

Purpose(s)
Bulk-forming laxative

USES
- relieves occasional constipation to help restore and maintain regularity
- this product generally produces bowel movement in 12 to 72 hours

WARNINGS
Choking:
Taking this product without adequate fluid may cause it to swell and block your throat or esophagus and may cause choking. Do not take this product if you have difficulty in swallowing. If you

experience chest pain, vomiting, or difficulty in swallowing or breathing after taking this product, seek immediate medical attention.

ASK A DOCTOR BEFORE USE IF YOU HAVE
- abdominal pain, nausea, or vomiting
- a sudden change in bowel habits that persists over a period of 2 weeks

ASK A DOCTOR OR PHARMACIST BEFORE USE IF YOU ARE
taking any other drug. Take this product 2 or more hours before or after other drugs. All laxatives may affect how other drugs work.

WHEN USING THIS PRODUCT
- do not use for more than 7 days unless directed by a doctor
- do not take more than 8 caplets in a 24 hour period unless directed by a doctor

STOP USE AND ASK A DOCTOR IF
rectal bleeding occurs or if you fail to have a bowel movement after use of this or any other laxative. These could be signs of a serious condition.

Keep out of reach of children.
In case of overdose, get medical help or contact a Poison Control Center right away.

DIRECTIONS
- take each dose of this product with at least 8 ounces (a full glass) of water or other fluid. Taking this product without enough liquid may cause choking. See Choking warning.
- FiberCon works naturally so continued use for one to three days is normally required to provide full benefit. Dosage may vary according to diet, exercise, previous laxative use or severity of constipation.

age	recommended dose	daily maximum
adults and children 12 years of age and over	2 caplets once a day	up to 4 times a day
children under 12 years	consult a physician	

OTHER INFORMATION
- **each caplet contains:** 140 mg calcium and 10 mg magnesium
- protect contents from moisture
- store at 20-25°C (68-77°F)

INACTIVE INGREDIENTS
caramel, crospovidone, hypromellose, magnesium stearate, microcrystalline cellulose, polyethylene glycol, silicon dioxide, sodium lauryl sulfate

QUESTIONS OR COMMENTS?
Call weekdays from 9 AM to 5 PM EST at **1-800-282-8805**

FLEET ENEMA (bisacodyl)
C.B. Fleet Company, Inc.

Active Ingredient(s) (in each 30-mL delivered dose)
Bisacodyl 10 mg......................Stimulant Laxative / Bowel Cleanser

USE
For relief of occasional constipation or bowel cleansing before rectal examination.

WARNINGS
For rectal use only.

ASK A DOCTOR BEFORE USING ANY LAXATIVE IF YOU HAVE
- abdominal pain, nausea, or vomiting
- a sudden change in bowel habits lasting more than 2 weeks
- already used a laxative for more than 1 week

STOP USE AND ASK A DOCTOR IF YOU HAVE
- rectal bleeding
- no bowel movement within 30 minutes of enema use

These symptoms may indicate a serious condition.

KEEP OUT OF REACH OF CHILDREN
If swallowed, get medical help or contact a Poison Control Center right away.

DIRECTIONS
Single Daily Dosage

adults and children 12 years and over	1 Bottle
children under 12 years	DO NOT USE

OTHER INFORMATION
- this product generally produces a bowel movement in 5-20 minutes
- store at temperatures not above 86F (30C)
- consult Physicians' Desk Reference for complete professional labeling
- carton sealed for safety. If seal with Fleet emblem on top or bottom flap is broken or missing, do not use

INACTIVE INGREDIENTS
carbomer 934P, glycerin, methylparaben, octoxynol-9, propylparaben, purified water, sodium hydroxide

QUESTIONS OR COMMENTS?
1-866-255-6960 or www.fleetlabs.com

FLEET ENEMA (monobasic sodium phosphate and dibasic sodium phosphate)
C.B. Fleet Company, Inc.

Active Ingredient(s) (in each 118-mL delivered dose)
Monobasic Sodium Phosphate 19 g.................Saline Laxative
Dibasic Sodium Phosphate 7 g........................Saline Laxative

USE
For relief of occasional constipation.

WARNINGS
For rectal use only.
Using more than one enema in 24 hours can be harmful.

ASK A DOCTOR BEFORE USING THIS PRODUCT IF THE CHILD
- is on a sodium-restricted diet
- has kidney disease

ASK A DOCTOR BEFORE USING ANY LAXATIVE IF THE CHILD HAS
- abdominal pain, nausea, or vomiting
- a sudden change in bowel habits lasting more than 2 weeks
- already used a laxative for more than 1 week

STOP USE AND CONSULT A DOCTOR IF THE CHILD HAS
- rectal bleeding
- no bowel movement within 30 minutes of enema use
- symptoms of dehydration (feeling thirsty, dizziness, vomiting or urinating less often than normal)
  These symptoms may indicate a serious condition.

KEEP OUT OF REACH OF CHILDREN
If swallowed, get medical help or contact a Poison Control Center right away.

DIRECTIONS
Single Daily Dosage
Do not use more unless directed by a doctor. See Warnings. Do not use if child is taking another sodium phosphates product.

children 5 to 11 years	1 bottle or as directed by a doctor
children 2 to under 5 years	one-half bottle (see below)
children under 2 years	DO NOT USE

One-half bottle preparation:
Unscrew cap and remove 2 tablespoons of liquid with a measuring spoon. Replace cap and follow directions.

OTHER INFORMATION
- each 118-mL delivered dose contains: sodium 4.4 g
- additional liquids by mouth are recommended while taking this product
- this product generally produces a bowel movement in 1-5 minutes
- carton sealed for safety. If seal with Fleet emblem on top or bottom flap is broken or missing, do not use
- for complete professional use warnings and precautions, consult Physicians' Desk Reference

INACTIVE INGREDIENTS
benzalkonium chloride, disodium EDTA, purified water

QUESTIONS OR COMMENTS?
1-866-255-6960 or www.pedia-lax.com

FLEET EXTRA (monobasic sodium phosphate and dibasic sodium phosphate)
C.B. Fleet Company, Inc.

Active Ingredient(s) (in each 197-mL delivered dose)
Monobasic Sodium Phosphate 19 g.................Saline Laxative
Dibasic Sodium Phosphate 7 g........................Saline Laxative

USE
For relief of occasional constipation.

WARNINGS
For rectal use only.
Using more than one enema in 24 hours can be harmful.

ASK A DOCTOR BEFORE USING THIS PRODUCT IF THE CHILD
- is on a sodium-restricted diet
- has kidney disease

ASK A DOCTOR BEFORE USING ANY LAXATIVE IF THE CHILD HAS
- abdominal pain, nausea, or vomiting
- a sudden change in bowel habits lasting more than 2 weeks
- already used a laxative for more than 1 week

STOP USE AND CONSULT A DOCTOR IF THE CHILD HAS
- rectal bleeding
- no bowel movement within 30 minutes of enema use
- symptoms of dehydration (feeling thirsty, dizziness, vomiting or urinating less often than normal)
  These symptoms may indicate a serious condition.

KEEP OUT OF REACH OF CHILDREN
If swallowed, get medical help or contact a Poison Control Center right away.

DIRECTIONS
Single Daily Dosage
Do not use more unless directed by a doctor. See Warnings. Do not use if child is taking another sodium phosphates product.

adults and children 12 years and over	1 bottle
children 2 to under 11 years	Use Pedia-Lax Enema
children under 2 years	DO NOT USE

children 5 to 11 years	1 bottle or as directed by a doctor
children 2 to under 5 years	one-half bottle (see below)
children under 2 years	DO NOT USE

One-half bottle preparation:
Unscrew cap and remove 2 tablespoons of liquid with a measuring spoon. Replace cap and follow directions.

OTHER INFORMATION
- each 197-mL delivered dose contains: sodium 4.4 g
- additional liquids by mouth are recommended while taking this product
- this product generally produces a bowel movement in 1-5 minutes
- carton sealed for safety. If seal with Fleet emblem on top or bottom flap is broken or missing, do not use
- for complete professional use warnings and precautions, consult Physicians' Desk Reference

INACTIVE INGREDIENTS
benzalkonium chloride, disodium EDTA, purified water

QUESTIONS OR COMMENTS?
1-866-255-6960 or www.pedia-lax.com

FLEET GLYCERIN SUPPOSITORY (glycerin)
C.B. Fleet Company, Inc.

Active Ingredient(s) (in each suppository)
Glycerin 2 g.................Hyperosmotic Laxative

USE
For relief of occasional constipation.

WARNINGS
For rectal use only.
May cause rectal discomfort or a burning sensation.

ASK A DOCTOR BEFORE USING ANY LAXATIVE IF YOU HAVE
• abdominal pain, nausea or vomiting
• a sudden change in bowel habits lasting more than 2 weeks
• already used a laxative for more than 1 week

STOP USE AND CONSULT A DOCTOR IF YOU HAVE
• rectal bleeding
• no bowel movement after using productThese symptoms may indicate a serious condition.

KEEP OUT OF REACH OF CHILDREN
If swallowed, get medical help or contact a Poison Control Center right away.

DIRECTIONS
Single daily dosage

adults and children 6 years and over	1 suppository, or as directed by a doctor
children 2 to under 6 years	use Pedia-Lax Glycerin Suppositories
children under 2 years	ask a doctor

Insert suppository well up into rectum. Suppository need not melt completely to produce laxative action.

OTHER INFORMATION
• This product generally produces a bowel movement in 1/4 to 1 hour.
• Store container tightly closed.
• Keep away from excessive heat.
• MOUTH OF JAR SEALED FOR SAFETY. IF FOIL IMPRINTED WITH GREEN FLEET EMBLEM IS BROKEN OR MISSING, DO NOT USE.

INACTIVE INGREDIENTS
edetate disodium, purified water, sodium hydroxide, stearic acid

QUESTIONS OR COMMENTS?
1-866-255-6960 or www.fleetlabs.com

FLEET LIQUID GLYCERIN SUPPOSITORIES
(glycerin)

C.B. Fleet Company, Inc.

Active Ingredient(s) (in each 5.4 mL average delivered dose)
Glycerin 5.4 g.................Hyperosmotic Laxative

USE
For relief of occasional constipation

WARNINGS
For rectal use only.
May cause rectal discomfort or a burning sensation.

ASK A DOCTOR BEFORE USING ANY LAXATIVE IF YOU HAVE
• abdominal pain, nausea or vomiting
• a sudden change in bowel habits lasting more than 2 weeks
• already used a laxative for more than 1 week

STOP USING THIS PRODUCT AND CONSULT A DOCTOR IF YOU HAVE
• rectal bleeding
• no bowel movement after use of a laxative
  These symptoms may indicate a serious condition.

KEEP OUT OF REACH OF CHILDREN
If swallowed, get medical help or contact a Poison Control Center right away.

DIRECTIONS
Single daily dosage

adults and children 6 years and over	1 suppository, or as directed by a doctor
children 2 to under 6 years	use Pedia-Lax Glycerin Suppositories
children under 2 years	ask a doctor

Insert suppository well up into rectum. Suppository need not melt completely to produce laxative action.

OTHER INFORMATION
• This product generally produces a bowel movement in 1/4 to 1 hour.
• Store container tightly closed. Keep away from excessive heat.
• MOUTH OF JAR SEALED FOR SAFETY. IF FOIL IMPRINTED WITH GREEN FLEET EMBLEM IS BROKEN OR MISSING, DO NOT USE.

INACTIVE INGREDIENTS
edetate disodium, purified water, sodium hydroxide, stearic acid

QUESTIONS OR COMMENTS?
1-866-255-6960

FLEET MINERAL OIL ENEMA (mineral oil)

C.B. Fleet Company, Inc.

Active Ingredient(s)
(in each 118-mL delivered dose)
Mineral Oil 100% ......Lubricant Laxative

USES
• for relief of fecal impaction
• for relief of occasional constipation
• for removal of residue after barium administration

WARNINGS
For rectal use only.
If pregnant or breast-feeding ask a health professional before use.

DIRECTIONS
Single daily dose

adults and children 12 years and over	1 bottle
children 2 to under 12 years	one-half bottle
children under 2 years	DO NOT USE

ASK A DOCTOR BEFORE USING ANY LAXATIVE IF YOU HAVE
• abdominal pain, nausea or vomiting?
• a sudden change in bowel habits lasting more than 2 weeks
• already used a laxative for more than 1 week

STOP USE AND ASK A DOCTOR IF YOU HAVE
• rectal bleeding
• no bowel movement after use

These symptoms may indicate a serious condition.

Keep out of reach of children
If swallowed, get medical help or contact a Poison Control Center right away.

OTHER INFORMATION
- sodium free
- this product generally produces a bowel movement in 2-15 minutes
- carton sealed for safety. If seal with Fleet emblem on top or bottom flap is missing, do not use
- consult Physicians' Desk Reference for complete professional labeling

QUESTIONS OR COMMENTS?
1-866-255-6960 or www.fleetlabs.com

FLEET SOF-LAX (docusate sodium)
C.B. Fleet Co., Inc.

DRUG FACTS

Active Ingredient(s) (in each softgel)	Purpose(s)
Docusate sodium 100 mg	Stool softener

USES
- for the prevention of dry, hard stools
- for relief of occasional constipation

WARNINGS
If pregnant or breast-feeding, ask a health care professional before use.
Keep out of reach of children. In case of overdose, get medical help or contact a Poison Control Center right away.

DO NOT USE
- if you are currently taking mineral oil, unless directed by a doctor
- when abdominal pain, nausea, or vomiting are present
- for longer than one week, unless directed by a doctor

ASK A DOCTOR BEFORE USE IF
- you notice a sudden change in bowel habits that persists over a period of 2 weeks

STOP USE AND ASK A DOCTOR IF
- you have rectal bleeding
- you fail to have a bowel movement after use

These symptoms may indicate a serious condition.

DIRECTIONS

Single daily dosage	
adults and children 12 years and over	1-3 softgels
children 2 to under 12 years	1 softgel
children under 2 years	ask a doctor

OTHER INFORMATION
- **each softgel contains:** sodium 5 mg
- this product generally produces a bowel movement within 12 to 72 hours
- mouth of bottle sealed for your safety. If foil imprinted "SEALED FOR YOUR PROTECTION" is broken or missing, do not use.

INACTIVE INGREDIENTS
edible white ink, FD&C red #40, FD&C yellow #6 gelatin, glycerin, mannitol, polyethylene glycol, polysorbate, propylene glycol, purified water and sorbitol.

QUESTIONS OR COMMENTS?
1-866-255-6960 or www.fleetlabs.com

FLINTSTONES WITH IRON CHEWABLES
(vitamins with iron)
Bayer Healthcare LLC

Serving Size: 1/2 tablet (2 & 3 years of age); 1 tablet (4 years of age and older)

	Amount Per Tablet	% DV (2 & 3 yrs)	% DV (Ages 4+)
Total Carbohydrate		**	
Sugars		**	**
Vitamin A (20% as beta-carotene)	2500 IU	50%	50%
Vitamin C	60 mg	75%	100%
Vitamin D	400 IU	50%	100%
Vitamin E	15 IU	75%	50%
Thiamin (B1)	1.05 mg	75%	70%
Riboflavin (B2)	1.2 mg	75%	71%
Niacin	13.5 mg	75%	68%
Vitamin B6	1.05 mg	75%	53%
Folic Acid	300 mcg	75%	75%
Vitamin B12	4.5 mcg	75%	75%
Iron	15 mg	75%	83%
Sodium	10 mg	**	
^ Percent Daily Values are based on a 2,000 calorie diet.			
** Daily Value not established.			

DIRECTIONS
Children 2 to 3 years of age - **Chew** one-half tablet daily, with food.
Adults and children 4 years of age and older - **Chew** one tablet daily, with food.

INGREDIENTS
sorbitol, mannitol, fructose, sodium ascorbate, ferrous fumarate, silicon dioxide, carrageenan, natural and artificial flavors, FD&C red #40 lake; less than 2% of: aspartame†, betacarotene, cholecalciferol, cyanocobalamin, D-calcium pantothenate, dl-alpha-tocopheryl acetate, FD&C blue #2 Lake, FD&C yellow #6 lake, folic acid, magnesium stearate, niacinamide, pyridoxine hydrochloride, riboflavin, soy lecithin, thiamine mononitrate, vitamin A acetate
Contains: Soy
† PHENYLKETONURICS: CONTAINS PHENYLALANINE

WARNING
Accidental overdose of iron-containing products is a leading cause of fatal poisoning in children under 6. Keep this product out of the reach of children. In case of accidental overdose, call a doctor or Poison Control Center immediately.

KEEP OUT OF REACH OF CHILDREN
CHILD RESISTANT CAP

FLORAJEN

American Lifeline, Inc.

INGREDIENTS
A freeze-dried strain of live 100% *Lactobacillus acidophilus*

OTHER INGREDIENTS
rice maltodextrin and gelatin capsules. Non-Dairy. *Does not* contain yeast, sugar, soy, eggs, corn, wheat, gluten, coloring or preservatives.

USAGE
Take 1 capsule daily unless a higher dosage is recommended by your health care professional, preferably on an empty stomach.

STORAGE
Refrigerate for maximum freshness and effectiveness. Can be stored at room temperature for up to two weeks while traveling and still maintain effectiveness.
Statements on this page have not been evaluated by the Food and Drug Administration. This product is not medicinal and is not intended to diagnose, treat, cure or prevent any disease.

FLORA Q

PharmaDerm A division of Fougera Pharmaceuticals Inc.

PRODUCT DESCRIPTION
Off-white capsules, each containing 180 mg* of a standardized, light-beige colored powder consisting of an aggregate of a minimum of 8 billion CFU (8 x 10^9 Colony Forming Units) freeze-dried cultures at time of manufacture of species listed below.
Guaranteed potency of no less than 4 billion CFU freeze-dried cultures at expiration date.
* Based on an estimated tapped density of 0.7 g/mL.
Also contains: maltodextrin, hypromellose, microcrystalline cellulose, sodium alginate, silicon dioxide, magnesium stearate, titanium dioxide, and FD&C Blue 2.
Each capsule, containing a proprietary probiotic blend and other ingredients, is equivalent to 230 mg per serving.
This product is free of the following allergens: wheat/gluten, milk/lactose, eggs, fish, crustacean shellfish, soybeans, tree nuts, and peanuts.
Contains no preservatives.
GENERIC NAME:
Lactobacillus acidophilus
Bifidobacterium
Lactobacillus paracasei
Streptococcus thermophilus
COMMON USES: This probiotic is used to help maintain the normal bacterial balance of the gastrointestinal tract.[†]
THE PROBIOTIC SPECIES IN FLORA˙Q®:
• Help maintain balance in the intestinal microflora.[†]
• Support the colonization of intestinal microflora.[†]
• Help support the modulation of intestinal microflora.[†]
• Promote gastrointestinal health.[†]

[†]These statements have not been evaluated by the Food and Drug Administration. This product is not intended to diagnose, treat, cure or prevent any disease.

HOW TO USE: Use this product as directed on the package, unless instructed differently by your doctor.
CAUTIONS: Before you begin taking any dietary supplement, check with your doctor or pharmacist.
KEEP OUT OF THE REACH OF CHILDREN.
POSSIBLE SIDE EFFECTS: Potential side effects that may dissipate include increased stomach gas. If this occurs and is bothersome, check with your doctor. Should you experience symptoms of an allergic reaction, including rash, itching, swelling, dizziness or trouble breathing, contact your doctor, nurse or pharmacist immediately.

DIRECTIONS
Take one capsule per day. May be taken with or without food.
HOW SUPPLIED: Off-white capsules imprinted **Flora˙Q®** are supplied in bottles of 30 (List 10337-400-30).

STORAGE
Potency guaranteed through expiration date on package when stored at room temperature (25° C/77° F) or below. DO NOT STORE IN THE BATHROOM. Keep container closed. No refrigeration needed.
Do not use if seal on bottle is broken or missing.
Manufactured for:
PharmaDerm®
A divisdion of
Fougera
PHARMEUTICALS INC.
Melville, New York 11747
www.pharmaderm.com
IL195B R11/11

FLORASTOR

BIOCODEX

SUPPLEMENT FACTS

Florastor		Florastor Kids	
Serving Size: 1 Capsule		Serving Size: 1 Powder Packet	
Amount per Capsule		**Amount per Packet**	
Saccharomyces boulardii lyo	250 mg*	*Saccharomyces boulardii lyo*	250 mg*
Lactose	33 mg*	Lactose	33 mg*
		Fructose	472 mg*
Other Ingredients: magnesium stearate, hydroxypropylmethylcellulose, titanium dioxide.		Other Ingredients: collodial anhydrous silica, tutti-frutti flavor.	
*Daily Value not established.		*Daily Value not established.	

Note: Florastor capsules and **Florastor Kids** powder packets will both be referred to as **Florastor** for the completion of product information.

CONTRAINDICATIONS
Florastor is contraindicated in patients with a central line. There are rare reported cases of fungemia due to accidental manual introduction of *Saccharomyces boulardii lyo* cells by individuals into the bloodstream via a central line. Should a patient develop fungemia, proper management practices include discontinuation of Florastor, treatment with appropriate antifungals and, when appropriate, removal of the central line. Central lines include short and long-term central venous catheters (CVCs), peripherally inserted central catheters (PICCs), and totally implantable devices (i.e. ports).
Florastor is contraindicated in patients with a known hypersensitivity to any of the components. *Saccharomyces boulardii lyo* is a single strain of yeast, therefore contraindicating use for any persons with a yeast allergy.

WARNINGS
Do not open **Florastor** capsules or packets in the vicinity of patients with central lines. Health care workers should follow standard good practices: always change gloves after handling

Florastor as to avoid any accidental transfer into a central line of any patient.

Nursing or Pregnant Mothers: In the absence of reliable animal teratogenesis data, it is preferable to check with your healthcare practitioner before using **Florastor.**

SUGGESTED USE OF FLORASTOR
Florastor helps support a healthy digestive system*. **Florastor** also acts to maintain the balance of intestinal flora*.

Length of Florastor Use
Long-term use of **Florastor** is not associated with complications. After repeated oral doses, **Florastor** transits through the digestive tract attaining steady-state levels that are maintained throughout the administration period. **Florastor** is no longer present in stools two to five days after discontinuation of treatment[3].

Recommended Serving
In general, taking one or two **Florastor** capsules or packets twice daily helps to protect your intestinal tract*.

For persons at least two months of age

Maintains the balance of intestinal flora*	One capsule or powder packet twice daily (500 mg)
Promotes intestinal health*	Two capsules or powder packets twice daily (1000 mg) for thirty days

ADMINISTRATION
Note: Do not mix **Florastor** in any carbonated, very hot (above 122°F), or alcohol-containing beverages or foods. Prepare only as needed for immediate administration as **Florastor** is viable for only thirty minutes after added to food or beverages.
- Swallow the capsule whole.
- Open the capsule or packet and empty the contents on your tongue. Follow immediately with a 4 oz. drink of water or juice.
- Open the capsule or packet and sprinkle over semi-solid food (i.e. applesauce, yogurt, etc.) for immediate administration.
- Open the capsule or packet and dissolve the contents in liquid (i.e. water, juice, milk, formula, etc.) for immediate administration.

FOOD OR DRUG INTERACTIONS
Food — Florastor can be taken with or without food, with no change in its efficacy.
Drugs — Florastor is not harmed by antibiotics because **Florastor** is a yeast (i.e. non-bacterial). Biocodex, Inc. does not recommend taking **Florastor** in conjunction with antifungals. **Florastor** does not have other known drug interactions.
Supplements — Florastor can be taken alone or with other dietary supplements, including bacterial probiotics.

SIDE-EFFECTS
Research has shown less than 1% of patients report constipation or thirst.
Note: **Florastor**, a non-pathogenic yeast, will not exacerbate or cause a yeast infection of Candida origin.

Restricted Diets
Lactose Intolerance — Florastor has 33 mg lactose (about the same as a 1/3 slice of cheese). Administration of **Florastor** is proven to increase lactase production, which helps with the digestion of lactose[4]*.
Gluten-Free Diet — Florastor is a gluten-free dietary supplement. It has no wheat, rye, oats, or barley in the capsule or part of its contents.
Vegan Diet — The lactose found in **Florastor** is sourced from milk collected for human consumption and is prepared without other ruminant materials than calf rennet.
Kosher — The factory is not inspected for kosher certification.

Allergens
Florastor DOES NOT include any of the following:
- corn,
- egg protein,
- fish,
- gluten,
- latex,
- meat,
- milk protein,
- nuts, or
- shellfish.

Note: Florastor may contain traces of soy.

Physical Description
Contents of **Florastor** and **Florastor Kids** packets when opened have a creamy color. Both have a yeast-like (i.e. sourdough bread) smell.

STORAGE CONDITIONS
Do not refrigerate. Florastor is produced via a manufacturing method, lyophilization, similar to freeze drying. The lyophilization of *Saccharomyces boulardii lyo* allows storage at room temperature (25°C or 77°F), away from excessive moisture, to guarantee an optimal level of living cells for a three-year shelf-life.

> [†]These statements have not been evaluated by the Food and Drug Administration. This product is not intended to diagnose, treat, cure or prevent any disease.

If you have any medical concerns or questions, we are available to help you at: 877-356-7787
info@biocodexusa.com
www.Florastor.com

FUNGI NAIL TOE AND FOOT MS (zinc undecylenate and undecylenic acid)

Kramer Laboratories

Undecylenic acid 5%
Zinc Undecylenate 20%
Antifungal
In case of accidental ingestion, contact a physician, emergency medical care facility or Poison Control Center immediately for advice.
Proven effective in the treatment of most athletes foot (tinea pedis) and ringworm (tinea corporis). Helps prevent most athlete's foot with daily use. for effective relief of itching, burning and cracking.

DIRECTIONS
Clean affected areas with soap and warm water and dry thoroughly. Apply a thin layer of Fungi-Nail Toe and Foot Anti-fungal ointment over affected area twice daily (morning and night) or as directed by doctor. Wear well-fitting ventilated shoes, and change shoes and socks at least once daily. For athletes foot pay special attention to spaces between the toes. For athletes foot and ringworm, use daily for 4 weeks. For toe fungus, apply under nail and around cuticle area. If condition persists longer, consult a doctor. This product is not effective on scalp or nails. Supervise children in the use of this product. Emulsifying wax NF, methylparaben, mineral oil, propylparaben, white petrolatum

WARNINGS
for external use only.
Do not use in children under 2 years of age unless directed by a doctor.
Avoid contact with eyes.

FUNGICURE MAXIMUM STRENGTH
(undecylenic acid)

Alva-Amco Pharmacal Companies, Inc.

Active Ingredient(s)
Undecylenic acid 25% w/v

Purpose(s)
Antifungal

USES
For the cure of most
- ringworm (tinea corporis)
- athlete's foot (tinea pedis)

For relief of
- itching
- scaling
- cracking
- burning
- redness
- soreness
- irritation
- discomforts which may accompany these conditions.

WARNINGS
For external use only

ASK A DOCTOR BEFORE USE
on children under 2 years of age.

WHEN USING THIS PRODUCT
avoid contact with the eyes.

STOP USE AND ASK A DOCTOR IF
- Irritation occurs
- There is no improvement within 4 weeks.

Keep out of reach of children. If swallowed, get medical help or contact a poison control center right away.

DIRECTIONS
- Read all package directions and warnings before using.
- Use only as directed.
- Clean the affected area with soap and warm water and dry thoroughly.
- Apply a thin layer of Fungicure over the affected area twice daily (morning and night), or as directed by a doctor.
- **This product is not effective on scalp or nails.**
- For athlete's foot, pay special attention to spaces between toes; wear well fitting, ventilated shoes and change shoes and socks at least once daily.
- For athlete's foot and ringworm, use daily for 4 weeks. If condition persists longer, consult a doctor.
- Intended for use by normally healthy adults only.
- Persons under 18 years of age or those with highly sensitive or allergic skin should use only as directed by a doctor.
- Supervise children in the use of this product.

OTHER INFORMATION
- Fungicure may be applied to cuticles, around nail edges and under nail tips where reachable with its applicator brush. This product is not intended to, nor will it, penetrate hard nail surfaces.
- While not all finger and toe fungal infections are curable with OTC topical medications, if you see improvement within 4 weeks of use, you may continue to use Fungicure until satisfactory results are obtained.
- You may report serious side effects to the phone number provided under *Questions?* below.

INACTIVE INGREDIENTS
aloe vera gel, fragrance, hypromellose, isopropyl alcohol (70% v/v), purified water and vitamin E.

QUESTIONS OR COMMENTS?
1-800-792-2582

FUNGICURE LIQUID GEL (undecylenic acid)
Alva-Amco

DRUGS FACTS

Active Ingredient(s)	Purpose(s)
Undecylenic acid 25% w/w	Antifungal

USES
For the cure of most:
- ringworm (tinea corporis)
- athlete's foot (tinea pedis).

For relief of:
- itching
- scaling
- cracking
- burning
- redness
- soreness
- irritation
- discomforts which may accompany these conditions

WARNINGS
For external use only

ASK A DOCTOR BEFORE USE
- on children under 2 years of age

WHEN USING THIS PRODUCT
- avoid contact with the eyes

STOP USE AND ASK A DOCTOR IF
- irritation occurs
- there is no improvement within 4 weeks

Keep out of reach of children. If swallowed, get medical help or contact a poison control center right away.

DIRECTIONS
- Read all package directions and warnings before using.
- Use only as directed.
- Clean the affected area with soap and warm water and dry thoroughly.
- Apply a thin layer of Fungicure over the affected area twice daily (morning and night), or as directed by a doctor.
- **This product is not effective on scalp or nails.**
- For athlete's foot, pay special attention to spaces between toes; wear well fitting, ventilated shoes, and change shoes and socks at least once daily.
- For athlete's foot and ringworm, use daily for 4 weeks. If condition persists longer, consult a doctor.
- Intended for use by normally healthy adults only.
- Persons under 18 years of age or those with highly sensitive or allergic skin should use only as directed by a doctor.
- Supervise children in the use of this product.

OTHER INFORMATION
- Fungicure may be applied to cuticles, around nail edges and under nail tips where reachable with its applicator brush.
- This product is not intended to, nor will it, penetrate hard nail surfaces.

- While not all finger and toe fungal infections are curable with OTC topical medications, if you see improvement within 4 weeks of use, you may continue to use Fungicure until satisfactory results are obtained.
- You may report serious side effects to the phone number provided under QUESTIONS OR COMMENTS below

INACTIVE INGREDIENTS
aloe vera gel, hydroxypropylcellulose, isopropyl alcohol (70% v/v), purified water and vitamin E

QUESTIONS OR COMMENTS?
1-800-792-2582
Some topical fungal infections may present themselves on the skin as ring-like formations with clear centers, commonly referred to as ringworm. Other such infections, when in the finger and toe areas, are often characterized by scaling of skin, burning, cracking, itching and related discomforts. When nails become infected, they may appear to become opaque (cloudy white), thickened, brittle, friable (easily broken) and in some cases, discolored (greenish/brown). NOTE: If you believe you may have any type of fungus infection, do not delay consulting a doctor for advice. You may wish to show him/her FUNGICURE Liquid Gel and discuss its use.
HOW FUNGICURE LIQUID GEL WORKS; PRODUCT DESCRIPTION AND ACTION:
MAXIMUM STRENGTH FUNGICURE Liquid Gel is an effective topical formulation containing the ACTIVE INGREDIENT: Undecylenic Acid 25% w/w INACTIVE INGREDIENTS: Aloe vera gel, hydroxypropylcellulose, isopropyl alcohol (70% v/v), purified water, vitamin E. Undecylenic acid in FUNGICURE Liquid Gel is a widely recognized, proven anti-fungal ingredient effective against 6 types of fungus including E. floccosum, T. mentagrophytes, M. canis, M gypseum, T. tonsurans and T. rubrum, which are known to cause topical infections of the body, hands and feet, including on and between fingers and toes, as well as on cuticles and skin around nails. FUNGICURE Liquid Gel acts promptly to target and destroy fungus at the site of infection while preventing its spread. FUNGICURE helps relieve associated burning, itching and discomforts by eliminating the fungus...allowing for the natural regrowth of healthy looking tissue.
WHY FUNGICURE LIQUID GEL IS SO EFFECTIVE IN NAIL AREA INFECTION:
Fungal infection of the nail areas can affect both the nail beds as well as the nail surfaces themselves, commonly referred to as the nail plates. While an actual intact nail plate, being a hard surface, is generally not readily penetrable by topical applications, there are instances where nail plates are not intact and are actually cracked open, breached or otherwise exposed, either partially or fully, including instances where a nail plate has actually lifted away and separated from its nail bed. There are other instances where fungus resides on skin around and adjacent to the nail plate, at the very edges, on the cuticles, and under the exposed quick of the nail.
In these instances where the nail itself and the nail bed, harboring fungus, are exposed, FUNGICURE Anti-Fungal Liquid Gel, with its powerful anti-fungal action, applied as directed, is able to reach the fungus by direct application or by related capillary action. Reaching the actual site where the fungus resides, FUNGICURE Anti-Fungal Liquid Gel eliminates the fungus, and in so doing, allows for the re-growth of healthy nail bed and nail plate tissue.
Fungal infections which are isolated beneath an intact nail plate or embedded within the nail plate itself may require consultation from a Doctor or Pharmacist for proper treatment. You may wish to show them FUNGICURE Liquid Gel and discuss its use.
PROMPT ACTION AND PROPER TREATMENT:
Recognizing and treating fungus infection early is very important for successful results. Therefore, it is wise to consult your doctor promptly for advice if you suspect you may have a fungal Infection. It is likewise important, for successful results, that once treatment is started with FUNGICURE it is continued uninterrupted, carefully following package directions, until

satisfactory results are achieved or advised by a doctor, as directed on the package.

FUNGICURE MANICURE PEDICURE
(clotrimazole)
Alva-Amco Pharmacal Companies, Inc.

Active Ingredient(s)
Clotrimazole, and 1% w/v)

Purpose(s)
Antifungal

USES
For the cure of most:
- Ringworm (tinea corporis)
- Athlete's foot (tinea pedis)

For relief of
- itching
- scaling
- cracking
- burning
- redness
- soreness
- irritation
- discomforts which may accompany these conditions. Inhibits the growth and reproduction of fungal cells.

WARNINGS FOR EXTERNAL USE ONLY.

ASK A DOCTOR BEFORE USE
on children under 2 years of age.

WHEN USING THIS PRODUCT
avoid contact with the eyes.

STOP USE AND ASK A DOCTOR IF
- irritation occurs
- there is no improvement within 4 weeks.

Keep out of reach of children. If swallowed, get medical help or contact a poison control center right away.

DIRECTIONS
- Read all package directions and warnings before use.
- Use only as directed.
- Clean the affected area with soap and warm water and dry thoroughly.
- Apply a thin layer of Fungicure Manicure & Pedicure Liquid over the affected area twice daily (morning and night), or as directed by a doctor.
- **This product is not effective on the scalp or nails.**
- Avoid applying to severely cracked or irritated areas.
- For athlete's foot: pay special attention to to spaces between toes; wear well fitting, ventilated shoes, and change shoes and socks at least once daily.
- For athlete's foot and ringworm, use daily for 4 weeks, If condition persists longer, consult a doctor.
- Intended for use by normally healthy adults only.
- Persons under 18 years of age or those with highly sensitive or allergic skin should use only as directed by a doctor.
- Supervise children in the use of this product.

OTHER INFORMATION
- Fungicure may be applied to cuticles, around nail edges and under nail tips where reachable with its applicator brush. This product is not intended to, nor will it, penetrate hard intact nail surfaces.
- While not all finger and toe fungal infections are curable with OTC topical medications, if you see improvement within 4 weeks of use, you may continue to use Fungicure until satisfactory results are obtained.

- You may report serious side effects to the phone number provided under *Questions?* below.

INACTIVE INGREDIENT
isopropyl alcohol

QUESTIONS OR COMMENTS?
1-800-792-2582

Maximum Strength
FUNGICURE Manicure & Pedicure
Anti-Fungal Treatment
- Easy Brush-On
- Instant Dry
- Odor Free
- Crystal Clear

The Manicure & Pedicure Fungi Specialist
A WORD ABOUT FUNGICURE Manicure & Pedicure Formula:
With your purchase of FUNGICURE Manicure & Pedicure Formula, you have chosen a highly effective and remarkably convenient treatment for common fungus infection of the finger and toe areas, including on cuticles and skin around and adjacent to nails edges and under nail tips where reachable with its convenient applicator brush.
Maintaining the appearance of your manicure and pedicure requires more than cosmetics. Proper hygiene is essential to help avoid potentially painful and unsightly fungus infections. FUNGICURE Manicure & Pedicure Formula is a maximum strength anti-fungal liquid, specifically formulated for the special needs of those who manicure, pedicure or use artificial nails-including manicure and nail care professionals.
FUNGICURE Manicure & Pedicure Formula is highly effective against common skin and cuticle area fungal infections, which can migrate to the nails. FUNGICURE Manicure & Pedicure Formula's convenient applicator brush allows for controlled, easily targeted application of anti-fungal medicine directly and neatly to the site of infection. FUNGICURE Manicure & Pedicure Formula dries fast and thoroughly, avoiding the mess and excess spreading so often associated with creams and "drop-on" liquids. With FUNGICURE, fingers need never touch infected areas. FUNGICURE Manicure & Pedicure Formula is crystal clear and leaves no residue or unpleasant medicinal odor.

WHAT IS FUNGUS INFECTION OF THE FINGER AND TOE AREAS?
Generally speaking, common fungus infections of the finger and toe areas (topical infections) are caused by a variety of fungi: actual living organisms (members of the yeast and mold family), which exist in the natural environment and tend to thrive in dark, damp conditions. These organisms may penetrate the skin surface through even the smallest crack or tear. They may be contracted by touching infected surfaces, animals or other people. Once infection starts, spreading may occur among body parts...one finger to another...one toe to another...from the skin and cuticle areas to the nails. There are a number of specific types of fungi, each of which can potentially infect body tissue and proceed to grow. Common topical fungi infectives generally fall into three categories: microsporum (hair and skin), epidermophyton (skin and nails), and trichophyton (hair, skin and nails). Among the more common fungi is E. floccosum which can cause ringworm infection on the body, hands and feet, on and in between the fingers and toes including the skin around the nails. Other common fungi are T. rubrum and T. mentagrophytes which can cause athlete's foot and infect the feet, on and between the toes including the skin around the toenails. Often such infections develop slowly and may be difficult to treat if not attended to promptly with an effective anti-fungal like FUNGICURE.
Fungal infections of the finger and toe areas present a special risk for those who manicure, pedicure or wear artificial nails. Many manicure procedures can enhance the risk of fungal infection. Certain types of artificial nails can trap moisture and fungi, providing a perfect environment in which fungus can grow and spread. Cutting cuticles can create opportunities for

fungal infections. Treating fungal infections on cuticles and nearby skin surfaces helps greatly reduce the risk of it spreading and attacking healthy nails. Stopping fungus before it infects healthy nails is the number one strategy for dealing with this potentially unsightly and very troublesome problem.
FUNGICURE Manicure & Pedicure Formula is a highly effective treatment, which helps eliminate fungus on cuticles and skin around and adjacent to the nails. Rely on FUNGICURE Manicure & Pedicure Formula liquid as an important anti-fungal defense.
HOW DO YOU KNOW IF YOU HAVE A TOPICAL FUNGUS INFECTION?
Some topical infections may present themselves on the skin as ringlike formations with clear centers, commonly referred to as ringworm. Other such infections, when in the finger and toe areas are often characterized by scaling of skin, burning, cracking, itching, and related discomforts. When nails become infected, they may appear to become opaque (cloudy white), thickened, brittle, friable (easily broken) and in some cases, discolored (greenish/brown). NOTE: If you believe you may have any type of fungus infection, do not delay consulting a doctor for advice. You may wish to show him/her FUNGICURE.
HOW FUNGICURE MANICURE & PEDICURE FORMULA LIQUID WORKS; PRODUCT DESCRIPTION AND ACTION:
FUNGICURE Manicure & Pedicure Formula is an effective topical formulation containing the ACTIVE INGREDIENT: Clotrimazole (1% w/v) INACTIVE INGREDIENT: Isopropyl alcohol.
The active ingredient Clotrimazole in FUNGICURE Manicure & Pedicure Formula is a widely recognized proven anti-fungal ingredient effective against fungi such as E. floccosum, T. mentagrophytes, and T. rubrum, which are known to cause topical infections of the body, hands and feet, including on and between fingers and toes, as well as on cuticles and skin around nails.
FUNGICURE Manicure & Pedicure Formula acts promptly to eliminate fungus at the site of infection while preventing its spread...plus helps relieve associated burning, itching and discomforts...allowing for the regrowth of healthy looking skin.
WHY FUNGICURE MANICURE & PEDICURE LIQUID IS SO EFFECTIVE IN NAIL AREA INFECTION:
Fungal infection of the nail areas can affect both the nail beds as well as the nail surfaces themselves, commonly referred to as the nail plates. While an actual intact nail plate, being a hard surface, is generally not penetrable by topical applications, there are instances where nail plates are not intact and are actually cracked open, breached or otherwise exposed, either partially or fully, including instances where a nail plate has actually lifted away and separated from its nail bed. There are other instances where fungus resides on skin around and adjacent to the nail plate at the very edges, on the cuticles, and under the exposed quick of the nail. In these instances where the nail itself is breached and the nail bed, harboring fungus, is exposed, FUNGICURE Manicure & Pedicure Anti-Fungal Liquid, with its powerful anti-fungal action, applied as directed, is able to reach the fungus by direct application or by related capillary action. Reaching the actual site where the fungus resides, FUNGICURE Manicure & Pedicure Anti-Fungal Liquid eliminates the fungus, and in so doing, allows for the re-growth of healthy nail bed and nail plate tissue.
Fungal infections which are isolated beneath an intact nail plate or embedded within the nail plate may require consultation from a Doctor or Pharmacist for proper treatment. You may wish to show them FUNGICURE Manicure & Pedicure Anti-Fungal Liquid and discuss its use.
PROMPT ACTION AND PROPER TREATMENT
Recognizing and treating fungus infection early is very important for successful results. Therefore, it is wise to consult your doctor promptly for advice if you suspect you may have a fungal infection. It is likewise important, for successful results, that once treatment is started with FUNGICURE Manicure & Pedicure Formula, it is continued uninterrupted, carefully following package directions, until satisfactory results are achieved or further advised by a doctor, as directed on the package. NOTE: Noticeable improvement may be expected

within 4 weeks in the case of ringworm (tinea corporis) and athlete's foot (tinea pedis). Consult your doctor for advice if noticeable improvement is not evident by this time or if condition persists or worsens.

HOW TO AVOID FUNGUS INFECTIONS AND REINFECTIONS:
• Since fungus enjoys and thrives on moisture, keep hands and feet meticulously clean and dry. Good personal hygiene is your first line of defense against recurring fungus infections.
• In cases where athlete's foot (tinea pedis) has been a problem, wear well ventilated shoes and change to clean socks at least once daily.
• All manicure and pedicure implements should be kept meticulously clean and sterilized after each use.
• Women who use artificial nails regularly should watch for changes in their nails. If nails become brittle, cracked or discolored it may be appropriate to avoid artificial nails for a period of time and a good idea to consult your doctor for advice.
• Avoid any practices that can tear or bruise the skin. Avoid trimming back cuticles too far, and cutting nails too close. Anything that tears or opens the skin invites infections. Be very observant for early signs of reinfections and don't hesitate to take prompt action with FUNGICURE Manicure & Pedicure Formula.

USES
For the cure of most: • ringworm (tinea corporis) • athlete's foot (tinea pedis). For relief of: • itching • scaling • cracking • burning • redness • soreness • irritation • discomforts which may accompany these conditions. Inhibits the growth and reproduction of fungal cells.

WARNINGS
For external use only.

ASK A DOCTOR BEFORE USE
on children under 2 years of age.

WHEN USING THIS PRODUCT
avoid contact with the eyes.

STOP USE AND ASK A DOCTOR IF
• irritation occurs • there is no improvement within 4 weeks.
Keep out of reach of children. If swallowed, get medical help or contact a poison control center right away.

DIRECTIONS
• Read all package directions and warnings before use. • Use only as directed. • Clean the affected area with soap and warm water and dry thoroughly. • Apply a thin layer of FUNGICURE Manicure & Pedicure Liquid over the affected area twice daily (morning and night) or as directed by a doctor. • **This product is not effective on the scalp or nails.** • Avoid applying to severely cracked or irritated areas. • For athlete's foot: pay special attention to spaces between toes; wear well fitting, ventilated shoes, and change shoes and socks at least once daily. • For athlete's foot and ringworm, use daily for 4 weeks. If condition persists longer consult a doctor. • Intended for use by normally healthy adults only. • Persons under 18 years of age or those with highly sensitive or allergic skin should use only as directed by a doctor. • Supervise children in the use of this product.

OTHER INFORMATION
• FUNGICURE may be applied to the cuticles, around nail edges and under nail tips where reachable with its applicator brush. This product is not intended to, nor will it, penetrate hard intact nail surfaces. • While not all finger and toe area fungal infections are curable with OTC topical medications, if you see improvement within 4 weeks of use, you may continue to use FUNGICURE until satisfactory results are obtained. • You may report serious side effects to the phone number provided under *Questions?* below.

INACTIVE INGREDIENT
isopropyl alcohol

QUESTIONS OR COMMENTS?
1-800-792-2582
How Supplied: As a topical liquid: net contents 1 fl. oz. (30 ml) in a bottle with brush applicator. **Storage:** Keep tightly closed when not in use. Store away from excessive heat and cold. When it comes to your manicure and pedicure, rely on FUNGICURE Manicure & Pedicure Formula Anti-Fungal Liquid - The Manicure & Pedicure Fungi Specialist - to help eliminate and prevent the spread of fungal infections of the finger and toe areas.

FUNGICURE FOR JOCK ITCH (sepia)
Alva-Amco Pharmacal Companies, Inc.

Active Ingredient(s)
Sepia 12x

Purpose(s)
Antifungal treatment

USES
For the treatment of most
• jock itch (tinea cruris)
• ringworm (tinea corporis)
• athlete's foot (tinea pedis)

For relief of:
• itching
• scaling
• cracking
• burning
• redness
• soreness
• irritation
• discomforts which may accompany these conditions.

WARNINGS
For external use only

ASK A DOCTOR BEFORE USE
on children under 2 years of age.

WHEN USING THIS PRODUCT
avoid contact with the eyes. If contact occurs rinse thoroughly with water.

STOP USE AND ASK A DOCTOR IF
• irritation occurs
• there is no improvement within 2 weeks (4 weeks for ringworm and athlete's foot).
Keep out of reach of children. If swallowed, get medical help or contact a poison control center right away.

DIRECTIONS
• Read all package directions and warnings before using.
• Use only as directed.
• Clean the affected area with Fungicure Anti-Fungal Soap for Jock Itch and Ringworm and warm water, rinse and dry thoroughly.
• For best results, leave on for 1-2 minutes before rinsing and drying.
• Use twice daily (morning and night), or as directed by a doctor.
• For jock itch, use daily for 2 weeks.
• For ringworm and athlete's foot, use daily for 4 weeks.

- For athlete's foot: pay special attention to spaces between the toes; wear well-fitting, ventilated shoes, and change shoes and socks at least once daily.
- Supervise children in the use of this product.
- Persons under 18 years of age or those with highly sensitive or allergic skin should use only as directed by a doctor.
- This product is not effective on the scalp or nails.

OTHER INFORMATION
You may report serious side effects to the phone number provided under *Questions?* below.

INACTIVE INGREDIENTS
lauramidopropyl betaine, panthenol, phospholipid EFA, purified water, sodium chloride, sodium C14 - 16 olefin sulfonate, tea tree oil.

QUESTIONS OR COMMENTS?
1-800-792-2582

FUNGICURE Anti-Fungal Soap for Jock Itch and Ringworm

Now Treat Jock Itch and Ringworm Infections in the Shower!

Eliminates Common Fungus That Can Attack Healthy Skin.

A WORD ABOUT FUNGICURE ANTI-FUNGAL SOAP FOR JOCK ITCH AND RINGWORM:

FUNGICURE Anti-Fungal Soap for Jock Itch and Ringworm provides a convenient way to treat most jock itch, ringworm, athlete's foot and other common fungus infections of the body, hands and feet while you bathe or shower. Use FUNGICURE Anti-Fungal Soap for Jock Itch and Ringworm as you would any other liquid soap, but with the added confidence that it is also effective for eliminating/washing away fungus. Use FUNGICURE Anti-Fungal Soap for Jock Itch and Ringworm alone or with other methods you may be using to control fungal infections.

WHAT IS FUNGUS INFECTION OF THE BODY, GROIN, AND HANDS and FEET AREAS?

Generally speaking, common fungus infections of the body, hands and feet areas (topical infections) are caused by a variety of fungi; actual living organisms (members of the yeast and mold family) which exist in varying degrees, at all times in nature, and tend to thrive in dark, damp and moist conditions...in the soil...on animals as well as humans. These organisms may penetrate the skin's surface through even the smallest crack or tear, may be spread from animals to humans and may be spread among humans. Common topical fungus infections generally fall into three categories: microsporum (hair and skin), epidermophyton (skin and nails), and trichophyton (hair, skin and nails). Among the more common fungi are T. rubrum which can cause jock itch, E. floccosum which can cause ringworm infection and affects the body, hands and feet, on and in between the fingers including the skin around the fingernails; also T. rubrum and T. mentagrophytes, which can cause athlete's foot and infect the feet, on and between the toes including the skin around the toenails. Often such infections develop slowly and may be difficult to treat if not attended to promptly and treated appropriately with an effective anti-fungal medicine.

HOW DO YOU KNOW IF YOU HAVE A TOPICAL FUNGUS INFECTION?

Topical fungal infections can affect anyone, but men typically experience a higher incidence of jock itch than women. The appearance of jock itch can be characterized as:

- A circular, reddish-brown, raised rash with elevated edges in the groin and/or thigh area.
- Itching, chafing, burning or skin redness.

- Flaking, peeling or cracking skin. Some topical fungus infections may present themselves on the skin as ring-like formations with clear centers, commonly referred to as ringworm. Other such infections, when on the feet, or finger and toe areas, are often characterized by scaling of the skin, burning, cracking, itching and related discomforts. When nails become infected, they may appear to become opaque (cloudy white), thickened, brittle, friable (easily broken) and in some cases, discolored (greenish/brown).

WHAT ARE CAUSES OF JOCK ITCH, RINGWORM AND OTHER FUNGAL INFECTIONS?

Jock itch and ringworm, like other fungal infections, can develop under a variety of conditions, including:

- Hot and humid weather conditions that can cause perspiration to accumulate.
- Friction caused by wearing tight, damp or perspiration-soaked clothing for an extended period of time (e.g. exercise or bathing suit garments).
- Sharing clothes or towels with others who have a fungal infection.

PRODUCT DESCRIPTION AND ACTION:

FUNGICURE Anti-Fungal Soap for Jock Itch is an effective homeopathic formulation containing the ACTIVE INGREDIENT: Sepia 12x

INACTIVE INGREDIENTS: lauramidopropyl betaine, panthenol, phospholipid EFA, purified water, sodium chloride, sodium C14-16 olefin sulfonate, tea tree oil.

PROMPT ACTION AND PROPER TREATMENT:

Recognizing and treating fungus infection early is very important for successful results, so it is wise to consult your doctor promptly for advice if you suspect you may have a fungal infection.

HOW TO AVOID RECURRENCE OF FUNGUS INFECTION:

- Good personal hygiene is your first line of defense against recurring fungus infections.
- Shower or bathe daily, as well as after physical activity that may cause sweating.
- Avoid sharing towels.
- Change and wear clean clothing, especially undergarments that are in contact with affected areas, daily.
- Avoid any practices that can tear or bruise skin. Anything that tears or opens the skin invites fungus to invade.
- If you have a fungal infection on another area of your body, such as ringworm, athlete's foot, or finger and toe area fungus, be sure to treat it right away to help prevent the fungus from spreading to the groin area. Regular use of FUNGICURE Anti-Fungal Soap for Jock Itch helps eliminate/wash away fungus and bacteria that can attack healthy skin.

USES
For the treatment of most: jock itch (tinea cruris), ringworm (tinea corporis), athlete's foot (tinea pedis). For relief of: itching, scaling, cracking, burning, redness, soreness, irritation, and discomforts which may accompany these conditions.

WARNINGS
For external use only.

ASK A DOCTOR BEFORE USE
on children under 2 years of age.

WHEN USING THIS PRODUCT
avoid contact with the eyes. If contact occurs rinse thoroughly with water.

STOP USE AND ASK A DOCTOR IF
irritation occurs or there is no improvement within 2 weeks (4
weeks for ringworm and athlete's foot).

Keep out of reach of children. If swallowed, get medical help
or contact a poison control center right away.

DIRECTIONS
Read all package directions and warnings before using. Use only
as directed. Clean the affected area with Fungicure Anti-Fungal
Soap for Jock Itch and Ringworm and warm water, rinse and
dry thoroughly. For best results, leave on for 1-2 minutes before
rinsing and drying. Use twice daily (morning and night), or as
directed by a doctor. For jock itch, use daily for 2 weeks. For
ringworm and athlete's foot, use daily for 4 weeks. For athlete's
foot: pay special attention to spaces between toes; wear well
fitting, ventilated shoes, and change shoes and socks at least
once daily. Supervise children in the use of this product. Persons
under 18 years of age or those with highly sensitive or allergic
skin should use only as directed by a doctor. This product is not
effective on the scalp or nails.

OTHER INFORMATION
You may report serious side effects to the phone number
provided under *Questions?* below.

QUESTIONS OR COMMENTS?
1-800-792-2582

How Supplied:
6 fluid ounces (177 ml) bottle

FUNGOID TINCTURE (miconazole nitrate)

Pedinol Pharmacal, Inc.

INGREDIENTS

Active Ingredient(s)
Miconazole Nitrate 2% USP.

INACTIVE INGREDIENTS
Acetic acid, benzyl alcohol, isopropyl alcohol (30%), laureth-4.
water.

INDICATIONS
Cures most athlete's foot (tinea pedis), and ringworm (tinea
corporis).

WARNINGS
**DO NOT USE ON CHILDREN UNDER TWO YEARS OF
AGE EXCEPT UNDER THE ADVICE AND SUPERVISION
OF A PHYSICIAN. FOR EXTERNAL USE ONLY. KEEP
OUT OF THE REACH OF CHILDREN.** In case of accidental
ingestion, seek professional assistance or contact a Poison
Control Center immediately. Avoid contact with eyes. If
irritation occurs or if there is no improvement within four
weeks, discontinue use and consult your PHYSICIAN or
PHARMACIST. Do not use if you are known to be sensitive to
any of the ingredients in this product. If you are diabetic or
have circulatory, renal or hepatic problems, consult a doctor or
pharmacist before using.

DIRECTIONS
1. Cleanse and dry affected areas.
2. Apply a thin application twice a day (morning and night) on
   skin under nails and surrounding cuticle areas or as
   recommended by your doctor. Remove Fungoid® Tincture from
   any untreated areas. Remove from all inanimate
   environmental surfaces.
Supervise children in the use of this product. For athlete's foot,
pay special attention to the spaces between the toes; wear well-
fitting, ventilated shoes, and change shoes and socks at least

once daily. For athlete's foot and ringworm, use daily for 4
weeks.
For fungal infection of the nail bed, if condition persists, consult
a doctor who may choose to debride or remove the nail to allow
application of Fungoid® Tincture to the skin of the nail bed.
This product is not effective on the scalp or nails.

HOW SUPPLIED
Available in a 1 fl. oz. (29.57 mL) bottle with brush applicator -
NDC 0884-0293-01.

RECOMMENDED STORAGE
Store at controlled room temperature 15°-30°C (59°-86°F).
Protect from freezing. If freezing occurs, warm to room
temperature.

GAS-X REGULAR STRENGTH CHEWABLE CHERRY (simethicone)

Novartis Consumer Health, Inc.

Active Ingredient(s)
Simethicone 80 mg

Purpose(s)
Antigas

USES
for the relief of
• pressure and bloating commonly referred to as gas

WARNINGS
Keep Out of Reach of Children

DIRECTIONS
• adults: chew 1 or 2 tablets as needed after meals and at
bedtime
• do not exceed 6 tablets in a 24 hours except under the advice
and supervision of a
physician

OTHER INFORMATION
• each tablet contains: calcium 30 mg
• store at controlled room temperature 20-25°C (68-77°F)
• protect from moisture

INACTIVE INGREDIENTS
calcium carbonate, D&C red 30 aluminum lake, dextrose,
flavors, maltodextrin, propylene glycol, soy protein isolate

QUESTIONS OR COMMENTS?
Call 1-800-452-0051 24 hours a day, 7 days a week

GAS-X EXTRA STRENGTH SOFTGELS (simethicone)

Novartis Consumer Health, Inc

Active Ingredient(s) (per softgel)
Simethicone 125 mg

Purpose(s)
Antigas

USE
for the relief of
• pressure, bloating, and fullness commonly referred to as gas

WARNINGS

KEEP OUT OF REACH OF CHILDREN.

DIRECTIONS
- adults: swallow with water 1 or 2 softgels as needed after meals and at bedtime
- do not exceed 4 softgels in 24 hours except under the advice and supervision of a physician

OTHER INFORMATION
- store at a controlled room temperature 20-25°C (68-77°F)
- protect from light, heat and moisture

INACTIVE INGREDIENTS
D&C yellow 10, FD&C blue 1, FD&C red 40, gelatin, glycerin, hypromellose, light mineral oil*, mannitol, medium chain triglycerides*, peppermint oil, purified water, sorbitol, soy lecithin*, titanium dioxide.
*may contain these ingredients

QUESTIONS OR COMMENTS?
call 1-800-452-0051

GAS-X THIN STRIPS (simethicone)
Novartis Consumer Healthcare, Inc.

Gas-X Thin Strips Cinnamon flavor

DRUG FACTS

Active Ingredient(s) (per strip) Purpose(s)
Simethicone 62.5 mg Antigas

USE
for the relief of
- pressure, bloating, and fullness commonly referred to as gas

WARNINGS
Keep out of reach of children

DIRECTIONS
- adults: allow 2 to 4 strips to dissolve on tongue as needed after meals and at bedtime
- do not exceed 8 strips in 24 hours except under the advice and supervision of a physician

OTHER INFORMATION
- store at a controlled room temperature 20-25°C (68-77°F)
- protect from moisture
- read all product information before using. Keep the box for important information.

INACTIVE INGREDIENTS
corn starch modified, ethyl alcohol, FD&C blue #1, flavor, hypromellose, maltodextrin, menthol, polyethylene glycol, sorbitol, sucralose, titanium dioxide, water

QUESTIONS OR COMMENTS?
call 1-800-452-0051

Gas-X Thin Strips Peppermint flavor

DRUG FACTS

Active Ingredient(s) (per strip) Purpose(s)
Simethicone 62.5 mg Antigas

USE
for the relief of
- pressure, bloating, and fullness commonly referred to as gas

WARNINGS
Keep out of reach of children

DIRECTIONS
- adults: allow 2 to 4 strips to dissolve on tongue as needed after meals and at bedtime
- do not exceed 8 strips in 24 hours except under the advice and supervision of a physician

OTHER INFORMATION
- store at a controlled room temperature 20-25°C (68-77°F)
- protect from moisture
- read all product information before using. Keep the box for important information.

INACTIVE INGREDIENTS
corn starch modified, ethyl alcohol, FD&C blue #1, flavor, hypromellose, maltodextrin, menthol, polyethylene glycol, sorbitol, sucralose, titanium dioxide, water

QUESTIONS OR COMMENTS?
call 1-800-452-0051

GAVISCON LIQUID (aluminum hydroxide and magnesium carbonate)
GlaxoSmithKline Consumer Healthcare LP

Active Ingredient(s) (in each 15mL tablespoonful) Regular Strength
Aluminum hydroxide 95mg
Magnesium carbonate 358mg

Active Ingredient(s) (in each 5mL teaspoonful) Extra Strength
Aluminum hydroxide 254mg
Magnesium carbonate 237.5mg

Purpose(s)
Antacid

USES
relieves
- heartburn
- acid indigestion
- sour stomach
- upset stomach associated with these symptoms

WARNINGS

DO NOT USE IF YOU HAVE KIDNEY DISEASE

ASK A DOCTOR OR PHARMACIST BEFORE USE IF YOU ARE
- taking a prescription drug. Antacids may interact with certain prescription drugs.
- if you are on a sodium-restricted diet

WHEN USING THIS PRODUCT (REGULAR STRENGTH)
- do not take more than 8 tablespoonfuls in 24 hours
- do not use the maximum dosage for more than 2 weeks
- laxative effect may occur

WHEN USING THIS PRODUCT (EXTRA STRENGTH)
- do not take more than 16 teaspoonfuls in 24 hours
- do not use the maximum dosage for more than 2 weeks
- laxative effect may occur

KEEP OUT OF REACH OF CHILDREN.
In case of overdose, get medical help or contact a Poison Control Center right away.

DIRECTIONS (REGULAR STRENGTH)
- shake well
- take 1-2 tablespoonfuls four times a day or as directed by a doctor
- take after meals and at bedtime
- dispense product only by spoon or other measuring device

DIRECTIONS (EXTRA STRENGTH)
- shake well
- take 2-4 teaspoonfuls four times a day or as directed by a doctor
- take after meals and at bedtime
- dispense product only by spoon or other measuring device

OTHER INFORMATION (REGULAR STRENGTH)
- **each tablespoon (15mL) contains:** magnesium 115mg, sodium 52mg
- store at up to 25°C (77°F); avoid freezing
- keep tightly closed

OTHER INFORMATION (EXTRA STRENGTH)
- **each teaspoon (5mL) contains:** magnesium 80mg, sodium 14mg
- store at up to 25°C (77°F); avoid freezing
- keep tightly closed

INACTIVE INGREDIENTS (REGULAR STRENGTH)
benzyl alcohol, D&C yellow #10, edetate disodium, FD&C blue #1, flavor, glycerin, saccharin sodium, sodium alginate, sorbitol solution, water, xanthan gum

INACTIVE INGREDIENTS (EXTRA STRENGTH)
benzyl alcohol, edetate disodium, flavor, glycerin, saccharin sodium, simethicone emulsion, sodium alginate, sorbitol solution, water, xanthan gum

QUESTIONS OR COMMENTS?
call toll-free (English/Spanish) **1-888-367-6471** weekdays
Distributed by:
GlaxoSmithKline Consumer Healthcare, L.P.
Moon Twp, PA 15108, Made in the U.S.A
©2010 GlaxoSmithKline
IMPORTANT:
Do not use if foil inner seal imprinted "SEALED FOR YOUR PROTECTION" is disturbed or missing.

GAVISCON EXTRA STRENGTH CHEWABLE TABLETS (aluminum hydroxide and magnesium carbonate)

GlaxoSmithKline Consumer Healthcare LP

Active Ingredient(s) (in each tablet) (Extra Strength)
Aluminum hydroxide 160mg
Magnesium carbonate 105mg

Active Ingredient(s) (in each tablet) (Regular Strength)
Dried aluminum hydroxide gel 80mg
Magnesium trisilicate 14.2mg

Purpose(s)
Antacid

USES (EXTRA STRENGTH)
relieves
- acid indigestion
- heartburn
- sour stomach
- upset stomach associated with these symptoms

USES (REGULAR STRENGTH)
temporarily relieves symptoms of:
- heartburn and acid indigestion due to acid reflux

WARNINGS (EXTRA STRENGTH)

ASK A DOCTOR OR PHARMACIST BEFORE USE IF YOU ARE
- taking a prescription drug. Antacids may interact with certain prescription drugs.
- if you are on a sodium-restricted diet

WHEN USING THIS PRODUCT
- do not take more than 16 tablets in 24 hours
- do not use the maximum dosage for more than 2 weeks

Keep out of reach of children.
In case of overdose, get medical help or contact a Poison Control Center right away.

WARNINGS (REGULAR STRENGTH)

DO NOT USE
- for peptic ulcers
- if you have trouble swallowing

ASK A DOCTOR BEFORE USE IF YOU HAVE
- kidney disease
- a sodium restricted diet

ASK A DOCTOR OR PHARMACIST IF YOU
- are taking a prescription drug. Antacids may interact with certain prescription drugs.

STOP USE AND ASK A DOCTOR IF
- heartburn or stomach pain continues
- you need to take this product for more than 14 days

Keep out of reach of children.
In case of overdose, get medical help or contact a Poison Control Center.

DIRECTIONS (EXTRA STRENGTH)
- chew 2-4 tablets four times a day or as directed by a doctor
- take after meals and at bedtime or as needed
- for best results follow by a half glass of water or other liquid
- DO NOT SWALLOW WHOLE

DIRECTIONS (REGULAR STRENGTH)
- **do not swallow tablets whole**
- chew 2 to 4 tablets after meals and at bedtime as needed (up to 4 times a day) or as directed by a doctor. For best results, drink a half glass of water or other liquid after each dose.
- do not take more than 16 tablets in 24 hours

OTHER INFORMATION (EXTRA STRENGTH)
- **Each tablet contains:** magnesium 35mg, sodium 20mg
- Store at up to 25°C (77°F) in a dry place

OTHER INFORMATION (REGULAR STRENGTH)
- **Each tablet contains:** magnesium 5mg, sodium 21 mg
- Store at up to 25°C (77°F) in a dry place

INACTIVE INGREDIENTS (EXTRA STRENGTH)
alginic acid, calcium stearate, flavor, sodium bicarbonate, and sucrose. May contain stearic acid. Contains sorbitol or mannitol. May contain starch.

INACTIVE INGREDIENTS (EXTRA STRENGTH CHERRY)
acesulfame k, alginic acid, artificial flavor, calcium stearate, corn starch, corn syrup solids, mannitol, sodium bicarbonate, stearic acid, sucrose

INACTIVE INGREDIENTS (REGULAR STRENGTH)
alginic acid, calcium stearate, flavor, sodium bicarbonate, starch (may contain corn starch) and sucrose

QUESTIONS OR COMMENTS?
call toll-free **1-888-367-6471** (English/Spanish) weekdays

GAVISCON EXTRA STRENGTH (aluminum hydroxide and magnesium carbonate)

GlaxoSmithKline Consumer Healthcare LP

Active Ingredient(s) (in each tablet) (Extra Strength)
Aluminum hydroxide 160mg
Magnesium carbonate 105mg

Active Ingredient(s) (in each tablet) (Regular Strength)
Dried aluminum hydroxide gel 80mg
Magnesium trisilicate 14.2mg

Purpose(s)
Antacid

USES (EXTRA STRENGTH)
relieves
• acid indigestion
• heartburn
• sour stomach
• upset stomach associated with these symptoms

USES (REGULAR STRENGTH)
temporarily relieves symptoms of:
• heartburn and acid indigestion due to acid reflux

WARNINGS (EXTRA STRENGTH)

ASK A DOCTOR OR PHARMACIST BEFORE USE IF YOU ARE
• taking a prescription drug. Antacids may interact with certain prescription drugs.
• if you are on a sodium-restricted diet

WHEN USING THIS PRODUCT
• do not take more than 16 tablets in 24 hours
• do not use the maximum dosage for more than 2 weeks

Keep out of reach of children.
In case of overdose, get medical help or contact a Poison Control Center right away.

WARNINGS (REGULAR STRENGTH)

DO NOT USE
• for peptic ulcers
• if you have trouble swallowing

ASK A DOCTOR BEFORE USE IF YOU HAVE
• kidney disease
• a sodium restricted diet

ASK A DOCTOR OR PHARMACIST IF YOU
• are taking a prescription drug. Antacids may interact with certain prescription drugs.

STOP USE AND ASK A DOCTOR IF
• heartburn or stomach pain continues
• you need to take this product for more than 14 days

Keep out of reach of children.
In case of overdose, get medical help or contact a Poison Control Center.

DIRECTIONS (EXTRA STRENGTH)
• chew 2-4 tablets four times a day or as directed by a doctor
• take after meals and at bedtime or as needed
• for best results follow by a half glass of water or other liquid
• DO NOT SWALLOW WHOLE

DIRECTIONS (REGULAR STRENGTH)
• **do not swallow tablets whole**
• chew 2 to 4 tablets after meals and at bedtime as needed (up to 4 times a day) or as directed by a doctor. For best results, drink a half glass of water or other liquid after each dose.
• do not take more than 16 tablets in 24 hours

OTHER INFORMATION (EXTRA STRENGTH)
• **Each tablet contains:** magnesium 35mg, sodium 20mg
• Store at up to 25°C (77°F) in a dry place

OTHER INFORMATION (REGULAR STRENGTH)
• **Each tablet contains:** magnesium 5mg, sodium 21 mg
• Store at up to 25°C (77°F) in a dry place

INACTIVE INGREDIENTS (EXTRA STRENGTH)
alginic acid, calcium stearate, flavor, sodium bicarbonate, and sucrose. May contain stearic acid. Contains sorbitol or mannitol. May contain starch.

INACTIVE INGREDIENTS (EXTRA STRENGTH CHERRY)
acesulfame k, alginic acid, artificial flavor, calcium stearate, corn starch, corn syrup solids, mannitol, sodium bicarbonate, stearic acid, sucrose

INACTIVE INGREDIENTS (REGULAR STRENGTH)
alginic acid, calcium stearate, flavor, sodium bicarbonate, starch (may contain corn starch) and sucrose

QUESTIONS OR COMMENTS?
call toll-free **1-888-367-6471** (English/Spanish) weekdays

GENTEAL MILD TO MODERATE (hypromellose)

Novartis Pharmaceuticals Corporation

Active Ingredient(s)
hypromellose (0.3%)

Purpose(s)
Lubricant

USES
• Relieves dryness of the eye.
• Temporarily relieves discomfort due to minor irritations of the eye or from exposure to wind or sun.
• As a protectant against further irritation.

WARNINGS

DO NOT USE
if solution changes color or becomes cloudy.
if you are sensitive to any ingredient in this product

WHEN USING THIS PRODUCT
do not touch tip of container to any surface. Replace cap after using.

STOP USE AND ASK A DOCTOR IF

you experience any of the following:
• eye pain
• changes in vision
• continued redness or irritation of the eye
• condition worsens or persists more than 72 hours

Keep out of reach of children.
If swallowed, get medical help or contact a Poison Control
Center right away.

DIRECTIONS

Put 1 or 2 drops in the affected eye(s) as needed.

OTHER INFORMATION

Store between 15°-25°C (59°-77°F).

INACTIVE INGREDIENTS

boric acid, phosphoric acid, potassium chloride, purified water,
sodium chloride and sodium perborate. May contain
hydrochloric acid and / or sodium hydroxide to adjust pH.

QUESTIONS OR COMMENTS?

call toll-free **1-866-393-6336**
MedInfo@AlconLabs.com
Serious side effects associated with use of this product may be
reported to this number.

GLUTOSE15 (dextrose)

Paddock Laboratories, Inc.

DIRECTIONS

**To treat a hypoglycemic reaction before unconsciousness oc-
curs:**
Twist tip off, squeeze entire contents of tube (15 grams of
glucose) into mouth and swallow. If no response within 15
minutes, repeat dosage. If no response within 30 minutes,
contact a healthcare provider.

WARNING

FOR ORAL USE ONLY. Do not administer to any person who
is unconscious or unable to swallow. Not recommended for
children under 2 years of age. Keep out of reach of children.

CAUTION:

Sealed tube. Do not use if tube has been opened or punctured.
Store at room temperature.
(02-06)
Paddock
Laboratories, Inc.
Minneapolis, MN 55427

Nutrition Facts	
Serving size 1.3 oz (1 tube)	
Servings per container 1	
Calories 60	
Amount/Serving	**% Daily Value***
Total Fat 0g	0%
Sodium 80mg	3%
Potassium 98mg	3%
Total Carbohydrates 15g	5%
Sugars 15g	
Protein 0g	
Not a significant source of other nutrients.	
*Percent Daily Values based on a 2,000 calorie diet.	

Ingredients:
purified water, dextrose (d-glucose) USP 40%, glycerin, lemon
flavoring, and preservatives in an oral gel base.

GOLD BOND FRICTION DEFENSE

Chattem, Inc.

USES

• Reduces Friction
• Soothes and Moisturizes Skin
• Non-Irritating - Gentle Enough For Even Sensitive Skin

WARNINGS

• For external use only.
• Keep out of reach of children.
• If swallowed, get medical help or contact a Poison Control
  Center immediately.
• Avoid contact with eyes.

AVAILABLE SIZE

1.75 oz. stick

DIRECTIONS

Apply liberally as often as needed to reduce friction and soothe
skin.

GOLD BOND INTENSIVE HEALING ANTI ITCH SKIN PROTECTANT (dimethicone and pramoxine hydrochloride)

Chattem, Inc.

Gold Bond Intensive Healing Anti-Itch Skin Protectant

Active Ingredient(s):
Dimethicone 6%

Purpose(s)
Skin protectant

Active Ingredient(s):
Pramoxine hydrochloride

Purpose(s)
Anti-itch

USES

for temporary relief of pain and itching associated with
• minor skin irritations,
• minor cuts
• minor burns
• minor sunburns
• rashes due to poison ivy, poison oak or poison sumac
• scrapes
• insect bites
• temporarily protects and helps relieve chapped or cracked skin

WARNINGS

For external use only

DO NOT USE ON

• deep or puncture wounds
• animal bites
• serious burns
• large areas of the body

WHEN USING THIS PRODUCT

• do not get into eyes or nose
• not for prolonged use

STOP USE AND ASK A DOCTOR IF
- condition worsens
- symptoms last for more than 7 days or clear up and occur again within a few days
- if redness, irritation, swelling or pain persists or increases

Keep out of reach of children.
If swallowed, get medical help or contact a Poison Control Center immediately.

DIRECTIONS
adults and children 2 years and older: apply to affected area up to 3 or 4 times daily
children under 2 years: consult a doctor

INACTIVE INGREDIENTS
water, glycerin, petrolatum, jojoba esters, cetyl alcohol, aloe barbadensis leaf juice, stearyl alcohol, distearyldimonium chloride, cetearyl alcohol, steareth-21, steareth-2, propylene glycol, chamomilla recutita (matricaria) flower extract, polysorbate 60, stearamidopropyl PG-dimonium chloride phosphate, methyl gluceth-20, tocopheryl acetate, magnesium ascorbyl phosphate, panthenol, retinyl palmitate, EDTA, potassium hydroxide, diazolidinyl urea, methylparaben, propylparaben, hydrolyzed jojoba esters, glyceryl stearate (283-069)
Distributed by CHATTEM, INC., P.O. Box 2219, Chattanooga, TN 37409-0219 USA ©2009 0041822-01
KEEP CARTON AS IT CONTAINS IMPORTANT PRODUCT INFORMATION www.goldbond.com

GOLD BOND ANTI ITCH CREAM (menthol and pramoxine hydrochloride)

Chattem, Inc.

DRUG FACTS

Active Ingredient(s)
Menthol 1%
Pramoxine hydrochloride 1%

Purpose(s)
Anti-itch, Pain relief

USES
for temporary relief of pain and itching associated with:
- minor skin irritations
- minor cuts
- minor burns
- minor sunburns
- rashes due to poison ivy, poison oak or poison sumac
- scrapes
- insect bites

WARNINGS
For external use only

DO NOT USE ON
- deep or puncture wounds
- animals bites
- serious burns
- large areas of the body

WHEN USING THIS PRODUCT
- do not get into eyes or nose
- not for prolonged use

STOP USE AND ASK A DOCTOR IF
- condition worsens
- symptoms last more than 7 days or clear up and occur again within a few days
- if redness, irritation, swelling or pain persists or increases

Keep out of reach of children.
If swallowed, get medical help or contact a Poison Control Center immediately.

DIRECTIONS
adults and children 2 years and older: apply to affected area up to 3 or 4 times daily
children under 2 years: consult a doctor

INACTIVE INGREDIENTS
water, propylene glycol, petrolatum, stearyl alcohol, aloe barbadensis leaf juice, sodium acrylates copolymer, steareth-21, mineral oil, steareth-2, tocopheryl acetate, thymol, eucalyptol, methyl salicylate, PPG-1 trideceth-6, diazolidinyl urea, disodium EDTA, triethanolamine, iodopropynyl butylcarbamate (240-022)

GOLD BOND MEDICATED ANTI-ITCH LOTION (dimethicone, menthol, and pramoxine hydrochloride)

Chattem, Inc.

USES
Temporarily relieves itching associated with:
- Minor burns
- Minor skin irritation
- Sunburn
- Eczema or psoriasis
- Rashes due to poison ivy, oak or sumac

Active Ingredient(s) / Purpose(s)
Dimethicone 5% / Skin Protectant
Menthol 0.5% / Anti-itch
Pramoxine hydrochloride 1% / Anti-itch

WARNINGS
For external use only. Avoid contact with eyes.

DO NOT USE ON
- Deep or puncture wounds
- Animal bites
- Serious burns

STOP USE AND ASK A DOCTOR IF
- Condition worsens.
- Symptoms persist for more than 7 days or clear up and occur again within a few days.
- Redness, irritation, swelling or pain persists or increases.

Keep out of reach of children. In case of accidental ingestion, get medical help or contact a Poison Control Center right away.

Available size:
5.5 oz. pump

DIRECTIONS
Adults and children 2 years and older: Apply freely to affected area 3 or 4 times daily.
Children under 2 years: Consult a doctor.

GOLD BOND EXTRA STRENGTH BODY LOTION (dimethicone and menthol)

Chattem, Inc.

DRUG FACTS - *EXTRA STRENGTH GOLD BOND BODY LOTION*

Active Ingredient(s)
Dimethicone 5%

Purpose(s)
Skin protectant

Active Ingredient(s)
Menthol 0.5%

Purpose(s)
Anti-itch

USES
temporarily relieves itching associated with
• minor skin irritation
• minor burns
• rashes due to poison ivy, oak or sumac
• insect bites
• sunburn
• temporarily protects and helps relieve chapped or cracked skin

WARNINGS
For external use only

DO NOT USE ON
• deep or puncture wounds
• animal bites
• serious burns

WHEN USING THIS PRODUCT
• avoid contact with eyes

STOP USE AND ASK A DOCTOR IF
• condition worsens
• symptoms persist for more than 7 days or clear up and occur again within a few days
• if redness, irritation, swelling or pain persists or increases

Keep out of reach of children.
If swallowed, get medical help or contact a Poison Control Center immediately.

DIRECTIONS
adults and children 2 years and older: apply freely to affected area 3 or 4 times daily
children under 2 years: consult a doctor

INACTIVE INGREDIENTS
water, glycerin, stearamidopropyl PG-dimonium chloride phosphate, petrolatum, emulsifying wax, aloe barbadensis leaf juice, cetyl alcohol, stearyl alcohol, distearyldimonium chloride, propylene glycol, steareth-21, steareth-2, tocopheryl acetate, disodium EDTA, imidazolidinyl urea, propylparaben, methylparaben, triethanolamine, fragrance (227-157)

GOLD BOND ORIGINAL STRENGTH BODY LOTION (dimethicone and menthol)

Chattem, Inc.

DRUG FACTS - *ORIGINAL STRENGTH GOLD BOND BODY LOTION*

Active Ingredient(s)
Dimethicone 5%

Purpose(s)
Skin protectant

Active Ingredient(s)
Menthol 0.15%

Purpose(s)
Anti-itch

USES
temporarily relieves itching associated with
• minor skin irritation
• minor burns
• rashes due to poison ivy, oak or sumac
• insect bites
• sunburn
• temporarily protects and helps relieve chapped or cracked skin

WARNINGS
For external use only

DO NOT USE ON
• deep or puncture wounds
• animal bites
• serious burns

WHEN USING THIS PRODUCT
• avoid contact with eyes

STOP USE AND ASK A DOCTOR IF
• condition worsens
• symptoms persist for more than 7 days or clear up and occur again within a few days
• if redness, irritation, swelling or pain persists or increases

Keep out of reach of children.
If swallowed, get medical help or contact a Poison Control Center immediately.

DIRECTIONS
adults and children 2 years and older: apply freely to affected area 3 or 4 times daily
children under 2 years: consult a doctor

INACTIVE INGREDIENTS
water, glycerin, stearamidopropyl PG-dimonium chloride phosphate, petrolatum, emulsifying wax, aloe barbadensis leaf juice, cetyl alcohol, stearyl alcohol, distearyldimonium chloride, propylene glycol, steareth-21, steareth-2, tocopheryl acetate, disodium EDTA, imidazolidinyl urea, propylparaben, methylparaben, triethanolamine, fragrance (227-156)

GOLD BOND EXTRA STRENGTH BODY POWDER (menthol and zinc oxide)

Chattem, Inc.

DRUG FACTS

Active Ingredient(s)
Menthol 0.8%

Purpose(s)
Anti-Itch

Active Ingredient(s)
Zinc Oxide 5.0%

Purpose(s)
Skin Protectant

USES
temporarily relieves the pain and itch associated with
• minor cuts
• sunburn
• insect bites
• scrapes
• prickly heat
• minor burns
• rashes
• minor skin irritations

WARNINGS
For external use only.

WHEN USING THIS PRODUCT
• avoid contact with eyes

STOP USE AND ASK A DOCTOR IF
• condition worsens
• symptoms do not get better within 7 days

Keep out of reach of children.
In case of accidental ingestion, get medical help or contact a Poison Control Center right away.

DIRECTIONS
• adults and children 2 years and older: apply freely up to 3 or 4 times daily
• under 2 years: ask a doctor
• for best results, dry skin thoroughly before applying

INACTIVE INGREDIENTS
talc, acacia, eucalyptol, methyl salicylate, salicylic acid, thymol, zinc stearate (227-072)

GOLD BOND ORIGINAL STRENGTH BODY POWDER (menthol and zinc oxide)

Chattem, Inc.

DRUG FACTS

Active Ingredient(s)
Menthol 0.15%

Purpose(s)
Anti-Itch

Active Ingredient(s)
Zinc Oxide 1.0%

Purpose(s)
Skin Protectant

USES
temporarily relieves the pain and itch associated with
• minor cuts
• sunburn
• insect bites
• scrapes
• prickly heat
• minor burns
• rashes
• minor skin irritations

WARNINGS
For external use only.

WHEN USING THIS PRODUCT
• avoid contact with eyes

STOP USE AND ASK A DOCTOR IF
• condition worsens
• symptoms do not get better within 7 days

Keep out of reach of children.
In case of accidental ingestion, get medical help or contact a Poison Control Center right away.

DIRECTIONS
• adults and children 2 years and older: apply freely up to 3 or 4 times daily
• under 2 years: ask a doctor
• for best results, dry skin thoroughly before applying

INACTIVE INGREDIENTS
talc, acacia, eucalyptol, methyl salicylate, salicylic acid, thymol, zinc stearate (227-073)

GOLD BOND FOOT POWDER MAXIMUM STRENGTH (menthol)

Chattem, Inc.

DRUG FACTS

Active Ingredient(s)
Menthol 1.0%

Purpose(s)
Anti-Itch

USES
temporarily relieves the pain and itch associated with minor skin irritations on the foot
• provides maximum strength itch relief
• absorbs excess moisture
• helps control foot odor and odor-causing bacteria
• cools and soothes irritated skin

WARNINGS
For external use only.

WHEN USING THIS PRODUCT
• avoid contact with eyes

STOP USE AND ASK A DOCTOR IF
• condition worsens
• symptoms do not get better within 7 days

Keep out of reach of children.
In case of accidental ingestion, get medical help or contact a Poison Control Center right away.

DIRECTIONS
- adults and children 2 years and older: apply freely up to 3 or 4 times daily.
- under 2 years: ask a doctor
- wash and dry feet, sprinkle powder liberally over feet, between toes, on bottoms of feet and in shoes

INACTIVE INGREDIENTS
talc, sodium bicarbonate, acacia, benzethonium chloride, eucalyptus oil, peppermint oil. (227-070)

GOLD BOND PAIN RELIEVING FOOT CREAM
(menthol)

Chattem, Inc.

USES
Temporarily relieves minor foot and ankle arches and pains associated with:
- Arthritis
- Muscle Aches
- Strains
- Sprains
- Muscle and Joint Pain

Active Ingredient(s) / Purpose(s)
Menthol 16% / Topical analgesic

WARNINGS
For external use only.

WHEN USING THIS PRODUCT
- Use only as directed.
- Do not bandage tightly or use with a heating pad.
- Avoid contact with eyes and mucous membranes.
- Do not apply to wounds or damaged skin.

STOP USE AND ASK A DOCTOR IF
- Condition worsens.
- Redness is present.
- Symptoms persist for more than 7 days or clear up and occur again within a few days.
- Irritation or burning develops.

If pregnant or breast-feeding, ask a health professional before use.
Keep out of reach of children. In case of accidental ingestion, get medical help or contact a Poison Control Center right away.

AVAILABLE SIZE
4 oz. tube

DIRECTIONS
Adults and children 12 years of age and older:
- Apply generously to affected area not more than 3 to 4 times daily.
- Massage gently for 30 seconds or until fully absorbed.
- Wash hands thoroughly after use.

Children under 12 years: Ask a doctor.

GOLD BOND THERAPEUTIC FOOT CREAM

Chattem, Inc.

USES
Helps heal dry, rough and cracked feet and heels:
- Relieves Dry, and Irritated Skin
- Soothes & Softens
- Cools & Revitalizes

KEY INGREDIENTS
Seven intensive moisturizers Vitamins A, C and E

DIRECTIONS
Apply liberally as often as needed. Reapply to extremely dry, rough or problem skin areas to help promote speed of healing and to increase level of moisturization.

GYNE-LOTRIMIN 3 (clotrimazole)

MSD Consumer Care, Inc.

DRUG FACTS

Active Ingredient(s)	Purpose(s)
Clotrimazole 2% (100 mg in each applicatorful)	Vaginal antifungal
Clotrimazole 2% (external cream)	Vaginal antifungal

USES
- treats vaginal yeast infections
- relieves external itching due to a vaginal yeast infection

WARNINGS
For vaginal use only
Do not use if you have never had a vaginal yeast infection diagnosed by a doctor

ASK A DOCTOR BEFORE USE IF YOU HAVE
- **vaginal itching and discomfort for the first time**
- **lower abdominal, back or shoulder pain, fever, chills, nausea, vomiting, or foul smelling vaginal discharge. You may have a more serious condition.**
- vaginal yeast infections often (such as once a month or 3 in 6 months). You could be pregnant or have a serious underlying medical cause for your symptoms, including diabetes or a weakened immune system.
- been exposed to the human immunodeficiency virus (HIV) that causes AIDS

WHEN USING THIS PRODUCT
- do not use tampons, douches, spermicides, or other vaginal products. Condoms and diaphragms may be damaged and fail to prevent pregnancy or sexually transmitted diseases (STDs).
- do not have vaginal intercourse
- mild increase in vaginal burning, itching or irritation may occur
- if you do not get complete relief ask a doctor before using another product

STOP USE AND ASK A DOCTOR IF
- **symptoms do not get better in 3 days**
- **symptoms last more than 7 days**
- **you get a rash or hives, abdominal pain, fever, chills, nausea, vomiting, or a foul smelling vaginal discharge**

If pregnant or breast-feeding, ask a health professional before use.
Keep out of the reach of children. If swallowed, get medical help or contact a Poison Control Center right away.

DIRECTIONS
- before using this product read the enclosed educational brochure for complete directions and information
- adults and children 12 years of age and over:
  - **vaginal cream:** insert one applicatorful of cream into the vagina at bedtime for 3 days in a row. Throw applicator away after use.

- **external cream:** use the same tube of cream if you have itching and irritation on the skin outside the vagina. Squeeze a small amount of cream onto your fingertip. Apply to itchy, irritated skin outside the vagina. Use 2 times daily for up to 7 days as needed.
- children under 12 years of age: ask a doctor

OTHER INFORMATION
- store between 20° to 25°C (68° to 77°F)
- see end panel of carton and tube crimp for lot number and expiration date
- **tamper-evident:** do not use if seal embossed with "S" over tube opening is missing, open or broken

INACTIVE INGREDIENTS
benzyl alcohol, cetostearyl alcohol, cetyl esters wax, 2-octyldodecanol, polysorbate 60, purified water, sorbitan monosterate

QUESTIONS OR COMMENTS?
call toll free **1-800-317-2165** between 8:00 AM and 5:00 PM Central Standard Time, Monday through Friday.

GYNE-LOTRIMIN 7 (clotrimazole)
MSD Consumer Care, Inc.

DRUG FACTS

Active Ingredient(s)	Purpose(s)
Clotrimazole 1% (50 mg in each applicatorful)	Vaginal antifungal
Clotrimazole 1% (external cream)	Vaginal antifungal

USES
- treats vaginal yeast infections
- relieves external itching due to a vaginal yeast infection

WARNINGS
- **For vaginal use only**

Do not use if you have never had a vaginal yeast infection diagnosed by a doctor

ASK A DOCTOR BEFORE USE IF YOU HAVE
- **vaginal itching and discomfort for the first time**
- **lower abdominal, back or shoulder pain, fever, chills, nausea, vomiting, or foul smelling vaginal discharge. You may have a more serious condition.**
- vaginal yeast infections often (such as once a month, or 3 in 6 months). You could be pregnant or have a serious underlying medical cause for your symptoms, including diabetes or a weakened immune system.
- been exposed to the human immunodeficiency virus (HIV) that causes AIDS

WHEN USING THIS PRODUCT
- do not use tampons, douches, spermicides, or other vaginal products. Condoms and diaphragms may be damaged and fail to prevent pregnancy or sexually transmitted diseases (STDs).
- do not have vaginal intercourse
- mild increase in vaginal burning, itching or irritation may occur
- if you do not get complete relief ask a doctor before using another product

STOP USE AND ASK A DOCTOR IF
- **symptoms do not get better in 3 days**
- **symptoms last more than 7 days**

- **you get a rash or hives, abdominal pain, fever, chills, nausea, vomiting, or a foul smelling vaginal discharge**

If pregnant or breast-feeding, ask a health professional before use.
Keep out of the reach of children. If swallowed, get medical help or contact a Poison Control Center right away.

DIRECTIONS
- before using this product read the enclosed educational brochure for complete directions and information
- adults and children 12 years of age and over:
  - **vaginal cream:** insert one applicatorful of cream into the vagina at bedtime for 7 days in a row. Wash applicator after each use.
  - **external cream:** use the same tube of cream if you have itching and irritation on the skin outside the vagina. Squeeze a small amount of cream onto your fingertip. Apply to itchy, irritated skin outside the vagina. Use 2 times daily for up to 7 days as needed.
- children under 12 years of age: ask a doctor

OTHER INFORMATION
- store between 20° to 25°C (68° to 77°F)
- see end panel of carton and tube crimp for lot number and expiration date
- **tamper-evident:** do not use if seal embossed with "S" over tube opening is missing, open or broken

INACTIVE INGREDIENTS
benzyl alcohol, cetostearyl alcohol, cetyl esters wax, 2-octyldodecanol, polysorbate 60, purified water, sorbitan monosterate

QUESTIONS OR COMMENTS?
call toll free **1-800-317-2165** between 8:00 AM and 5:00 PM Central Standard Time, Monday through Friday.

HALFPRIN LOW DOSE (aspirin)
Kramer Laboratories

Aspirin 162 mg
Pain reliever
Keep out of reach of children. In case of overdose, get medical help or contact a Poison Control Center right away.
For the temporary relief of minor aches and pains or as recommended by your doctor. If immediate relief is needed, chew the tablet for quicker absorption.

DIRECTIONS
drink a full glass of water with each dose; adults and children 12 years and over: take 2 to 4 tablets every 4 hours not to exceed 24 tablets in 24 hours unless directed by a doctor
Children under 12 years - consult a doctor
Corn Starch, croscarmellose Sodium, DandC yellow no. 10, FDandC RED NO. 40, FDandC YELLOW NO. 6, Hypromellose, HYPROMELLOSE PHTHALATE, CELLULOSE, MICROCRYSTALLINE, Mineral Oil, Polysorbate 80, POLYETHYLENE GLYCOL, Titanium Dioxide
Reye's syndrome: Children and teenagers who have or are recovering from chicken pox or flu-like symptoms should not use this product. When using this product, if changes in behavior with nausea and vomiting occur, consult a doctor because these symptoms could be an early sign of Reye's syndrome, a rare but serious illness.

Allergy Alert: Aspirin may cause a severe allergic reaction which may include:
- hives • facial swelling • asthma (wheezing) • shock

Stomach bleeding warning: This product contains an NSAID, which may cause severe stomach bleeding. The chance is higher if you • are age 60 or older • have had stomach ulcers or bleeding problems • take a blood thinning (anticoagulant) or steroid drug • take other drugs containing prescription or nonprescription NSAIDs (aspirin, ibuprofen, naproxen, or others) • have 3 or more alcoholic drinks every day while using this product • take more or for a longer time than directed.

Do not use if you are allergic to aspirin or any other pain reliever/fever reducer.

HALLS DEFENSE VITAMIN C SUPPLEMENT DROPS

Mondelēz International

SUPPLEMENT FACTS

Serving Size 1 Drop

	Amount per Serving	%Daily Value*
Calories	15	
Sodium	10 mg	<1%*
Total Carbohydrate	4 g	1%*
Sugars	3 g	†
Vitamin C	60 mg	100%

Percent Daily Values (DV) are based on a 2,000 calorie diet.

† *Daily Value (DV) not established.*

OTHER INGREDIENTS
Assorted Citrus:
sugar, glucose syrup, sodium ascorbate, citric acid, natural flavoring, ascorbic acid, color added (with soy lecithin), and red 40.
Strawberry:
sugar, glucose syrup, sodium ascorbate, citric acid, ascorbic acid, natural and artificial flavoring, blue 2, red 40.
Watermelon:
sugar, glucose syrup, sodium ascorbate, citric acid, malic acid, ascorbic acid, potassium citrate, artificial flavor, red 40.

HALLS DEFENSE® HARVEST CHERRY SUPPLEMENT DROPS

Mondelēz International

SUPPLEMENT FACTS

Serving Size 1 Drop

	Amount per Serving	%Daily Value*
Calories	15	
Sodium	10 mg	<1%*
Total Carbohydrate	4 g	1%*
Sugars	3 g	†
Vitamin C	60 mg	100%
Zinc	1.5 mg	10%
Standardized Echinacea Root Extract	15 mg	†

Percent Daily Values (DV) are based on a 2,000 calorie diet.

† *Daily Value (DV) not established.*

OTHER INGREDIENTS
Harvest Cherry:
Sugar, glucose syrup, sodium ascorbate, citric acid, partially hydrogenated cottonseed oil, natural flavoring, ascorbic acid, zinc sulfate, red 40, oils of angelica root, anise star, ginger, lemon grass, sage and white thyme, blue 1.

SUGGESTED USE:
As a dietary supplement for adults, take 1 drop 4 times per day.

WARNINGS:
Do not use for more than 8 weeks consecutively. Do not use if you have a severe systemic illness such as tuberculosis, leukosis, collagen disease, multiple sclerosis or similar condition. Do not use if you have allergies to the daisy family (Asteraceae). Do not use if you are pregnant or breast feeding. Keep out of reach of children.

HERPECIN (dimethicone, meradimate, octinoxate, octisalate, and oxybenzone)

Chattem, Inc.

DRUG FACTS

Active Ingredient(s)
Dimethicone 1%

Purpose(s)
Skin protectant

Active Ingredient(s)
Meradimate 5%
Octinoxate 7.5%
Octisalate 5%
Oxybenzone 6%

Purpose(s)
Sunscreens

USES
• helps prevent sunburn on lips
• relieves dry chapped lips
• helps treat and relieve cold sores/fever blisters

WARNINGS
Skin Cancer/Skin Aging Alert: Spending time in the sun increases your risk of skin cancer and early skin aging. This product has been shown only to help prevent sunburn where applied on lips, not skin cancer or early skin aging.

For external use only

DO NOT USE
- on broken skin
- if you are allergic to any ingredient in this product

WHEN USING THIS PRODUCT
- keep out of eyes. Rinse with water to remove.
- apply only to affected areas
- avoid applying directly inside your mouth
- do not share this product with anyone since this may spread infection

STOP USE AND ASK A DOCTOR IF
- rash occurs, condition worsens or does not improve within 7 days

Keep out of reach of children.
If swallowed, get medical help or contact a Poison Control Center right away.

DIRECTIONS
adults and children 12 years or over:
- apply liberally and evenly to affected area on lips at first sign of cold sore and 15 minutes before sun exposure
- rub in gently but completely
- for cracking or dryness continue to cover lips until absorbed
- reapply liberally as often as needed and at least every 2 hours when in sun
- use a water resistant sunscreen on lips if swimming or sweating

children under 12 years: ask a doctor

OTHER INFORMATION
- protect the product in this container from excessive heat and direct sun

INACTIVE INGREDIENTS
helianthus annuus (hybrid sunflower) oil, petrolatum, ozokerite, mineral oil, microcrystalline wax, talc, titanium dioxide, beeswax, melissa officinalis (balm mint) extract, cetyl lactate, glyceryl laurate, flavor, lysine HCl, ascorbyl palmitate, tocopheryl acetate, pyridoxine HCl, panthenol, BHT (244-014)

ICYHOT PAIN RELIEVING STICK
ICYHOT PAIN RELIEVING BALM
(menthol and methyl salicylate)
McNeil Consumer Healthcare Div. McNeil-PPC, Inc

DRUG FACTS
Stick:

Active Ingredient(s)	Purpose(s)
Menthol 10%	Topical analgesic
Methyl salicylate 30%	Topical analgesic

Balm:

Active Ingredient(s)	Purpose(s)
Menthol 7.6%	Topical analgesic
Methyl salicylate 29%	Topical analgesic

USES
temporarily relieves minor pain associated with:
- arthritis
- simple backache
- muscle strains
- sprains
- bruises
- cramps

WARNINGS
For external use only

SEE INSIDE LABEL FOR COMPLETE DRUG FACTS
Allergy Alert: If prone to allergic reaction from aspirin or salicylates, consult a doctor before use.

WHEN USING THIS PRODUCT
- use only as directed
- do not bandage tightly or use with a heating pad
- avoid contact with eyes or mucous membranes
- do not apply to wounds or damaged, broken or irritated skin

STOP USE AND ASK A DOCTOR IF
- condition worsens
- redness is present
- irritation develops
- symptoms persist for more than 7 days or clear up and occur again within a few days

If pregnant or breast-feeding, ask a health care professional before use.
Keep out of reach of children. If swallowed, get medical help or contact a Poison Control Center right away.

DIRECTIONS
adults and children over 12 years:
- apply generously to affected area
- massage into painful area until thoroughly absorbed into skin
- repeat as necessary, but not more than 4 times daily

children 12 years or younger: ask a doctor

INACTIVE INGREDIENTS
Stick: ceresin, cyclomethicone, hydrogenated castor oil, microcrystalline wax, paraffin, PEG-150 distearate, propylene glycol, stearic acid, stearyl alcohol
Balm: paraffin, white petrolatum

ICYHOT (menthol and methyl salicylate)
Chattem, Inc.

ICYHOT® PAIN RELIEVING CREAM

DRUG FACTS

Active Ingredient(s)
Menthol 10%
Methyl salicylate 30%

Purpose(s)
Topical analgesic

USES
temporarily relieves minor pain associated with:
- arthritis
- simple backache
- muscle strains
- sprains
- bruises
- cramps

WARNINGS
For external use only
Allergy Alert: If prone to allergic reaction from aspirin or salicylates, consult a doctor before use.

WHEN USING THIS PRODUCT
- use only as directed
- do not bandage tightly or use with a heating pad
- avoid contact with eyes or mucous membranes
- do not apply to wounds or damaged, broken or irritated skin

STOP USE AND ASK A DOCTOR IF
- condition worsens
- symptoms persist for more than 7 days or clear up and occur again within a few days
- redness is present
- irritation develops

If pregnant or breast-feeding,
ask a health care professional before use.

Keep out of reach of children.
If case of accidental ingestion, get medical help or contact a Poison Control Center right away.

DIRECTIONS
adults and children over 12 years:
- apply generously to affected area
- massage into painful area until thoroughly absorbed into skin
- repeat as necessary, but not more than 4 times daily

children 12 years or younger: ask a doctor

INACTIVE INGREDIENTS
carbomer, cetyl esters, emulsifying wax, oleth-3 phosphate, stearic acid, triethanolamine, water (245-110)
Close cap tightly after use.

ICYHOT NATURALS (menthol)
Chattem, Inc.

DRUG FACTS

Active Ingredient(s)
Menthol 7.5%

Purpose(s)
Topical analgesic

USES
temporarily relieves minor pain associated with:
- arthritis
- simple backache
- muscle strains
- sprains
- bruises
- cramps

WARNINGS
For external use only

WHEN USING THIS PRODUCT
- use only as directed
- do not bandage tightly or use with a heating pad
- avoid contact with eyes and mucous membranes
- do not apply to wounds or damaged, broken or irritated skin
- a transient burning sensation may occur upon application but generally disappears in several days
- if severe burning sensation occurs, discontinue use immediately
- do not expose the area treated with product to heat or direct sunlight

STOP USE AND ASK A DOCTOR IF
- condition worsens
- redness is present
- irritation develops
- symptoms persist for more than 7 days or clear up and occur again within a few days

If pregnant or breast-feeding,
ask a health professional before use.

Keep out of reach of children.
if swallowed, get medical help or contact a Poison Control Center right away.

DIRECTIONS
adults and children over 12 years:
- apply generously to affected area
- massage into painful area until thoroughly absorbed into skin
- repeat as necessary, but no more than 3 to 4 times daily
- WASH HANDS WITH SOAP AND WATER AFTER APPLYING

children 12 years or younger: ask a doctor

INACTIVE INGREDIENTS
aloe barbadensis leaf juice, beeswax, benzyl alcohol, capsaicin, cetearyl alcohol, cetyl alcohol, cetyl esters, cetyl palmitate, citrus paradise (grapefruit) peel oil, di-PEG-2 soyamine IPDI, disodium EDTA, distearyldimonium chloride, eucalyptus globules leaf oil, glycerin, hydrogenated olive oil, jojoba esters, melaleuca alternifolia (tea tree) leaf oil, menthe viridis (spearmint) leaf oil, olea europaea (olive) fruit oil, olea europaea (olive) oil unsaponifiables, polysorbate 60, potassium hydroxide, propanediol, sorbitan olivate, sorbitan palmitate, steareth-2, steareth-21, stearyl alcohol, water (283-109)
Close cap tightly after use. Keep carton as it contains important information about this product.

ICYHOT MEDICATED NO MESS APPLICATOR (menthol)
Chattem, Inc.

IcyHot® - Medicated No Mess Applicator

Active Ingredient(s)
Menthol 16%

Purpose(s)
Topical analgesic

USES
temporarily relieves minor pain associated with:
- arthritis
- simple backache
- muscle strains
- sprains
- bruises
- cramps

WARNINGS
For external use only

WHEN USING THIS PRODUCT
- use only as directed
- do not bandage tightly or use with a heating pad
- avoid contact with eyes and mucous membranes
- do not apply to wounds or damaged, broken or irritated skin
- a transient burning sensation may occur upon application but generally disappears in several days
- if severe burning sensation occurs, discontinue use immediately
- do not expose the area treated with product to heat or direct sunlight

STOP USE AND ASK A DOCTOR IF
- condition worsens
- redness is present
- irritation develops
- symptoms persist for more than 7 days or clear up and occur again within a few days

Flammable
- keep away from fire or flame

If pregnant or breast-feeding
ask a health professional before use.

Keep out of reach of children
If swallowed, get medical help or contact a Poison Control Center right away.

DIRECTIONS
adults and children over 12 years:
- apply generously to affected area
- massage into painful area until thoroughly absorbed into skin
- repeat as necessary, but no more than 3-4 times daily
- **IF MEDICINE COMES IN CONTACT WITH HANDS, WASH WITH SOAP AND WATER**

children 12 years or younger: ask a doctor

INACTIVE INGREDIENTS
acrylates/C10-30 alkyl acrylate crosspolymer, capsaicin, glycerin, isopropyl myristate, propylene glycol, SD alcohol 40 (30%), water (245-256)

Close cap tightly after use. Keep carton as it contains important information.
Distributed by Chattem, Inc.
P.O. Box 2219
Chattanooga, TN 37409-0219
U.S.A ©2010 www.icyhot.com Recyclable Carton

ICYHOT ARM, NECK & LEG AND SMALL AREAS
ICYHOT BACK AND LARGE AREAS
ICYHOT XL BACK AND LARGE AREAS
(menthol)

Chattem, Inc.

IcyHot® - Medicated Patch
ARM, NECK & LEG & SMALL AREAS

Active Ingredient(s)
Menthol 5%

Purpose(s)
Topical analgesic

USES
- temporarily relieves minor pain associated with:
  - arthritis
  - simple backache
  - bursitis
  - tendonitis
  - muscle strains
  - sprains
  - bruises
  - cramps

WARNINGS
For external use only

WHEN USING THIS PRODUCT
- use only as directed
- do not bandage tightly or use with a heating pad
- avoid contact with eyes and mucous membranes

- do not apply to wounds or damaged skin, broken or irritated skin

STOP USE AND ASK A DOCTOR IF
- condition worsens
- redness is present
- irritation develops
- symptoms persist for more than 7 days or clear up and occur again within a few days

If pregnant or breast-feeding
ask a health professional before use.

Keep out of reach of children.
If swallowed, get medical help or contact a Poison Control Center right away.

DIRECTIONS
adults and children over 12 years.
- remove backing from patch by grasping both ends firmly and gently pulling until backing separates in middle
- carefully remove smaller portion of backing from patch and apply exposed portion of patch to affected area
- once exposed portion of patch is positioned, carefully remove remaining backing to completely apply patch to affected area
- apply one patch to affected area
- wear one IcyHot Patch up to 8 hours
- repeat as necessary, but no more than 4 times daily

children 12 years or younger: ask a doctor

INACTIVE INGREDIENTS
acrylic acid, aluminum hydroxide, carmellose sodium, 2-ethylhexyl acrylate, glycerin, isopropyl myristate, methyl acrylate, nonoxynol-30, polyacrylate, polyacrylic acid, polysorbate 80, sorbitan sesquioleate, starch, talc, tartaric acid, titanium dioxide, water
KEEP CARTON AS IT CONTAINS IMPORTANT INFORMATION FOR USAGE OF THE PRODUCT.
Distributed by Chattem, Inc.
P.O. Box 2219
Chattanooga, TN 37409-0219 USA
©2007 www.icyhot.com
Made in Japan. 0049602-01

IcyHot® - Medicated Patch
BACK & LARGE AREAS

Active Ingredient(s)
Menthol 5%

Purpose(s)
Topical analgesic

USES
- temporarily relieves minor pain associated with:
  - arthritis
  - simple backache
  - bursitis
  - tendonitis
  - muscle strains
  - sprains
  - bruises
  - cramps

WARNINGS
For external use only

WHEN USING THIS PRODUCT
- use only as directed
- do not bandage tightly or use with a heating pad
- avoid contact with eyes and mucous membranes
- do not apply to wounds or damaged skin

STOP USE AND ASK A DOCTOR IF
- condition worsens
- redness is present
- irritation develops
- symptoms persist for more than 7 days or clear up and occur again within a few days

If pregnant or breast-feeding
ask a health professional before use.

Keep out of reach of children.
If swallowed, get medical help or contact a Poison Control Center right away.

DIRECTIONS
adults and children over 12 years.
- remove backing from patch by grasping both ends firmly and gently pulling until backing separates in middle
- carefully remove backing from patch
- apply one patch to affected area
- wear one IcyHot Patch up to 8 hours
- repeat as necessary, but no more than 4 times daily

children 12 years or younger: ask a doctor

INACTIVE INGREDIENTS
acrylic acid, aluminum hydroxide, carmellose sodium, 2-ethylhexyl acrylate, glycerin, isopropyl myristate, methyl acrylate, nonoxynol-30, polyacrylate, polyacrylic acid, polysorbate 80, sorbitan sesquioleate, starch, talc, tartaric acid, titanium dioxide, water
Visit us on the web at www.icyhot.com Made in Japan

IcyHot® - Medicated Patch
XL BACK & LARGE AREAS

Active Ingredient(s)
Menthol 5%

Purpose(s)
Topical analgesic

USES
- temporarily relieves minor pain associated with:
  - arthritis
  - simple backache
  - bursitis
  - tendonitis
  - muscle strains
  - sprains
  - bruises
  - cramps

WARNINGS
For external use only

WHEN USING THIS PRODUCT
- use only as directed
- do not bandage tightly or use with a heating pad
- avoid contact with eyes and mucous membranes
- do not apply to wounds or damaged skin, broken or irritated skin

STOP USE AND ASK A DOCTOR IF
- condition worsens
- redness is present
- irritation develops
- symptoms persist for more than 7 days or clear up and occur again within a few days

If pregnant or breast-feeding
ask a health professional before use.

Keep out of reach of children.
If swallowed, get medical help or contact a Poison Control Center right away.

DIRECTIONS
adults and children over 12 years.
- remove backing from patch by grasping both ends firmly and gently pulling until backing separates
- carefully remove smaller portion of backing from patch and apply exposed portion of patch to affected area
- once exposed portion of patch is positioned, carefully remove remaining backing to completely apply patch to affected area
- apply one patch to affected area
- wear one IcyHot Patch up to 8 hours
- repeat as necessary, but no more than 4 times daily

children 12 years or younger: ask a doctor

INACTIVE INGREDIENTS
acrylic acid, aluminum hydroxide, carmellose sodium, 2-ethylhexyl acrylate, glycerin, isopropyl myristate, methyl acrylate, nonoxynol-30, polyacrylate, polyacrylic acid, polysorbate 80, sorbitan sesquioleate, starch, talc, tartaric acid, titanium dioxide, water
KEEP CARTON AS IT CONTAINS IMPORTANT INFORMATION FOR USAGE OF THE PRODUCT.
Made in Japan. Visit us on the web at www.icyhot.com

ICYHOT MEDICATED ROLL MEDIUM AND LARGE (menthol)

Chattem, Inc.

ICYHOT® - MEDICATED ROLL MEDIUM
Wrist, Ankle, Shoulder

Active Ingredient(s)
Menthol 7.5%

Purpose(s)
Topical analgesic

USES
temporarily relieves minor pain associated with:
- arthritis
- simple backache
- muscle strains
- sprains
- bruises
- cramps

WARNINGS
For external use only

WHEN USING THIS PRODUCT
- use only as directed
- do not bandage tightly or use with a heating pad
- do not overwrap or wrap strips over themselves
- do not wrap around neck
- do not apply over large areas of the body or apply in strips longer than 6 inches
- avoid contact with eyes and mucous membranes
- do not apply to wounds or damaged skin, broken or irritated skin

STOP USE AND ASK A DOCTOR IF
- condition worsens
- redness is present
- irritation develops
- symptoms persist for more than 7 days or clear up and occur again within a few days

If pregnant or breast-feeding
ask a health professional before use.

Keep out of reach of children.
If swallowed, get medical help or contact a Poison Control Center right away.

DIRECTIONS
adults and children over 12 years.
- tear or cut roll to desired size
- carefully remove backing from one end of strip and place on affected area
- remove remaining backing and press into place
- wear one IcyHot Medicated Roll up to 8 hours
- repeat as necessary, but no more than 3 to 4 times daily

children 12 years or younger: ask a doctor

INACTIVE INGREDIENTS
caprylic/capric triglyceride, 2,6-di-tert-butyl-4-(4,6-bis(octylthio)-1,3,5-triazin-2-ylamino)
phenol, mineral oil, petroleum resins, polyisobutene, polyisoprene, styrene/isoprene copolymer, terpene polymer (245-286)
Keep carton as it contains important information for usage of this product.
Distributed by Chattem, Inc.
P.O. Box 2219
Chattanooga, TN 37409-0219 USA
©2009 www.icyhot.com
Chattem ®
ROLL MADE IN JAPAN Recyclable Carton 0044605-04

ICYHOT® - MEDICATED ROLL LARGE
Knee, Shoulder, Back

Active Ingredient(s)
Menthol 7.5%

Purpose(s)
Topical analgesic

USES
temporarily relieves minor pain associated with:
- arthritis
- simple backache
- muscle strains
- sprains
- bruises
- cramps

WARNINGS
For external use only

WHEN USING THIS PRODUCT
- use only as directed
- do not bandage tightly or use with a heating pad
- do not overwrap or wrap strips over themselves
- do not wrap around neck
- do not apply over large areas of the body or apply in strips longer than 6 inches
- avoid contact with eyes and mucous membranes
- do not apply to wounds or damaged skin, broken or irritated skin

STOP USE AND ASK A DOCTOR IF
- condition worsens
- redness is present
- irritation develops
- symptoms persist for more than 7 days or clear up and occur again within a few days

If pregnant or breast-feeding
ask a health professional before use.

Keep out of reach of children.
If swallowed, get medical help or contact a Poison Control Center right away.

DIRECTIONS
adults and children over 12 years.
- tear or cut roll to desired size
- carefully remove backing from one end of strip and place on affected area
- remove remaining backing and press into place
- wear one IcyHot Medicated Roll up to 8 hours
- repeat as necessary, but no more than 3 to 4 times daily

children 12 years or younger: ask a doctor

INACTIVE INGREDIENTS
caprylic/capric triglyceride, 2,6-di-tert-butyl-4-(4,6-bis(octylthio)-1,3,5-triazin-2-ylamino)
phenol, mineral oil, petroleum resins, polyisobutene, polyisoprene, styrene/isoprene copolymer, terpene polymer (245-286)
Keep carton as it contains important information for usage of this product.
Distributed by Chattem, Inc.
P.O. Box 2219
Chattanooga, TN 37409-0219 USA
©2009 www.icyhot.com
Chattem ®
ROLL MADE IN JAPAN Recyclable Carton 0044614-04

ICYHOT MEDICATED SLEEVE (menthol)
Chattem, Inc.

DRUG FACTS
IcyHot Medicated Sleeve - Small

Active Ingredient(s)
Menthol 16%

Purpose(s)
Topical analgesic

USES
temporarily relieves minor pain associated with:
- arthritis
- bursitis
- tendonitis
- muscle strains
- sprains
- bruises
- cramps

WARNINGS
For external use only

WHEN USING THIS PRODUCT
- use only as directed
- do not bandage tightly over sleeve or use with a heating pad
- avoid contact with eyes and mucous membranes
- do not apply to wounds or damaged skin

STOP USE AND ASK A DOCTOR IF
- condition worsens
- redness is present
- irritation develops
- symptoms persist for more than 7 days or clear up and occur again within a few days

If pregnant or breast-feeding,
ask a health professional before use.

Keep out of reach of children.
If swallowed, get medical help or contact a Poison Control Center right away.

DIRECTIONS
adults and children over 12 years:
- remove plastic insert and discard
- pull ICYHOT® SLEEVE onto ankle, elbow or wrist - **note:** medicine is away from skin
- carefully pull ICYHOT® SLEEVE over itself, medicine will then be touching the skin

note: the drawing (above) should help you understand how to do this
- apply one ICYHOT® SLEEVE to affected area
- repeat as necessary, but no more than 4 times daily
- sleeve should feel snug but not tight

children 12 years or younger: ask a doctor

INACTIVE INGREDIENTS
cetyl alcohol, diethylene glycol monoethyl ether, diisopropyl adipate, disodium EDTA, glycerin, glyceryl dilaurate, glyceryl stearate, menthyl lactate, methylparaben, PEG-150 stearate, phenoxyethanol, polysorbate 80, soya sterol, water, xanthan gum (may contain citric acid) (245-39)

DRUG FACTS

IcyHot Medicated Sleeve - Large

Active Ingredient(s)
Menthol 16%

Purpose(s)
Topical analgesic

USES
temporarily relieves minor pain associated with:
- arthritis
- bursitis
- tendonitis
- muscle strains
- sprains
- bruises
- cramps

WARNINGS
For external use only

WHEN USING THIS PRODUCT
- use only as directed
- do not bandage tightly over sleeve or use with a heating pad
- avoid contact with eyes and mucous membranes
- do not apply to wounds or damaged skin

STOP USE AND ASK A DOCTOR IF
- condition worsens
- redness is present
- irritation develops
- symptoms persist for more than 7 days or clear up and occur again within a few days

If pregnant or breast-feeding,
ask a health professional before use.

Keep out of reach of children.
If swallowed, get medical help or contact a Poison Control Center right away.

DIRECTIONS
adults and children over 12 years:
- remove plastic insert and discard
- pull ICYHOT® SLEEVE onto ankle, elbow or knee - **note**: medicine is away from skin
- carefully pull ICYHOT® SLEEVE over itself, medicine will then be touching the skin
  note: the drawing (above) should help you understand how to do this
- apply one ICYHOT® SLEEVE to affected area
- repeat as necessary, but no more than 4 times daily
- sleeve should feel snug but not tight

children 12 years or younger: ask a doctor

INACTIVE INGREDIENTS
cetyl alcohol, citric acid, diethylene glycol monoethyl ether, diisopropyl adipate, disodium EDTA, ethoxydiglycol, glycerin, glyceryl dilaurate, glyceryl stearate, glycine soya sterols, menthyl lactate, methylparaben, PEG-150 stearate, phenoxyethanol, polysorbate 80, water, xanthan gum (245-39)

ICYHOT MEDICATED SPRAY (menthol)
Chattem, Inc.

ICYHOT® - MEDICATED SPRAY

Active Ingredient(s)
Menthol 16%

Purpose(s)
Topical analgesic

USES
temporarily relieves minor pain associated with:
- arthritis
- simple
- backache
- muscle
- strains
- sprains
- bruises
- cramps

WARNINGS
For external use only

WHEN USING THIS PRODUCT
- use only as directed
- do not bandage tightly or use with a heating pad
- avoid contact with eyes and mucous membranes
- do not apply to wounds or damaged, broken or irritated skin
- do not spray onto face
- avoid inhaling spray mist and fumes

STOP USE AND ASK A DOCTOR IF
- condition worsens
- redness is present
- irritation develops
- symptoms persist for more than 7 days or clear up and occur again within a few days

Flammable
- do not use near heat or flame or while smoking
- avoid long term storage above 104ºF (40ºC)
- do not puncture or incinerate. Contents under pressure.
- do not store at temperatures above 120ºF (49ºC)

If pregnant or breast-feeding
ask a health professional before use.

Keep out of reach of children
If swallowed, get medical help or contact a Poison Control Center right away.

DIRECTIONS
adults and children over 12 years:
- spray affected area with desired amount of product
- product will dry quickly on its own, and does not need to be rubbed in
- repeat as necessary, but no more than 3-4 times daily

children 12 years or younger: ask a doctor

INACTIVE INGREDIENTS
glycerin, propylene glycol, SD alcohol 40-2 (55%), water (283-016)
Dist. by Chattem, Inc., P.O. Box 2219
Chattanooga, TN 37409-0219
USA ©2009 www.icyhot.com

ICYHOT VANISHING SCENT (menthol)

Chattem, Inc.

DRUG FACTS

Active Ingredient(s)
Menthol 2.5%

Purpose(s)
Topical analgesic

USES
temporarily relieves minor pain associated with:
- arthritis
- simple backache
- muscle strains
- sprains
- bruises
- cramps

WARNINGS
For external use only

WHEN USING THIS PRODUCT
- use only as directed
- do not bandage tightly or use with a heating pad
- avoid contact with eyes or mucous membranes
- do not apply to wounds or damaged, broken or irritated skin

STOP USE AND ASK A DOCTOR IF
- condition worsens
- symptoms persist for more than 7 days or clear up and occur again within a few days
- redness is present
- irritation develops

If pregnant or breast-feeding, ask a health care professional before use.

Keep out of reach of children. If swallowed, get medical help or contact a Poison Control Center right away.

DIRECTIONS
adults and children over 12 years:
- apply generously to affected area
- squeeze desired amount of IcyHot® pain relieving gel onto affected area
- using the sponge-top applicator, massage dispensed gel into painful area until thoroughly absorbed
- repeat as necessary, but not more than 4 times daily

children 12 years or younger: ask a doctor

INACTIVE INGREDIENTS
allantoin, aloe barbadensis leaf juice, carbomer, DMDM hydantoin, glycerin, methylparaben, phenoxyethanol, propylparaben, SD alcohol 40-2 (15.47%), steareth-2, steareth-21, triethanolamine, water (245-135)
Keep carton as it contains important information. Close cap tightly after use.

IMODIUM A-D (loperamide hydrochloride)

McNeil Consumer Healthcare Div McNeil-PPC, Inc.

DRUG FACTS

Active Ingredient(s) (in each caplet)
Loperamide HCl 2 mg

Purpose(s)
Anti-diarrheal

USE
controls symptoms of diarrhea, including Travelers' Diarrhea

WARNINGS
Allergy alert

DO NOT USE
if you have ever had a rash or other allergic reaction to loperamide HCl
Do not use if you have bloody or black stool

ASK A DOCTOR BEFORE USE IF YOU HAVE
- fever
- mucus in the stool
- a history of liver disease

ASK A DOCTOR OR PHARMACIST BEFORE USE IF YOU ARE
taking antibiotics

WHEN USING THIS PRODUCT
tiredness, drowsiness or dizziness may occur. Be careful when driving or operating machinery.

STOP USE AND ASK A DOCTOR IF
- symptoms get worse
- diarrhea lasts for more than 2 days
- you get abdominal swelling or bulging. These may be signs of a serious condition.

If pregnant or breast-feeding, ask a health professional before use.
Keep out of reach of children. In case of overdose, get medical help or contact a Poison Control Center right away. (1-800-222-1222)

DIRECTIONS
- drink plenty of clear fluids to help prevent dehydration caused by diarrhea
- find right dose on chart. If possible, use weight to dose; otherwise, use age.

adults and children 12 years and over	2 caplets after the first loose stool; 1 caplet after each subsequent loose stool; but no more than 4 caplets in 24 hours
children 9-11 years (60-95 lbs)	1 caplet after the first loose stool; 1/2 caplet after each subsequent loose stool; but no more than 3 caplets in 24 hours
children 6-8 years (48-59 lbs)	1 caplet after the first loose stool; 1/2 caplet after each subsequent loose stool; but no more than 2 caplets in 24 hours
children under 6 years (up to 47 lbs)	ask a doctor

OTHER INFORMATION
- each caplet contains: calcium 10 mg
- store between 20-25°C (68-77°F)
- do not use if carton or blister unit is open or torn
- see side panel for lot number and expiration date

INACTIVE INGREDIENTS
colloidal silicon dioxide, dibasic calcium phosphate dihydrate, D&C yellow no. 10 aluminum lake, FD&C blue no. 1 aluminum lake, magnesium stearate, microcrystalline cellulose

QUESTIONS OR COMMENTS?
call 1-877-895-3665

IMODIUM A-D EZ CHEWS (loperamide hydrochloride)
McNeil Consumer Healthcare Div McNeil-PPC, Inc.

DRUG FACTS

Active Ingredient(s) (in each tablet)
Loperamide HCl 2 mg

Purpose(s)
Anti-diarrheal

USE
controls symptoms of diarrhea, including Travelers' Diarrhea

WARNINGS
Allergy alert

DO NOT USE
if you have ever had a rash or other allergic reaction to loperamide HCl
Do not use if you have bloody or black stool

ASK A DOCTOR BEFORE USE IF YOU HAVE
• fever
• mucus in the stool
• a history of liver disease

ASK A DOCTOR OR PHARMACIST BEFORE USE IF YOU ARE
taking antibiotics

WHEN USING THIS PRODUCT
tiredness, drowsiness or dizziness may occur. Be careful when driving or operating machinery.

STOP USE AND ASK A DOCTOR IF
• symptoms get worse
• diarrhea lasts for more than 2 days
• you get abdominal swelling or bulging. These may be signs of a serious condition.

If pregnant or breast-feeding, ask a health professional before use.
Keep out of reach of children. In case of overdose, get medical help or contact a Poison Control Center right away. (1-800-222-1222)

DIRECTIONS
• **drink plenty of clear fluids to help prevent dehydration caused by diarrhea**
• take only on an empty stomach (1 hour before or 2 hours after a meal)
• find right dose on chart. If possible, use weight to dose; otherwise, use age.

adults and children 12 years and over	chew 2 tablets after the first loose stool; chew 1 tablet after each subsequent loose stool; but no more than 4 tablets in 24 hours
children 9-11 years (60-95 lbs)	chew 1 tablet after the first loose stool; chew ½ tablet after each subsequent loose stool; but no more than 3 tablets in 24 hours
children 6-8 years (48-59 lbs)	chew 1 tablet after the first loose stool; chew ½ tablet after each subsequent loose stool; but no more than 2 tablets in 24 hours
children under 6 years (up to 47 lbs)	ask a doctor

OTHER INFORMATION
• **contains milk**
• store between 20-25° C (68-77° F)
• **do not use if carton is open or if printed foil seal under bottle cap is open or torn**
• see bottom panel for lot number and expiration date

INACTIVE INGREDIENTS
acesulfame potassium, basic polymethacrylate, cellulose acetate, confectioner's sugar, crospovidone, D&C yellow #10 aluminum lake, dextrose excipient, FD&C blue #1 aluminum lake, flavors, magnesium stearate, microcrystalline cellulose, milk powder, sucralose

QUESTIONS OR COMMENTS?
call **1-877-895-3665**

IMODIUM A-D LIQUID FOR USE IN CHILDREN (loperamide hydrochloride)
McNeil Consumer Healthcare Div McNeil-PPC, Inc.

USES
Controls symptoms of diarrhea, including Traveler's Diarrhea.

AVAILABLE AS
• liquid

DIRECTIONS
• **Drink plenty of clear fluids to help prevent dehydration caused by diarrhea.**
• Find right dose on chart. If possible, use weight to dose; otherwise, use age.
• Shake well before using.
• Only use attached measuring cup to dose product.

AGE/WEIGHT	IMODIUM® A-D LIQUID FOR USE IN CHILDREN
Adults & Children 12 years & over	30 mL (6 tsp) after first loose stool; 15 mL (3 tsp) after each subsequent loose stool; but no more than 60 mL (12 tsp) in 24 hours
Children 9 - 11 years (60-95 lbs)	15 mL (3 tsp) after first loose stool; 7.5 mL (1 ½ tsp) after each subsequent loose stool; but no more than 45 mL (9 tsp) in 24 hours
Children 6 - 8 years (48-59 lbs)	15 mL (3 tsp) after first loose stool; 7.5 mL (1 ½ tsp) after each subsequent loose stool; but no more than 30 mL (6 tsp) in 24 hours
Children under 6 years (up to 47 lbs)	Ask a doctor.

INGREDIENTS

	ACTIVE INGREDIENTS	INACTIVE INGREDIENTS
IMODIUM® A-D Liquid	Loperamide HCl 1 mg (in each 7.5 mL)	Carboxymethyl-cellulose sodium, citric acid, D&C yellow #10, FD&C blue #1, glycerin, flavor, microcrystalline cellulose, propylene glycol, simethicone emulsion, sodium benzoate, sucralose, titanium dioxide, xanthan gum.

WARNINGS
Allergy alert: Do not use if you have ever had a rash or other allergic reaction to loperamide HCl.

DO NOT USE
if you have bloody or black stool.

ASK A DOCTOR BEFORE USE IF YOU HAVE
- fever.
- Mucus in the stool.
- A history of liver disease.

ASK A DOCTOR OR PHARMACIST BEFORE USE IF YOU ARE
taking antibiotics.

WHEN USING THIS PRODUCT
tiredness, drowsiness, or dizziness may occur. Be careful when driving or operating machinery.

STOP USE AND ASK A DOCTOR IF
- Symptoms get worse.
- Diarrhea lasts for more than 2 days.
- You get abdominal swelling or bulging. These may be signs of a serious condition.

If pregnant or breast-feeding, ask a health professional before use.
Keep out of the reach of children.
In case of overdose, get medical help or contact a Poison Control Center right away. (1-800-222-1222)

OTHER INFORMATION
- Each 30 mL (6 tsp) contains: sodium 16 mg
- Store between 20 and 25°C (68-77°F).
- Do not use if printed inner or outer neckband is broken or missing.

IMODIUM A-D (loperamide hydrochloride)
McNeil Consumer Healthcare Div McNeil-PPC, Inc.

DRUG FACTS
Active Ingredient(s) (in each 7.5 mL)
Loperamide HCl 1 mg

Purpose(s)
Anti-diarrheal

USE
controls symptoms of diarrhea, including Travelers' Diarrhea

WARNINGS
Allergy alert

DO NOT USE
if you have ever had a rash or other allergic reaction to loperamide HCl
Do not use if you have bloody or black stool

ASK A DOCTOR BEFORE USE IF YOU HAVE
- fever
- mucus in the stool
- a history of liver disease

ASK A DOCTOR OR PHARMACIST BEFORE USE IF YOU ARE
taking antibiotics

WHEN USING THIS PRODUCT
tiredness, drowsiness or dizziness may occur. Be careful when driving or operating machinery.

STOP USE AND ASK A DOCTOR IF
- symptoms get worse
- diarrhea lasts for more than 2 days
- you get abdominal swelling or bulging. These may be signs of a serious condition.

If pregnant or breast-feeding, ask a health professional before use.
Keep out of reach of children. In case of overdose, get medical help or contact a Poison Control Center right away. (1-800-222-1222)

DIRECTIONS
- drink plenty of clear fluids to help prevent dehydration caused by diarrhea
- find right dose on chart. If possible, use weight to dose; otherwise use age.
- shake well before using
- only use attached measuring cup to dose product

adults and children 12 years and over	30 mL (6 tsp) after the first loose stool; 15 mL (3 tsp) after each subsequent loose stool; but no more than 60 mL (12 tsp) in 24 hours
children 9-11 years (60-95 lbs)	15 mL (3 tsp) after first loose stool; 7.5 mL (1 1/2 tsp) after each subsequent loose stool; but no more than 45 mL (9 tsp) in 24 hours
children 6-8 years (48-59 lbs)	15 mL (3 tsp) after first loose stool; 7.5 mL (1 1/2 tsp) after each subsequent loose stool; but no more than 30 mL (6 tsp) in 24 hours
children under 6 years (up to 47 lbs)	ask a doctor

OTHER INFORMATION
- each 30 mL (6 tsp) contains: **sodium 16 mg**
- store between 20-25°C (68-77°F)
- **do not use if printed inner or outer neckband is broken or missing**
- see side panel for lot number and expiration date

INACTIVE INGREDIENTS
carboxymethylcellulose sodium, citric acid, D&C yellow #10, FD&C blue #1, glycerin, flavor, microcrystalline cellulose, propylene glycol, purified water, simethicone emulsion, sodium benzoate, sucralose, titanium dioxide, xanthan gum

QUESTIONS OR COMMENTS?
call **1-877-895-3665**

IMODIUM MULTI-SYMPTOM RELIEF
(loperamide hydrochloride and simethicone)
McNeil Consumer Healthcare Div McNeil-PPC, Inc.

DRUGS FACTS

Active Ingredient(s) (in each caplet)	Purpose(s)
Loperamide HCl 2 mg	Anti-diarrheal
Simethicone 125 mg	Anti-gas

USES
relieves symptoms of diarrhea plus bloating, pressure and cramps, commonly referred to as gas

WARNINGS
Allergy alert
Do not use if you have ever had a rash or other allergic reaction to loperamide HCl
Do not use if you have bloody or black stool

ASK A DOCTOR BEFORE USE IF YOU HAVE
- fever
- mucus in the stool
- a history of liver disease

ASK A DOCTOR OR PHARMACIST BEFORE USE IF YOU ARE
- taking antibiotics

WHEN USING THIS PRODUCT
- tiredness, drowsiness or dizziness may occur. Be careful when driving or operating machinery.

STOP USE AND ASK A DOCTOR IF
- symptoms get worse
- diarrhea lasts for more than 2 days
- you get abdominal swelling or bulging. These may be signs of a serious condition.

If pregnant or breast-feeding, ask a health professional before use.
Keep out of reach of children. In case of overdose, get medical help or contact a Poison Control Center right away. (1-800-222-1222)

DIRECTIONS
- **drink plenty of clear fluids to help prevent dehydration caused by diarrhea**
- take only on an empty stomach (1 hour before or 2 hours after a meal)
- find right dose on chart below. If possible, use weight to dose; otherwise, use age.

adults and children 12 years and over	2 caplet after the first loose stool; 1 caplet after each subsequent loose stool; but no more than 4 caplets in 24 hours
children 9-11 years (60-95 lbs)	1 caplet after the first loose stool; ½ caplet after each subsequent loose stool; but no more than 3 caplets in 24 hours
children 6-8 years (48-59 lbs)	1 caplet after the first loose stool; ½ caplet after each subsequent loose stool; but no more than 2 caplets in 24 hours
children under 6 years (up to 47 lbs)	ask a doctor

OTHER INFORMATION
- each caplet contains: calcium 165 mg, sodium 4 mg
- store between 20-25°C (68-77°F). Protect from light.
- do not use if carton is open or if blister unit is open or torn
- see side panel for expiration date and lot number

INACTIVE INGREDIENTS
acesulfame potassium, croscarmellose sodium, dibasic calcium phosphate, flavor, microcrystalline cellulose, stearic acid

QUESTIONS OR COMMENTS?
call 1-877-895-3665

INSTA-GLUCOSE
Valeant Pharmaceuticals

INGREDIENTS
- Liquid glucose
- Purified water
- Artificial cherry flavor
- Methylparaben
- Potassium sorbate

- Sodium benzoate
- Propylparaben

INSTRUCTIONS
- Use under medical supervision
- Twist off cap and discard
- Bring tube to mouth and squeeze slowly and evenly, swallowing entire contents
- If no response after 10 minutes, repeat with another tube

STORAGE
- 25° C (77° F)
- Excursions permitted: 15-30° C (59-86° F)
- Safe for travel

IVY-DRY BUGBITE

Ivy-Dry, Inc.

Ivy-Dry® BugBite temporary relieves the pain and itching associated with minor skin irritations, inflammation and rashes due to insect bites and stings, poison ivy, oak or sumac and minor skin irritations. It's convenient size and easy spray cap allows you to use it on the go, wherever you may experience the urge to itch. It also contains Zin Complex which allows emollients to remain on the skin longer without causing irritation, further reducing the chances of irritation and redness. This new forumal helps **Ivy-Dry® BugBite** fight itching, redness and irritation more effectively!
Ideal for:
- Bug Bites
- Poison Ivy
- Bug Stings

Any questions on any of our products, please call Toll Free 1-800-443-8856

IVY DRY CREAM (benzyl alcohol, camphor, and menthol)

Ivy Dry, Inc.

Active Ingredient(s)
Benzyl Alcohol 10%
Camphor 0.6%
Menthol 0.4%

Purpose(s)
External Analgesic

USES
for the temporary relief of itching associated with insect bites and minor skin irritations.

WARNINGS
For external use only.

DO NOT USE
- face or genital areas
- on a reas of blistered or broken skin
- with a compress after application

WHEN USING THIS PRODUCT
do not get into eyes if contact occurs, flush eyes with water

STOP USE AND ASK A DOCTOR IF
- condition worsens
- symptoms last more than 7 days or clear up and occur again within a few days.

If pregnant or breastfeeding
ask a health professional before use.

Keep out of reach of children.
If swallowed, get medical help or contact Poison Control Center right away.

DIRECTIONS
- Apply to affected area not more than 3 times daily.
- Children under 2 years of age: do not use, ask a doctor.
- Severe reactions to Urushiol (the chemical released by the plant, which causes the irritation) can look like chemical burns and have a thick leathery appearance. Additional applications may be necessary.
- Test product on small patch of skin before applying to the entire body.

OTHER INFORMATION
- Store at room temperature.
- You may report a serious adverse reaction to Report Reaction, LLC. PO Box 22, Plainsboro, NJ 08536-0222.

INACTIVE INGREDIENTS
water, structure XL, cutina GMS, phenoxol T, cremaphor CO 40, butylene glycol, zinc acetate, steareth-2, steareth-20, steareth 100, proaqua ISL, pelemol IPM, estol 1543, glydant plus, dimethicone, VE acetate, allantoin.
Made in the U.S.A. for:
IVY-DRY, INC.
299-B Fairfield Ave.
Fairfield, NJ 07070
©2012 Ivy-Dry, Inc.

QUESTIONS OR COMMENTS?
www.ivydry.com

IVY-DRY SOAP

Ivy-Dry, Inc.

Quickly washes away the itch from Poison-Ivy, Oak and Sumac
Simpler to use and less expensive than the competition. One of the main problems when treating poison ivy is reoccurrences or reinfections and most times this is caused by not completely removing the Urushiol (the toxin that causes poison ivy) from your skin or your environs. Creams and Scrubs work on small areas, but Ivy Dry Soap is made to treat larger areas and as a total body wash. You can even use the soap to wash your clothes, pets and tools. The goal is to remove Urushiol from your body and your surrounding as quickly as possible.
Ivy Dry® Soap is a complete body wash. Many people recontaminate themselves by touching the items that initially came in contact with the poison ivy (clothes, tools, pets, etc.). By washing your entire body and these objects thoroughly, you will reduce the chance of missing an area that hasn't manifested yet. Patent pending.
Ideal for:
- Poison Ivy
- Poison Sumac
- Poison Oak

Any questions on any of our products, please call Toll Free 1-800-443-8856

IVY-DRY SUPER (benzyl alcohol, camphor, and menthol)

Ivy-Dry, Inc.

Active Ingredient(s)
Benzyl Alcohol 10%
Camphor 0.5%
Menthol 0.25%

Purpose(s)
External Analgesic

USES
- for the temporary relief of itching associated with insect bites and minor skin irritations

For external use only.

DO NOT USE
- on face or genital areas
- on areas of blistered or broken skin
- with a compress after application

WHEN USING THIS PRODUCT
- do not get into eyes
- if contact occurs, flush eyes with water

STOP USE AND ASK A DOCTOR IF
- condition worsens
- symptoms last more than 7 days or clear up and occur again within a few days.

If pregnant or breast-feeding,
ask a doctor before use.

Keep out of reach of children.
If swallowed, get medical help or contact Poison Control Center right away.

DIRECTIONS
- Apply to affected area not more than 3 times daily.
- Children under 6 years of age: do not use, ask a doctor.
- Severe reactions to Urushiol (the chemical released by the plant, which causes the irritation) can look like chemical burns and have a thick leathery appearance. Additional applications may be necessary.
- Test product on small patch of skin before applying to the entire body.

OTHER INFORMATION
Store at room temperature
You may report a serious adverse reaction to Report Reaction LLC, PO Box 22, Plainsboro, NJ 08536-0222

INACTIVE INGREDIENTS
water, isopropanol, zinc acetate, isoceteth-20, zinc lactate

IVY-DRY SUPER (benzyl alcohol, camphor, and menthol)

Ivy-Dry, Inc.

Active Ingredient(s)
Benzyl Alcohol 10%
Camphor 0.5%
Menthol 0.25%

Purpose(s)
External Analgesic

USES
- for the temporary relief of itching associated with insect bites and minor skin irritations

For external use only.

DO NOT USE
- on face or genital areas
- on areas of blistered or broken skin
- with a compress after application

WHEN USING THIS PRODUCT
- do not get into eyes
- if contact occurs, flush eyes with water

STOP USE AND ASK A DOCTOR IF
- condition worsens
- symptoms last more than 7 days or clear up and occur again within a few days.

If pregnant or breast-feeding,
ask a doctor before use.

Keep out of reach of children.
If swallowed, get medical help or contact Poison Control Center right away.

DIRECTIONS
- Apply to affected area not more than 3 times daily.
- Children under 6 years of age: do not use, ask a doctor.
- Severe reactions to Urushiol (the chemical released by the plant, which causes the irritation) can look like chemical burns and have a thick leathery appearance. Additional applications may be necessary.
- Test product on small patch of skin before applying to the entire body.

OTHER INFORMATION
Store at room temperature
You may report a serious adverse reaction to Report Reaction, LLC PO Box 22 Plainsboro, NJ 08536-0222

INACTIVE INFORMATION
water, isopropanol, zinc acetate, isoceteth-20, zinc lactate.

KANKA MOUTH PAIN (benzocaine)

Blistex

DRUG FACTS

Active Ingredient(s)	Purpose(s)
Benzocaine 20.0% (w/w)	Oral anesthetic/analgesic

USES
- for the temporary relief of pain due to canker sores, minor irritation of the mouth and gums caused by dentures or orthodontic appliances, or minor injury of the mouth or gums

WARNINGS
For oral use only
Allergy alert: do not use this product if you have a history of allergy to local anesthetics such as procaine, butacaine, benzocaine, or other "caine" anesthetics.

WHEN USING THIS PRODUCT
- do not use for more than 7 days unless directed by a dentist or doctor. If sore mouth symptoms do not improve in 7 days; if irritation, pain or redness persists or worsens; or if swelling, rash or fever develops, see your doctor or dentist promptly. Do not exceed recommended dosage.

Keep out of reach of children.
If swallowed, get medical help or contact a Poison Control Center right away.

DIRECTIONS
- to assure formation of a long-lasting film coating, dry affected area and apply medication undiluted with applicator
- allow a few seconds for coating to form
- use up to 4 times daily, or as directed by a dentist or doctor
- children under 2 years of age: consult a dentist or doctor
- children under 12 years of age should be supervised in the use of this product

OTHER INFORMATION
- do not purchase if package has been opened
- store at 20-25°C (68-77°F)
- cap tightly after use to avoid evaporation
- avoid contact with the eyes
- avoid contact with clothing and household/furniture surfaces to prevent possible staining
- this is a personal care item, and should be used by one individual only

INACTIVE INGREDIENTS
benzyl alcohol, cetylpyridinium chloride, compound benzoin tincture, dimethyl isosorbide, ethylcellulose, flavor, octylacrylamide/acrylates/butylaminoethyl methacrylate copolymer, oleth-10, PEG-6, propylene glycol, ricinus communis (castor) seed oil, SD alcohol 38-B (29.6% v/v), sodium saccharin, sucralose, tannic acid

---

KAOPECTATE REGULAR STRENGTH VANILLA FLAVOR ANTI DIARRHEAL (bismuth subsalicylate)

Physicians Total Care, Inc.

ACTIVE INGREDIENT(S) (PER 15ML):
Bismuth subsalicylate 262 mg

PURPOSE(S)
Anti-diarrheal
Upset stomach reliever

USES
- relieves diarrhea
- relieves nausea and upset stomach associated with this symptom

WARNINGS
Reye's Syndrome:
Children and teenagers who have or are recovering from chicken pox or flu-like symptoms should not use this product. When using this product, if changes in behavior with nausea and vomiting occur, consult a doctor because these symptoms could be an early sign of Reye's syndrome, a rare but serious illness.

Allergy Alert: Contains salicylate.

Do not take if you are
- allergic to salicylates (including aspirin)
- taking other salicylate products

DO NOT USE IF YOU HAVE
- an ulcer
- a bleeding problem
- bloody or black stool

ASK A DOCTOR BEFORE USE IF YOU HAVE
- fever
- mucus in the stool

ASK A DOCTOR OR PHARMACIST BEFORE USE IF YOU ARE TAKING ANY DRUG FOR
- diabetes
- gout
- arthritis
- anticoagulation (thinning the blood)

WHEN USING THIS PRODUCT
a temporary, but harmless, darkening of the stool and/or tongue may occur

STOP USE AND ASK A DOCTOR IF
- symptoms get worse
- ringing in the ears or loss of hearing occurs
- diarrhea lasts more than 2 days

If pregnant or breast-feeding,
ask a health professional before use.

Keep out of reach of children.
In case of overdose, get medical help or contact a Poison Control Center right away.

DIRECTIONS
- **shake well immediately before each use**
- adults and children 12 years of age and older: 30 mL or 2 tablespoonfuls
- for accurate dosing, use convenient pre-measured dose cup
- repeat dose every 1/2 hour to 1 hour as needed
- do not exceed 8 doses in 24 hours
- use until diarrhea stops but not more than 2 days
- children under 12 years: ask a doctor
- drink plenty of clear fluids to help prevent dehydration caused by diarrhea

OTHER INFORMATION
- **each 15 mL tablespoonful contains:** sodium 4 mg
- **each 15 mL tablespoonful contains:** total salicylates 130 mg
- **do not use if inner seal is broken or missing**
- **low sodium**

INACTIVE INGREDIENTS
caramel, carboxymethylcellulose sodium, flavor, microcrystalline cellulose, sodium salicylate, sorbic acid, sucrose, water, xanthan gum (245-241)
Dist. by CHATTEM, INC.
P.O. Box 2219
Chattanooga, TN 37409 USA
© 2008 Chattem, Inc.
Made in Canada
CHATTEM® www.chattem.com
Additional barcode labeling by:
Physicians Total Care, Inc.
Tulsa, Oklahoma 74146

KERASAL DF: DUAL MOISTURIZING FOOT CREAM

ALTERNA LLC

DRUGS FACTS

INGREDIENTS
water, urea, mineral oil, ammonium lactate, petrolatum, propylene glycol, glyceryl stearate SE, glyceryl stearate, glycerin, cetyl alcohol, PEG-100 stearate, steareth-2, xanthan gum, disodium EDTA, phenoxyethanol, methylparaben, butylparaben, ethylparaben, propylparaben, isobutylparaben.

OVERVIEW

Kerasal DF is an effective two-step system for promoting diabetic foot health. The Dual Moisturizing Foot Cream contains both urea and ammonium lactate in effective concentrations that are also safe for the diabetic foot. Diabetic patients should use Kerasal DF Foaming Foot Cleanser followed by the DF Moisturizing Foot Cream as a daily regimen to keep feet clean and hydrated.

BENEFITS

- Excellent moisturizing benefits for severely dry skin
- Provides beneficial healing and protection by penetrating and rehydrating skin cells
- Combines two very effective moisturizers — Urea 20% and Ammonium Lactate 5% into one easy-to-use formulation

DIRECTIONS

Wash your feet with soap and warm water and dry completely before applying – or– use a foot cleanser like Kerasal's DF Foaming Foot Cleanser. Squeeze out a dime size dose into the palm of your hand and gently massage into the skin until fully absorbed. Apply to the top and bottom of both feet. Do not apply in between toes. Apply to affected dry, rough, cracked areas and areas of thickened skin. Daily applications preferably at bedtime allow your feet to absorb product more fully.

WARNINGS

For external use only. Seek professional help if ingested. Do not use on irritated, infected skin or open wounds of any kind. Do not apply between toes. When using this product do not get into the eyes. If eye contact occurs, rinse thoroughly with water. Stop use and ask a doctor if redness, discomfort or irritation occur following use of this product. Sunburn alert: this product contains an alpha hydroxyl acid (AHA) that may increase your skin's sensitivity to the sun and particularly the possibility of sunburn. Use a sunscreen and limit sun exposure while using this product and for a week afterwards. Keep out of reach of children.

KERASAL ULTRA20 (urea and ammonium lactate)

Alterna, LLC

DRUG FACTS

Active Ingredient(s)
Urea 20%
Ammonium lactate 5%

DIRECTIONS

- Wash your feet with cleanser and warm water and dry before applying.
- Apply to the top and bottom of both feet and gently massage into the skin until fully absorbed.
- Do not apply in between toes.
- Apply to affected rough, dry areas and areas of thickened skin.
- Daily applications leave skin softer and more resilient.

INACTIVE INGREDIENTS

water, urea, mineral oil, ammonium lactate, petrolatum, propylene glycol, glyceryl stearate SE, glyceryl stearate, glycerin, cetyl alcohol, PEG-100 stearate, steareth-2, xanthan gum, disodium EDTA, phenoxyethanol, methylparaben, butylparaben, ethylparaben, propylparaben, isobutylparaben

KONSYL BALANCE (inulin and psyllium husk)

Konsyl Pharmaceuticals, Inc.

Active Ingredient(s)

Inulin (a natural vegetable fiber), refined psyllium husk (a water soluble fiber)

INACTIVE INGREDIENTS

maltodextrin, citric acid, flavor, aspartame, silicon dioxide, FD&C yellow #6

DIRECTIONS

Stir 1 rounded teaspoon of Balance into 8 oz. of water. Stir well until thoroughly mixed. Not recommended for use in carbonated beverages.
12 years to Adult: 1 rounded tsp up to 3 times daily
7 to 11 years: 1/2 adult dose up to 3 times daily
Under 6 years: Ask your doctor
Notice: This product should be used with at least a full glass of liquid. Using this product without enough liquid may cause choking. Do not use this product if you have difficulty swallowing.

WARNINGS

- Phenylketonurics: Contains phenylalanine
- Do not use if printed seal is broken or missing. Keep out of reach of children. If you are pregnant or nursing a baby, ask a health professional before use.

Allergy alert
Inhaled or ingested psyllium powder may cause an allergic reaction to people sensitive to psyllium.

KONSYL EASY MIX (psyllium hydrophilic mucilloid)

Konsyl Pharmaceuticals, Inc.

Active Ingredient(s) (in each dose)

Psyllium Hydrophilic Mucilloid 4.3 grams . . . .
Purpose(s)
Bulk-Forming Laxative

USE

For relief of occasional constipation and to induce regularity. This product generally produces bowel movements within 12 to 72 hours.

WARNINGS ALLERGY ALERT

As with any natural grain product, Inhaled or ingested psyllium powder may cause an allergic reaction in people sensitive to psyIllum.
Choking Taking this product without adequate fluid may cause it to swell and block your throat or esophagus and may cause choking. Do not take this product if you have difficulty in swallowing. If you experience chest pain, vomiting or difficulty in swallowing or breathing after taking this product, seek immediate medical attention.

DO NOT USE

laxative products when abdominal pain, nausea or vomiting are present unless directed by a doctor.

ASK A DOCTOR BEFORE USE IF YOU HAVE

a sudden change in bowel habits that persists over a period of two weeks

STOP USE AND ASK A DOCTOR IF

you experience rectal bleeding - you fail to have a bowel movement

Keep out of reach of children. In case of overdose, get medical help or contact a Poison Control Center right away.

DIRECTIONS
Mix this product (child or adult dose) with at least 8 ounces (a full glass) of water or other fluid. Taking this product without enough fluid may cause choking. See choking warnings.
Adults and children 12 years and older: sprinkle one teaspoonful into a glass with 8 oz. of juice, water or other fluid; stir briskly 3-5 seconds; drinks promptly; if mixture thickens, add more fluid, stir; follow with additional fluid to aid product action; take 1-3 times daily.
Children 6 years to under 12 years: 1/2 adult dose, in 8 oz. of fluid; 1-3 times daily.
Children under 6 years: ask a doctor.

OTHER INFORMATION
each 6g dose contains: Calcium 8 mg, Potassium 37 mg, Sodium 7 mg. - laxatives, including bulk fibers, may affect how other medicines work, wait 1-2 hours before or after taking other medicines - tamper-evident bottle mouth sealed for your protection - do not use if imprinted inner seal is broken or missing - store below 86 degree F (30 degree Centigrade) - keep container tightly closed - protect from moisture Heart Healthy - Diets low in saturated fat and cholesterol that include 7 grams of soluble fiber per day from psyllium husk may reduce the risk of Corinary Heart Disease (CHD) by lowering cholesterol. One adult dose of this product contains 2 grams of this soluble fiber.

INACTIVE INGREDIENTS
maltodextrin, silicon dioxide

QUESTIONS OR COMMENTS?
Call Konsyl Pharmaceuticals, Inc. at 1-800-356-6795 8:30 a.m. to 5 p.m. ET.

KONSYL FIBER CAPLETS (calcium polycarbophil)
Konsyl Pharmaceuticals, Inc.

INDICATIONS
For relief of constipation/irregularity. Helps restore and maintain regularity, promotes normal bowel function by increasing bulk volume and water content of the stool. Generally produces a bowel movement 12 - 72 hours after ingesting.

Active Ingredient(s) (in each caplet)
calcium polycarbophil 625 mg equivalent to 500 mg polycarbophil.

INACTIVE INGREDIENTS
(May contain the following): calcium carbonate, caramel, crospovidone, hypromellose, hydroxypropyl methylcellulose, maltodextrin, microcrystalline cellulose, magnesium stearate, polyethylene glycol, silicon dioxide, sodium lauryl sulfate.

DIRECTIONS
TAKE THIS PRODUCT (CHILD OR ADULT DOSE) WITH AT LEAST 8 OUNCES (A FULL GLASS) OF WATER OR OTHER FLUID. TAKING THIS PRODUCT WITHOUT ENOUGH LIQUID MAY CAUSE CHOKING, SEE LABEL WARNINGS.
DOSAGE: Adults: 2 caplets 1 to 4 times a day.
Children 6 to 12 years: 1 caplet 1 to 3 times a day.
Under 6 years consult a physician.
Dosage will vary according to diet, exercise, previous laxative use or severity of constipation. The recommended adult starting dose is 2 to 4 tablets daily. May be increased up to 8 tablets daily.

WARNINGS
Choking
Taking this product without adequate fluid may cause it to swell and block your throat or esophagus and may cause choking. Do not take this product if you have difficulty in swallowing. If you experience chest pain, vomiting, or difficulty in swallowing or breathing after taking this product, seek immediate medical attention.

DO NOT USE
if you are taking any form of tetracycline antibiotic.

ASK A DOCTOR BEFORE USE IF YOU HAVE
stomach pain, nausea or vomiting or a sudden change in bowel habits that persists over 2 weeks.

ASK A DOCTOR OR PHARMACIST BEFORE USE IF YOU ARE
taking any other drug. Take this product 2 or more hours before or after other drugs. All laxatives may affect how other drugs work.

WHEN USING THIS PRODUCT
Do not use for more than 7 days unless directed by a doctor. Do not take caplets more than 4 times in a 24 hour period unless directed by a doctor.

STOP USE AND ASK A DOCTOR IF YOU
fail to have a bowel movement or have rectal bleeding. These could be signs of a serious condition.
If pregnant or breast feeding, ask a health professional before use.
Keep out of reach of childern. In case of overdose, get medical help or contact a Poison Control Center right away.

KONSYL ORANGE FLAVOR (psyllium husk)
Konsyl Pharmaceuticals, Inc.

Active Ingredient(s) (in each dose)
Psyllium Hydrophilic Mucilloid 3.4 grams
Purpose(s)
Bulk-Forming Laxative

USE
For relief of occasional constipation. Generally produces effect in 12-72 hours. Naural bulk producing fiber encourages normal elimination without chemical stimulants.

WARNINGS ALLERGY ALERT
Inhaled or ingested psyllium powder may cause an allergic reaction in people sensitive to psyllium. Choking Taking this product without adequate fluid may cause it ot swell and block your throat or esophagus and may cause choking. Do not take this product if you have difficulty in swallowing. If you experience chest pain, vomiting or difficulty in swallowing or breathing after taking this product, seek immediate medical attention.

DO NOT USE
laxative products when abdominal pain, nausea or vomiting are present unless directed by a doctor.

ASK A DOCTOR BEFORE USE IF YOU HAVE
- a sudden change in bowel habits that persists over a period of two weeks.

WHEN USING THIS PRODUCT
- do not take for a period longer than 1 week, unless directed by a doctor

STOP USE AND ASK A DOCTOR IF
- you experience rectal bleeding - you fail to have a bowel movement
Keep out of reach of children. In case of overdose, get medical help or contact a Poison Control Center right away.

DIRECTIONS
Mix this product (child or adult dose) with at least 8 ounces (a full glass) of water or other fluid. Taking this product without enough liquid may cause choking. See choking warnings. Adults and children 12 years and over: sprinkle one dose, 1 rounded tablespoonful (12g), in 8 oz of liquid, 1-3 times daily. Children 6 years to under 12 years: 1/2 the adult dose in 8 oz of liquid, up to 3 times daily. Children under 6 years: Consult a doctor.

OTHER INFORMATION
each 12 g dose contains: Calcium 6 mg, Potassium 31 mg, Sodium 3 mg - store below 86 Degree F (30 Degree Centigrade) - keep container tightly closed - protect from excessive moisture - tamper-evident bottle mouth sealed for your protection - do not use if imprinted inner seal is broken or missing - laxatives, including bulk fibers, may affect how other medicines work, wait 1-2 hours before or after taking other medicines. - can be taken 1 to 3 times daily, before or after meals, mornings, or evenings - maximum daily dose (3 tablespoonfuls) is very low sodium - do not discard Konsyl Orange powder into any plumbing systems - note to diabetics: this product contains 66% sugar (sucrose) - each dose provides 3 grams total dietary fiber - each dose contains 35 calories

INACTIVE INGREDIENTS
citric acid, D and C yellow no. 10 and FD and C yellow no. 6 (sunset yellow), flavoring, sucrose.

QUESTIONS OR COMMENTS?
Call Konsyl Pharmaceuticals, Inc. at 1-800-36-6795 8:30 a.m to 5 p.m. ET.

WHEN USING THIS PRODUCT
physicians recommend a gradual increase in dietary fiber. If minor gas or bloating occurs, begin with a increase the dose over several days. Always follow with 8 oz. of fluid.
Manufactured by Konsyl Pharmaceuticals, Inc. Easton, MD 21601 www.konsyl.com Konsyl Pharmaceuticals, Inc. 33792 0810 Dietary Fiber Supplement Diets low in saturated fat and cholesterol that include 7 grams of soluble fiber per day from psyllium hust may reduce the risk of Coronary Heart Disease (CHD) by lowering cholesterol. ONE ADULT DOSE OF THIS PRODUCT CONTAINS 2.0 GRAMS PF THIS SOLUBLE FIBER = 3.4 G OF PSYLLIUM Dosage Adults 12 years and older: 1 Rounded teaspoonful in 8 oz. of fluid 2 TIMES DAILY, follow with additional fluid to aid product action, before or after meals, mornings or evenings. Children under 12 years: Consult a doctor. Notice Ask a doctor before use if you consider taking this product as part of a cholesterol-lowering program. See directions for use before taking this product.

SUPPLEMENTS FACTS
Serving size (dose): 1 rounded teaspoonful psyllium 3.4g Serving per container 45 Amount Per Serving %DV* Calories (Available) 35 Sodium 0% Carbohydrates (Available) 8g 3% Dietary Fiber 3g 11% Soluble Fiber 2g - Sugars 8g - Calcium 0% Iron 6% *Percent Daily Values (DV) are based on a 2,000 calorie diet. - Daily Value (DV) not established.

KONSYL ORANGE FLAVOR PACKETS
(psyllium husk)

Konsyl Pharmaceuticals, Inc.

INDICATIONS
Konsyl Orange Fiber Supplement is effective in relieving occasional constipation and restoring regularity.
Use as a Fiber Supplement: An easy way to increase your daily fiber intake
Use as a Laxative: Generally produces a bowel movement in 12 to 72 hours

Active Ingredient(s)
Per Rounded Tablespoonful: Psyllium Hydrophilic Mucilloid 3.4 g.

INACTIVE INGREDIENTS
sucrose, citric acid, FD&C yellow #6, D&C yellow #10, flavoring

DIRECTIONS
Mix this product (child or adult dose) with at least 8 ounces (a full glass) of water or other fluid. Taking this product without enough liquid may cause choking.
See choking warnings.
Adults and children 12 years and older: put 1 dose (1 rounded tablespoon) into shaker cup or closed container; add at least 8 oz. of juice, water or other beverage; shake 3 to 5 seconds; drink promptly. If mixture thickens, add more fluid, stir. Follow with additional fluid to aid product action; take 1-3 times daily.
Children 6 years to under 12 years: 1/2 adult dose, in 8 oz. of fluid; 1-3 times daily
Children under 6: ask a doctor.

WHEN USING THIS PRODUCT
physicians recommend a gradual increase in dietary fiber. If minor gas or bloating occurs, begin with a half-dose of Konsyl Orange and slowly increase the dose over several days. Always follow with 8 oz. of fluid.
Laxatives, including bulk fibers, may affect how other medicines work. Wait 1-2 hours before or after taking other medicines. Can be taken before or after meals, mornings or evening.

WARNINGS
Read entire package label before use.

Choking
Taking this product without adequate fluid may cause it to swell and block your throat or esophagus and may cause choking. Do not take this product if you have difficulty in swallowing. If you experience chest pain, vomiting or difficulty in swallowing or breathing after taking this product, seek immediate medical attention.

Allergy Alert
This product may cause allergic reaction in people sensitive to inhaled or ingested psyllium.

DO NOT USE
laxative products when abdominal pain, nausea or vomiting are present unless directed by a doctor.

ASK A DOCTOR BEFORE USE IF YOU HAVE
a sudden change in bowel habits that persists over 2 weeks.

STOP USE AND ASK A DOCTOR IF
- You experience rectal bleeding.
- You fail to have a bowel movement.
- Keep out of reach of children.
  In case of overdose, get medical help or contact a Poison Control Center right away.

KONSYL ORANGE SUGAR FREE (psyllium husk)
Konsyl Pharmaceuticals, Inc.

Active Ingredient(s) (in each dose)
Psyllium Hydrophilic Mucilloid 3.5 g
Purpose(s)
Bulk-forming laxative

USE
For relief of occasional constipation (irregularity). Generally produces bowel movement in 12-72 hours. Natural bulk producing fiber encourages normal elimination without chemical stimulants.

WARNINGS
Allergy alert: Inhaled or ingested psyllium powder may cause an allergic reaction in people sensitive to psyllium.
Choking
Taking this product without adequate fluid may cause it to swell and block your throat or esophagus and may cause choking. Do not take this product if you have difficulty in swallowing. If you experience chest pain, vomiting or difficulty in swallowing or breathing after taking this product, seek immediate medical attention.

DO NOT USE
laxative products when abdominal pain, nausea or vomiting are present unless directed by a doctor.

ASK A DOCTOR BEFORE USE IF YOU HAVE
a sudden change in bowel habits that persists over a period of two weeks.

WHEN USING THIS PRODUCT
do not take for a period longer than 1 week, unless directed by a doctor

STOP USE AND ASK A DOCTOR IF
- you experience rectal bleeding
- you fail to have a bowel movement
Keep out of reach of children. In case of overdose, get medical help or contact a Poison Control Center right away.

DIRECTIONS
Mix this product (child or adult dose) with at least 8 ounces (a full glass) of water or other fluid. Taking this product without enough liquid may cause choking. See choking warnings.

adults and children 12 years and over	1 rounded tablespoonful(11g) mixed in 8 oz of liquid, 1-3 times daily, at the first sign of irregularity.
children 6 to under 12 years	1/2 the adult dose in 8 oz of liquid, up to 3 times daily.
children under 6 years	Consult a doctor.

OTHER INFORMATION
each 11 g dose contains: Calcium 6mg, Potassium 31 mg, Sodium 3 mg
- note to diabetics: this product contains sugar (sucrose)
- store below 30°C (86°F)
- keep tightly closed to protect from humidity
- tamper-evident bottle mouth sealed for your protection
- do not use if imprinted inner seal is broken or missing
- maximum daily dose (3 tablespoonfuls) is very low sodium
- each dose provides 3 grams total dietary fiber
- each dose contains 35 calories

INACTIVE INGREDIENTS
aspartae, citric acid, FD and C yellow no. 6 (sunset yellow), flavoring, maltodextrin, silicon dioxide.

QUESTIONS OR COMMENTS?
Call Konsyl Pharmaceuticals, Inc. at 1-800-356-6795 8:30 a.m. to 5 p.m. ET.
Diets low in saturated fat and cholesterol that include 7 grams of soluble fiber per day from psyllium husk may reduce the risk of Coronary Heart Disease (CHD) by lowering cholesterol. ONE ADULT DOSE OF THIS PRODUCT CONTAINS 2 GRAMS OF THIS SOLUBLE FIBER = 3.4 GRAMS OF PSYLLIUM.

KONSYL ORANGE SUGAR FREE PACKETS
(psyllium husk)
Konsyl Pharmaceuticals, Inc.

INDICATIONS
Konsyl Orange Sugar Free Fiber Supplement is effective in relieving occasional constipation and restoring regularity.
Use as a Fiber Supplement: An easy way to increase your daily fiber intake
Use as a Laxative: Generally produces a bowel movement in 12 to 72 hours

Active Ingredient(s)
Per packet: Psyllium Hydrophilic Mucilloid 3.4g.

INACTIVE INGREDIENTS
aspartame, citric acid, FD&C yellow #6, flavoring, maltodextrin, silicon dioxide

DIRECTIONS
Mix this product (child or adult dose) with at least 8 ounces (a full glass) of water or other fluid. Taking this product without enough liquid may cause choking. See choking warnings.
Adults and children 12 years and older: put 1 dose (1 packet) into a shaker cup or closed container; add at least 8 oz. of juice, water or other beverage; shake 3 to 5 seconds; drink promptly; if mixture thickens, add more fluid, sitr; follow with addicional fluid to aid product action; take 1-3 times daily.
Children 6 years to under 12 years: 1/2 adult dose, in 8 oz. of fluid; 1-3 times daily.
Children under 6: ask a doctor.

WHEN USING THIS PRODUCT
physicians recommend a gradual increase in dietary fiber. If minor gas or bloating occurs, begin with a half-dose of Knosyl Orange Sugar Free and slowly increase the dose over several days. Always follow with 8 oz. of fluid. Laxatives, including bulk fibers, may affect how other medicines work, wait 1-2 hours before or after taking other medicines. Can be taken before or after meals, mornings or evening.

WARNINGS
Read entire package label before use.

Choking
Taking this product without adequate fluid may cause it to swell and block your throat or esophagus and may cause choking. Do not take this product if you have difficulty in swallowing. If you experience chest pain, vomiting or difficulty in swallowing or breathing after taking this product, seek immediate medical attention.

Allergy Alert
This product may cause allergic reaction in people sensitive to inhaled or ingested psyllium.

DO NOT USE
laxative products when abdominal pain, nausea or vomiting are present unless directed by a doctor.

ASK A DOCTOR BEFORE USE IF YOU HAVE
a sudden change in bowel habits that persists over 2 weeks.

STOP USE AND ASK A DOCTOR IF
• You experience rectal bleeding
• You fail to have a bowel movement

Keep out of reach of children. In case of overdose, get medical help or contact a Poison Control Center right away.

KONSYL ORIGINAL FORMULA (psyllium husk)

Konsyl Pharmaceuticals, Inc.

INDICATIONS
Konsyl Original Natural Fiber Supplement: Effective in relieving occasional constipation and restoring regularity
Use as a Fiber Supplement: An easy way to increase your daily fiber intake. Diets low in saturated fat and cholesterol that include 7 grams of soluble fiber per day from psyllium husk, as in Konsyl, may reduce the risk of heart disease by lowering cholesterol. One adult dose of Konsyl Original Formula provides 3 grams of this soluble fiber = 6 grams of psyllium.
Use as a Laxative: For relief of occasional constipation and to induce regularity, generally produces bowel movement in 12 to 72 hours.

Active Ingredient(s)
Per Rounded Teaspoonful: Psyllium Hydrophilic Mucilloid 6g.

DIRECTIONS
Mix this product (child or adult dose) with at least 8 ounces (a full glass) of water or other fluid. Taking this product without enough liquid may cause choking. See choking warnings.
Adults and children 12 years and older: put 1 dose (1 rounded teaspoonful) into a shaker cup or closed container; add at least 8 oz. of juice, water or other beverage; shake 3 to 5 seconds; drink promptly; if mixture thickens, add more fluid, stir; follow with additional fluid to aid product action; take 1-3 times daily.
Children 6 years to under 12 years: 1/2 adult dose, in 8 oz. of fluid; 1-3 times daily.
Children under 6: ask a doctor.

WHEN USING THIS PRODUCT
physicians recommend a gradual increase in dietary fiber. If minor gas or bloating occurs, begin with a half-dose of Konsyl and slowly increase the dose over several days. Always follow with 8 oz. of fluid.
Laxatives, including bulk fibers, may affect how other medicines work, wait 1-2 hours before or after taking other medicines. Can be taken before or after meals, mornings or evening.

WARNINGS
Read entire package label beofre use.
Choking
Taking this product without adequate fluid may cause it to swell and block your throat or esophagus and may cause choking. Do not take this product if you have difficulty in swallowing. If you experience chest pain, vomiting or difficulty in swallowing or breathing after taking this product, seek immediate medical attention.
Allergy Alert
This product may cause allergic reaction in people sensitive to inhaled or ingested psyllium.

DO NOT USE
laxative products when abdominal pain, nausea or vomiting are present unless directed by a doctor.

ASK A DOCTOR BEFORE USE IF YOU HAVE
a sudden change in bowel habits that persists over 2 weeks.

STOP USE AND ASK A DOCTOR IF
You experience rectal bleeding
You fail to have a bowel movement
Keep out of reach of children. In case of overdose, get medical help or contact a Poison Control Center right away.

KONSYL PACKETS (psyllium hydrophilic mucilloid)

Konsyl Pharmaceuticals, Inc.

INDICATIONS
Konsyl Original Natural Fiber Supplement: Effective in relieving occasional constipation and restoring regularity
Use as a Fiber Supplement: An easy way to increase your daily fiber intake. Diets low in saturated fat and cholesterol that include 7 grams of soluble fiber per day from psyllium husk, as in Konsyl, may reduce the risk of heart disease by lowering cholesterol. One adult dose of Konsyl Original Formula provides 3 grams of this soluble fiber = 6 grams of psyllium.
Use as a Laxative: For relief of occasional constipation and to induce regularity, generally produces bowel movement in 12 to 72 hours.

Active Ingredient(s)
Per packet: Pysllium Hydrophilic Mucilloid 6g.

DIRECTIONS
Mix this product (child or adult dose) with at least 8 ounces (a full glass) of water or other fluid. Taking this product without enough liquid may cause choking. See choking warnings.
Adults and children 12 years and older: put 1 dose (1 packet) into a shaker cup or closed container; add at least 8 oz. of juice, water or other beverage; shake 3 to 5 seconds; drink promptly; if mixture thickens, add more fluid, stir; follow with additional fluid to aid product action; take 1-3 times daily.
Children 6 years to under 12 years: 1/2 adult dose, in 8 oz. of fluid; 1-3 times daily.
Children under 6: ask a doctor.

WHEN USING THIS PRODUCT
physicians recommend a gradual increase in dietary fiber. If minor gas or bloating occurs, begin with a half-dose of Konsyl and slowly increase the dose over several days. Always follow with 8 oz. of fluid.
Laxatives, including bulk fibers, may affect how other medicines work, wait 1-2 hours before or after taking other medicines. Can be taken before or after meals, mornings or evening.

WARNINGS
Read entire package label before use.
Choking
Taking this product without adequate fluid may cause it to swell and block your throat or esophagus and may cause choking. Do not take this product if you have difficulty in swallowing. If you experience chest pain, vomiting or difficulty in swallowing or breathing after talking this prodct, seek immediate medical attention.
Allergy Alert
This product may cause allergic reaction in people sensitive to inhaled or ingested psyllium.

DO NOT USE
laxative products when abdominal pain, nausea or vomiting are present unless directed by a docor.

ASK A DOCTOR BEFORE USE IF YOU HAVE
a sudden change in bowel habits that persists over 2 weeks.

STOP USE AND ASK A DOCTOR IF
You experience rectal bleeding
You fail to have a bowel moevement

Keep out of reach of children. In case of overdose, get medical help or contact a Poison Control Center right away.

KONSYL 100 PERCENT NATURAL PSYLLIUM FIBER (psyllium husk)
Konsyl Pharmaceuticals, Inc.

Active Ingredient(s) (in each dose)
Psyllium husk approx. 520 mg
Purpose(s)
Bulk-forming laxative

USES
- for relief of occasional constipation (irregularity) - this product generally produces bowel movement in 12 to 72 hours

WARNINGS ALLERGY ALERT
This product may cause an allergic reaction in people sensitive to inhaled or ingested psyllium. Choking: Taking this product without adequate fluid may cause it to swell and block your throat or esophagus and may cause choking. Do not take this product if you have difficulty in swallowing. If you experience chest pain, vomiting, or difficulty in swallowing or breathing after taking this product, seek immediate medical attention.

ASK A DOCTOR BEFORE USE IF YOU HAVE
- stomach pain, nausea, or vomiting - a sudden change in bowel habits that persists over 2 weeks

STOP USE AND ASK A DOCTOR IF
- you fail to have a bowel movement or have rectal bleeding. These could be sings of a serious condition. - you need to use a laxative for more than 1 week If pregnant or breast-feeding, ask a health professional before use.
Keep out of reach of children. In case of overdose, get medical help or contact a Poison Control Center right away.

DIRECTIONS
- Take this product (child or adult dose) with at least 8 ounces (a full glass0 of water or other fluid. Taking this product without enough liquid may cause choking. See choking warning. - follow dosage below or use as directed by a doctor. - drink a full glass (8 oz) of water or other liquid with each dose - continued use for 1 to 3 days is normally required to provide full benefit

| adults and children 12 years and over | 5 capsules one to three times days |
| Children under 12 years | consult a doctor |

LOT: EXP:

OTHER INFORMATION
- keep tightly closed - store at room temperature - contains a 100% natural therapeutic fiber

INACTIVE INGREDIENTS
FDandC yellow #6, gelatin. polyethylene glycol. polysorbate 80

SUPPLEMENTS FACTS
Serving Size: 6 capsules Servings per Container:16 Amount Per Serving %DV* Calories 10 Total Carb. 3g.....1% Dietary Fiber 3g.......11% Soluble Fiber 2g........+ Protein less than 1 gram.........+ Iron 0.4 mg.......2% *Percent Daily Values (DV) are based on a 2.000 calorie diet. not equal to + Daily Value (DV) not established

USES
An easy way to increase your daily fiber intake. Diets low in saturated fat and cholesterol that include 7 grams of soluble fiber per day from psyllium husk may reduce the risk of heart disease by lowering cholesterol. One serving of this product provides 2.4 grams of this soluble fiber. Consult a doctor if you intend to use this product as part of a cholesterol-lowering program

DIRECTIONS
Adults 12 yrs. and older: 2-6 capsules for increasing daily fiber intake: 6 capsules for cholesterol lowering use. Take product with 8 oz of liquid (swallow 1 capsule at a time) up to 3 times daily. NOTICE: Take this product with at least 8 oz (a full glass) of liquid. Taking without enough liquid may cause choking. Do not take if you have difficulty swallowing.

QUESTIONS OR COMMENTS?
1-800-356-6795 8:30 a.m. to 5 p.m ET Manufactured By: Konsyl Pharmaceuticals, Inc. Easton, MD 21601 www.konsyl.com Konsyl Pharmaceuticals, Inc. 34076 0710 3 0224-1847-10 0

KONSYL OVERNIGHT RELIEF SENNA PROMPT (psyllium and sennosides)
Konsyl Pharmaceuticals, Inc.

DRUG FACTS
Active Ingredient(s) (in each capsule) Purpose(s)
Psyllium 500 mg........................ ....Bulk-forming laxative
Sennosides 9 mg... .Stimulant laxative

USES
- for relief of occasional constipation (irregularity) - this product generally produces bowel movement in 6 to 12 hours

WARNINGS ALLERGY ALERT
This product may cause an allergic reaction in people sensitive to inhaled or ingested psyllium. Choking: Taking this product without adequate fluid may cause it to swell and block your throat or esophagus and may cause choking. Do not take this product if you have difficulty in swallowing. If you experience chest pain, vomiting, or difficulty in swallowing or breathing after taking this product, seek immediate medical attention.

ASK A DOCTOR BEFORE USE IF YOU HAVE
- abdominal pain, nausea, or vomiting - a sudden change in bowel habits that persists over 2 weeks If pregnant or breast-feeding, ask a health professional before use.

STOP USE AND ASK A DOCTOR IF
- you fail to have a bowel movement or have rectal bleeding. These could be signs of a serious condition. - you need to use a laxative for more than 1 week
Keep out of reach of children. In case of overdose, get medical help or contact a Poison Control Center right away.

DIRECTIONS
- Take this product (child or adult dose) with at least 8 ounces (a full glass) of water or other fluid. Taking this product without enough liquid may cause choking. See choking warning. - follow dosage below or use as directed by a doctor

| adults and children 12 years and over | 1-5 capsules one or two times daily |
| children under 12 years | consult a doctor |

INACTIVE INGREDIENTS
D and C yellow #10 al. lake, FD and C blue #1 al. lake, gelatin, polyethylene glycol, polysorbate 80.

OTHER INFORMATION
- keep tightly closed - store at room temperature
Manufactured By: 34708 Konsyl Pharmaceuticals, Inc.
Easton, MD 21601 1-800-356-6795 www.konsyl.com
0710 3 0224 1 86090 1

KONSYL NATURALLY SWEETENED (psyllium husk)

Konsyl Pharmaceuticals, Inc.

INDICATIONS
Konsyl-D is effective in relieving occasional constipation and restoring regularity.
Use as a Fiber Supplement: An easy way to increase your daily fiber intake.
Use as a Laxative: Generally produces a bowl movement in 12 to 72 hours.

Active Ingredient(s)
Per Rounded Teaspoonful: Psyllium Hydrophilic Mucilloid 3.4g.

INACTIVE INGREDIENT
dextrose

DIRECTIONS
Mix this product (child or adult dose) with at least 8 ounces (a full glass) of water or other fluid. Taking this product without enough liquid may cause choking. See choking warnings.
- **Adults and children 12 years and older:** put 1 dose (1 rounded teaspoonful) into a shaker cup or closed container; add at least 8 oz. of juice, water or other beverage; shake 3 to 5 seconds; drink promptly; if mixture thickens, add more fluid, stir; follow with additional fluid to aid product action; take 1-3 times daily.
- **Children 6 years to under 12 years:** 1/2 adult dose, in 8 oz of fluid; 1-3 times daily
- **Children under 6:** ask a doctor.

WHEN USING THIS PRODUCT
physicians recommend a gradual increase in dietary fiber. If minor gas or bloating occurs, begin with half-dose of Konsyl-D and slowly increase the dose over several days.
Always follow with 8 oz. of fluid
Laxatives, including bulk fibers, may affect how other medicines work. Wait 1-2 hours before or after taking other medicines.
Can be taken before or after meals, mornings or evening.

WARNINGS
Read entire package label, before use.

Choking
Taking this product without adequate fluid may cause it to swell and block your throat or esophagus and may cause choking. Do not take this product if you have difficulty in swallowing. If you experience chest pain, vomiting or difficulty in swallowing or breathing after taking this product, seek immediate medical attention.

Allergy Alert
This product may cause allergic reaction in people sensitive to inhaled or ingested psyllium.

DO NOT USE
laxative products when abdominal pain, nausea or vomiting are present unless directed by a doctor

ASK A DOCTOR BEFORE USE IF YOU HAVE
a sudden change in bowel habits that persists over 2 weeks..

STOP USE AND ASK A DOCTOR IF
- You experience rectal bleeding.
- You fail to have a bowel movement.

Keep out of reach of children. In case of overdose, get medical help or contact a Poison Control Center right away.

LACTINEX

Becton, Dickinson and Company

- **What is lactobacillus? What does the bacterium do?**
Lactobacilli are bacteria that normally live in the human small intestine and vagina. *Lactobacillus acidophilus* is generally considered to be beneficial because it produces vitamin K, lactase, and antimicrobial substances such as acidolin, acidolphilin, lactocidin, and bacteriocin.[1] *Lactobacillus acidophilus* is the most commonly used probiotic, or "friendly" bacteria. Such healthy bacteria inhabit the intestines and vagina and protect against the entrance and proliferation of "bad" organisms that can cause disease. This is accomplished through a variety of mechanisms. For example, the breakdown of food by *L. acidophilus* leads to production of lactic acid, hydrogen peroxide, and other byproducts that make the environment hostile for undesired organisms. *L. acidophilus* also produces lactase, the enzyme that breaks down milk sugar (lactose) into simple sugars.
- **Is Lactinex the same as acidophilus?**
Lactinex products are a blend of *Lactobacillus acidophilus* and *Lactobacillus helveticus (bulgaricus)*.
- **How is Lactinex supplied?**
Each salable unit of the Lactinex Lactobacillus Granules (cat no. 236712) is one carton, which contains 12 packets. Each salable unit of the Lactinex Lactobacillus Tablets (cat. no. 236850) is one bottle, which contains 50 tablets.
- **How do tablets and granules differ? What is the concentration of each?**
The tablet may be taken orally (chewed), followed by a small amount of liquid, while the granules can be added to other foods (i.e. cereal) or beverages. At the time of manufacture, each format contains a cumulative colony forming unit count (CFU) of: 1,000,000 CFU/tablet and 100,000,000 CFU/packet; therefore, 100 tablets = 1 package of granules.
- **What other ingredients are in Lactinex?**
One packet of Lactinex Lactobacillus Granules (cat no. 236712) contains 380 mg lactose, 24 mg glucose, 34 mg sucrose, 5.0 mg calcium, 5.0 mg sodium, and 20 mg potassium. One tablet of Lactinex Lactobacillus Tablets (cat. no. 236850) contains 240 mg lactose, 12 mg glucose, 125 mg sucrose, 1.3 mg calcium, 1.4 mg sodium and 5.0 mg potassium. Other ingredients are milk, whey powder, soy peptone, talc (tablet) and mineral oil (tablet). For details, please refer to the Lactinex Product Information Sheet.
- **What is the recommended dosage?**
The product information sheet recommends taking 4 tablets 3 or 4 times a day of the Lactinex Tablets (cat. no. 236850), or one packet 3 or 4 times a day of the Lactinex Granules (cat. no. 236712).
- **How do I take it?**
As the product information sheet recommends, the Lactinex tablets can be chewed and swallowed, and may be followed by a small amount of milk, fruit juice or water. The Lactinex granules can be added to cereal, food or milk.
- **Does Lactinex have any calcium?**
One packet of Lactinex Lactobacillus Granules (cat no. 236712) contains 5.0 mg calcium. One tablet of Lactinex Lactobacillus Tablets (cat. no. 236850) contains 1.3 mg calcium.
- **Does Lactinex have sugar?**
One packet of Lactinex Lactobacillus Granules (cat no. 236712) contains 24 mg glucose. One tablet of Lactinex Lactobacillus Tablets (cat. no. 236850) contains 12 mg glucose.
- **Does Lactinex have gluten?**
No, both Lactinex products are gluten free.

- **Can individuals sensitive to milk products use Lactinex?**
  Milk products are present in Lactinex. Do not use if sensitive to milk products. A person who exhibits intolerance to lactose may experience some gastrointestinal distress after taking Lactinex.
- **Can individuals sensitive to soy products use Lactinex?**
  Soy products are present in Lactinex. Do not use if sensitive to soy products.
- **How does Lactinex compare to an ounce of buttermilk in *Lactobacillus* content?**
  We have no equivalency data on the *Lactobacillus* content of buttermilk changes as it ages. However, there are approximately 4,000,000 cells of the (mixed) lactobacilli in 4 tablets at time of manufacture and a package of granules contains 100 million cells at time of manufacture.
- **What is the stability (shelf life) of Lactinex tablets or granules if not stored at 2-8 °C?**
  While 2-8 °C (refrigerated) storage is strongly recommended, it may not always be realistic, especially during times of transport. Internal studies have shown that organism counts are relatively unaffected during shipment for distribution (24 - 48 hrs) at ambient temperature, if product is refrigerated immediately upon arrival. Product should be stored at refrigerator temperatures to retain maximum stability. We have no claims or stability data for the product if it has been left outside of this storage condition for extended periods of time.
- **Are *Lactobacillus* resistant to antibiotics?**
  No, the *Lactobacillus* cultures in Lactinex are not resistant to antibiotics. Consult with your healthcare provider if you are on antibiotic therapy and are considering Lactinex as a dietary supplement.
- **Can Lactinex be used as a source of *L. acidophilus* to treat vaginal infections taken orally or inserted vaginally?**
  Lactinex is not recommended as a source of *L. acidophilus* to treat this condition.
- **Can Lactinex be given to an infant or child? If so, how much?**
  A pediatrician should always be consulted prior to the use of Lactinex in infants or children.
- **Can pregnant women take Lactinex?**
  A pregnant woman should consult with her physician before using Lactinex.
- **Can Lactinex be used as a starter for yogurt?**
  This is not recommended. There is no data to support this.
- **Is Lactinex useful in preventing or treating cold sores?**
  Use of this product in treatment of fever blisters and cold sores was based on reports published between 1958 and 1965. There have been unsolicited testimonials to add additional support. More recently, well-controlled evaluations have not produced substantial evidence of its effectiveness. Accordingly, BD discontinued this claim in late 1986 and the labeling was changed.
- **Does Lactinex have tamper-proof packaging?**
  Each Lactinex product has safety seals. The tablets have a foil seal over the mouth of the bottle, and the granules are packaged inside foil-sealed pouches. Both types are "tamper evident".
- **Where can I buy it?**
  Most drug stores carry Lactinex products. Please note that as Lactinex products require refrigeration, therefore Lactinex is not accessible directly to consumers from the shelf. You need to ask your pharmacist to obtain Lactinex.
- **Is there an NDC number for Lactinex?**
  As Lactinex is considered a dietary supplement or food supplement by the FDA, there is no valid National Drug Code (NDC) for any of the Lactinex products.
- **Can I take it with food or on an empty stomach?**
  The product information sheet recommends taking the Lactinex granules with cereal, food, or milk, and chewing the Lactinex tablets, and may be followed by a small amount of milk, fruit juice or water.

- **Where can I find the expiry?**
  Product expiry is clearly printed on each bottle of the Lactinex Lactobacillus Tablets (cat. no. 236850), and on each packet of the Lactinex Lactobacillus Granules (cat no. 236712).
- **Are there other precautions?**
  If you are allergic to milk, soy or sensitive to lactose, you should avoid the use of Lactinex.
- **What about allergies?**
  People who have known allergies or asthma may be at an increased risk for a reaction from any new treatment. The physician should always know a patient's allergy history. Signs of an allergic reaction are skin rash, hives or itching.
- **How long should I take lactobacillus?**
  The Lactinex products are generally harmless. Consult with your physician for extended period of use.
- **How about side effects?**
  There are no known side effects of lactobacillus.
- **Who is responsible for ensuring the safety and efficacy of dietary supplements?**
  Manufacturers of dietary supplements are responsible for making sure their products are safe before they go to market. They are also responsible for determining that the claims on their labels are accurate and truthful. Dietary supplement products are not reviewed by the government before they are marketed, but FDA has the responsibility to take action against any unsafe dietary supplement product that reaches the market. If FDA can prove that claims on marketed dietary supplement products are false and misleading, the agency may take action against products with such claims. (www.cfsan.fda.gov/~dms/ds-savvy.html (http://www.cfsan.fda.gov/~dms/ds-savvy.html))

[1]Cited from Mayo Clinic: http://www.mayoclinic.com/health/lactobacillus/NS_patient-acidophilus

Lactinex Product Information

Product	Lactinex Granule Packet	Lactinex Tablet
Manufacture Cat. No.	236712	236850
Product Configuration	12 packets/carton	50 tablets/bottle
Storage Condition	Refrigerated (2 - 8 °C)	Refrigerated (2 - 8 °C)
Unit Weight	1.0 g	0.5 g
Cultures	*Lactobacillus acidophilus (gasseri); Lactobacillus helveticus (bulgaricus)*	*Lactobacillus acidophilus (gasseri); Lactobacillus helveticus (bulgaricus)*
Live cells at time of manufacture	100 million	1 million
Other Ingredients	Milk, whey powder, soy peptone	Milk, whey powder, talc, mineral oil, soy peptone
Sodium	5 mg	1.4 mg
Calcium	5.0 mg	1.3 mg
Potassium	20 mg	5 mg
Glucose	24 mg	12 mg
Lactose	380 mg	240 mg
Sucrose	34 mg	125 mg
Serving size	1 packet, 3 - 4 times daily	4 tablets, 3 - 4 times daily
Equivalency	1	100

LAMISIL AT CREAM (terbinafine hydrochloride)
Novartis Consumer Health, Inc.

DRUG FACTS

Active Ingredient(s)
Terbinafine hydrochloride 1%

Purpose(s)
Antifungal

USES
- cures most athlete's foot (tinea pedis)
- cures most jock itch (tinea cruris) and ringworm (tinea corporis)
- relieves itching, burning, cracking and scaling which accompany these conditions

WARNINGS
For external use only

DO NOT USE
- on nails or scalp
- in or near the mouth or eyes
- for vaginal yeast infections

WHEN USING THIS PRODUCT
do not get into eyes. If eye contact occurs, rinse thoroughly with water.

STOP USE AND ASK A DOCTOR IF
too much irritation occurs or gets worse
Keep out of reach of children. If swallowed, get medical help or contact a poison control center right away.

DIRECTIONS
- adults and children 12 years and over:
  - use the tip of the cap to break the seal and open the tube
  - wash the affected skin with soap and water and dry completely before applying
  - **for athlete's foot** wear well-fitting, ventilated shoes. Change shoes and socks at least once daily.
    - **between the toes only:** apply twice a day (morning and night) for **1 week** or as directed by a doctor
    - **on the bottom or sides of the foot:** apply twice a day (morning and night) for **2 weeks** or as directed by a doctor
  - **for jock itch and ringworm:** apply once a day (morning or night) for **1 week** or as directed by a doctor
  - wash hands after each use
- children under 12 years: ask a doctor

OTHER INFORMATION
- do not use if seal on tube is broken or is not visible
- store at controlled room temperature 20-25°C (68-77°F)

INACTIVE INGREDIENTS
benzyl alcohol, cetyl alcohol, cetyl palmitate, isopropyl myristate, polysorbate 60, purified water, sodium hydroxide, sorbitan monostearate, stearyl alcohol

QUESTIONS OR COMMENTS?
call **1-800-452-0051**
Distributed by: **Novartis Consumer Health, Inc.**
Parsippany, NJ 07054-0622

LAMISIL AF DEFENSE (tolnaftate)
Novartis Consumer Health, Inc.

Active Ingredient(s)
Tolnaftate

Purpose(s)
Antifungal

USES
- treats and prevents most athlete's foot (tinea pedis), and ringworm (tinea corporis)
- prevents most athlete's foot (tinea pedis) with daily use
- relieves itching, burning, cracking and scaling which accompany these conditions

WARNINGS
For external use only

DO NOT USE
- on children under 2 years of age unless directed by a doctor
- in or near the mouth or the eyes
- on nails or scalp

WHEN USING THIS PRODUCT
do not get into eyes. If eye contact occurs, rinse eyes thoroughly with water.

STOP USE AND ASK A DOCTOR IF
- irritation occurs or gets worse
- no improvement in athlete's foot within 4 weeks

KEEP OUT OF REACH OF CHILDREN
If swallowed, get medical help or contact a Poison Control Center right away.

DIRECTIONS
- adults and children 2 years of age and over
  - to open tube, peel off foil seal
  - wash the affected area and dry thoroughly
  - apply a thin layer over affected area twice daily (morning and night) or as directed by a doctor
  - **for athlete's foot** pay special attention to spaces between the toes
    - wear well-fitting, ventilated shoes
    - change shoes and socks at least once daily
  - use daily for 4 weeks; if condition persists longer, consult a doctor
  - **to prevent athlete's foot,** apply once or twice daily (morning and/or night)
  - supervise children in the use of this product
  - wash hands after each use
- children under 2 years of age: ask a doctor

OTHER INFORMATION
- do not use if seal on tube is broken or is not visible
- store at controlled room temperature 20°C- 25°C (68°F- 77°F)

INACTIVE INGREDIENTS
acrylates/C10-30 acrylate cross polymer, carbomer, corn starch, cyclomethicone, edetate disodium, ethyl alcohol, fragrance, isopropyl mysristate, propylene glycol, purified water, strong ammonia solution

QUESTIONS OR COMMENTS?
call **1-800-452-0051**
Distr. By: **Novartis Consumer Health, Inc.**
Parsippany, NJ 07054-0622 ©2008

LAMISIL AT ANTIFUNGAL GEL (terbinafine)

Novartis Consumer Health, Inc.

Active Ingredient(s)
Terbinafine1%

Purpose(s)
Antifungal

USES
- cures most athlete's foot (tinea pedis) between the toes.
- Effectiveness on the bottom or sides of foot is unknown.
- cures most jock itch (tinea cruris) and ringworm (tinea corporis)
- relieves itching, burning, cracking and scaling which accompany these conditions

WARNINGS
For external use only

DO NOT USE
- on nails or scalp
- in or near the mouth or eyes
- for vaginal yeast infections

WHEN USING THIS PRODUCT
do not get into eyes. If eye contact occurs, rinse thoroughly with water.

STOP USE AND ASK A DOCTOR
do not get into eyes. If eye contact occurs, rinse thoroughly with water.

KEEP OUT OF REACH OF CHILDREN
If swallowed, get medical help or contact a poison control center right away.

DIRECTIONS
- adults and children 12 years and over
  - use the tip of the cap to break the seal and open the tube
  - wash the affected skin with soap and water and dry completely before applying
  - **for athlete's foot**
  - **between the toes:** apply once a day at bedtime for 1 week or as directed by a doctor. Wear well-fitting, ventilated shoes. Change shoes and socks at least once daily
  - **for jock itch and ringworm:** apply once a day (morning or night) **for 1 week** or as directed by a doctor.
  - wash hands after each use
- children under 12 years: ask a doctor

OTHER INFORMATION
- do not use if seal on tube is broken or is not visible
- store at or below 30°C (86°F)

INACTIVE INGREDIENTS
benzyl alcohol, butylated hydroxytoluene, carbomer 974 P, ethanol, isopropyl myristate, polysorbate 20, purified water, sodium hydroxide, sorbitan monolaurate

QUESTIONS OR COMMENTS?
call **1-800-452-0051**
Distributed by:
Novartis Consumer Health, Inc.
Parsippany, NJ 07054-0622

LAMISIL AT SPRAY PUMP (terbinafine hydrochloride)

Novartis Consumer Health, Inc.

Active Ingredient(s)
Terbinafine hydrochloride

Purpose(s)
Antifungal

USES
- cures most jock itch (tinea cruris)
- relieves itching, burning, cracking, and scaling which accompany this condition

WARNINGS
For external use only

DO NOT USE
- on nails or scalp
- in or near the mouth or the eyes
- for vaginal yeast infections

WHEN USING THIS PRODUCT
do not get into eyes. If contact occurs, rinse eyes thoroughly with water.

STOP USE AND ASK A DOCTOR
if too much irritation occurs or gets worse.

KEEP OUT OF REACH OF CHILDREN
If swallowed, get medical help or contact a poison control center right away.

DIRECTIONS
- adults and children 12 years and over
  - wash the affected area with soap and water and dry completely before applying
  - spray affected area once a day (morning **or** night) for 1 week or as directed by a doctor
  - wash hands after each use
- children under 12 years: ask a doctor

OTHER INFORMATION
store at 8 - 25° C (46 - 77° F)

ADDITIONAL INFORMATION
Full Prescription Strength
For Effective Relief of: ° Itching ° Burning
Distr. By:
- **Novartis Consumer Health, Inc.**
- Parsippany, NJ 07054-0622 ©2006

INACTIVE INGREDIENTS
cetomacrogol, ethanol, propylene glycol, purified water USP

QUESTIONS OR COMMENTS?
call **1-800-452-0051** 24 hours a day, 7 days a week

LAMISIL AT CREAM FOR JOCK ITCH
(terbinafine hydrochloride)

Novartis Consumer Health, Inc.

Active Ingredient(s)
Terbinafine hydrochloride

Purpose(s)
Antifungal

USES
- cures most jock itch (tinea cruris)
- relieves itching, burning, cracking and scaling which accompany this condition

WARNINGS
For external use only

DO NOT USE
- on nails or scalp
- in or near the mouth or eyes
- for vaginal yeast infections

WHEN USING THIS PRODUCT
do not get into eyes. If eye contact occurs, rinse thoroughly with water.

STOP USE AND ASK DOCTOR
if too much irritation occurs or gets worse

KEEP OUT OF REACH OF CHILDREN
If swallowed, get medical help or contact a poison control center right away.

DIRECTIONS
- adults and children 12 years and over:
  - use the tip of the cap to break the seal and open the tube
  - wash the affected skin with soap and water and dry completely before applying
  - apply once a day (morning **or** night) for **1 week** or as directed by a doctor
  - wash hands after each use
- children under 12 years: ask a doctor

OTHER INFORMATION
- do not use if seal on tube is broken or is not visible
- store at controlled room temperature 20-25°C (68-77°F)

INACTIVE INGREDIENTS
benzyl alcohol, cetyl alcohol, cetyl palmitate, isopropyl myristate, polysorbate 60, purified water, sodium hydroxide, sorbitan monostearate, stearyl alcohol

QUESTIONS OR COMMENTS?
call **1-800-452-0051**
Novartis Consumer Health, Inc.
Parsippany, NJ 07054-0622 ©2008

LAMISIL AT SPRAY FOR JOCK ITCH
(terbinafine hydrochloride)

Novartis Consumer Health, Inc.

DRUG FACTS

Active Ingredient(s)
Terbinafine hydrochloride

Purpose(s)
Antifungal

USES
- cures most jock itch (tinea cruris)
- relieves itching, burning, cracking and scaling which accompany this condition

WARNINGS
For external use only

DO NOT USE
- on nails or scalp
- in or near the mouth or eyes
- for vaginal yeast infections

WHEN USING THIS PRODUCT
do not get into eyes. If eye contact occurs, rinse thoroughly with water.

STOP USE AND ASK A DOCTOR
if too much irritation occurs or gets worse.
Keep out of reach of children. If swallowed, get medical help or contact a poison control center right away.

DIRECTIONS
- adults and children 12 years and over:
  - wash the affected area with soap and water and dry completely before applying
  - spray affected area once a day (morning or night) for **1 week** or as directed by a doctor
  - wash hands after each use
- children under 12 years: ask a doctor

OTHER INFORMATION
- store at 8°-25°C (46-77°F)

INACTIVE INGREDIENTS
cetomacrogol, ethanol, propylene glycol, purified water USP

QUESTIONS OR COMMENTS?
call **1-800-452-0051**

LANACANE MAXIMUM STRENGTH ANTI-ITCH (benzethonium chloride and benzocaine)

Reckitt Benckiser LLC

DRUG FACTS

Active Ingredient(s)	Purpose(s)
Benzethonium chloride 0.2%	First-aid antiseptic
Benzocaine 20%	Pain relief cream

USES
- first aid for the temporary relief of pain and itching and to help prevent infection in minor cuts, scrapes and burns

WARNINGS
For external use only

DO NOT USE
- in the eyes
- over large areas of the body

ASK A DOCTOR BEFORE USE IF YOU HAVE
- deep or puncture wounds
- animal bites
- serious burns

STOP USE AND ASK A DOCTOR IF
- condition worsens
- needed for longer than 1 week

Keep out of reach children. If swallowed, get medical help or contact a Poison Control Center right away.

DIRECTIONS
- adults and children 2 years of age and older: clean the affected area and apply a small amount to the affected area not more than 1 to 3 times daily
- children under 2: ask a doctor
- may be covered with a sterile bandage

OTHER INFORMATION
- store at 20-25°C (68-77°F)
- retain carton for future reference

INACTIVE INGREDIENTS
acetylated lanolin alcohol, aloe, cetyl acetate, cetyl alcohol, cholecalciferol, corn oil, dimethicone, dl-alpha tocopherol acetate, fragrance, glycerin, glyceryl monostearate, isopropyl myristate, methylparaben, mineral oil, PEG-100 stearate, polyvinylpyrrolidone/eicosene copolymer, propylparaben, pyrithione zinc, sorbitan monostearate, stearamidopropyl PG-dimonium chloride phosphate, vitamin A palmitate, water

QUESTIONS OR COMMENTS?
1-866-252-5327
You may also report side effects to this phone number.
Distributed by Reckitt Benckiser
Parsippany, NJ 07054-0224

LANACANE ANTI-CHAFING GEL
Reckitt Benckiser LLC

HELPS PREVENT CHAFING
Help Prevent Chafing before you have to treat it:
- Helps prevent chafing caused by friction such as repeated rubbing of skin on skin or skin on clothing.
- A little goes a long way, lasts all day. Just a dab gives skin a lasting silkiness that helps prevents chafing.
- Use anywhere repeated motion rubs skin raw: shoulders, waistline, under arms, inner thighs, chest...even feet!
- Non-greasy, dries on contact and provides long-lasting comfort.
- Fragrance-free, hypoallergenic, moisture-proof, and won't stain clothes.

Treating the chafed area:
- Just a dab will provide a silky, invisible barrier which helps prevent the chafed area from becoming more sore by helping to prevent friction acting on the raw skin
- Use where skin is sore due to skin rubbing on skin and skin rubbing on clothing

Lanacane Anti-Chafing Gel dries on contact, has a silky, smooth feel and lasts as long as you need it to so you're allowed the comfort and freedom to carry on doing all the things you want to do.

LANACANE FIRST AID SPRAY (benzethonium chloride and benzocaine)
Reckitt Benckiser LLC

DRUGS FACTS

Active Ingredient(s)	Purpose(s)
Benzethonium chloride 0.2%	First-aid antiseptic
Benzocaine 20%	Pain relief spray

USES
first aid for the temporary relief of pain and itching and to help prevent infection in minor cuts, scrapes and burns

WARNINGS
For external use only

Flammable
do not use near heat, flame or fire or while smoking

DO NOT USE
- in the eyes
- over large areas of the body

WHEN USING THIS PRODUCT
- do not puncture or incinerate. Content under pressure. Do not store at temperatures above 120 F°.
- intentional misuse by deliberately concentrating and inhaling the contents can be harmful or fatal

ASK A DOCTOR BEFORE USE IF YOU HAVE
- deep or puncture wounds
- animal bites
- serious burns

STOP USE AND ASK A DOCTOR IF
- condition worsens
- needed for longer than 1 week

Keep out of reach of children. If swallowed, get medical help or contact a Poison Control Center right away.

DIRECTIONS
- adults and children 2 years of age and older: clean the affected area and spray a small amount on the affected area not more than 1 to 3 times daily
- children under 2 years of age: ask a doctor
- may be covered with a sterile bandage
- if bandaged, let dry first

OTHER INFORMATION
store at 20-25°C (68-77°F)

INACTIVE INGREDIENTS
alcohol (24.5% v/v), aloe, cyclomethicone, dipropylene glycol, dl-alpha tocopherol acetate, isobutane

QUESTIONS OR COMMENTS?
1-866-252-5327
Distributed by Reckitt Benckiser
Parsippany, NJ 07054-0224

LICEMD (dimethicone)
Reckitt Benckiser LLC

DRUGS FACTS

Active Ingredient(s)	Purpose(s)
Piperonyl butoxide (4%)	Lice treatment
Pyrethrum extract (equivalent to pyrethrins 0.33%)	Lice treatment

USES
treats head, pubic (crab), and body lice

WARNINGS
For external use only

DO NOT USE
- near eyes
- inside nose, mouth or vagina
- on lice in eyebrows or eyelashes. See a doctor if lice are present in these areas.

ASK A DOCTOR BEFORE USE IF YOU
- are allergic to ragweed. May cause breathing difficulty or an asthmatic attack.

WHEN USING THIS PRODUCT
- keep eyes tightly closed and protect eyes with a washcloth or towel
- if product gets in eyes, flush with water right away
- scalp itching or redness may occur

STOP USE AND ASK A DOCTOR IF
- breathing difficulty occurs
- eye irritation occurs
- skin or scalp irritation continues or infection occurs

Keep out of reach of children.
If swallowed, get medical help or contact a Poison Control center right away.

DIRECTIONS
- **Important: Read warnings before use.**
  Read leaflet inside carton for complete directions before use.
  Adults and children 2 years and over:

Inspect
- check each household member with a magnifying glass in bright light for lice/nits (eggs)
- look for tiny nits near scalp, beginning at back of neck and behind ears
- examine small sections of hair at a time
- unlike dandruff which moves when touched, nits stick to the hair
- if either lice or nits are found, treat with this product

Treat
- apply this product thoroughly to dry hair or other affected area. For head lice, first apply behind ears and to back of neck.
- allow this product to remain on hair or other affected area for 10 minutes, but no longer
- wash area thoroughly with warm water and soap or shampoo
- for head lice, towel dry hair and comb out tangles

Remove lice and their eggs (nits)
- use a fine-tooth comb or the special lice/nit comb. Remove any remaining nits by hand (using a throw-away glove).
- hair should remain slightly damp while removing nits
- if hair dries during combing, dampen slightly with water
- for head lice, part hair into sections. Do one section at a time starting on top of head. Longer hair may take 1 to 2 hours.
- lift a 1 to 2 inch wide strand of hair. Place comb as close to scalp as possible and comb with a firm, even motion away from scalp.
- pin back each strand of hair after combing
- clean comb often. Wipe nits away with tissue and discard in a plastic bag. Seal bag and discard to prevent lice from coming back.
- after combing, thoroughly recheck for lice/nits. Repeat combing if necessary.
- check daily for any lice/nits that you missed
- a second treatment with this product must be done in 7 to 10 days to kill any newly hatched lice
- if infestation continues, see a doctor for other treatments

Children under 2 years: ask a doctor

OTHER INFORMATION
- store at 20-25°C (68-77°F). Avoid excessive heat.
- keep carton for important product information
- see leaflet inside carton for additional information

INACTIVE INGREDIENTS
butylated hydroxytoluene, carboxymethylcellulose sodium, dimethicone, fragrance, hydroxyethylcellulose, methylchloroisothiazolinone, methylisothiazolinone, petroleum distillates, water

QUESTIONS OR COMMENTS?
1-866-252-5327.
You may also report side effects to this phone number.

LICEFREEE EVERYDAY (natrum muriaticum)
Tec Laboratories, Inc.

DRUG FACTS

Active Ingredient(s)	Purpose(s)
Natrum muriaticum 1X	Pediculosis remedy and prophylactic

USE
- for the prevention and treatment of head lice infestations

WARNINGS
- For external use only.
- Ask a doctor before use if you have infestation of eyebrows or eyelashes, or if you are pregnant.

WHEN USING THIS PRODUCT
- do not use in or near the eyes, close eyes while product is being applied
- do not permit contact with mucous membranes, such as inside the nose as irritation or stinging may occur

STOP USE AND ASK A DOCTOR IF
- skin irritation or infection is present or develops
- keep out of reach of children
- if swallowed, get medical help or contact a Poison Control Center right away

DIRECTIONS
Adults and children 6 months and older:
- Apply a generous amount of shampoo to wet hair, work into a lather while massaging into scalp. Rinse.
- Repeat, this time leaving the shampoo on the hair for at least 3 minutes.
- To treat a head lice infestation, use the shampoo daily for at least 2 weeks.
- For prevention, use daily.

Children under 6 months:
Do not use, consult a doctor.

OTHER INFORMATION
Store at 59-86°F (15-30°C)

INACTIVE INGREDIENTS
benzyl alcohol, cocamidopropyl betaine, caprylic / capric triglycerides, coconut oil, disodium EDTA, fragrances, purified water, sodium laureth sulfate, tea tree oil

LITTLE REMEDIES DECONGESTANT NOSE DROPS (phenylephrine hydrochloride)
Medtech Products Inc.

DRUG FACTS

Active Ingredient(s)	Purpose(s)
Phenylephrine hydrochloride USP 0.125%	Nasal decongestant

USES
- temporarily relieves nasal congestion due to common cold, hay fever or other upper respiratory allergies
- helps clear nasal passages; shrinks swollen membranes
- temporarily restores freer breathing through the nose
- helps decongest sinus openings and passages; temporarily relieves sinus congestion and pressure

WARNINGS
Do not exceed recommended dosage.

DO NOT USE
- **with any other products containing decongestants**

ASK A DOCTOR BEFORE USE IF YOURR CHILD HAS
- heart disease
- high blood pressure
- thyroid disease
- diabetes

WHEN USING THIS PRODUCT
- temporary discomfort such as burning, stinging, sneezing or an increase in nasal discharge may occur
- the use of this dispenser by more than one person may spread infection
- use only as directed

STOP USE AND ASK A DOCTOR IF
- nervousness, dizziness, or sleeplessness occurs
- symptoms persist. Do not use for more than 3 days. Use only as directed. Frequent or prolonged use may cause nasal congestion to recur or worsen.

Keep out of reach of children.
In case of overdose, get medical help or contact a Poison Control Center (1-800-222-1222) right away.

DIRECTIONS
- (nasal use only)
- children 2 to under 6 years (with adult supervision): 2 to 3 drops in each nostril, not more often than every 4 hours
- children under 2 years of age: Consult a doctor

OTHER INFORMATION
- **Do not use if plastic neck band on cap is broken or missing.**
- Do not use if solution is brown or contains a precipitate.
- Protect from light.
- Store at 20-25°C (68-77°F).
- See bottle or box for lot number and expiration date.

INACTIVE INGREDIENTS
benzalkonium chloride, glycerin, polyethylene glycol, potassium phosphate monobasic, purified water, sodium EDTA, sodium phosphate dibasic

QUESTIONS OR COMMENTS?
For further information you may contact us at: **1-800-7-LITTLE**
Mon. – Fri. 8:00 a.m. to 8:00 p.m. EST. or visit us online at **www.LittleRemedies.com**

LITTLE REMEDIES DECONGESTANT PLUS COUGH (dextromethorphan and phenylephrine HCl)
Medtech Products Inc.

DRUG FACTS

Active Ingredient(s)	Purpose(s)
Dextromethorphan HBr 5mg	Cough suppressant
Phenylephrine HCl 2.5 mg	Nasal decongestant

USES TEMPORARILY RELIEVES:
- cough due to minor throat & bronchial irritation as may occur with the common cold
- nasal congestion due to the common cold, hay fever or other respiratory allergies

WARNINGS

DO NOT USE
- With any other products containing decongestants or cough suppressants. Ask a doctor or pharmacist before using with other drugs if you are not sure. Drug Interaction Precaution:
- Do not give this product to a child who is taking a prescription monoamine oxidase inhibitor (MAOI) (certain drugs for depression, psychiatric, or emotional condition, or Parkinson's disease), or for 2 weeks after stopping the MAOI drug. If you are uncertain whether your child's prescription drug contains an MAOI, as a doctor or pharmacist before giving this product.

ASK A DOCTOR BEFORE USE IF THE CHILD HAS
- heart or thyroid disease
- high blood pressure or diabetes
- a cough accompanied by excessive phlegm (mucus) or has a persistent or chronic cough such as occurs with asthma

WHEN USING THIS PRODUCT
- **DO NOT EXCEED RECOMMENDED DOSING.**

STOP USE AND ASK A DOCTOR IF
- your child becomes nervous, dizzy or sleepless
- symptoms do not get better within 7 days, or are accompanied by fever
- cough persists for more than 7 days, tends to recur, or is accompanied by high fever, rash or persistent headaches. These could be signs of a serious condition.

Keep out of reach of children. In case of overdose get medical help or contact a Poison Control Center (1-800-222-1222) right away.

DIRECTIONS
- Give this medicine by mouth only.
- Only use the enclosed dropper.
- **Do not use any other dropper, spoon or dosing device when giving this medicine to your child.**
- Fill the enclosed dropper to the prescribed level and slowly dispense the liquid into your child's mouth (towards the inner cheek).
- Do not give more than 6 doses in any 24-hour period (see overdose warning).
- If needed, repeat dose every 4 hours or as directed by a doctor.

Age (yr)	Dose
Under 4	**Do not use**
4 to under 6	1 mL
6 to under 12	2 mL

OTHER INFORMATION
- Store at 68°-77°F (20-25°C).
- Protect from moisture.
- Oral dosing device enclosed.
- Check expiration date on bottle or box before using.

INACTIVE INGREDIENTS
citric acid, glycerin, high fructose corn syrup, natural grape flavor, purified water, sodium benzoate, sucralose

QUESTIONS OR COMMENTS?
1-800-754-8853 Mon.-Fri. 8 am to 8 pm EST
LittleRemedies.com

LITTLE REMEDIES FOR COLDS HONEY ELIXIR

Medtech Products Inc.

SUPPLEMENT FACTS

Serving Size: 1 teaspoon (tsp)

Each Serving Contains	Amount Per Serving	% DV Children ages 1 to 4	% DV Adults & Children ages over 4
Calories	20		
Carbohydrate	4 g	†	2%*
Sugars	4 g	†	†
Honey	5.2 g	†	†
* Percent daily values are based on a 2,000 calorie diet			
† DV not established			

USE
- to soothe cough and sore throat

DO NOT USE
- In children younger than 12 months because of the risk of botulism. Ask a doctor or pharmacist before using if you are not sure.

ASK A DOCTOR BEFORE USE IF THE CHILD HAS
- cough that occurs with too much phlegm (mucus)
- cough that lasts or is chronic such as occurs with asthma or chronic bronchitis
- high blood pressure or diabetes

STOP USE AND ASK A DOCTOR IF
- cough persists for more than 7 days, tends to recur, or is accompanied by high fever, rash or persistent headaches. These could be signs of a serious condition.

Keep out of reach of children.

DIRECTIONS
Give recommended serving size every 2-4 hours using the measuring cup provided
- Children ages 1 to 4: 1 tsp
- Adults and children over age 4: 2 tsp

OTHER INFORMATION
- Store at 59°-77°F (15°-25°C)
- See bottom panel on bottle or box for Lot Number and Expiration Date

INACTIVE INGREDIENTS
honey (wildflower), purified water, glycerin, sodium benzoate (preservative)

QUESTIONS OR COMMENTS?
1-800-754-8853 Mon.-Fri. 8 am to 8 pm EST
LittleRemedies.com

LITTLE REMEDIES FOR COLDS HONEY POPS

Medtech Products Inc.

SUPPLEMENT FACTS

Serving Size: 1 Lollipop

Each Serving Contains	Amount Per Serving	% DV Children ages 1 to 4	% DV Adults & Children ages over 4
Calories	20		
Carbohydrate	4 g	†	2%*
Sugars	4 g	†	†
* Percent daily values are based on a 2,000 calorie diet			
† DV not established			

USE
- to soothe cough and sore throat

WARNINGS
- **CHOKING HAZARD:** Not for children under 3 years
- Contains natural honey, which is not recommended for children under one year.

ASK A DOCTOR BEFORE USE IF YOUR CHILD HAS
- cough that occurs with too much phlegm (mucus)
- cough that lasts or is chronic such as occurs with asthma or chronic bronchitis
- high blood pressure or diabetes

STOP USE AND ASK A DOCTOR IF
- cough persists for more than 7 days, tends to recur, or is accompanied by high fever, rash or persistent headaches. These could be signs of a serious condition.

Keep out of reach of children.

DIRECTIONS
- give one Honey POP every 2-4 hours

OTHER INFORMATION
- Store at 68°-77°F (20°-25°C) in a dry place
- See bottom panel on box or foil pouch for Lot Number and Expiration Date

INACTIVE INGREDIENTS
caramel color, corn syrup, honey, natural flavor, sucrose, water

QUESTIONS OR COMMENTS?
1-800-754-8853 Mon.-Fri. 8 am to 8 pm EST
LittleRemedies.com

LITTLE REMEDIES FOR COLDS HYDRATION CRYSTALS

Medtech Products Inc.

SUPPLEMENT FACTS

Serving Size: 1 packet (1 tsp)

Each Serving Contains	Amount Per Serving	% DV Children ages 1 to 4	% DV Adults & Children ages over 4
Calories	10		
Sodium	120 mg	†	5%**
Potassium	90 mg	†	3%**
Carbohydrate	2 g	†	0%**
Sugars	2 g	†	†
Vitamin C	9 mg	23%	15%
** Percent daily values are based on a 2,000 calorie diet			
† DV not established			

USES

Keep your little ones hydrated and support their immune systems with anti-oxidants like Vitamin C and Elderberry

DO NOT USE

- For children under 12 months, consult a doctor regarding hydration needs. Ask a doctor or pharmacist before using if you are not sure.

STOP USE AND ASK A DOCTOR IF

- Vomiting or diarrhea persists for more than 24 hours. These could be signs of a serious condition.

Keep out of reach of children

DIRECTIONS

- Add one pack of Little Remedies® Hydration Crystals to 4 fl oz of water in child's *sippy cup or bottle* throughout the day. Blend packs with water only.
- Stir to dissolve.
- To help maintain proper hydration, the child should consume 4-8 servings (16-32 fl oz) per day
- If there is vomiting or fever, or if diarrhea continues beyond 24 hours, consult a doctor.

OTHER INFORMATION

- Store unused mixed product in sealed container in refrigerator for up to 24 hours
- Store packets at 59°-77°F (15°-25°C)
- See bottom panel on box for Lot Number and Expiration Date

INACTIVE INGREDIENTS

dextrose, malic acid, sodium chloride, citric acid, potassium bicarbonate, sodium bicarbonate, natural flavor, sucralose, ascorbic acid, elderberry extract, grape seed extract

QUESTIONS OR COMMENTS?

1-800-754-8853 Mon.-Fri. 8 am to 8 pm EST
LittleRemedies.com

LITTLE REMEDIES FOR COLDS MULTI-SYMPTOM COLD FORMULA

(acetaminophen, dextromethorphan, and phenylephrine)
Medtech Products Inc.

DRUG FACTS

Active Ingredient(s) (in each 1.0 mL)	Purpose(s)
Acetaminophen 80 mg	Pain reliever/fever reducer
Dextromethorphan HBr 2.5 mg	Cough suppressant
Phenylephrine HCl USP 1.25 mg	Nasal decongestant

USES

Temporarily:
- relieves minor aches and pains which may be associated with the common cold, sore throats or headache
- reduces fever
- relieves cough and nasal congestion due to minor throat/bronchial irritation, the common cold, hay fever or other respiratory allergies

WARNINGS

Liver warning: This product contains acetaminophen. Severe liver damage may occur if your child takes
- more than 5 doses in 24 hours, which is the maximum daily amount
- with other drugs containing acetaminophen

Sore throat warning: If sore throat is severe, persists for more than 2 days, or is accompanied or followed by fever, headache, rash, nausea or vomiting, consult a doctor promptly.
Drug Interaction Precaution: Do not give this product to a child who is taking prescription monoamine oxidase inhibitor (MAOI) (certain drugs for depression, psychiatric or emotional conditions, or Parkinson's disease), or for 2 weeks after stopping the MAOI drug. If you are uncertain whether your child's prescription drug contains an MAOI, ask a doctor or pharmacist before giving this product.

DO NOT USE

- with any other products containing acetaminophen, (prescription or non-prescription). If you are not sure whether a drug contains acetaminophen, ask a doctor or pharmacist.

ASK A DOCTOR BEFORE USE IF THE CHILD HAS

- liver, heart or thyroid disease
- high blood pressure or diabetes
- a cough accompanied by excessive phlegm (mucus) or has a persistent or chronic cough such as occurs with asthma

ASK A DOCTOR OR A PHARMACIST BEFORE USE IF YOUR CHILD

- **is taking the blood thinning drug warfarin**

WHEN USING THIS PRODUCT

- **DO NOT EXCEED RECOMMENDED DOSAGE**

STOP USE AND ASK A DOCTOR IF

- your child becomes nervous, dizzy or sleepless
- new symptoms occur
- fever gets worse or lasts more than 3 days
- pain, cough or nasal congestion gets worse or lasts more than 5 days

- cough tends to recur or is accompanied by high fever, rash or persistent headaches
- redness or swelling is present

These could be signs of a serious condition.
Keep out of reach of children.

OVERDOSE WARNING *
- Taking more than the recommended dose (overdose) can cause serious liver damage. In case of overdose, get medical help or contact a Poison Control Center (1800-222-1222) right away. **Prompt medical attention is critical even if you do not notice any signs or symptoms.**

DIRECTIONS
- **this product does not contain directions or complete warnings for adult use**
- give this medicine by mouth only
- only use the enclosed dropper. Do not use any other dropper, spoon or dosing device when giving this medicine to your child.
- fill the enclosed dropper to the prescribed level and slowly dispense the liquid into your child's mouth (towards the inner cheek)
- do not give more than 5 times in any 24-hour period (see overdose warning)
- if needed, repeat dose every 4 hours or as directed by a doctor

Age (yr)	Dose
Under 4	Do not use
4 to under 6	2 mL
6 to under 12	4 mL

OTHER INFORMATION
- store at 68°-77°F (20°-25°C)
- AccuSafe® Oral dosing device enclosed
- check expiration date on bottle or box before using

INACTIVE INGREDIENTS
citric acid, glycerin, natural flavor, potassium sorbate, povidone, propylene glycol, purified water, sodium citrate, sucralose, sucrose, xanthan gum

QUESTIONS OR COMMENTS?
1-800-754-8853 Mon.-Fr. 8 am to 8 pm EST
LittleRemedies.com

LITTLE REMEDIES FOR COLDS SOOTHING SYRUP

Medtech Products Inc.

SUPPLEMENT FACTS

Serving Size: 1 teaspoon (tsp)

Each Serving Contains	Amount Per Serving	% DV Children ages 1 to 4	% DV Adults & Children ages over 4
Calories	20		
Carbohydrate	4 g	†	2% **
Sugars	4 g	†	†
Elderberry extract	575 mg	†	†
* Percent daily values are based on a 2,000 calorie diet			
† DV not established			

USE
To soothe sore throat and boost immune system

DO NOT USE
- In children younger than 12 months because of the risk of botulism. Ask a doctor or pharmacist before using if you are not sure.

ASK A DOCTOR BEFORE USE IF YOUR CHILD HAS
- cough that occurs with too much phlegm (mucus)
- cough that lasts or is chronic such as occurs with asthma or chronic bronchitis
- high blood pressure or diabetes

STOP USE AND ASK A DOCTOR IF
- cough persists for more than 7 days, tends to recur, or is accompanied by high fever, rash or persistent headaches. These could be signs of a serious condition.

Keep out of reach of children.

DIRECTIONS
Give recommended serving size every 2-4 hours using the measuring cup provided
- Children ages 1 to 4: 1 tsp
- Adults and children over age 4: 2 tsp

OTHER INFORMATION
- Store at 59°-77°F (15°-25°C)
- See bottom panel on bottle or box for Lot Number and Expiration Date
- The product color may change over time. This is normal and does not affect the product or its taste.

INACTIVE INGREDIENTS
purified water, sugar, honey, ascorbic acid, sodium benzoate, sodium citrate, natural flavor, xantham gum

QUESTIONS OR COMMENTS?
1-800-754-8853 Mon.-Fri. 8 am to 8 pm EST
LittleRemedies.com

LITTLE REMEDIES FOR FEVERS CHILDREN'S FEVER/PAIN RELIEVER (acetaminophen)

Medtech Products Inc.

DRUG FACTS

Active Ingredient(s) (in each 5 mL)	Purpose(s)
Acetaminophen 160 mg	Pain reliever/ fever reducer

USES
Temporarily:
- reduces fever
- relieves minor aches and pains which may be associated with the common cold, flu, headache, sore throat or toothache

WARNINGS
Liver warning: This product contains acetaminophen. Severe liver damage may occur if your child takes:
- more than 5 doses in 24 hours, which is the maximum daily amount
- with other drugs containing acetaminophen

Sore throat warning: If sore throat is severe, persists for more than 2 days, or is accompanied or followed by fever, headache, rash, nausea, or vomiting, consult a doctor promptly

ASK A DOCTOR BEFORE USE IF THE CHILD HAS
• liver disease

ASK A DOCTOR OR PHARMACIST BEFORE USE IF THE CHILD
• is taking the blood thinning drug warfarin

DO NOT USE
• With any other products containing acetaminophen, (prescription or non-prescription). If you are not sure whether a drug contains acetaminophen, ask a doctor or pharmacist.
• If your child is allergic to acetaminophen or any of the inactive ingredients in this product.

WHEN USING THIS PRODUCT
• **DO NOT EXCEED RECOMMENDED DOSE (see overdose warning)**

STOP USE AND ASK A DOCTOR IF
• new symptoms occur
• fever gets worse or lasts more than 3 days
• pain gets worse or lasts more than 5 days
• redness or swelling is present

These could be signs of a serious condition
Keep out of reach of children.

OVERDOSE WARNING
Taking more than the recommended dose (overdose) can cause serious liver damage. In case of overdose, get medical help or contact a Poison Control Center (1-800-222-1222) right away. **Prompt medical attention is critical even if you do not notice any signs or symptoms.**

DIRECTIONS
This product does not contain directions or complete warnings for adult use
• **Do not give more than directed (see overdose warning)**
• **Shake well before using**
• Find the right dose on the chart below. Use weight to determine dose; otherwise, use age.
• Pour liquid into AccuSafe® dosing cup to the appropriate amount of your child's weight and/or age
• Only use the enclosed AccuSafe® dosing cup
• If needed, repeat dose every 4 hours while symptoms last
• Do not give more than 5 times in any 24 hour period (see overdose warning)
• Do not give for more than 5 days unless directed by a doctor
• Replace cap tightly to maintain child resistance

Weight (lbs)	Age (yrs)	Dose
Under 24	Under 2	Ask a doctor
24-35	2-under 4	5 mL
36-47	4-under 6	7.5 mL
48-59	6-under 9	10 mL
60-71	9-under 11	12.5 mL
72-95	11-under 12	15 mL

OTHER INFORMATION
• store at 68°-77°F (20°-25°C)
• AccuSafe® dosing cup enclosed
• check expiration date on bottle or box before using

INACTIVE INGREDIENTS
citric acid, glycerin, natural cherry flavor, potassium sorbate, povidone, propylene glycol, purified water, sodium citrate, sucralose, sucrose, xanthan gum

QUESTIONS OR COMMENTS?
1-800-754-8853 Mon.-Fri. 8 am to 8 pm EST
LittleRemedies.com

LITTLE REMEDIES FOR FEVERS INFANT FEVER/PAIN RELIEVER (acetaminophen)
Medtech Products Inc.

DRUG FACTS

Active Ingredient(s) (in each 5.0 mL)	Purpose(s)
Acetaminophen 160 mg	Pain reliever/Fever reducer

USES
Temporarily:
• reduces fever
• relieves minor aches and pains which may be associated with the common cold, flu, headache, sore throat or toothache

WARNINGS
Liver warning: This product contains acetaminophen. Severe liver damage may occur if your child takes:
• more than 5 doses in 24 hours, which is the maximum daily amount
• with other drugs containing acetaminophen

Sore throat warning: If sore throat is severe, persists for more than 2 days, or is accompanied or followed by fever, headache, rash, nausea, or vomiting, consult a doctor promptly.

DO NOT USE
• with any other products containing acetaminophen, (prescription or non-prescription). If you are not sure whether a drug contains acetaminophen, ask a doctor or pharmacist.
• if your child is allergic to acetaminophen or any of the inactive ingredients in this product.

ASK A DOCTOR BEFORE USE IF THE CHILD HAS
• liver disease

ASK A DOCTOR OR PHARMACIST BEFORE USE IF THE CHILD
• is taking the blood thinning drug warfarin.

WHEN USING THIS PRODUCT
• **DO NOT EXCEED RECOMMENDED DOSE (see overdose warning)**

STOP USE AND ASK A DOCTOR IF
• new symptoms occur
• fever gets worse or lasts more than 3 days
• pain gets worse or lasts more than 5 days
• redness or swelling is present

These could be signs of a serious condition.
Keep out of reach of children

OVERDOSE WARNING
Taking more than the recommended dose (overdose) can cause serious liver damage. In case of overdose, get medical help or contact a Poison Control Center (1-800-222-1222) right away. **Prompt medical attention is critical even if you do not notice any signs or symptoms.**

DIRECTIONS
This product does not contain directions or complete warnings for adult use.
• **Shake well before using**
• Find the right dose on the chart on the side panel. (If possible, use weight to determine dose; otherwise, use age.)
• Only use the enclosed AccuSafe® syringe
• **Do not use any other syringe, dropper, spoon or dosing device when giving this medicine to your child.**

- Remove cap, attach syringe to flow restrictor and invert bottle
- Pull back syringe until filled to the prescribed level and slowly dispense the liquid into your child's mouth (toward the inner cheek)
- If needed, repeat dose every 4 hours while symptoms last
- Do not give more than 5 times in any 24-hour period (see overdose warning)
- Replace cap tightly to maintain child resistance.

Weight (lbs)	Age (yrs)	Dose
Under 24	**Under 2**	**Ask a doctor**
24-35	2-3	5 mL

OTHER INFORMATION
- store at 68°-77°F (20°-25°C)
- AccuSafe® Oral dosing device enclosed
- check expiration date on bottle or box before using

INACTIVE INGREDIENTS
citric acid, glycerin, natural flavor, potassium sorbate, povidone, propylene glycol, purified water, sodium citrate, sucralose, sucrose, xanthan gum

QUESTIONS OR COMMENTS?
1-800-754-8853 Mon.-Fri. 8 am to 8 pm EST
LittleRemedies.com

LITTLE REMEDIES LITTLE TUMMYS LAXATIVE DROPS (sennosides)

Medtech Products Inc.

DRUG FACTS

Active Ingredient(s) (in each 1.0 mL)	Purpose(s)
Sennosides 8.8 mg	Stimulant laxative

USES
- For relief of occasional constipation (irregularity)
- Generally produces bowel movement in 6-12 hours

WARNINGS
Do not give laxative products to your child for a period longer than 1 week unless directed by a doctor.

ASK A DOCTOR BEFORE USE IF YOUR CHILD HAS
- stomach pain
- nausea
- vomiting
- a sudden change in bowel movements that continues over a period of 2 weeks

STOP USE AND ASK A DOCTOR IF THE CHILD
- has rectal bleeding or failure to have a bowel movement after use of a laxative. These symptoms may indicate a serious condition.

Keep out of reach of children. In case of overdose, get medical help or contact a Poison Control Center (1-800-222-1222) right away.

DIRECTIONS
- Best given to the child at bedtime or as directed by doctor
- Use chart below to find correct dose
- Only use enclosed dropper
- Fill dropper to prescribed level and dispense liquid slowly into child's mouth, toward inner cheek
- **Do not exceed the recommended maximum dose**

Age (yr)	Starting Dose	Maximum Dose
Under 2	Consult Doctor	Consult Doctor
2 to under 6	0.5 mL to 0.75 mL Once a day	0.75 mL Twice a day
6 to under 12	1 mL to 1.5 mL Once a day	1.5 mL Twice a day

OTHER INFORMATION
- Store at 68°-77°F (20°-25°C)
- Do not freeze
- Bottle is child resistant only if the original cap or dropper is in place.
- See bottle or box for lot number and expiration date

INACTIVE INGREDIENTS
ascorbic acid, natural chocolate flavor, methyl- paraben, polysorbate 20, potassium sorbate, propyl gallate, propylene glycol, purified water, sorbitol, soya lecithin, sucralose

QUESTIONS OR COMMENTS?
1-800-754-8853 Mon.-Fri. 8 am to 8 pm EST
LittleRemedies.com

LITTLE REMEDIES SALINE SPRAY/DROPS

Medtech

DRUGS FACTS

Ingredients
water, sodium chloride, glycerin, disodium phosphate, potassium phosphate, benzalkonium, chloride, disodium EDTA

USES
- Moisturizes dry, irritated, or crusty nasal passages due to low humidity, heated environments, air travel, allergies or colds.
- Helps loosen mucus secretions to aid aspiration and removal from nose and sinuses, allowing for easier breathing. For newborns/infants this can be assisted with the use of our specially designed "Soft Tip" Nasal Aspirator.

WARNINGS
Keep out of reach of children.
- **The use of this dispenser by more than one person may spread infection.**
- Wipe nozzle clean after each use.

DIRECTIONS
(For nasal use only)
- Newborns/Infants: 2 to 6 drops in each nostril as often as needed or as directed by your doctor.
- Children & Adults: 2 to 6 sprays/drops into each nostril as often as needed or as directed by a doctor.

OTHER INFORMATION
- This product is non-medicated and can be used as often as needed without the worry of any harmful side effects or drug interactions. The specially buffered formula is alcohol free and will not sting or burn delicate nasal membranes.
- Store at 68°-77°F (20°-25°C).
- See bottle or box for Lot No. and Exp. Date.

QUESTIONS OR COMMENTS?
1-800-754-8853 Mon - Fri. 8 am to 8 pm EST
LittleRemedies.com

LOTRIMIN AF ATHLETE'S FOOT ANTIFUNGAL CREAM (clotrimazole)

MSD Consumer Care, Inc.

DRUG FACTS

Active Ingredient(s)
Clotrimazole 1%

Purpose(s)
Antifungal

USES
• cures most athlete's foot, jock itch, and ringworm
• relieves itching, burning, cracking, scaling and discomfort which accompany these conditions

WARNINGS
For external use only

DO NOT USE
on children under 2 years of age unless directed by a doctor.

WHEN USING THIS PRODUCT
avoid contact with the eyes

STOP USE AND ASK A DOCTOR IF
• irritation occurs
• there is no improvement within 4 weeks (for athlete's foot and ringworm) or 2 weeks (for jock itch)

Keep out of reach of children. If swallowed, get medical help or contact a Poison Control Center right away.

DIRECTIONS
• wash affected area and dry thoroughly
• apply a thin layer over affected area twice daily (morning and night)
• supervise children in the use of this product
• for athlete's foot: pay special attention to spaces between the toes, wear well-fitting, ventilated shoes and change shoes and socks at least once daily
• for athlete's foot and ringworm, use daily for 4 weeks; for jock itch, use daily for 2 weeks
• if condition persists longer, ask a doctor
• this product is not effective on the scalp or nails

OTHER INFORMATION
store between 20° to 25°C (68° to 77°F)

INACTIVE INGREDIENTS
benzyl alcohol, cetyl alcohol, cetyl esters wax, octyldodecanol, polysorbate 60, sorbitan monostearate, stearyl alcohol, water

QUESTIONS OR COMMENTS?
866-360-3226
Distributed by MSD Consumer Care, Inc., PO Box 377, Memphis, TN 38151 USA, a subsidiary of Merck & Co., Inc., Whitehouse Station, NJ USA.

LOTRIMIN AF ATHLETE'S FOOT ANTIFUNGAL POWDER (miconazole nitrate)

MSD Consumer care, Inc.

DRUG FACTS

Active Ingredient(s)
Miconazole nitrate 2%

Purpose(s)
Antifungal

USES
• Cures most athlete's foot (tinea pedis), jock itch (tinea cruris) and ringworm (tinea corporis)
• relieves itching, cracking, burning and scaling

WARNINGS
For external use only
Avoid contact with the eyes

STOP USE AND ASK A DOCTOR IF
irritation occurs or if there is no improvement within 4 weeks (for athlete's foot and ringworm) or 2 weeks (for jock itch)

DO NOT USE
on children under 2 years of age unless directed by a doctor.
Keep out of reach of children. If swallowed, get medical help or contact a Poison Control Center right away.

DIRECTIONS
• wash affected area and dry thoroughly
• sprinkle a thin layer over affected area twice daily (morning and night)
• supervise children in the use of this product
• for athlete's foot: pay special attention to spaces between the toes; wear well-fitting, ventilated shoes and change shoes and socks at least once daily
• for athlete's foot and ringworm, use daily for 4 weeks; for jock itch, use daily for 2 weeks
• if condition persists longer, ask a doctor
• this product is not effective on the scalp or nails

OTHER INFORMATION
store between 20° to 25°C (68° to 77°F)

INACTIVE INGREDIENTS
benzethonium chloride, corn starch, kaolin, sodium bicarbonate, starch/acrylates/acrylamide copolymer, zinc oxide
© Copyright & Distributed by MSD Consumer Care, Inc., PO Box 377, Memphis, TN 38151 USA, a subsidiary of Merck & Co., Inc., Whitehouse Station, NJ USA.

LOTRIMIN AF ATHLETE'S FOOT DEODORANT POWDER SPRAY (miconazole nitrate)

MSD Consumer care, Inc.

DRUG FACTS

Active Ingredient(s)
Miconazole nitrate 2%

Purpose(s)
Antifungal

USES
• proven clinically effective in the treatment of most athlete's foot (tinea pedis), jock itch (tinea cruris) and ringworm (tinea corporis)
• for effective relief of itching, cracking, burning, scaling and discomfort

WARNINGS
For external use only

Flammable
Do not use while smoking or near heat or flame

WHEN USING THIS PRODUCT
- avoid contact with the eyes
- use only as directed. Intentional misuse by deliberately concentrating and inhaling contents can be harmful or fatal.
- contents under pressure. Do not puncture or incinerate. Do not store at temperature above 120°F.

STOP USE AND ASK A DOCTOR IF
- irritation occurs
- there is no improvement within 4 weeks (for athlete's foot and ringworm) or 2 weeks (for jock itch)

Do not use on children under 2 years of age except under the advice and supervision of a doctor.

Keep out of reach of children. If swallowed, get medical help or contact a Poison Control Center right away.

DIRECTIONS
- wash affected area and dry thoroughly
- shake can well and spray a thin layer over affected area twice daily (morning and night)
- supervise children in the use of this product
- for athlete's foot: pay special attention to spaces between the toes; wear well-fitting, ventilated shoes and change shoes and socks at least once daily
- for athlete's foot and ringworm, use daily for 4 weeks; for jock itch, use daily for 2 weeks
- if condition persists longer, ask a doctor
- this product is not effective on the scalp or nails
- in case of clogging, clean nozzle with a pin

OTHER INFORMATION
store between 20° to 25°C (68° to 77°F)

INACTIVE INGREDIENTS
alcohol denat. (8% v/v), fragrance, isobutane, stearalkonium hectorite, talc

QUESTIONS OR COMMENTS?
1-866-360-3266
Distributed by MSD Consumer Care, Inc., PO Box 377, Memphis, TN 38151 USA, a subsidiary of Merck & Co., Inc., Whitehouse Station, NJ USA.

LOTRIMIN AF ATHLETE'S FOOT LIQUID SPRAY (miconazole nitrate)

MSD Consumer care, Inc.

DRUG FACTS

Active Ingredient(s)
Miconazole nitrate 2%

Purpose(s)
Antifungal

USES
- proven clinically effective in the treatment of most athlete's foot (tinea pedis), jock itch (tinea cruris) and ringworm (tinea corporis)
- for effective relief of itching, cracking, burning, scaling and discomfort

WARNINGS
For external use only

Flammable
Do not use while smoking or near heat or flame

WHEN USING THIS PRODUCT
- avoid contact with the eyes
- use only as directed. Intentional misuse by deliberately concentrating and inhaling contents can be harmful or fatal

---

- contents under pressure. Do not puncture or incinerate. Do not store at temperature above 120°F.

STOP USE AND ASK A DOCTOR IF
- irritation occurs
- there is no improvement within 4 weeks (for athlete's foot and ringworm) or 2 weeks (for jock itch)

Do not use on children under 2 years of age except under the advice and supervision of a doctor.

Keep out of reach of children. If swallowed, get medical help or contact a Poison Control Center right away.

DIRECTIONS
- wash affected area and dry thoroughly
- shake can well and spray a thin layer over affected area twice daily (morning and night)
- supervise children in the use of this product
- for athlete's foot: pay special attention to spaces between the toes; wear well-fitting, ventilated shoes and change shoes and socks at least once daily
- for athlete's foot and ringworm, use daily for 4 weeks; for jock itch, use daily for 2 weeks
- if condition persists longer, ask a doctor
- this product is not effective on the scalp or nails

OTHER INFORMATION
store between 20° to 25°C (68° to 77°F)

INACTIVE INGREDIENTS
alcohol denat. (13% v/v), cocamide DEA, isobutane, propylene glycol, tocopherol (vitamin E)

QUESTIONS OR COMMENTS?
1-866-360-3266
© Copyright & Distributed by MSD Consumer Care, Inc., PO Box 377, Memphis, TN 38151 USA, a subsidiary of Merck & Co., Inc., Whitehouse Station, NJ USA.

LOTRIMIN AF ATHLETE'S FOOT POWDER SPRAY (miconazole nitrate)

MSD Consumer care, Inc.

DRUG FACTS

Active Ingredient(s)
Miconazole nitrate 2%

Purpose(s)
Antifungal

USES
- proven clinically effective in the treatment of most athlete's foot (tinea pedis), jock itch (tinea cruris) and ringworm (tinea corporis)
- for effective relief of itching, cracking, burning, scaling and discomfort

WARNINGS
For external use only
Flammable: Do not use while smoking or near heat or flame

WHEN USING THIS PRODUCT
- avoid contact with the eyes
- use only as directed. Intentional misuse by deliberately concentrating and inhaling contents can be harmful or fatal
- contents under pressure. Do not puncture or incinerate. Do not store at temperature above 120°F.

STOP USE AND ASK A DOCTOR IF
- irritation occurs
- there is no improvement within 4 weeks (for athlete's foot and ringworm) or 2 weeks (for jock itch)

DO NOT USE
on children under 2 years of age except under the advice and supervision of a doctor.
Keep out of reach of children. If swallowed, get medical help or contact a Poison Control Center right away.

DIRECTIONS
- wash affected area and dry thoroughly
- shake can well and spray a thin layer over affected area twice daily (morning and night)
- supervise children in the use of this product
- for athlete's foot: pay special attention to spaces between the toes; wear well-fitting, ventilated shoes and change shoes and socks at least once daily
- for athlete's foot and ringworm, use daily for 4 weeks; for jock itch, use daily for 2 weeks
- if condition persists longer, ask a doctor
- this product is not effective on the scalp or nails
- in case of clogging, clean nozzle with a pin

OTHER INFORMATION
store between 20° to 25°C (68° to 77°F)

INACTIVE INGREDIENTS
alcohol denat. (8% v/v), isobutane, stearalkonium hectorite, talc

QUESTIONS OR COMMENTS?
1-866-360-3266
Distributed by MSD Consumer Care, Inc., PO Box 377, Memphis, TN 38151 USA, a subsidiary of Merck & Co., Inc., Whitehouse Station, NJ USA.

LOTRIMIN AF JOCK ITCH ANTIFUNGAL CREAM (clotrimazole)

MSD Consumer care, Inc.

DRUG FACTS

Active Ingredient(s)
Clotrimazole 1%

Purpose(s)
Antifungal

USES
- cures most jock itch
- relieves itching, burning, scaling, chafing and discomfort associated with jock itch

WARNINGS
For external use only

DO NOT USE
on children under 2 years of age unless directed by a doctor.

WHEN USING THIS PRODUCT
avoid contact with the eyes

STOP USE AND ASK A DOCTOR IF
- irritation occurs
- there is no improvement within 2 weeks

Keep out of reach of children. If swallowed, get medical help or contact a Poison Control Center right away.

DIRECTIONS
- wash affected area and dry thoroughly
- apply a thin layer over affected area twice daily (morning and night)
- supervise children in the use of this product
- use daily for 2 weeks
- if condition persists longer, ask a doctor
- this product is not effective on the scalp or nails

OTHER INFORMATION
store between 20° to 25°C (68° to 77°F)

INACTIVE INGREDIENTS
benzyl alcohol, cetyl alcohol, cetyl esters wax, octyldodecanol, polysorbate 60, sorbitan monostearate, stearyl alcohol, water

QUESTIONS OR COMMENTS?
1-866-360-3266
Distributed by MSD Consumer Care, Inc., PO Box 377, Memphis, TN 38151 USA,
a subsidiary of Merck & Co., Inc., Whitehouse Station, NJ USA.

LOTRIMIN AF JOCK ITCH ANTIFUNGAL POWDER SPRAY (miconazole nitrate)

MSD Consumer care, Inc.

DRUG FACTS

Active Ingredient(s)
Miconazole nitrate 2%

Purpose(s)
Antifungal

USES
- proven clinically effective in the treatment of most jock itch (tinea cruris)
- for effective relief of itching, burning, scaling and discomfort, and chafing associated with jock itch

WARNINGS
For external use only
Flammable: Do not use while smoking or near heat or flame

WHEN USING THIS PRODUCT
- avoid contact with the eyes
- use only as directed. Intentional misuse by deliberately concentrating and inhaling contents can be harmful or fatal
- contents under pressure. Do not puncture or incinerate. Do not store at temperature above 120°F.

STOP USE AND ASK A DOCTOR IF
- irritation occurs
- there is no improvement within 2 weeks

Do not use on children under 2 years of age except under the advice and supervision of a doctor.
Keep out of reach of children. If swallowed, get medical help or contact a Poison Control Center right away.

DIRECTIONS
- wash affected area and dry thoroughly
- shake can well and spray a thin layer over affected area twice daily (morning and night)
- supervise children in the use of this product
- use daily for 2 weeks
- if condition persists longer, ask a doctor
- this product is not effective on the scalp or nails
- in case of clogging, clean nozzle with a pin

OTHER INFORMATION
store between 20° to 25°C (68° to 77°F)

INACTIVE INGREDIENTS
alcohol denat. (8% v/v), isobutane, stearalkonium hectorite, talc

QUESTIONS OR COMMENTS?
1-866-360-3266
© Copyright & Distributed by MSD Consumer Care, Inc., PO Box 377, Memphis, TN 38151 USA, a subsidiary of Merck & Co., Inc., Whitehouse Station, NJ USA.

LOTRIMIN AF RINGWORM CREAM
(clotrimazole)

MSD Consumer Care, Inc.

DRUG FACTS

Active Ingredient(s)
Clotrimazole 1%

Purpose(s)
Antifungal

USES
• cures most ringworm
• relieves itching, redness, irritation and discomfort which accompany this condition

WARNINGS
For external use only

WHEN USING THIS PRODUCT
avoid contact with the eyes

STOP USE AND ASK A DOCTOR IF
• irritation occurs
• there is no improvement within 4 weeks

DO NOT USE
on children under 2 years of age unless directed by a doctor.
Keep out of reach of children. If swallowed, get medical help or contact a Poison Control Center right away.

DIRECTIONS
• wash affected area and dry thoroughly
• apply a thin layer over affected area twice daily (morning and night)
• supervise children in the use of this product
• use daily for 4 weeks
• if condition persists longer, ask a doctor
• this product is not effective on the scalp or nails

OTHER INFORMATION
store between 20° to 25°C (68° to 77°F)

INACTIVE INGREDIENTS
benzyl alcohol, cetyl alcohol, cetyl esters wax, octyldodecanol, polysorbate 60, sorbitan monostearate, stearyl alcohol, water

QUESTIONS OR COMMENTS?
1-866-360-3266
Distributed by MSD Consumer Care, Inc., PO Box 377, Memphis, TN 38151 USA, a subsidiary of Merck & Co., Inc., Whitehouse Station, NJ USA.

LOTRIMIN ULTRA ATHLETE'S FOOT CREAM
(butenafine hydrochloride)

MSD Consumer Care, Inc.

DRUG FACTS

Active Ingredient(s)
Butenafine hydrochloride 1%

Purpose(s)
Antifungal

USES
• cures most athlete's foot between the toes. Effectiveness on the bottom or sides of foot is unknown.
• cures most jock itch and ringworm
• relieves itching, burning, cracking, and scaling which accompany these conditions

WARNINGS
For external use only

DO NOT USE
• on nails or scalp
• in or near the mouth or the eyes
• for vaginal yeast infections

WHEN USING THIS PRODUCT
do not get into the eyes. If eye contact occurs, rinse thoroughly with water.

STOP USE AND ASK A DOCTOR IF
too much irritation occurs or irritation gets worse
Keep out of reach of children. If swallowed, get medical help or contact a Poison Control Center right away.

DIRECTIONS
• adults and children 12 years and older:
  • use the tip of the cap to break the seal and open the tube
  • wash the affected skin with soap and water and dry completely before applying
  • **for athlete's foot between the toes**: apply to affected skin between and around the toes twice a day for 1 week (morning and night), or once a day for 4 weeks, or as directed by a doctor. Wear well-fitting, ventilated shoes. Change shoes and socks as least once daily.
  • **for jock itch and ringworm**: apply once a day to affected skin for 2 weeks or as directed by a doctor
  • wash hands after each use
• children under 12 years: ask a doctor

OTHER INFORMATION
• do not use if seal on tube is broken or not visible
• store between 20° to 25°C (68° to 77°F)

INACTIVE INGREDIENTS
benzyl alcohol, cetyl alcohol, diethanolamine, glycerin, glyceryl monostearate SE, polyoxyethylene (23) cetyl ether, propylene glycol dicaprylate, purified water, sodium benzoate, stearic acid, white petrolatum

QUESTIONS OR COMMENTS?
866-360-3226
Distributed by MSD Consumer Care, Inc., PO Box 377, Memphis, TN 38151 USA, a subsidiary of Merck & Co., Inc., Whitehouse Station, NJ USA.

LOTRIMIN ULTRA JOCK ITCH CREAM
MSD Consumer Care, Inc.

- Lotrimin Ultra® Jock Itch Cream uses a prescription strength active ingredient to cure most jock itch while providing effective relief from these symptoms:
  - Itching
  - Burning
  - Cracking
  - Scaling
  - Chafing
  - Discomfort
- Lotrimin Ultra® penetrates to kill the fungus right where it starts

MAALOX ADVANCED MAXIMUM STRENGTH - CHEWABLE - ASSORTED FRUIT
(calcium carbonate and simethicone)

Novartis Consumer Health, Inc.

DRUG FACTS

Active Ingredient(s) (in each tablet)	Purpose(s)
Calcium Carbonate 1000mg	Antacid
Simethicone 60mg	Antigas

USES
for the relief of:
- acid indigestion
- heartburn
- sour stomach
- upset stomach associated with these symptoms
- bloating and pressure commonly referred to as gas

WARNINGS
Do not take more than 8 tablets in 24 hours or use the maximum dosage for more than 2 weeks except under the advice and supervision of a doctor

ASK A DOCTOR BEFORE USE IF YOU HAVE
- kidney stones
- a calcium-restricted diet

ASK A DOCTOR OR PHARMACIST BEFORE USE IF YOU ARE
presently taking a prescription drug. Antacids may interact with certain prescription drugs.

WHEN USING THIS PRODUCT
- at maximum dose, constipation may occur

STOP USE AND ASK A DOCTOR IF
symptoms last for more than 2 weeks
Keep out of reach of children.

DIRECTIONS
- adults and children 12 years and older: chew 1 to 2 tablets as symptoms occur or as directed by a doctor
- do not take more than 8 tablets in 24 hours or use the maximum dosage for more than 2 weeks except under the advice and supervision of a doctor

OTHER INFORMATION
- **each tablet contains:** calcium 400 mg
- store at controlled room temperature 20-25°C (68-77°F)

- keep tightly closed and dry
- keep tightly closed and avoid freezing

INACTIVE INGREDIENTS
acesulfame K, colloidal silicon dioxide, croscarmellose sodium, D&C red 30 aluminum lake, D&C yellow 10 aluminum lake, dextrose, FD&C red 40 aluminum lake, FD&C yellow 6 aluminum lake, flavors, magnesium stearate, maltodextrin, mannitol, pregelatinized starch

QUESTIONS OR COMMENTS?
Call **1-800-452-0051**

MAALOX ADVANCED REGULAR STRENGTH - LIQUID - MINT (aluminum hydroxide, magnesium hydroxide, and simethicone)

Novartis Consumer Health, Inc.

DRUG FACTS

Active Ingredient(s) (in each 5 mL=1 teaspoonful)	Purpose(s)
Aluminum hydroxide (equiv. to dried gel, USP) 200 mg	Antacid
Magnesium hydroxide 200 mg	Antacid
Simethicone 20 mg	Antigas

USES
for the relief of:
- acid indigestion
- heartburn
- sour stomach
- upset stomach due to these symptoms
- pressure and bloating commonly referred to as gas

WARNINGS
Do not take more than 16 teaspoonsful in a 24-hour period or use the maximum dosage for more than 2 weeks except under the advice and supervision of a physician

ASK A DOCTOR BEFORE USE IF YOU HAVE
- kidney disease
- a magnesium-restricted diet

ASK A DOCTOR OR PHARMACIST BEFORE USE IF YOU ARE
presently taking a prescription drug. Antacids may interact with certain prescription drugs.

STOP USE AND ASK A DOCTOR IF
symptoms last more than 2 weeks
Keep out of reach of children

DIRECTIONS
- shake well before using
- adults and children 12 years and older: take 2 to 4 teaspoonsful four times a day or as directed by a physician
- do not take more than 16 teaspoonsful in 24 hours or use the maximum dosage for more than 2 weeks
- children under 12 years: consult a physician

OTHER INFORMATION
- **each tablet contains:** magnesium 75 mg, potassium 5 mg
- store at controlled room temperature 20-25°C (68-77°F)
- protect from freezing

INACTIVE INGREDIENTS

butylparaben, carboxymethylcellulose sodium, flavor, glycerin, hypromellose, microcrystalline cellulose, propylene glycol, propylparaben, purified water, saccharin sodium, sorbitol

QUESTIONS OR COMMENTS?
Call 1-800-452-0051

MAALOX REGULAR STRENGTH - CHEWABLE - WILD BERRY (calcium carbonate)

Novartis Consumer Health, Inc.

DRUG FACTS

Active Ingredient(s) (in each tablet)	Purpose(s)
Calcium carbonate 600 mg	Antacid

USES
for the relief of:
- acid indigestion
- heartburn
- sour stomach
- upset stomach due to these symptoms

WARNINGS

ASK A DOCTOR BEFORE USE IF YOU HAVE
- kidney stones
- a calcium-restricted diet

ASK A DOCTOR OR PHARMACIST BEFORE USE IF YOU ARE
presently taking a prescription drug. Antacids may interact with certain prescription drugs.

STOP USE AND ASK A DOCTOR IF
symptoms last more than 2 weeks
Keep out of reach of children

DIRECTIONS
- chew 1 to 2 tablets as symptoms occur or as directed by a doctor
- do not take more than 12 tablets in 24 hours or use the maximum dosage for more than 2 weeks except under the advice and supervision of a doctor

OTHER INFORMATION
- **each tablet contains:** calcium 240 mg
- store at controlled room temperature 20-25°C (68-77°F)
- keep tightly closed and dry

INACTIVE INGREDIENTS
aspartame, colloidal silicon dioxide, croscarmellose sodium, D&C red #30, dextrose, flavors, magnesium stearate, maltodextrin, mannitol, pregelatinized starch

QUESTIONS OR COMMENTS?
Call 1-800-452-0051

MAALOX TOTAL RELIEF - LIQUID - STRAWBERRY (bismuth subsalicylate)

Novartis Consumer Health, Inc.

DRUG FACTS

Active Ingredient(s) (in each 15 mL, 1 tablespoonful)	
Bismuth Subsalicylate 525 mg	Upset Stomach Reliever/ Antidiarrheal

USES
for the relief of:
- upset stomach associated with nausea, heartburn, and gas due to overindulgence in food
- diarrhea

WARNINGS
Reye's syndrome: Children and teenagers who have or are recovering from chicken pox or flu-like symptoms should not use this product. When using this product, if changes in behavior with nausea and vomiting occur, consult a doctor because these symptoms could be an early sign of Reye's syndrome, a rare but serious illness.
Allergy alert: Contains salicylate. Do not take if you are
- allergic to salicylates (including aspirin)
- taking other salicylate products

DO NOT USE IF YOU HAVE
- bloody or black stool
- an ulcer
- a bleeding problem

ASK A DOCTOR BEFORE USE IF YOU HAVE
- fever
- mucus in the stool

ASK A DOCTOR OR PHARMACIST BEFORE USE IF YOU ARE TAKING ANY DRUG FOR
- anticoagulation (blood thinning)
- diabetes
- gout
- arthritis

WHEN USING THIS PRODUCT
a temporary, but harmless, darkening of the stool and/or tongue may occur.

STOP USE AND ASK A DOCTOR IF
- diarrhea or other symptoms get worse or last more than 2 days
- ringing in the ears or a loss of hearing occurs
If pregnant or breast-feeding, ask a health professional before use.
Keep out of reach of children. In case of overdose, get medical help or contact a Poison Control Center right away.

DIRECTIONS
- shake well before using
- adults and children 12 years and older: 2 tablespoonfuls (30 mL) every hour, as required, not to exceed 8 tablespoonfuls (120 mL) in 24 hours
- use until diarrhea stops but not more than 2 days
- drink plenty of clear fluids to help prevent dehydration caused by diarrhea
- children under 12 years: ask a doctor

OTHER INFORMATION
- **each tablespoonful contains:** sodium 6 mg
- **each tablespoonful contains:** salicylate 232 mg
- store at controlled room temperature 20-25°C (68-77°F)
- keep tightly closed and avoid freezing

INACTIVE INGREDIENTS
flavors[1], methylparaben, microcrystalline cellulose, propylene glycol, propylparaben, purified water, salicylic acid, sodium salicylate, sorbitol, sucralose, xanthan gum
[1]contains ethyl alcohol

QUESTIONS OR COMMENTS?
Call **1-800-452-0051** 24 hours a day, 7 days a week.

METAMUCIL CLEAR & NATURAL (inulin)
Procter & Gamble

METAMUCIL CLEAR & NATURAL INULIN FIBER SUPPLEMENT POWDER INGREDIENTS
Inulin fiber is:
- 100% natural
- Harvested from chicory roots, a natural vegetable fiber
- Completely dissolvable in most beverages and foods, making it clear-mixing

INGREDIENT: Inulin (100% natural vegetable fiber)

METAMUCIL CLEAR & NATURAL INULIN FIBER SUPPLEMENT POWDER INFORMATION AND FACTS

Serving Size: 1 heaping tsp (5.8g)	
Servings Per Container: [34] [57]	
Amount Per Serving	%DV*
Calories 25	
Total Carb. 6 g	2%*
Dietary Fiber 5 g	20%*
Soluble Fiber 5 g	†
Sugars 0 g	†
* Percent Daily Values (DV) are based on a 2,000 calorie diet.	
† Daily Value (DV) not established.	

METAMUCIL CLEAR & NATURAL INULIN FIBER SUPPLEMENT POWDER DIRECTIONS

DIRECTIONS
1 heaping teaspoon, up to three times daily. Each heaping teaspoon contains 5 grams of fiber.
Mix in Liquid: Stir 1 heaping teaspoon briskly in 8 oz. or more of water or other beverage. Product dissolves best in room-temperature or warmer liquid, and dissolves more slowly in cold liquid. Not recommended for carbonated beverages.
New Users: Start with one serving per day as your body adjusts to the extra fiber in your diet, and gradually increase up to three servings per day.
Cooking and Baking: Add desired amount directly to foods as you prepare them. For best results, use in moist foods or recipes.
Cooking and Baking: Add desired amount directly to foods as you prepare them. For best results, use in moist foods or recipes.
Adults 12 years and older: 1 heaping teaspoon, up to three times daily
6 to 11 years: 1/2 adult serving, up to three times daily
Younger than 6 years: Consult a doctor.

METAMUCIL CLEAR & NATURAL INULIN FIBER SUPPLEMENT OTHER INFORMATION
- **Do not use if printed inner seal is broken or missing.**
- Fill controlled by weight, not volume. Contents may settle during shipping and handling.
- Store at room temperature with lid tightly closed.
- See bottom for Best If Used by Date.

QUESTIONS OR COMMENTS?
1-800-525-2855

METAMUCIL FIBER MULTIGRAIN WAFERS
Procter & Gamble

METAMUCIL MULTIGRAIN WAFERS INGREDIENTS
Apple MultiGrain Wafers: Wheat Flour, Corn Oil, Sucrose, Psyllium Husk, Fructose, Oat Hull Fiber, Brown Sugar, Corn Starch, Soy Lecithin, Cinnamon, Natural and Artificial Flavors, Molasses, Sodium Bicarbonate, Ascorbic Acid (Preservative)
Cinnamon MultiGrain Wafers: Wheat Flour, Sucrose, Corn Oil, Psyllium Husk, Oats, Fructose, Oat Hull Fiber, Corn Starch, Soy Lecithin, Cinnamon, Molasses, Natural and Artificial Flavors, Nutmeg, Sodium Bicarbonate, Ascorbic Acid (Preservative)

METAMUCIL MULTIGRAIN WAFERS FIBER SUPPLEMENT INFORMATION AND FACTS
Helps Your Natural Cleansing Process
- Metamucil provides 100% natural fiber, in the form of psyllium husk, to help promote and maintain regularity.
- Can be used for occasional constipation.

Excellent Source of Dietary Fiber
- Provides 20% of your recommended daily amount of dietary fiber per serving.
- Contains 4.5 g total fat per serving.

Apple Crisp MultiGrain Wafers

Serving Size 1 packet (2 wafers)	
Servings Per Container 12	
Amount Per Serving	
Calories 100	Calories from Fat 40
	% Daily Value*
Total Fat 4.5g	7%
Saturated Fat 0.5g	3%
Trans Fat 0g	†
Cholesterol 0mg	0%
Sodium 20mg	0%
Potassium 55mg	2%
Total Carbohydrate 16g	5%
Dietary Fiber 5g	20%
Soluble Fiber 3g	†
Sugars 6g	†
Protein 1g	
Vitamin A 0%	Vitamin C 35%
Calcium 2%	Iron 8%
* Percent Daily Values are based on a 2,000 calorie diet. Your daily values may be higher or lower depending on your calorie needs:	

	Calories	2,000	2,500
Total Fat	Less than	65g	80g
Sat Fat	Less than	20g	25g
Cholesterol	Less than	300g	300g
Sodium	Less than	2,400mg	2,400mg
Total Carbohydrate		300g	375g
Dietary Fiber		25g	30g

†Daily Value not established.

Cinnamon Spice MultiGrain Wafers

Serving Size 1 packet (2 wafers)	
Servings Per Container 12	
Amount Per Serving	
Calories 100	Calories from Fat 40
	% Daily Value*
Total Fat 4.5g	7%
Saturated Fat 0.5g	3%
Trans Fat 0g	†
Cholesterol 0mg	0%
Sodium 20mg	0%
Potassium 55mg	2%
Total Carbohydrate 16g	5%
Dietary Fiber 5g	20%
Soluble Fiber 3g	†
Sugars 6g	†
Protein 1g	
Vitamin A 0%	Vitamin C 40%
Calcium 2%	Iron 4%

* Percent Daily Values are based on a 2,000 calorie diet. Your daily values may be higher or lower depending on your calorie needs:

	Calories	2,000	2,500
Total Fat	Less than	65g	80g
Sat Fat	Less than	20g	25g
Cholesterol	Less than	300g	300g
Sodium	Less than	2,400mg	2,400mg
Total Carbohydrate		300g	375g
Dietary Fiber		25g	30g

†Daily Value not established.

METAMUCIL WAFERS FIBER SUPPLEMENT DIRECTIONS
SERVING SUGGESTION: FOR ADULTS 12 AND OLDER
- Enjoy 1 serving (2 wafers) with at least 8 oz of your favorite hot or cold beverage.
- Metamucil Fiber Wafers are a great-tasting, easy way to increase your daily fiber intake.
- Each adult serving (2 wafers) provides 5 grams of 100% natural fiber.
- Eat up to 3 servings per day.

METAMUCIL WAFERS FIBER SUPPLEMENT WARNINGS
- **Choking:** Metamucil Fiber Wafers should be eaten with at least a full glass (8 oz) of liquid. Eating this product without enough liquid may cause choking. Do not eat Fiber Wafers if you have difficulty in swallowing. Eat in an upright position. If you experience chest pain, vomiting, or difficulty in swallowing or breathing after taking this product, seek immediate medical attention.

- **Allergy Alert:** May cause an allergic reaction in people sensitive to inhaled or ingested psyllium.
- This product may affect how well medicines work. If you are taking a prescription medicine by mouth, eat this product at least 2 hours before or 2 hours after the prescribed medicine.
- **New Users:** Start with 1 dose per day; gradually increase to 3 doses per day as necessary. As your body adjusts to increased fiber intake, you may experience changes in bowel habits or minor bloating.
- Ask a doctor before use if you have a sudden change in bowel habits persisting for 2 weeks, abdominal pain, nausea, or vomiting.
- Stop use and ask a doctor if you have constipation lasting more than 7 days or rectal bleeding occurs. These may be signs of a serious condition.
- **Keep out of reach of children.** In case of accidental ingestion, contact your doctor or a Poison Control Center right away.

OTHER INFORMATION
- Store at room temperature.

QUESTIONS OR COMMENTS?
1-800-983-4237

METAMUCIL FIBER SINGLES (psyllium husk)
Procter & Gamble

ORANGE FIBER SINGLES INGREDIENTS
Sucrose, Psyllium Husk, Citric Acid, Natural and Artificial Orange Flavor, Yellow 6
Active Ingredient(s) (in each serving)
Psyllium Husk, Approximately 3.4 g

INACTIVE INGREDIENTS
citric acid, FD&C yellow no. 6, natural and artificial orange flavor, sucrose
Orange Sugar Free Fiber Singles Ingredients
psyllium husk, maltodextrin, citric acid, natural and artificial orange flavor, aspartame, yellow 6
Active Ingredient(s) (in each serving)
Psyllium Husk, Approximately 3.4 g

INACTIVE INGREDIENTS
aspartame, citric acid, FD&C yellow no. 6, maltodextrin, natural and artificial orange flavor

PSYLLIUM FIBER SINGLES

SUPPLEMENT FACTS
Rely on Metamucil for these important multiple health benefits:
- Helps lower cholesterol to promote heart health*
- Promotes digestive health†
- Low glycemic index*†
- Gluten free (less than 20 ppm gluten)*

Daily fiber supplement. Each serving adds 3 grams of fiber to your diet.

Orange Fiber Singles:

SUPPLEMENT FACTS	
Serving Size: 1 packet (12g)	
Servings Per Container: 30	
Amount Per Serving	%DV*
Calories 45	
Total Carb. 12 g	4%*
Dietary Fiber 3 g	12%*
Soluble Fiber 2 g	†
Sugars 9 g	†
Iron 0.8 mg	4%
Sodium 5 mg	<1%
Potassium 30 mg	<1%
* Percent Daily Values (%DV) are based on a 2,000 calorie diet.	
† Daily Value (DV) not established.	

Orange Sugar Free Fiber Singles:

SUPPLEMENT FACTS	
Serving Size: 1 packet (5.85g)	
Servings Per Container: 30	
Amount Per Serving	%DV*
Calories 20	
Total Carb. 5 g	2%*
Dietary Fiber 3 g	12%*
Soluble Fiber 2 g	†
Sugars 0 g	†
Iron 0.8 mg	4%
Sodium 5 mg	<1%
Potassium 30 mg	<1%
* Percent Daily Values (%DV) are based on a 2,000 calorie diet.	
† Daily Value (DV) not established.	

PSYLLIUM FIBER SINGLES SUPPLEMENT DIRECTIONS

Adults 12 years and older:
- 1 packet in 8 oz of liquid 3 times daily for daily fiber supplement.
- 1 packet in 8 oz of liquid 3 times daily for cholesterol lowering to promote heart health.

Under 12 years:
- Consult a doctor. See mixing directions in **Therapy for Regularity Directions**.

NOTICE: Mix this product with at least 8 oz (a full glass) of liquid. Taking without enough liquid may cause choking. Do not take if you have difficulty swallowing.

PSYLLIUM FIBER SINGLES THERAPY FOR REGULARITY DIRECTIONS
Purpose
- Fiber laxative

USES
- Effective in treating occasional constipation and restoring regularity

Put one dose into an empty glass. Mix this product (child or adult dose) with at least 8 ounces (a full glass) of water or other fluid. Taking this product without enough liquid may cause choking. See choking warning. Stir briskly and drink promptly. If mixture thickens, add more liquid and stir.
- **Adults 12 years and older:** 1 packet in 8 oz of liquid at the first sign of irregularity. Can be taken up to 3 times daily. Generally produces effect in 12 to 72 hours.

- **6 to 11 years:** 1/2 adult dose in 8 oz of liquid, up to 3 times daily.
- **Under 6 years:** Consult a doctor

Bulk-forming fibers like psyllium husk may affect how well other medicines work. If you are taking a prescription medicine by mouth, take this product at least 2 hours before or 2 hours after the prescribed medicine. As your body adjusts to increased fiber intake, you may experience changes in bowel habits or minor bloating.
New Users: Start with 1 dose per day; gradually increase to 3 doses per day as necessary.

PSYLLIUM FIBER SINGLES WARNINGS
Choking: Taking this product without adequate fluid may cause it to swell and block your throat or esophagus and may cause choking. Do not take this product if you have difficulty swallowing. If you experience chest pain, vomiting, or difficulty in swallowing or breathing after taking this product, seek immediate medical attention.
Allergy alert:
This product may cause allergic reaction in people sensitive to inhaled or ingested psyllium.

ASK A DOCTOR BEFORE USE IF YOU HAVE
- A sudden change in bowel habits persisting for 2 weeks
- Abdominal pain, nausea, or vomiting

STOP USE AND ASK A DOCTOR IF
- Constipation lasts more than 7 days
- Rectal bleeding occurs

These may be signs of a serious condition.
Keep out of reach of children.
In case of overdose, get medical help or contact a Poison Control Center right away.

PSYLLIUM FIBER SINGLES OTHER INFORMATION
- Each packet contains: potassium 30 mg; sodium 5 mg.
- PHENYLKETONURICS: CONTAINS PHENYLALANINE, 25 mg per packet
- See side of carton and individual packets for expiration date.
- Contains 100% natural, therapeutic fiber

QUESTIONS OR COMMENTS?
1-800-983-4237
* Psyllium fiber, as in Metamucil powders and capsules, is recognized by the FDA to treat occasional constipation and help lower cholesterol. Diets low in saturated fat and cholesterol that include 7 grams of soluble fiber per day from psyllium husk may reduce the risk of heart disease by lowering cholesterol. One adult dose of Metamucil has at least 2.1 grams of this soluble fiber. Use as directed. May contain trace amounts of gluten. If you have specific dietary needs, you should consult your doctor before consuming this product. This Metamucil product has a low glycemic index, a measure of the effect of dietary carbohydrates on blood sugar levels.
† THESE STATEMENTS HAVE NOT BEEN EVALUATED BY THE FOOD AND DRUG ADMINISTRATION. THIS PRODUCT IS NOT INTENDED TO DIAGNOSE, TREAT, CURE, OR PREVENT ANY DISEASE.

METAMUCIL THERAPY FOR REGULARITY
(psyllium husk)

Procter & Gamble

DRUG FACTS

Active Ingredient(s) (in each tablespoon)
Psyllium husk approximately 3.4 g

Purpose(s)
Fiber therapy for regularity

USES
- effective in treating occasional constipation and restoring regularity

WARNINGS
Choking
Taking this product without adequate fluid may cause it to swell and block your throat or esophagus and may cause choking. Do not take this product if you have difficulty in swallowing. If you experience chest pain, vomiting, or difficulty in swallowing or breathing after taking this product, seek immediate medical attention.

Allergy alert
This product may cause allergic reaction in people sensitive to inhaled or ingested psyllium.

ASK A DOCTOR BEFORE USE
if you have
- a sudden change in bowel habits persisting for 2 weeks
- abdominal pain, nausea or vomiting

STOP USE AND ASK A DOCTOR IF
- constipation lasts more than 7 days
- rectal bleeding occurs

These may be signs of a serious condition.
Keep out of reach of children. In case of overdose, contact a doctor or a Poison Control Center right away.

DIRECTIONS
Put one dose into an empty glass. Mix this product (child or adult dose) with at least 8 ounces (a full glass) of water or other fluid. Taking this product without enough liquid may cause choking. See choking warning. Stir briskly and drink promptly. If mixture thickens, add more liquid and stir.

Adults 12 yrs. & older	1 rounded **TABLESPOON** in 8 oz of liquid at the first sign of irregularity. Can be taken up to 3 times daily. Generally produces effect in 12 - 72 hours.
6 - 11 yrs.	½ adult dose in 8 oz of liquid, up to 3 times daily
Under 6 yrs.	Consult a doctor

Bulk-forming fibers like psyllium husk may affect how well other medicines work. If you are taking a prescription medicine by mouth, take this product at least 2 hours before or 2 hours after the prescribed medicine. As your body adjusts to increased fiber intake, you may experience changes in bowel habits or minor bloating.

New Users
Start with 1 dose per day; gradually increase to 3 doses per day as necessary.

OTHER INFORMATION
- **each teaspoon contains:** potassium 35 mg; sodium 5 mg
- store at room temperature tightly closed to protect from humidity
- see bottom of canister for expiration date
- contains a 100% natural, therapeutic fiber

INACTIVE INGREDIENTS
citric acid, FD&C yellow No. 6, natural and artificial orange flavor, sucrose

QUESTIONS OR COMMENTS?
1-800-983-4237
Dist. by Procter & Gamble,
Cincinnati OH 45202

METAMUCIL PSYLLIUM FIBER CAPSULES
(psyllium husk)

Procter & Gamble

Fit more fiber into your daily routine with Metamucil® Capsules, containing 100% natural psyllium fiber.** Look for these convenient capsules in two varieties, with and without calcium, in the fiber supplement aisle where you shop.
Rely on Metamucil for these important multiple health benefits:
- Helps lower cholesterol to promote heart health*
- Promotes digestive health†
- Low glycemic index*†
- Gluten free (less than 20 ppm gluten)*

Metamucil Psyllium Fiber Capsules
100% natural psyllium fiber to help reduce your risk of heart disease by lowering your cholesterol.*
Metamucil Psyllium Fiber Capsules Plus Calcium
100% natural psyllium fiber plus calcium to help strengthen bones and promote your digestive health.†
* Diets low in saturated fat and cholesterol that include 7 grams of soluble fiber per day from psyllium husk may reduce the risk of heart disease by lowering cholesterol. One adult dose of Metamucil has at least 2.1 grams of this soluble fiber. Use as directed. May contain trace amounts of gluten. If you have specific dietary needs, you should consult your doctor before consuming this product. This Metamucil product has a low glycemic index, a measure of the effect of dietary carbohydrates on blood sugar levels.
† THESE STATEMENTS HAVE NOT BEEN EVALUATED BY THE FOOD AND DRUG ADMINISTRATION. THIS PRODUCT IS NOT INTENDED TO DIAGNOSE, TREAT, CURE, OR PREVENT ANY DISEASE.
** Take Capsules with 8 oz of water.

MEXSANA MEDICATED (topical starch)

MSD Consumer Care, Inc.

DRUG FACTS

Active Ingredient(s)	Purpose(s)
Topical starch 83.7%	Skin protectant

USES
- temporarily protects and helps relieve minor skin irritation

WARNINGS
For external use only

DO NOT USE
- On broken skin

Keep out of reach of children. If swallowed, get medical help or contact a Poison Control Center right away.

WHEN USING THIS PRODUCT
- do not get into eyes
- keep away from face and mouth to avoid breathing it

STOP USE AND ASK A DOCTOR IF
- conditions worsens
- symptoms last more than 7 days or clear up and occur again within a few days

DIRECTIONS
- apply as needed

INACTIVE INGREDIENTS
benzethonium chloride, camphor, eucalyptus globulus leaf oil, fragrance, kaolin, lemon oil, zinc oxide

QUESTIONS OR COMMENTS?
1-866-360-3226

MICATIN (miconazole nitrate)

WellSpring Pharmaceutical Corporation

Active Ingredient(s)
Miconazole nitrate 2%

Purpose(s)
Antifungal

USES
- proven clinically effective in the treatment of most athlete's foot, jock itch and ringworm
- for effective relief of itching, scaling, burning and discomfort that can company these conditions

WARNINGS
For external use only

DO NOT USE
on children less than 2 years of age unless directed by a doctor

WHEN USING THIS PRODUCT
avoid contact with the eyes

STOP USE AND ASK A DOCTOR IF
- irritation occurs
- condition persists
- there is no improvement of athlete's foot or ringworm within 4 weeks or jock itch within 2 weeks

Keep out of reach of children.
If swallowed, get medical help or contact a Poison Control Center right away. (1-800-222-1222)

DIRECTIONS
- clean the affected area and dry thoroughly
- apply a thin layer of the product over affected area twice daily (morning and night) or as directed by a doctor
- supervise children in the use of this product
- for athlete's foot, pay special attention to the spaces between the toes; wear well-fitting, ventilated shoes, and change shoes and socks at least once daily
- for athlete's foot and ringworm, use daily for 4 weeks
- for jock itch, use daily for 2 weeks
- not effective on the scalp or nails

OTHER INFORMATION
- do not use if seal on tube is punctured or not visible
- to puncture the seal, reverse the cap and place the puncture-top onto the tube. Push down firmly until the seal is open. To close, screw the top back on the the tube.
- store at 20° to 25°C (68° to 77°F)
- see carton back panel and tube crimp for lot number and expiration date.

INACTIVE INGREDIENTS
benzoic acid, butylated hydroxyanisole, mineral oil, peglicol 5 oleate, pegoxol 7 stearate, purified water

QUESTIONS OR COMMENTS?
1-866-337-4500 info@wellspringpharm.com

DISTRIBUTED BY
WellSpring Pharmaceutical Corporation
Sarasota, FL 34243 USA
© WellSpring 2010
Made in Canada

MIDOL COMPLETE (acetaminophen, caffeine, and pyrilamine maleate)

Bayer HealthCare LLC

Active Ingredient(s) (in each caplet)
Acetaminophen 500 mg. Pain reliever
Caffeine 60 mg. Diuretic
Pyrilamine maleate 15 mg. Antihistamine

USES
for the temporary relief of these symptoms associated with menstrual periods:
- cramps
- bloating
- water-weight gain
- headache
- backache
- muscle aches
- fatigue

WARNINGS
Liver warning
This product contains acetaminophen. Severe liver damage may occur if you take
- more than 6 caplets in 24 hours, which is the maximum daily amount for this product
- with other drugs containing acetaminophen
- 3 or more alcoholic drinks every day while using this product

DO NOT USE
- with any other drug containing acetaminophen (prescription or nonprescription). If you are not sure whether a drug contains acetaminophen, ask a doctor or pharmacist.
- if you have ever had an allergic reaction to this product or any of its ingredients

ASK A DOCTOR BEFORE USE IF YOU HAVE
- liver disease
- glaucoma
- difficulty in urination due to enlargement of the prostate gland
- a breathing problem such as emphysema or chronic bronchitis

ASK A DOCTOR OR PHARMACIST BEFORE USE IF YOU ARE
- taking the blood thinning drug warfarin
- taking sedatives or tranquilizers

WHEN USING THIS PRODUCT
- you may get drowsy
- avoid alcoholic drinks
- excitability may occur, especially in children
- alcohol, sedatives, and tranquilizers may increase drowsiness
- be careful when driving a motor vehicle or operating machinery
- limit the use of caffeine-containing medications, foods, or beverages because too much caffeine may cause nervousness, irritability, sleeplessness, and, occasionally, rapid heartbeat. The recommended dose of this product contains about as much caffeine as a cup of coffee.

STOP USE AND ASK A DOCTOR IF
- new symptoms occur
- redness or swelling is present

- pain gets worse or lasts more than 10 days
- fever gets worse or lasts more than 3 days

If pregnant or breast-feeding, ask a health professional before use.

Keep out of reach of children. In case of overdose, get medical help or contact a Poison Control Center right away. Quick medical attention is critical for adults as well as for children even if you do not notice any signs or symptoms.

DIRECTIONS
- do not take more than the recommended dose
- adults and children 12 years and older:
  - take 2 caplets with water
  - repeat every 6 hours, as needed
  - do not exceed 6 caplets per day
- children under 12 years: consult a doctor.

OTHER INFORMATION
store at room temperature

INACTIVE INGREDIENTS
carnauba wax, croscarmellose sodium, FD&C blue #2 aluminum lake, hypromellose, magnesium stearate, microcrystalline cellulose, pregelatinized starch, propylene glycol, shellac, titanium dioxide, triacetin

QUESTIONS OR COMMENTS?
1-800-331-4536 (Mon - Fri 9AM - 5PM EST) or www.midol.com

MIDOL EXTENDED RELIEF (naproxen sodium)
Bayer HealthCare LLC, Consumer Care

DRUG FACTS

Active Ingredient(s) (in each caplet)
Naproxen sodium 220 mg (naproxen 200 mg) (NSAID)[1]
[1]nonsteroidal anti-inflammatory drug

Purpose(s)
Pain reliever/fever reducer

USES
temporarily relieves minor aches and pains due to:
- menstrual cramps
- muscle aches
- headache
- backache
- minor pain of arthritis
- toothache
- the common cold
- temporarily reduces fever

WARNINGS
Allergy alert
Naproxen sodium may cause a severe allergic reaction, especially in people allergic to aspirin. Symptoms may include:
- hives
- facial swelling
- asthma (wheezing)
- shock
- skin reddening
- rash
- blisters

If an allergic reaction occurs, stop use and seek medical help right away.

Stomach bleeding warning
This product contains an NSAID, which may cause severe stomach bleeding. The chance is higher if you:
- are age 60 or older
- have had stomach ulcers or bleeding problems
- take a blood thinning (anticoagulant) or steroid drug

- take other drugs containing prescription or nonprescription NSAIDs (aspirin, ibuprofen, naproxen, or others)
- have 3 or more alcoholic drinks every day while using this product
- take more or for a longer time than directed

DO NOT USE
- if you have ever had an allergic reaction to any other pain reliever/fever reducer
- right before or after heart surgery

ASK A DOCTOR BEFORE USE IF
- the stomach bleeding warning applies to you
- you have a history of stomach problems, such as heartburn
- you have high blood pressure, heart disease, liver cirrhosis, or kidney disease
- you are taking a diuretic
- you have problems or serious side effects from taking pain relievers or fever reducers
- you have asthma

ASK A DOCTOR OR PHARMACIST BEFORE USE IF YOU ARE
- under a doctor's care for any serious condition
- taking any other drug

WHEN USING THIS PRODUCT
- take with food or milk if stomach upset occurs
- the risk of heart attack or stroke may increase if you use more than directed or for longer than directed.

STOP USE AND ASK A DOCTOR IF
- you experience any of the following signs of stomach bleeding:
  - feel faint
  - vomit blood
  - have bloody or black stools
  - have stomach pain that does not get better
- pain gets worse or lasts more than 10 days
- fever gets worse or lasts more than 3 days
- you have difficulty swallowing
- it feels like the pill is stuck in your throat
- redness or swelling is present in the painful area
- any new symptoms appear

If pregnant or breast-feeding, ask a health professional before use. It is especially important not to use naproxen sodium during the last 3 months of pregnancy unless definitely directed to do so by a doctor because it may cause problems in the unborn child or complications during delivery.
Keep out of reach of children. In case of overdose, get medical help or contact a Poison Control Center right away.

DIRECTIONS
- **do not take more than directed**
- **the smallest effective dose should be used**
- drink a full glass of water with each dose

under 12 years	ask a doctor
adults and children 12 years and older	take 1 caplet every 8 to 12 hours while symptoms last. For the first dose you may take 2 caplets within the first hour. Do not exceed 2 caplets in any 8- to 12-hour period. Do not exceed 3 caplets in a 24-hour period.

OTHER INFORMATION
- **each caplet contains:** sodium 20 mg
- store at 20-25°C (68-77°F). Avoid high humidity and excessive heat above 40°C (104°F).

INACTIVE INGREDIENTS
FD&C blue #2 lake, hypromellose, magnesium stearate, microcrystalline cellulose, polyethylene glycol, povidone, talc, titanium dioxide

QUESTIONS OR COMMENTS?
1-800-331-4536
(Mon-Fri 9-5 EST) or www.midol.com

MIDOL (ibuprofen)

Bayer HealthCare LLC - Consumer Care

DRUG FACTS

Active Ingredient(s) (in each capsule)
Ibuprofen 200 mg (NSAID)[1]
[1]nonsteroidal anti-inflammatory drug

Purpose(s)
Pain reliever/fever reducer

USES
- temporarily relieves minor aches and pains due to:
  - menstrual cramps
  - headache
  - muscular aches
  - backache
  - minor pain of arthritis
  - toothache
  - the common cold
- temporarily reduces fever

WARNINGS
Allergy alert
Ibuprofen may cause a severe allergic reaction, especially in people allergic to aspirin. Symptoms may include:
- hives
- facial swelling
- asthma (wheezing)
- shock
- skin reddening
- rash
- blisters

If an allergic reaction occurs, stop use and seek medical help right away.

Stomach bleeding warning
This product contains an NSAID, which may cause severe stomach bleeding. The chance is higher if you:
- are age 60 or older
- have had stomach ulcers or bleeding problems
- take a blood thinning (anticoagulant) or steroid drug
- take other drugs containing prescription or nonprescription NSAIDs (aspirin, ibuprofen, naproxen, or others)
- have 3 or more alcoholic drinks every day while using this product
- take more or for a longer time than directed

DO NOT USE
- if you have ever had an allergic reaction to any other pain reliever/fever reducer
- right before or after heart surgery

ASK A DOCTOR BEFORE USE IF
- the stomach bleeding warning applies to you
- you have a history of stomach problems, such as heartburn
- you have high blood pressure, heart disease, liver cirrhosis, or kidney disease
- you are taking a diuretic
- you have problems or serious side effects from taking pain relievers or fever reducers
- you have asthma

ASK A DOCTOR OR PHARMACIST BEFORE USE IF YOU ARE
- under a doctor's care for any serious condition
- taking aspirin for heart attack or stroke, because ibuprofen may decrease this benefit of aspirin
- taking any other drug

WHEN USING THIS PRODUCT
- take with food or milk if stomach upset occurs
- the risk of heart attack or stroke may increase if you use more than directed or for longer than directed

STOP USE AND ASK A DOCTOR IF
- you experience any of the following signs of stomach bleeding:
  - feel faint
  - vomit blood
  - have bloody or black stools
  - have stomach pain that does not get better
- pain gets worse or lasts more than 10 days
- fever gets worse or lasts more than 3 days
- redness or swelling is present in the painful area
- any new symptoms appear

If pregnant or breast-feeding, ask a health professional before use. It is especially important not to use ibuprofen during the last 3 months of pregnancy unless definitely directed to do so by a doctor because it may cause problems in the unborn child or complications during delivery.
Keep out of reach of children. In case of overdose, get medical help or contact a Poison Control Center right away.

DIRECTIONS
- **do not take more than directed**
- **the smallest effective dose should be used**
- adults and children 12 years and over:
  - take 1 capsule every 4 to 6 hours while symptoms persist
  - if pain or fever does not respond to 1 capsule, 2 capsules may be used
  - do not exceed 6 capsules in 24 hours, unless directed by a doctor
- children under 12 years; consult a doctor

OTHER INFORMATION
- store at 20°-25°C (68°-77°F)
- avoid high humidity and excessive heat above 40°C (104°F)
- read all warnings and directions before use. Keep carton.

INACTIVE INGREDIENTS
FD&C Blue #1, gelatin, hypromellose, mannitol, polyethylene glycol, propylene glycol, povidone, purified water, sorbitan, sorbitol, titanium dioxide, vitamin E polyethylene glycol succinate.

QUESTIONS OR COMMENTS?
1-800-331-4536 or www.midol.com
Distributed by:
Bayer HealthCare LLC
Consumer Care
P.O. Box 1910
Morristown, NJ 07962-1910 USA

MIDOL PM (acetaminophen and diphenhydramine citrate)

Bayer HealthCare LLC

Active Ingredient(s) (in each caplet)
Acetaminophen 500 mg. Pain reliever
Diphenhydramine citrate 38 mg. Nighttime sleep-aid

USE
for relief of occasional sleeplessness when associated with minor aches and pains from premenstrual and menstrual periods (dysmenorrhea).

WARNINGS
Liver warning
This product contains acetaminophen. Severe liver damage may occur if you take
- more than 8 caplets in 24 hours, which is the maximum daily amount
- with other drugs containing acetaminophen
- 3 or more alcoholic drinks every day while using this product

DO NOT USE
- with any other drug containing acetaminophen (prescription or nonprescription). If you are not sure whether a drug contains acetaminophen, ask a doctor or pharmacist.
- in children under 12 years of age
- with any other product containing diphenhydramine, even one used on skin

ASK A DOCTOR BEFORE USE IF YOU HAVE
- liver disease
- a breathing problem such as emphysema or chronic bronchitis
- glaucoma
- trouble urinating due to an enlarged prostate gland

ASK A DOCTOR OR PHARMACIST BEFORE USE IF YOU ARE
- taking the blood thinning drug warfarin
- taking sedatives or tranquilizers

WHEN USING THIS PRODUCT
- drowsiness will occur
- avoid alcoholic drinks
- do not drive a motor vehicle or operate machinery

STOP USE AND ASK A DOCTOR IF
- sleeplessness persists continuously for more than 2 weeks. Insomnia may be a symptom of serious underlying medical illness.
- pain gets worse or lasts more than 10 days
- fever gets worse or lasts more than 3 days
- new symptoms occur
- redness or swelling is present

If pregnant or breast-feeding, ask a health professional before use.
Keep out of reach of children. In case of overdose, get medical help or contact a Poison Control Center right away. Quick medical attention is critical for adults as well as for children even if you do not notice any signs or symptoms.

DIRECTIONS
- do not take more than the recommended dose
- adults and children 12 years and older: take 2 caplets at bedtime if needed, or as directed by a doctor
- children under 12 years: do not use

OTHER INFORMATION
store at room temperature

INACTIVE INGREDIENTS
carnauba wax, corn starch, croscarmellose sodium, FD&C blue #1 aluminum lake, FD&C blue #2 aluminum lake, hypromellose, microcrystalline cellulose, povidone, propylene glycol, shellac, stearic acid, titanium dioxide

QUESTIONS OR COMMENTS?
1-800-331-4536 (Mon - Fri 9AM - 5PM EST) or www.midol.com

MIDOL TEEN FORMULA (acetaminophen and pamabrom)

Bayer HealthCare LLC

Active Ingredient(s) (in each caplet)
Acetaminophen 500 mg. Pain reliever
Pamabrom 25 mg. Diuretic

USES
for the temporary relief of these symptoms associated with menstrual periods:
- cramps
- bloating
- water-weight gain
- headache
- backache
- muscle aches

WARNINGS
Liver warning
This product contains acetaminophen. Severe liver damage may occur if you take
- more than 6 caplets in 24 hours, which is the maximum daily amount for this product
- with other drugs containing acetaminophen
- 3 or more alcoholic drinks every day while using this product

DO NOT USE
- with any other drug containing acetaminophen (prescription or nonprescription). If you are not sure whether a drug contains acetaminophen, ask a doctor or pharmacist.
- if you have ever had an allergic reaction to this product or any of its ingredients

ASK A DOCTOR BEFORE USE IF YOU HAVE
liver disease

ASK A DOCTOR OR PHARMACIST BEFORE USE IF YOU ARE
taking the blood thinning drug warfarin

STOP USE AND ASK A DOCTOR IF
- new symptoms occur
- redness or swelling is present
- pain gets worse or lasts more than 10 days
- fever gets worse or lasts more than 3 days

If pregnant or breast-feeding, ask a health professional before use.
Keep out of reach of children. In case of overdose, get medical help or contact a Poison Control Center right away. Quick medical attention is critical for adults as well as for children even if you do not notice any signs or symptoms.

DIRECTIONS
- do not take more than the recommended dose
- adults and children 12 years and older:
  - take 2 caplets with water
  - repeat every 6 hours, as needed
  - do not exceed 6 caplets per day
- children under 12 years: consult a doctor

OTHER INFORMATION
store at room temperature

INACTIVE INGREDIENTS
carnauba wax, croscarmellose sodium, D&C red #7 calcium lake, FD&C blue #2 aluminum lake, hypromellose, magnesium stearate, microcrystalline cellulose, pregelatinized starch, propylene glycol, shellac, titanium dioxide, triacetin

MIRACLE FOOT REPAIR CREAM (menthol)
Winning Solutions

Active Ingredient(s): MENTHOL 0.1%
Purpose(s): External Analgesic

WARNINGS
For external use only.
Keep out of reach of children: In case of accidental ingestion, get medical help or contact a Poison Control center right away.

DIRECTIONS
adults and children 2 years and older apply as needed under 2 years ask a doctor. wash and dry skin apply liberally over attached area and massage until absorbed.

USES
Temporary protects and helps relieve chapped or cracked skin

INACTIVE INGREDIENTS
aloe barabardensis leaf juice, water, mineral oil, glyceryl stearate, PEG-100 stearte, cetyl alcohol, cetearyl alcohol, polysorbate 60, propylene glycol, stearic acid, hydrogenated polyisobutene, dimethicone, triethanolamine, salicylic acid, imidazolidinyl urea, chondrus crispus (carrageenan), methylparaben, propylparaben, mentha piperita (peppermint oil), chloroxylenol, dmdm hydantoin

MIRALAX (polyethylene glycol 3350)
MSD Consumer Care, Inc.

DRUG FACTS

Active Ingredient(s) (in each dose) (Bottle Only)
Polyethylene Glycol 3350, 17 g (cap filled to line)

Purpose(s)
Osmotic Laxative

Active Ingredient(s) (in each dose) (Packet Only)
Polyethylene Glycol 3350, 17 g

Purpose(s)
Osmotic Laxative

USE
• relieves occasional constipation (irregularity)
• generally produces a bowel movement in 1 to 3 days

WARNINGS
Allergy alert
Do not use if you are allergic to polyethylene glycol

DO NOT USE
if you have kidney disease, except under the advice and supervision of a doctor

ASK A DOCTOR BEFORE USE IF YOU HAVE
• nausea, vomiting or abdominal pain
• a sudden change in bowel habits that lasts over 2 weeks
• irritable bowel syndrome

ASK A DOCTOR OF PHARMACIST BEFORE USE IF YOU ARE
taking a prescription drug

WHEN USING THIS PRODUCT
you may have loose, watery, more frequent stools

STOP USE AND ASK A DOCTOR IF
• you have rectal bleeding or you nausea, bloating or cramping or abdominal pain gets worse. These may be signs of a serious condition.
• you get diarrhea
• you need to use a laxative for longer than 1 week

If pregnant or breast-feeding, ask a health professional before use.
Keep out of the reach of children. In case of overdose, get medical help or contact a Poison Control Center right away.

DIRECTIONS (BOTTLE ONLY)
• **do not take more than directed unless advised by your doctor**
• the bottle top is a measuring cap marked to contain 17 grams of powder when filled to the indicated line (white section in cap)
• adults and children 17 years of age and older:
  • fill to top of white section in cap which is marked to indicate the correct dose (17 g)
  • stir and dissolve in any 4 to 8 ounces of beverage (cold, hot or room temperature) then drink
  • use once a day
  • use no more than 7 days
• children 16 years of age or under: ask a doctor

DIRECTIONS (PACKET ONLY)
• **do not take more than directed unless advised by your doctor**
• adults and children 17 years of age and older:
  • stir and dissolve one packet of powder (17 g) in any 4 to 8 ounces of beverage (cold, hot or room temperature) then drink
  • use once a day
  • use no more than 7 days
• children 16 years of age or under: ask a doctor

OTHER INFORMATION (BOTTLE ONLY)
• store at 20°-25°C (68°-77°F)
• tamper-evident: do not use if foil seal under cap, printed with "SEALED for YOUR PROTECTION" is missing, open or broken

OTHER INFORMATION (PACKET ONLY)
• store at 20°-25°C (68°-77°F)
• tamper-evident: do not use if foil is open or broken

INACTIVE INGREDIENTS
none

QUESTIONS OR COMMENTS?
1-800-MiraLAX (1-800-647-2529) or www.MiraLAX.com

INFANTS MOTRIN (ibuprofen)
McNeil Consumer Healthcare Div McNeil-PPC, Inc

DRUG FACTS

Active Ingredient(s) (in each 1.25 mL)
Ibuprofen 50 mg (NSAID)[1]
[1]nonsteroidal anti-inflammatory drug

Purpose(s)
Pain reliever/fever reducer

USES
temporarily:
- reduces fever
- relieves minor aches and pains due to the common cold, flu, sore throat, headaches and toothaches

WARNINGS
Allergy alert
Ibuprofen may cause a severe allergic reaction, especially in people allergic to aspirin.
Symptoms may include:
- hives
- facial swelling
- asthma (wheezing)
- shock
- skin reddening
- rash
- blisters

If an allergic reaction occurs, stop use and seek medical help right away.

Stomach bleeding warning
This product contains an NSAID, which may cause severe stomach bleeding. The chance is higher if your child:
- has had stomach ulcers or bleeding problems
- takes a blood thinning (anticoagulant) or steroid drug
- takes other drugs containing prescription or nonprescription NSAIDs (aspirin, ibuprofen, naproxen, or others)
- takes more or for a longer time than directed

Sore throat warning
Severe or persistent sore throat or sore throat accompanied by high fever, headache, nausea, and vomiting may be serious. Consult doctor promptly. Do not use more than 2 days or administer to children under 3 years of age unless directed by doctor.

DO NOT USE
- if the child has ever had an allergic reaction to any other pain reliever/fever reducer
- right before or after heart surgery

ASK A DOCTOR BEFORE USE IF
- stomach bleeding warning applies to your child
- child has a history of stomach problems, such as heartburn
- child has problems or serious side effects from taking pain relievers or fever reducers
- child has not been drinking fluids
- child has lost a lot of fluid due to vomiting or diarrhea
- child has high blood pressure, heart disease, liver cirrhosis, or kidney disease
- child has asthma
- child is taking a diuretic

ASK A DOCTOR OR PHARMACIST BEFORE USE IF THE CHILD IS
- under a doctor's care for any serious condition
- taking any other drug

WHEN USING THIS PRODUCT
- take with food or milk if stomach upset occurs
- the risk of heart attack or stroke may increase if you use more than directed or for longer than directed

STOP USE AND ASK A DOCTOR IF
- child experiences any of the following signs of stomach bleeding
  - feels faint
  - vomits blood
  - has bloody or black stools
  - has stomach pain that does not get better
- the child does not get any relief within first day (24 hours) of treatment
- fever or pain gets worse or lasts more than 3 days

- redness or swelling is present in the painful area
- any new symptoms appear

Keep out of reach of children. In case of overdose, get medical help or contact a Poison Control Center right away. (1-800-222-1222)

DIRECTIONS
- **this product does not contain directions or complete warnings for adult use**
- **do not give more than directed**
- shake well before using
- find right dose on chart below. If possible, use weight to dose; otherwise use age.
- measure with the dosing device provided. Do not use with any other device.
- dispense liquid slowly into the child's mouth, toward the inner cheek
- if needed, repeat dose every **6-8 hours**
- do not use more than **4 times a day**

Dosing Chart		
Weight (lb)	Age (mos)	Dose (mL)
under 6 mos	ask a doctor	
12-17 lbs	6-11 mos	1.25 mL
18-23 lbs	12-23 mos	1.875 mL

OTHER INFORMATION
- store between 20-25°C (68-77°F)
- **Tamper evident statement**
- see bottom panel for lot number and expiration date

INACTIVE INGREDIENTS
anhydrous citric acid, caramel, FD&C red no. 40, flavors, glycerin, polysorbate 80, pregelatinized starch, purified water, sodium benzoate, sorbitol solution, sucrose, xanthan gum

QUESTIONS OR COMMENTS?
Call **1-877-895-3665**: weekdays 8:00 AM to 8:00 PM EST

CHILDREN'S MOTRIN (ibuprofen)
McNeil Consumer Healthcare Div. McNeil-PPC, Inc

DRUG FACTS

Active Ingredient(s) (in each 5 mL = 1 teaspoon)
Ibuprofen 100 mg (NSAID)[1]

[1] nonsteroidal anti-inflammatory drug
Purpose(s)
Pain reliever/fever reducer

USES
temporarily:
- relieves minor aches and pains due to the common cold, flu, sore throat, headache and toothache
- reduces fever

WARNINGS
Allergy alert
Ibuprofen may cause a severe allergic reaction, especially in people allergic to aspirin. Symptoms may include:
- hives
- facial swelling
- asthma (wheezing)
- shock
- skin reddening
- rash
- blisters

If an allergic reaction occurs, stop use and seek medical help right away.

Stomach bleeding warning
This product contains an NSAID, which may cause severe stomach bleeding. The chance is higher if your child:
- has had stomach ulcers or bleeding problems
- takes a blood thinning (anticoagulant) or steroid drug
- takes other drugs containing an NSAID (aspirin, ibuprofen, naproxen, or others)
- takes more or for a longer time than directed

Sore throat warning
Severe or persistent sore throat or sore throat accompanied by high fever, headache, nausea, and vomiting may be serious. Consult doctor promptly. Do not use more than 2 days or administer to children under 3 years of age unless directed by doctor.

DO NOT USE
- if the child has ever had an allergic reaction to any other pain reliever/fever reducer
- right before or after heart surgery

ASK A DOCTOR BEFORE USE IF
- stomach bleeding warning applies to your child
- child has a history of stomach problems, such as heartburn
- child has problems or serious side effects from taking pain relievers or fever reducers
- child has not been drinking fluids
- child has lost a lot of fluid due to vomiting or diarrhea
- child has high blood pressure, heart disease, liver cirrhosis, or kidney disease
- child has asthma
- child is taking a diuretic

ASK A DOCTOR OR PHARMACIST BEFORE USE IF THE CHILD IS
- under a doctor's care for any serious condition
- taking any other drug

WHEN USING THIS PRODUCT
- take with food or milk if stomach upset occurs
- the risk of heart attack or stroke may increase if you use more than directed or for longer than directed

STOP USE AND ASK A DOCTOR IF
- child experiences any of the following signs of stomach bleeding:
  - feels faint
  - vomits blood
  - has bloody or black stools
  - has stomach pain that does not get better
- the child does not get any relief within first day (24 hours) of treatment
- fever or pain gets worse or lasts more than 3 days
- redness or swelling is present in the painful area
- any new symptoms appear

Keep out of reach of children. In case of overdose, get medical help or contact a Poison Control Center right away. (1-800-222-1222)

DIRECTIONS
- **this product does not contain directions or complete warnings for adult use**
- **do not give more than directed**
- shake well before using
- do not give longer than 10 days, unless directed by a doctor (see Warnings)
- find right dose on chart below (if possible, use weight to dose; otherwise use age)
- use only enclosed measuring cup
- if needed, repeat dose every **6-8 hours**
- do not use more than **4 times a day**
- replace original bottle cap to maintain child resistance

Dosing Chart		
Weight (lbs)	**Age (years)**	**Dose (tsp or mL)**
	under 2 years	ask a doctor
24-35 lbs	2-3 years	1 tsp or 5 mL
36-47 lbs	4-5 years	1½ tsp or 7.5 mL
48-59 lbs	6-8 years	2 tsp or 10 mL
60-71 lbs	9-10 years	2½ tsp or 12.5 mL
72-95 lbs	11 years	3 tsp or 15 mL

OTHER INFORMATION
- **each teaspoon contains:** sodium 2 mg
- store between 20-25°C (68-77°F)
- Tamper evident packaging
  - Carton: do not use if carton is opened or if carton tape imprinted "Safety Seal®" or bottle wrap imprinted "Safety Seal®" is broken or missing
  - Bottle: do not use if bottle wrap imprinted "Safety Seal®" and "USE WITH ENCLOSED DOSING DEVICE ONLY" is broken or missing

INACTIVE INGREDIENTS
Berry Flavor
acesulfame potassium, anhydrous citric acid, D&C yellow no.10, FD&C red no.40, flavors, glycerin, polysorbate 80, pregelatinized starch, purified water, sodium benzoate, sucrose, xanthan gum
Dye-Free Berry Flavor
acesulfame potassium, anhydrous citric acid, flavors, glycerin, polysorbate 80, pregelatinized starch, purified water, sodium benzoate, sucrose, xanthan gum

QUESTIONS OR COMMENTS?
Call **1-877-962-5357**

MOTRIN IB (ibuprofen)
McNeil Consumer Healthcare Div McNeil-PPC, Inc

DRUG FACTS

Active Ingredient(s) (in each caplet)
Ibuprofen 200 mg (NSAID)[1]
[1]nonsteroidal anti-inflammatory drug

Purpose(s)
Pain reliever/fever reducer

USES
- temporarily relieves minor aches and pains due to:
  - headache
  - muscular aches
  - minor pain of arthritis
  - toothache
  - backache
  - the common cold
  - menstrual cramps
- temporarily reduces fever

WARNINGS
Allergy alert
Ibuprofen may cause a severe allergic reaction, especially in people allergic to aspirin. Symptoms may include:
- hives
- facial swelling
- asthma (wheezing)
- shock
- skin reddening

- rash
- blisters

If an allergic reaction occurs, stop use and seek medical help right away.

Stomach bleeding warning
This product contains an NSAID, which may cause severe stomach bleeding. The chance is higher if you:
- are age 60 or older
- have had stomach ulcers or bleeding problems
- take a blood thinning (anticoagulant) or steroid drug
- take other drugs containing prescription or nonprescription NSAIDs (aspirin, ibuprofen, naproxen, or others)
- have 3 or more alcoholic drinks every day while using this product
- take more or for a longer time than directed

DO NOT USE
- if you have ever had an allergic reaction to any other pain reliever/fever reducer
- right before or after heart surgery

ASK A DOCTOR BEFORE USE IF
- you have problems or serious side effects from taking pain relievers or fever reducers
- the stomach bleeding warning applies to you
- you have a history of stomach problems, such as heartburn
- you have high blood pressure, heart disease, liver cirrhosis, or kidney disease
- you have asthma
- you are taking a diuretic

ASK A DOCTOR OR PHARMACIST BEFORE USE IF YOU ARE
- taking aspirin for heart attack or stroke, because ibuprofen may decrease this benefit of aspirin
- under a doctor's care for any serious condition
- taking any other drug

WHEN USING THIS PRODUCT
- take with food or milk if stomach upset occurs
- the risk of heart attack or stroke may increase if you use more than directed or for longer than directed

STOP USE AND ASK A DOCTOR IF
- you experience any of the following signs of stomach bleeding
  - feel faint
  - vomit blood
  - have bloody or black stools
  - have stomach pain that does not get better
- pain gets worse or lasts more than 10 days
- fever gets worse or lasts more than 3 days
- redness or swelling is present in the painful area
- any new symptoms appear

If pregnant or breast-feeding, ask a health professional before use. It is especially important not to use ibuprofen during the last 3 months of pregnancy unless definitely directed to do so by a doctor because it may cause problems in the unborn child or complications during delivery.
Keep out of reach of children. In case of overdose, get medical help or contact a Poison Control Center right away. (1-800-222-1222)

DIRECTIONS
- **do not take more than directed**
- **the smallest effective dose should be used**

adults and children 12 years and older	take 1 caplet every 4 to 6 hours while symptoms persist if pain or fever does not respond to 1 caplet, 2 caplets may be used do not exceed 6 caplets in 24 hours, unless directed by a doctor
children under 12 years	ask a doctor

OTHER INFORMATION
- store between 20-25°C (68-77°F)
- **do not use if neck wrap or foil inner seal imprinted "SAFETY SEAL®" is broken or missing**
- see end panel for lot number and expiration date

INACTIVE INGREDIENTS
carnauba wax, colloidal silicon dioxide, corn starch, FD&C yellow no. 6, hypromellose, iron oxide, magnesium stearate, polydextrose, polyethylene glycol, pregelatinized starch, propylene glycol, shellac, stearic acid, titanium dioxide

QUESTIONS OR COMMENTS?
Call **1-877-962-5357:** weekdays 8:00 AM to 8:00 PM EST

MOTRIN PM (ibuprofen and diphenhydramine citrate)
McNeil Consumer Healthcare Div McNeil-PPC, Inc

DRUG FACTS

Active Ingredient(s) (in each caplet)	Purpose(s)
Diphenhydramine citrate 38 mg	Nighttime sleep-aid
Ibuprofen 200 mg (NSAID)*	Pain reliever
*nonsteroidal anti-inflammatory drug	

USES
- for relief of occasional sleeplessness when associated with minor aches and pains
- helps you fall asleep and stay asleep

WARNINGS
Allergy alert
Ibuprofen may cause a severe allergic reaction, especially in people allergic to aspirin. Symptoms may include:
- hives
- facial swelling
- asthma (wheezing)
- shock
- skin reddening
- rash
- blisters

If an allergic reaction occurs, stop use and seek medical help right away.

Stomach bleeding warning
This product contains an NSAID, which may cause severe stomach bleeding. The chance is higher if you:
- are age 60 or older
- have had stomach ulcers or bleeding problems
- take a blood thinning (anticoagulant) or steroid drug
- take other drugs containing prescription or nonprescription NSAIDs (aspirin, ibuprofen, naproxen, or others)
- have 3 or more alcoholic drinks every day while using this product
- take more or for a longer time than directed

DO NOT USE
- if you have ever had an allergic reaction to any other pain reliever/fever reducer
- unless you have time for a full night's sleep
- in children under 12 years of age
- right before or after heart surgery
- with any other product containing diphenhydramine, even one used on skin
- if you have sleeplessness without pain

ASK A DOCTOR BEFORE USE IF
- the stomach bleeding warning applies to you
- you have a history of stomach problems, such as heartburn
- you have high blood pressure, heart disease, liver cirrhosis, or kidney disease
- you are taking a diuretic
- you have a breathing problem such as emphysema or chronic bronchitis
- you have asthma
- you have glaucoma
- you have trouble urinating due to an enlarged prostate gland

ASK A DOCTOR OR PHARMACIST BEFORE USE IF YOU ARE
- taking sedatives or tranquilizers, or any other sleep-aid
- under a doctor's care for any continuing medical illness
- taking any other antihistamines
- taking aspirin for heart attack or stroke, because ibuprofen may decrease this benefit of aspirin
- taking any other drug

WHEN USING THIS PRODUCT
- drowsiness will occur
- avoid alcoholic drinks
- do not drive a motor vehicle or operate machinery
- take with food or milk if stomach upset occurs
- the risk of heart attack or stroke may increase if you use more than directed or for longer than directed

STOP USE AND ASK A DOCTOR IF
- you experience any of the following signs of stomach bleeding:
  - feel faint
  - vomit blood
  - have bloody or black stools
  - have stomach pain that does not get better
- sleeplessness persists continuously for more than 2 weeks. Insomnia may be a symptom of a serious underlying medical illness.
- redness or swelling is present in the painful area
- any new symptoms appear

If pregnant or breast-feeding, ask a health professional before use. It is especially important not to use ibuprofen during the last 3 months of pregnancy unless definitely directed to do so by a doctor because it may cause problems in the unborn child or complications during delivery.

Keep out of reach of children. In case of overdose, get medical help or contact a Poison Control Center right away. (1-800-222-1222)

DIRECTIONS
- **do not take more than directed**
- **do not take longer than 10 days, unless directed by a doctor (see Warnings)**
- adults and children 12 years and over: take 2 caplets at bedtime
- do not take more than 2 caplets in 24 hours

OTHER INFORMATION
- read all warnings and directions before use. Keep carton.
- store at 20°-25°C (68°-77°F)
- avoid excessive heat above 40°C (104°F)

INACTIVE INGREDIENTS
colloidal silicon dioxide, croscarmellose sodium, glyceryl behenate, hydroxypropyl cellulose, lactose monohydrate, magnesium stearate, microcrystalline cellulose, polyethylene glycol, polyvinyl alcohol, pregelatinized starch, talc, titanium dioxide

QUESTIONS OR COMMENTS?
1-800-962-5357

CHILDREN'S MUCINEX CHEST CONGESTION GRAPE (guaifenesin)

Reckitt Benckiser LLC

DRUG FACTS

Active Ingredient(s) (in each 5 mL)	Purpose(s)
Guaifenesin 100 mg	Expectorant

USES
- helps loosen phlegm (mucus) and thin bronchial secretions to rid the bronchial passageways of bothersome mucus and make coughs more productive

ASK A DOCTOR BEFORE USE IF THE CHILD HAS
- cough that occurs with too much phlegm (mucus)
- persistent or chronic cough such as occurs with asthma

STOP USE AND ASK A DOCTOR IF
- cough lasts more than 7 days, comes back, or occurs with fever, rash, or persistent headache. These could be signs of a serious illness.

Keep out of reach of children. In case of overdose, get medical help or contact a Poison Control Center right away.

DIRECTIONS
- do not take more than 6 doses in any 24-hour period

Age	Dose
children 6 years to under 12 years	1-2 teaspoonfuls every 4 hours
children 4 years to under 6 years	½-1 teaspoonful every 4 hours
children under 4 years	do not use

OTHER INFORMATION
- each 5 mL contains: **sodium 3 mg**
- tamper evident: do not use if seal under bottle cap printed "SEALED for YOUR PROTECTION" is torn or missing.
- store between 20-25°C (68-77°F)
- do not refrigerate
- dosing cup provided

INACTIVE INGREDIENTS
citric acid anhydrous, dextrose, FD&C blue #1, FD&C red #40, flavor, glycerin, methylparaben, potassium sorbate, propylene glycol, propylparaben, purified water, saccharin sodium, sodium hydroxide, sucralose, xanthan gum

CHILDREN'S MUCINEX CHEST CONGESTION CHERRY (dextromethorphan and guaifenesin)

Reckitt Benckiser LLC

DRUG FACTS

Active Ingredient(s) (in each 5 mL tsp)	Purpose(s)
Dextromethorphan HBr 5 mg	Cough suppressant
Guaifenesin 100 mg	Expectorant

USES
- helps loosen phlegm (mucus) and thin bronchial secretions to rid the bronchial passageways of bothersome mucus and make coughs more productive
- temporarily relieves:
  - cough due to minor throat and bronchial irritation as may occur with the common cold or inhaled irritants
  - the intensity of coughing
  - the impulse to cough to help your child get to sleep

DO NOT USE
- in a child who is taking a prescription monoamine oxidase inhibitor (MAOI) (certain drugs for depression, psychiatric, or emotional conditions, or Parkinson's disease), or for 2 weeks after stopping the MAOI drug. If you do not know if your child's prescription drug contains an MAOI, ask a doctor or pharmacist before giving this product.

ASK A DOCTOR BEFORE USE IF THE CHILD HAS
- cough that occurs with too much phlegm (mucus)
- persistent or chronic cough such as occurs with asthma

STOP USE AND ASK A DOCTOR IF
- cough lasts more than 7 days, comes back, or occurs with fever, rash, or persistent headache. These could be signs of a serious illness.

Keep out of reach of children. In case of overdose, get medical help or contact a Poison Control Center right away.

DIRECTIONS
- do not take more than 6 doses in any 24-hour period

Age	Dose
children 6 years to under 12 years	1-2 teaspoonfuls every 4 hours
children 4 years to under 6 years	½-1 teaspoonful every 4 hours
children under 4 years	do not use

OTHER INFORMATION
- each 5 mL teaspoonful contains: **sodium 3 mg**
- tamper evident: do not use if seal under bottle cap printed "SEALED for YOUR PROTECTION" is torn or missing
- store between 20-25°C (68-77°F)
- do not refrigerate
- dosing cup provided

INACTIVE INGREDIENTS
citric acid anhydrous, dextrose, D&C red #33, FD&C red #40, flavors, glycerin, methylparaben, potassium sorbate, propylene glycol, propylparaben, purified water, saccharin sodium, sodium hydroxide, sucralose, xanthan gum

CHILDREN'S MUCINEX MULTI-SYMPTOM COLD & FEVER LIQUID (BERRY BLAST FLAVOR) (dextromethorphan, guaifenesin, and phenylephrine)

Reckitt Benckiser LLC

DRUG FACTS

Active Ingredient(s) (in each 10 mL)	Purpose(s)
Dextromethorphan HBr 10 mg	Cough suppressant
Guaifenesin 200 mg	Expectorant
Phenylephrine HCl 5 mg	Nasal decongestant

USES
- temporarily relieves these common cold and flu symptoms:
  - nasal congestion
  - stuffy nose
  - cough due to minor throat and bronchial irritation
  - the intensity of coughing
  - the impulse to cough to help your child get to sleep
  - minor aches and pains
  - sore throat
  - headache
- temporarily reduces fever
- helps loosen phlegm (mucus) and thin bronchial secretions to rid the bronchial passageways of bothersome mucus and make coughs more productive

WARNINGS
Liver warning: This product contains acetaminophen. Severe liver damage may occur if your child takes
- more than 5 doses in 24 hours, which is the maximum daily amount
- with other drugs containing acetaminophen

Sore throat warning: If sore throat is severe, persists for more than 2 days, is accompanied or followed by fever, headache, rash, nausea or vomiting, consult a doctor promptly.

DO NOT USE
- **with any other drug containing acetaminophen** (prescription or nonprescription). If you are not sure whether a drug contains acetaminophen, ask a doctor or pharmacist.
- in a child who is taking a prescription monoamine oxidase inhibitor (MAOI) (certain drugs for depression, psychiatric, or emotional conditions, or Parkinson's disease), or for 2 weeks after stopping the MAOI drug. If you do not know if your child's prescription drug contains an MAOI, ask a doctor or pharmacist before giving this product.

ASK A DOCTOR BEFORE USE IF YOUR CHILD HAS
- liver disease
- heart disease
- high blood pressure
- thyroid disease
- diabetes
- a breathing problem such as chronic bronchitis
- persistent or chronic cough such as occurs with asthma
- cough that occurs with too much phlegm (mucus)

ASK A DOCTOR OR PHARMACIST BEFORE USE IF
- your child is taking the blood thinning drug warfarin

WHEN USING THIS PRODUCT
- do not use more than directed (see Overdose warning)

STOP USE AND ASK A DOCTOR IF
- nervousness, dizziness or sleeplessness occur
- pain, nasal congestion or cough gets worse or lasts more than 5 days
- fever gets worse or lasts more than 3 days
- redness or swelling is present
- new symptoms occur
- cough comes back, or occurs with rash or headache that lasts. These could be signs of a serious condition.

Keep out of reach of children.

OVERDOSE WARNING
Taking more than the recommended dose (overdose) may cause liver damage. In case of overdose, get medical help or contact a Poison Control Center right away. Quick medical attention is critical even if you do not notice any signs or symptoms.

DIRECTIONS
- **this product does not contain directions or complete warnings for adult use**
- **do not give more than directed (see Overdose warning)**
- do not give more than 5 doses in any 24-hour period
- if needed, repeat dose every 4 hours while symptoms last
- do not give more than 5 days unless directed by a doctor
- **shake well before using**
- measure only with dosing cup provided
- do not use dosing cup with other products
- dose as follows or as directed by a doctor
- mL = milliliter
- **Children 6 to under 12 years of age:**   10 mL in dosing cup provided
- **Children under 6 years of age:** do not use

OTHER INFORMATION
- each 10 mL contains: **sodium 6 mg**
- tamper evident: do not use if neckband on bottle cap is broken or missing.
- store between 15-30°C (59-86°F)
- do not refrigerate
- dosing cup provided

INACTIVE INGREDIENTS
anhydrous citric acid, edetate disodium, FD&C Blue #1, FD&C Red #40, flavors, glycerin, propylene glycol, propyl gallate, purified water, sodium benzoate, sorbitol, sucralose, trisodium citrate dihydrate,* xanthan gum *may contain this ingredient

QUESTIONS OR COMMENTS?
1-866-MUCINEX (1-866-682-4639)
You may also report side effects to this phone number.

CHILDRENS MUCINEX MULTI-SYMPTOM COLD (dextromethorphan hydrobromide, guaifenesin, and phenylephrine hydrochloride)

Reckitt Benckiser LLC

DRUG FACTS

Active Ingredient(s) (in each 5 mL)	Purpose(s)
Dextromethorphan HBr 5 mg	Cough suppressant
Guaifenesin 100 mg	Expectorant
Phenylephrine HCl 2.5 mg	Nasal decongestant

USES
- helps loosen phlegm (mucus) and thin bronchial secretions to rid the bronchial passageways of bothersome mucus and make coughs more productive

- temporarily relieves:
  - cough due to minor throat and bronchial irritation as may occur with the common cold or inhaled irritants
  - the intensity of coughing
  - the impulse to cough to help your child get to sleep
  - nasal congestion due to a cold
  - stuffy nose

WARNINGS

DO NOT USE
in a child who is taking a prescription monoamine oxidase inhibitor (MAOI) (certain drugs for depression, psychiatric, or emotional conditions, or Parkinson's disease), or for 2 weeks after stopping the MAOI drug. If you do not know if your child's prescription drug contains an MAOI, ask a doctor or pharmacist before giving this product.

ASK A DOCTOR BEFORE USE IF THE CHILD HAS
- heart disease
- high blood pressure
- thyroid disease
- diabetes
- cough that occurs with too much phlegm (mucus)
- persistent or chronic cough such as occurs with asthma

WHEN USING THIS PRODUCT
- **do not use more than directed**

STOP USE AND ASK A DOCTOR IF
- your child gets nervous, dizzy or sleepless
- symptoms do not get better within 7 days or occur with fever
- cough lasts more than 7 days, comes back, or occurs with fever, rash, or persistent headache. These could be signs of a serious illness.

Keep out of reach of children
In case of overdose, get medical help or contact a Poison Control Center right away.

DIRECTIONS
- do not take more than 6 doses in any 24-hour period
- measure only with dosing cup provided
- do not use dosing cup with other products
- dose as follows or as directed by a doctor
- mL = milliliter

Age	Dose
children 6 years to under 12 years	10 mL every 4 hours
children 4 years to under 6 years	5 mL every 4 hours
children under 4 years	do not use

OTHER INFORMATION
- each 5 mL contains: **sodium 3 mg**
- tamper evident: do not use if neckband on bottle cap is broken or missing
- store between 20-25°C (68-77°F)
- do not refrigerate
- dosing cup provided

INACTIVE INGREDIENTS
anhydrous citric acid, D&C red #33, dextrose, FD&C blue #1, FD&C red #40, flavors, glycerin, methylparaben, potassium sorbate, propyl gallate, propylene glycol, propylparaben, purified water, saccharin sodium, sodium hydroxide, sorbitol, sucralose, xanthan gum

QUESTIONS OR COMMENTS?
1-866-MUCINEX (1-866-682-4639)
You may also report side effects to this phone number.

MUCINEX COLD LIQUID (MIXED BERRY FLAVOR) (guaifenesin and phenylephrine HCl)
Reckitt Benckiser LLC

DRUG FACTS

Active Ingredient(s) (in each 5 mL tsp)	Purpose(s)
Guaifenesin 100 mg	Expectorant
Phenylephrine HCl 2.5 mg	Nasal decongestant

USES
- helps loosen phlegm (mucus) and thin bronchial secretions to rid the bronchial passageways of bothersome mucus and make coughs more productive
- temporarily relieves:
  - nasal congestion due to a cold
  - stuffy nose

DO NOT USE
- in a child who is taking a prescription monoamine oxidase inhibitor (MAOI) (certain drugs for depression, psychiatric, or emotional conditions, or Parkinson's disease), or for 2 weeks after stopping the MAOI drug. If you do not know if your child's prescription drug contains an MAOI, ask a doctor or pharmacist before giving this product.

ASK A DOCTOR BEFORE USE IF THE CHILD HAS
- heart disease
- high blood pressure
- thyroid disease
- diabetes
- cough that occurs with too much phlegm (mucus)
- persistent or chronic cough such as occurs with asthma

WHEN USING THIS PRODUCT
- **do not use more than directed**

STOP USE AND ASK A DOCTOR IF
- you get nervous, dizzy or sleepless
- symptoms do not get better within 7 days or occur with fever
- cough lasts more than 7 days, comes back, or occurs with fever, rash, or persistent headache. These could be signs of a serious illness.

Keep out of reach of children. In case of overdose, get medical help or contact a Poison Control Center right away.

DIRECTIONS
- do not take more than 6 doses in any 24-hour period

Age	Dose
children 6 years to under 12 years	2 teaspoonfuls every 4 hours
children 4 years to under 6 years	1 teaspoonful every 4 hours
children under 4 years	do not use

OTHER INFORMATION
- each 5 mL teaspoonful contains: **sodium 3 mg**
- tamper evident: do not use if seal under bottle cap printed "SEALED for YOUR PROTECTION" is torn or missing.
- store between 20-25°C (68-77°F)
- do not refrigerate
- dosage cup provided

INACTIVE INGREDIENTS
citric acid anhydrous, dextrose, D&C red #33, FD&C blue #1, FD&C red #40, flavors, glycerin, methylparaben, potassium sorbate, propyl gallate, propylene glycol, propylparaben, purified water, saccharin sodium, sodium hydroxide, sorbitol solution, sucralose, xanthan gum

MUCINEX COUGH MINI-MELTS (ORANGE CREME FLAVOR) (dextromethorphan HBr and guaifenesin)
Reckitt Benckiser LLC

DRUGS FACTS

Active Ingredient(s) (in each packet)	Purpose(s)
Dextromethorphan HBr 5 mg	Cough suppressant
Guaifenesin 100 mg	Expectorant

USES
- helps loosen phlegm (mucus) and thin bronchial secretions to rid the bronchial passageways of bothersome mucus and make coughs more productive
- temporarily relieves:
  - cough due to minor throat and bronchial irritation as may occur with the common cold or inhaled irritants
  - the intensity of coughing
  - the impulse to cough to help you get to sleep

WARNINGS
Do not use if you are now taking a prescription monoamine oxidase inhibitor (MAOI) (certain drugs for depression, psychiatric, or emotional conditions, or Parkinson's disease), or for 2 weeks after stopping the MAOI drug. If you do not know if your prescription drug contains an MAOI, ask a doctor or pharmacist before taking this product.

ASK A DOCTOR BEFORE USE IF YOU HAVE
- persistent or chronic cough such as occurs with smoking, asthma, chronic bronchitis, or emphysema
- cough that occurs with too much phlegm (mucus)

STOP USE AND ASK A DOCTOR IF
- cough lasts more than 7 days, comes back, or occurs with fever, rash, or persistent headache. These could be signs of a serious illness.

If pregnant or breast-feeding, ask a healthcare professional before use.
Keep out of reach of children. In case of overdose, get medical help or contact a Poison Control Center right away.

DIRECTIONS
- empty entire contents of packet onto tongue and swallow
- for best taste, do not chew granules
- do not take more than 6 doses in any 24-hour period

adults and children 12 years and over	2 to 4 packets every 4 hours
children 6 years to under 12 years	1 to 2 packets every 4 hours
children 4 years to under 6 years	1 packet every 4 hours
children under 4 years	do not use

OTHER INFORMATION
- **each packet contains:** magnesium 6 mg and sodium 3 mg
- **phenylketonurics:** contains phenylalanine 2 mg per packet
- store between 15-25°C (59-77°F)
- tamper evident: do not use if carton is open or if packets are torn or open

INACTIVE INGREDIENTS
aspartame, butylated methacrylate copolymer, carbomer homopolymer, creme flavor, magnesium stearate, microcrystalline cellulose, orange flavor, povidone, sodium bicarbonate, sodium carboxymethylcellulose, sorbitol, stearic acid, talc, triethyl citrate

MUCINEX FOR KIDS (guaifenesin)

Reckitt Benckiser, Inc.

DRUG FACTS

Active Ingredient(s) (in each packet)
Guaifenesin, USP 50 mg

Purpose(s)
Expectorant

USES
helps loosen phlegm (mucus) and thin bronchial secretions to rid the bronchial passageways of bothersome mucus and make coughs more productive

WARNINGS

ASK A DOCTOR BEFORE USE IF THE CHILD HAS
- persistent or chronic cough such as occurs with asthma or chronic bronchitis
- cough that occurs with too much phlegm (mucus)

STOP USE AND ASK A DOCTOR IF
cough lasts more than 7 days, comes back, or occurs with fever, rash, or persistent headache. These could be signs of a serious illness.
Keep out of reach of children. In case of overdose, get medical help or contact a Poison Control Center right away.

DIRECTIONS
- empty entire contents of packet onto tongue and swallow
- for best taste, do not chew granules
- do not take more than 6 doses in any 24-hour period

Age	Dose
children 6 years to under 12 years	2 to 4 packets every 4 hours
children 4 years to under 6 years	1 to 2 packets every 4 hours
children under 4 years	do not use

OTHER INFORMATION
- **each packet contains:** magnesium 6 mg and sodium 2 mg
- **phenylketonurics:** contains phenylalanine 0.6 mg per packet
- store between 15-25°C (59-77°F)
- tamper evident: do not use if carton is open or if packets are torn or open

INACTIVE INGREDIENTS
aspartame, butylated methacrylate copolymer, carbomer, carboxymethylcellulose sodium, grape flavor, magnesium stearate, microcrystalline cellulose, povidone, raspberry flavor, sodium bicarbonate, sorbitol, stearic acid, talc, triethyl citrate

QUESTIONS OR COMMENTS?
1-866-MUCINEX (1-866-682-4639) or www.mucinex.com
Made in Germany
Distributed by:
Reckitt Benckiser Inc.
Parsippany, NJ
07054-0224
© RBI 2009

MUCINEX D (guaifenesin and pseudoephedrine hydrochloride)

Reckitt Benckiser LLC

DRUG FACTS

Active Ingredient(s) (in each extended-release bi-layer tablet)	Purpose(s)
Guaifenesin 600 mg	Expectorant
Pseudoephedrine HCl 60 mg	Nasal Decongestant

USES
- helps loosen phlegm (mucus) and thin bronchial secretions to rid the bronchial passageways of bothersome mucus and make coughs more productive
- temporarily relieves nasal congestion due to:
  - common cold
  - hay fever
  - upper respiratory allergies
- temporarily restores freer breathing through the nose
- promotes nasal and/or sinus drainage
- temporarily relieves sinus congestion and pressure

WARNINGS

DO NOT USE
if you are now taking a prescription monoamine oxidase inhibitor (MAOI) (certain drugs for depression, psychiatric or emotional conditions, or Parkinson's disease), or for 2 weeks after stopping the MAOI drug. If you do not know if your prescription drug contains an MAOI, ask a doctor or pharmacist before taking this product.

ASK A DOCTOR BEFORE USE IF YOU HAVE
- heart disease
- high blood pressure
- thyroid disease
- diabetes
- trouble urinating due to an enlarged prostate gland
- persistent or chronic cough such as occurs with smoking, asthma, chronic bronchitis, or emphysema
- cough accompanied by too much phlegm (mucus)

WHEN USING THIS PRODUCT
- **do not use more than directed**

STOP USE AND ASK A DOCTOR IF
- you get nervous, dizzy, or sleepless
- symptoms do not get better within 7 days, come back or occur with a fever, rash, or persistent headache. These could be signs of a serious illness.

If pregnant or breast-feeding, ask a health professional before use.
Keep out of reach of children. In case of overdose, get medical help or contact a Poison Control Center right away.

DIRECTIONS
- do not crush, chew, or break tablet
- take with a full glass of water
- this product can be administered without regard for timing of meals
- adults and children 12 years and older: 2 tablets every 12 hours; not more than 4 tablets in 24 hours
- children under 12 years of age: do not use

OTHER INFORMATION
- tamper evident: do not use if carton is open or if printed seal on blister is broken or missing
- store at 20-25°C (68-77°F)

INACTIVE INGREDIENTS
carbomer homopolymer type B; FD&C yellow #6 aluminum lake; hypromellose, USP; magnesium stearate, NF; microcrystalline cellulose, NF; sodium starch glycolate, NF

QUESTIONS OR COMMENTS?
1-866-MUCINEX (1-866-682-4639) You may also report side effects to this phone number.
Distributed by:
Reckitt Benckiser
Parsippany, NJ 07054-0224
© 2012 RB

MUCINEX DM (guaifenesin and dextromethorphan hydrobromide)

Reckitt Benckiser LLC

600 mg guaifenesin & 30 mg dextromethorphan HBr extended-release bi-layer tablets
EXPECTORANT & COUGH SUPPRESSANT

DRUG FACTS

Active Ingredient(s) (in each extended-release bi-layer tablet)	Purpose(s)
Dextromethorphan HBr 30 mg	Cough suppressant
Guaifenesin 600 mg	Expectorant

USES
- helps loosen phlegm (mucus) and thin bronchial secretions to rid the bronchial passageways of bothersome mucus and make coughs more productive
- temporarily relieves:
  - cough due to minor throat and bronchial irritation as may occur with the common cold or inhaled irritants
  - the intensity of coughing
  - the impulse to cough to help you get to sleep

WARNINGS

DO NOT USE
- for children under 12 years of age
- if you are now taking a prescription monoamine oxidase inhibitor (MAOI) (certain drugs for depression, psychiatric or emotional conditions, or Parkinson's disease), or for 2 weeks after stopping the MAOI drug. If you do not know if your prescription drug contains an MAOI, ask a doctor or pharmacist before taking this product.

ASK A DOCTOR BEFORE USE IF YOU HAVE
- persistent or chronic cough such as occurs with smoking, asthma, chronic bronchitis, or emphysema
- cough accompanied by too much phlegm (mucus)

WHEN USING THIS PRODUCT
- do not use more than directed

STOP USE AND ASK A DOCTOR IF
- cough lasts more than 7 days, comes back, or occurs with fever, rash, or persistent headache. These could be signs of a serious illness.

If pregnant or breast-feeding, ask a health professional before use.
Keep out of reach of children. In case of overdose, get medical help or contact a Poison Control Center right away.

DIRECTIONS
- do not crush, chew, or break tablet
- take with a full glass of water
- this product can be administered without regard for timing of meals
- adults and children 12 years and older: 1 or 2 tablets every 12 hours; not more than 4 tablets in 24 hours
- children under 12 years of age: do not use

OTHER INFORMATION
- tamper evident: do not use if carton is open or if printed seal on blister is broken or missing
- store at 20-25°C (68-77°F)

INACTIVE INGREDIENTS
carbomer homopolymer type B; D&C yellow #10 aluminum lake; hypromellose, USP; magnesium stearate, NF; microcrystalline cellulose, NF; sodium starch glycolate, NF

QUESTIONS OR COMMENTS?
1-866-MUCINEX (1-866-682-4639) You may also report side effects to this phone number.
Distributed by:
Reckitt Benckiser
Parsippany, NJ 07054-0224
©2012 RB

MUCINEX EXPECTORANT (guaifenesin)

Reckitt-Benckiser LLC

DRUG FACTS

Active Ingredient(s) (in each extended-release bi-layer tablet)	Purpose(s)
Guaifenesin 600 mg	Expectorant

USES
helps loosen phlegm (mucus) and thin bronchial secretions to rid the bronchial passageways of bothersome mucus and make coughs more productive

WARNINGS

DO NOT USE
- for children under 12 years of age

ASK A DOCTOR BEFORE USE IF YOU HAVE
- persistent or chronic cough such as occurs with smoking, asthma, chronic bronchitis, or emphysema
- cough accompanied by too much phlegm (mucus)

STOP USE AND ASK A DOCTOR IF
- cough lasts more than 7 days, comes back, or occurs with fever, rash, or persistent headache. These could be signs of a serious illness.

If pregnant or breast-feeding, ask a health professional before use.

Keep out of reach of children. In case of overdose, get medical help or contact a Poison Control Center right away.

DIRECTIONS
- do not crush, chew, or break tablet
- take with a full glass of water
- this product can be administered without regard for the timing of meals
- adults and children 12 years of age and over: 1 or 2 tablets every 12 hours. Do not exceed 4 tablets in 24 hours.
- children under 12 years of age: do not use

OTHER INFORMATION
- tamper evident: do not use if carton is open or if seal on bottle printed "SEALED for YOUR PROTECTION" is broken or missing
- store between 20-25°C (68-77°F)

INACTIVE INGREDIENTS
carbomer 934P, NF; FD&C blue #1 aluminum lake; hypromellose, USP; magnesium stearate, NF; microcrystalline cellulose, NF; sodium starch glycolate, NF

MUCINEX FAST-MAX COLD, FLU AND SORE THROAT (acetaminophen, dextromethorphan hydrobromide, guaifenesin, and phenylephrine hydrochloride)

Reckitt Benckiser LLC

DRUG FACTS

Active Ingredient(s) (in each 20 mL)	Purpose(s)
Acetaminophen 650 mg	Pain reliever/fever reducer
Dextromethorphan HBr 20 mg	Cough suppressant
Guaifenesin 400 mg	Expectorant
Phenylephrine HCl 10 mg	Nasal decongestant

USES
- temporarily relieves these common cold and flu symptoms:
  - nasal congestion
  - sinus congestion and pressure
  - cough due to minor throat and bronchial irritation
  - minor aches and pains
  - sore throat
  - headache
- temporarily reduces fever
- temporarily promotes nasal and/or sinus drainage
- helps loosen phlegm (mucus) and thin bronchial secretions to rid the bronchial passageways of bothersome mucus and make coughs more productive

WARNINGS
Liver warning
This product contains acetaminophen. Severe liver damage may occur if you take:
- more than 6 doses in 24 hours, which is the maximum daily amount
- with other drugs containing acetaminophen
- 3 or more alcoholic drinks daily while using this product

Sore throat warning
if sore throat is severe, persists for more than 2 days, is accompanied or followed by fever, headache, rash, nausea or vomiting, consult a doctor promptly.

DO NOT USE
- **with any other drug containing acetaminophen** (prescription or nonprescription). If you are not sure whether a drug contains acetaminophen, ask a doctor or pharmacist.
- for children under 12 years of age
- if you are now taking a prescription monoamine oxidase inhibitor (MAOI) (certain drugs for depression, psychiatric, or emotional conditions, or Parkinson's disease), or for 2 weeks after stopping the MAOI drug. If you do not know if your prescription drug contains an MAOI, ask a doctor or pharmacist before taking this product.

ASK A DOCTOR BEFORE USE IF YOU HAVE
- liver disease
- heart disease
- high blood pressure
- thyroid disease
- diabetes
- trouble urinating due to an enlarged prostate gland
- persistent or chronic cough such as occurs with smoking, asthma, chronic bronchitis or emphysema
- cough that occurs with too much phlegm (mucus)

ASK A DOCTOR OR PHARMACIST BEFORE USE IF
- you are taking the blood thinning drug warfarin

WHEN USING THIS PRODUCT
- do not use more than directed

STOP USE AND ASK A DOCTOR IF
- nervousness, dizziness or sleeplessness occur
- pain, nasal congestion or cough gets worse or lasts more than 7 days
- fever gets worse or lasts more than 3 days
- redness or swelling is present
- new symptoms occur
- cough comes back, or occurs with rash or persistent headache. These could be signs of a serious condition.

If pregnant or breast-feeding, ask a health professional before use.
Keep out of reach of children.

OVERDOSE WARNING
Taking more than the recommended dose (overdose) may cause liver damage. In case of overdose, get medical help or contact a Poison Control Center right away. Quick medical attention is critical for adults as well as for children even if you do not notice any signs or symptoms.

DIRECTIONS
- **do not take more than directed (see Overdose warning)**
- do not take more than 6 doses in any 24-hour period
- measure only with dosing cup provided
- do not use dosing cup with other products
- dose as follows or as directed by a doctor
- mL = milliliter
- **Adults and children 12 years and older:** 20 mL in dosing cup provided every 4 hours.
- **Children under 12 years of age:** Do not use.

OTHER INFORMATION
- each 20 mL contains: **sodium 12 mg**
- tamper evident: do not use if neckband on bottle cap is broken or missing
- store between 15-30°C (59-86°F)
- do not refrigerate
- dosing cup provided

INACTIVE INGREDIENTS
anhydrous citric acid, edetate disodium, FD&C blue #1, FD&C red #40, flavors, glycerin, propylene glycol, propyl gallate,

purified water, sodium benzoate, sorbitol, sucralose, trisodium citrate dihydrate[1], xanthan gum
[1]may contain this ingredient

QUESTIONS OR COMMENTS?
1-866-MUCINEX
 (1-866-682-4639)
You may also report side effects to this phone number.
Dist. by: Reckitt Benckiser
Parsippany, NJ 07054-0224

MYLANTA GAS MAXIMUM STRENGTH CHEWABLE TABLETS (simethicone)

McNeil Consumer Pharmaceuticals Co.

DRUGS FACTS

Active Ingredient(s) (in each tablet)	Purpose(s)
Simethicone 125 mg	Antigas

USES
• relieves bloating, pressure, and discomfort of gas which can be caused by certain foods (such as beans, bran, and broccoli) or air swallowing

WARNINGS
Keep out of reach of children.

DIRECTIONS
• thoroughly chew 1-2 tablets as needed after meals and at bedtime
• do not exceed 4 tablets per day unless directed by a physician

OTHER INFORMATION
• **each tablet contains:** calcium 66 mg
• store between 20-25°C (68-77°F). Avoid high humidity.
• **do not use if carton or any blister unit is open or broken**

INACTIVE INGREDIENTS
D&C red no. 7 calcium lake, dextrates, flavors, magnesium stearate, modified starch, silicon dioxide, tribasic calcium phosphate

QUESTIONS OR COMMENTS?
call 1-800-469-5268 (toll-free) or 215-273-8755 (collect)

MYLANTA MAXIMUM STRENGTH (aluminum hydroxide, magnesium hydroxide, and simethicone)

McNeil Consumer Pharmaceuticals Co.

Active Ingredient(s) (in each 5 mL teaspoon)	Purpose(s)
Aluminum hydroxide 400 mg (equivalent to dried gel, USP)	Antacid
Magnesium hydroxide 400 mg	Anacid
Simethicone 40 mg	Anti-gas

INACTIVE INGREDIENTS
Mint Flavor:
butylparaben, D&C yellow #10, FD&C green #3, FD&C yellow #6, flavors, glycerin, hydroxyethyl cellulose, propylparaben, propylene glycol, purified water, sodium saccharin, sorbitol.
Cherry Flavor:
butylparaben, FD&C red #40, flavors, glycerin, hydroxyethyl cellulose, propylparaben, propylene glycol, purified water, sodium saccharin, sorbitol.
Original Flavor:
butylparaben, carboxymethylcellulose sodium, flavors, hypromellose, microcrystalline cellulose, propylparaben, purified water, sorbitol.

USES
Use this remedy to relieve the following symptoms:
• heartburn
• acid indigestion
• sour stomach
• upset stomach due to these symptoms
• pressure and bloating commonly referred to as gas

WARNINGS
• Ask a doctor before use if you have kidney disease.
• Ask a doctor or pharmacist before use if you are **taking a prescription drug. Antacids may interact with certain prescription drugs.**
• Stop use and ask a doctor if symptoms last for more than 2 weeks.
• Keep out of reach of children.

DIRECTIONS
Shake well.
Adults and children over 12 years: take 2-4 teaspoonfuls between meals, at bedtime, or as directed by a doctor.
Do not take more than 12 teaspoonfuls in a 24-hour period or use the maximum dosage for more than 2 weeks.
Children under 12 years: Ask a doctor.

OTHER INFORMATION
Do not use if breakaway band on plastic cap is broken or missing.
Do not freeze.
See back panel for lot number and expiration date.
Each teaspoon contains: sodium 2 mg (does not apply to Classic formula).
Does not meet USP requirements for preservative effectiveness.

MYLANTA REGULAR STRENGTH (aluminum hydroxide, magnesium hydroxide, and simethicone)

McNeil Consumer Pharmaceuticals Co.

Active Ingredient(s) (in each 5 mL teaspoon)	Purpose(s)
Aluminum hydroxide 200 mg (equivalent to dried gel, USP)	Antacid
Magnesium hydroxide 200 mg	Antacid
Simethicone 20 mg	Antigas

INACTIVE INGREDIENTS
Original Flavor:
butylparaben, carboxymethylcellulose sodium, flavors, hypromellose, microcrystalline cellulose, propylparaben, purified water, sorbitol.
Mint Flavor:
butylparaben, carboxymethlcellulose sodium, flavors, hypromellose, microcrystalline cellulose propylparaben, purified water, saccharin sodium, sorbitol.

USES
Use this remedy to relieve the following symptoms:
- heartburn
- acid indigestion
- sour stomach
- upset stomach due to these symptoms
- pressure and bloating commonly referred to as gas

WARNINGS
- Ask a doctor before use if you have kidney disease.
- Ask a doctor or pharmacist before use if you are **taking a prescription drug.** Antacids may interact with certain prescription drugs.
- Stop use and ask a doctor if **symptoms last for more than 2 weeks.**
- Keep out of reach of children.

DIRECTIONS
Shake well.
Adults and children over 12 years: take 2-4 teaspoonfuls between meals, at bedtime, or as directed by a doctor.
Do not take more than 24 teaspoonfuls in a 24-hour period or use the maximum dosage for more than 2 weeks.
Children under 12 years: Ask a doctor.

OTHER INFORMATION
Do not use if breakaway band on plastic cap is broken or missing.
Do not freeze.
See back panel for lot number and expiration date.
Does not meet USP requirements for preservative effectiveness.

MYLANTA SUPREME (calcium carbonate and magnesium hydroxide)
McNeil Consumer Pharmaceuticals Co.

Active Ingredient(s) (in each 5 mL teaspoon)	Purpose(s)
Calcium carbonate 400 mg	Antacid
Magnesium hydroxide 135 mg	Antacid

INACTIVE INGREDIENTS
Cherry Flavor:
benzyl alcohol, flavors, hydroxyethyl cellulose, purified water, simethicone, sodium carbonate, sodium saccharin, sorbitol, xanthan gum.

USES
Use this remedy to relieve the following symptoms:
- heartburn
- acid indigestion
- sour stomach
- associated symptoms of upset stomach
- overindulgence in food and drink

WARNINGS
- Ask a doctor before use if you have **kidney disease.**
- Ask a doctor or pharmacist before use if you are taking a prescription drug. Antacids may interact with certain prescription drugs.
- Stop use and ask a doctor if **symptoms last for more than 2 weeks.**
- Keep out of reach of children. **In case of overdose, get medical help or contact a poison control center right away.**

DIRECTIONS
Shake well.
Take 2-4 teaspoonfuls between meals, at bedtime, or as directed by a physician.
Do not take more than 18 teaspoonfuls in a 24-hour period, or use the maximum dosage for more than 2 weeks.

OTHER INFORMATION
Do not freeze.

MYLANTA ULTIMATE STRENGTH LIQUID
(aluminum hydroxide and magnesium hydroxide)
McNeil Consumer Pharmaceuticals Co.

Active Ingredient(s) (in each 5 mL teaspoon)	Purpose(s)
Aluminum hydroxide 500 mg	Antacid
Magnesium hydroxide 500 mg	Antacid

INACTIVE INGREDIENTS
Cherry Flavor:
butylparaben, carboxymethylcellulose sodium, FD&C red #40, flavors, hypromellose, microcrystalline cellulose, propylparaben, purified water, sodium sacchann, sorbitol.

USES
Relieves:
heartburn, acid indigestion, sour stomach, upset stomach due to these symptoms.

WARNINGS
- Ask a doctor before use if you have: kidney disease or a magnesium-restricted diet.
- Ask a doctor or pharmacist if you are taking a prescription drug. Antacids may interact with certain prescription drugs.
- **Stop use and ask your doctor if your symptoms persist more than 2 weeks.**
- **Keep out of reach of children.**

DIRECTIONS
- Shake well.
- Adults/children 12 years and older: take 2 -4 teaspoons between meals, at bedtime or as directed by a doctor.
- Do not take more than 9 teaspoons in a 24-hour period, or use the maximum dosage for more than 2 weeks.
- Children under 12 years: ask your doctor.

OTHER INFORMATION
Each teaspoon contains: magnesium 171 mg; sodium 2 mg, do not use if breakaway band on plastic cap is broken or missing.
Does not meet USP requirements for preservative effectiveness.
Do not freeze.

NAPHCON A (naphazoline hydrochloride and pheniramine maleate)
Alcon Laboratories, INC.

For the temporary relief of the minor eye symptoms of itching and redness caused by ragweed, pollen, grass, animal dander and hair.

DESCRIPTION
Active: Naphazoline Hydrochloride 0.025%, Pheniramine Maleate 0.3%. **Preservative:** Benzalkonium Chloride 0.01%.

Inactive: Boric Acid, Edetate Disodium 0.01%, Purified Water, Sodium Borate, Sodium Chloride, Sodium Hydroxide and/or Hydrochloric Acid (to adjust pH). The sterile ophthalmic solution has a pH of about 6 and a tonicity of about 270 mOsm/Kg.

DIRECTIONS
Put 1 or 2 drops in the affected eye(s) up to 4 times every day.

WARNINGS
To avoid contamination, do not touch tip of container to any surface. Replace cap after using.
If solution changes color or becomes cloudy, do not use.

STOP USE AND ASK A DOCTOR IF
you feel eye pain, changes in vision occur, redness or irritation of the eye(s) gets worse or lasts more than 72 hours.

WHEN USING THIS PRODUCT,
pupils may become enlarged temporarily. Overuse may cause more redness of the eye(s). If you are sensitive to any ingredient in this product, do not use.

DO NOT USE
this product if you have heart disease, high blood pressure, narrow angle glaucoma or trouble urinating unless directed by a physician. Accidental swallowing by infants and children may lead to coma and marked reduction in body temperature. Before using in children under 6 years of age, consult your physician. Keep this and all drugs out of the reach of children. If swallowed, get medical help or contact a Poison Control Center right away. Remove contact lenses before using.
Store at 20°- 25°C (68°- 77°F). Protect from light. Use before the expiration date marked on the carton or bottle.
ALCON LABORATORIES, INC.
FORT WORTH, TX 76134 USA
© 2002, 2004, 2005 Alcon, Inc.

NASAFLO NETI POT
NeilMed Pharmaceuticals Inc.

USES
- Nasal Allergies, Dryness & Hay Fever
- Sinus Pressure & Nasal Stuffiness
- Nasal Symptoms from Flu & Cold
- Nasal Irritation from Occupational & House Dust, Fumes, Animal Dander, Grass, Pollen, Smoke, etc.
- Post Nasal Drip & Nasal Congestion

WARNINGS
Use only as directed, if symptoms persist see your doctor/healthcare professional. Always read the label.
IMPORTANT: NeilMed® SINUS RINSE™ Mixture Packets should be used with NeilMed® 240 mL (8 fl oz) NASAFLO® to achieve the best results. You may use NeilMed® packets with other irrigation devices, as long as you mix with the correct volume of water. Our recommendation is to replace Neti Pot every three months.
Rinse your nasal passages only with NeilMed® SINUS RINSE™ packets. Our packets contain a mixture of USP grade sodium chloride and sodium bicarbonate. These ingredients are the purest quality available to make the dry powder mixture.
Rinsing your nasal passages with only plain water will result in a severe burning sensation. Use distilled, micro-filtered (through 0.2 micron), commercially bottled or previously boiled & cooled down water at lukewarm or body temperature, properly mixed with NeilMed® SINUS RINSE™ packets. Do not use tap or faucet water for dissolving the mixture unless it has been previously boiled and cooled down. Do not rinse if nasal passages are completely blocked or if you have an ear infection or blocked ears. If you have had recent ear or sinus surgery, contact your physician prior to irrigation. If you experience any pressure in the ears or burning in the nasal passages, stop irrigation and get further directions from your physician. Keep out of reach of children. Read and retain this enclosed brochure for instructions and other important information. Inside components of this unit are not for individual sale.
Do not discard this printed box and any enclosed printed material. The inside final product may not have all the details you require for the ongoing use of the product.
Saline is considered safe.
The U.S. FDA is recommending that common cough and cold over the counter medicines not be given to babies and toddlers, and that antihistamines should not be given to children under age 6.

DIRECTIONS
Step 1
Please wash your hands and rinse the device. Fill the NASAFLO® with 240 mL (8 fl oz) of lukewarm distilled, filtered or previously boiled water. Please do not use tap or faucet water to dissolve the mixture unless it has been previously boiled and cooled down. You may warm the water in a microwave, but we recommend that you warm it in increments of 5 to 10 seconds to avoid overheating, damaging the device or scalding your nasal passage.

Step 2
Cut the SINUS RINSE™ mixture packet at the corner and pour contents into the pot. Tighten the lid on the device securely. Place one finger over the hole of the cap and shake the device gently to dissolve the mixture.

Step 3
Standing in front of a sink, bend forward to your comfort level and tilt your head to one side. Keeping your mouth open, and without holding your breath, apply the tip of the device snugly against your nasal passage and ALLOW THE SOLUTION TO GENTLY FLOW until the solution starts draining from the opposite nasal passage. Use roughly half the solution in the NASAFLO® (120 mL / 4 fl oz).
It should not enter your mouth unless you are tilting your head backwards. To adjust or stop the flow, you may place your finger over the hole of the cap, and depending on the seal, you may be able to control the flow.

Step 4
Blow your nose very gently, without pinching nose completely to avoid pressure on eardrums. If tolerable, sniff in gently any residual solution remaining in the nasal passage once or twice, because this may clean out the posterior nasopharyngeal area, which is the area at the back of your nasal passage. At times, some solution will reach the back of your throat, so please spit it out.
For NASAFLO® users, to help drain any residual solution, blow your nose gently while tilting your head forward and to the same side of the nasal passage you just rinsed.

Step 5
Now repeat steps 3 & 4 on your other nasal passage,
If there is any solution left over, please discard it. We recommend you make a fresh solution each time you rinse. Rinse once or twice daily OR as directed by your physician. NeilMed® NASAFLO®: Please clean with soap & water and let air dry.

OTHER INFORMATION
Contains:
- 1 custom 8oz. (240ml) Neti Pot
- 50 regular premixed packets of pH balanced sodium chloride & sodium bicarbonate mixture (USP grade, natural ingredients, isotonic, preservative & iodine free)
- Educational brochure
- Instructions in English, Spanish or French

STORE OR KEEP IN A COOL & DRY PLACE
The NasaFLO® Neti Pot allows for a smooth gravity flow that does not create any pressure in the nasal passage, ears or sinuses. For adults & children 4 years and up.

QUESTIONS OR COMMENTS?
Call Toll Free in USA & Canada only: +1 877 477 8633, TEL: +1 707 525 3784 or Email to questions@neilmed.com

NEOSPORIN ORIGINAL (bacitracin, neomycin, and polymyxin B)

Johnson & Johnson Consumer Products Company, and Division of Johnson & Johnson Consumer Companies, Inc.

DRUG FACTS

Active Ingredient(s) (in each gram)	Purpose(s)
Bacitracin 400 units	First aid antibiotic
Neomycin 3.5 mg	First aid antibiotic
Polymyxin B 5,000 units	First aid antibiotic

USE
first aid to help prevent infection in minor:
• cuts
• scrapes
• burns

WARNINGS
For external use only.

DO NOT USE
• if you are allergic to any of the ingredients
• in the eyes
• over large areas of the body

ASK A DOCTOR BEFORE USE IF YOU HAVE
• deep or puncture wounds
• animal bites
• serious burns

STOP USE AND ASK A DOCTOR IF
• you need to use longer than 1 week
• condition persists or gets worse
• rash or other allergic reaction develops

Keep out of reach of children. If swallowed, get medical help or contact a Poison Control Center right away.

DIRECTIONS
• clean the affected area
• apply a small amount of this product (an amount equal to the surface area of the tip of a finger) on the area 1 to 3 times daily
• may be covered with a sterile bandage

OTHER INFORMATION
• store at 20° to 25°C (68° to 77° F)

INACTIVE INGREDIENTS
cocoa butter, cottonseed oil, olive oil, sodium pyruvate, vitamin E, white petrolatum

QUESTIONS OR COMMENTS?
call **1-800-223-0182**

Dist: Johnson & Johnson Consumer
Products Company Division of
Johnson & Johnson
Consumer Companies, Inc.
Skillman, NJ 08558 USA

NEOSPORIN PLUS PAIN RELIEF NEO TO GO
(bacitracin zinc, neomycin sulfate, polymyxin B sulfate, and pramoxine hydrochloride)

Johnson & Johnson Consumer Products Company and Division of Johnson & Johnson Consumer Companies, Inc.

DRUG FACTS

Active Ingredient(s) (in each gram)	Purpose(s)
Bacitracin 500 units	First aid antibiotic
Neomycin 3.5 mg	First aid antibiotic
Polymyxin B 10,000 units	First aid antibiotic
Pramoxine HCl 10 mg	External analgesic

USES
first aid to help prevent infection and for temporary relief of pain or discomfort in minor:
• cuts
• scrapes
• burns

WARNINGS
For external use only.

DO NOT USE
• if you are allergic to any of the ingredients
• in the eyes
• over large areas of the body

ASK A DOCTOR BEFORE USE IF YOU HAVE
• deep or puncture wounds
• animal bites
• serious burns

STOP USE AND ASK A DOCTOR IF
• you need to use longer than 1 week
• condition persists or gets worse
• symptoms persist for more than 1 week, or clear up and occur again within a few days
• rash or other allergic reaction develops

Keep out of reach of children. If swallowed, get medical help or contact a Poison Control Center right away.

DIRECTIONS
• adults and children 2 years of age and older:
  • clean the affected area
  • apply a small amount of this product (an amount equal to the surface area of the tip of a finger) on the area 1 to 3 times daily
  • may be covered with a sterile bandage
• children under 2 years of age: ask a doctor

OTHER INFORMATION
• store at 20° to 25°C (68° to 77° F)

INACTIVE INGREDIENT
white petrolatum

QUESTIONS OR COMMENTS?
call toll-free **800-223-0182** or **215-273-8755** (collect)

NEO-SYNEPHRINE COLD & SINUS MILD STRENGTH SPRAY (phenylephrine hydrochloride)

Bayer HealthCare

DRUG FACTS

Active Ingredient(s)	Purpose(s)
Phenylephrine hydrochloride 0.25%	Nasal decongestant

USES
- temporarily relieves nasal congestion:
  - due to common cold
  - due to hay fever or other upper respiratory allergies (allergic rhinitis)
- temporarily relieves stuffy nose
- helps clear nasal passages; shrinks swollen membranes
- temporarily restores freer breathing through the nose
- helps decongest sinus openings and passages; temporarily relieves sinus congestion and pressure

ASK A DOCTOR BEFORE USE IF YOU HAVE
- heart disease
- high blood pressure
- thyroid disease
- diabetes
- difficulty in urination due to enlargement of the prostate gland

WHEN USING THIS PRODUCT
- **do not exceed recommended dosage**
- do not use more than 3 days. Use only as directed. Frequent or prolonged use may cause nasal congestion to recur or worsen.
- temporary discomfort may occur such as burning, stinging, sneezing, or an increase in nasal discharge
- use of this container by more than one person may spread infection

STOP USE AND ASK A DOCTOR IF
- symptoms persist for more than 3 days

If pregnant or breast-feeding, ask a health professional before use.
Keep out of reach of children. If swallowed, get medical help or contact a Poison Control Center right away.

DIRECTIONS
- use only as directed
- to spray, squeeze bottle quickly and firmly

adults and children 6 to under 12 years (with adult supervision)	2 or 3 sprays in each nostril not more often than every 4 hours
children under 6 years	ask a doctor

OTHER INFORMATION
- store at room temperature
- protect from light

INACTIVE INGREDIENTS
anhydrous citric acid, benzalkonium chloride, purified water, sodium chloride, sodium citrate

QUESTIONS OR COMMENTS?
1-800-986-0369 (Mon-Fri 9AM-5PM EST) or www.bayercare.com

NEO-SYNEPHRINE COLD & SINUS EXTRA STRENGTH SPRAY (phenylephrine hydrochloride)

Bayer HealthCare LLC

Active Ingredient(s)
Phenylephrine hydrochloride 1.0%. Nasal decongestant

USES
- temporarily relieves nasal congestion:
  - due to common cold
  - due to hay fever or other upper respiratory allergies (allergic rhinitis)
- temporarily relieves stuffy nose
- helps clear nasal passages; shrinks swollen membranes
- temporarily restores freer breathing through the nose
- helps decongest sinus openings and passages; temporarily relieves sinus congestion and pressure

WARNINGS

ASK A DOCTOR BEFORE USE IF YOU HAVE
- heart disease
- high blood pressure
- thyroid disease
- diabetes
- difficulty in urination due to enlargement of the prostate gland

WHEN USING THIS PRODUCT
- **do not exceed recommended dosage.**
- do not use more than 3 days. Use only as directed. Frequent or prolonged use may cause nasal congestion to recur or worsen
- temporary discomfort may occur such as burning, stinging, sneezing, or an increase in nasal discharge
- use of this container by more than one person may spread infection

STOP USE AND ASK A DOCTOR IF
symptoms persist for more than 3 days
If breast-feeding, ask a health professional before use.
Keep out of reach of children. If swallowed, get medical help or contact a Poison Control Center right away.

DIRECTIONS
- use only as directed
- to spray, squeeze bottle quickly and firmly

adults and children 12 years and older
- 2 or 3 sprays in each nostril not more often than every 4 hours

children under 12 years
- ask a doctor

OTHER INFORMATION
- store at room temperature
- protect from light

INACTIVE INGREDIENTS
anhydrous citric acid, benzalkonium chloride, purified water, sodium chloride, sodium citrate

QUESTIONS OR COMMENTS?
1-800-986-0369 (Mon-Fri 9AM-5PM EST) or www.bayercare.com

NEO-SYNEPHRINE NASAL SPRAY REGULAR STRENGTH SPRAY (phenylephrine hydrochloride)

Bayer HealthCare LLC

Active Ingredient(s)
Phenylephrine hydrochloride 0.5%. Nasal decongestant

USES
- temporarily relieves nasal congestion:
  - due to common cold
  - due to hay fever or other upper respiratory allergies (allergic rhinitis)
- temporarily relieves stuffy nose
- helps clear nasal passages; shrinks swollen membranes
- temporarily restores freer breathing through the nose
- helps decongest sinus openings and passages; temporarily relieves sinus congestion and pressure

WARNINGS

ASK A DOCTOR BEFORE USE IF YOU HAVE
- heart disease
- high blood pressure
- thyroid disease
- diabetes
- difficulty in urination due to enlargement of the prostate gland

WHEN USING THIS PRODUCT
- **do not exceed recommended dosage.**
- do not use more than 3 days. Use only as directed. Frequent or prolonged use may cause nasal congestion to recur or worsen
- temporary discomfort may occur such as burning, stinging, sneezing, or an increase in nasal discharge
- use of this container by more than one person may spread infection

STOP USE AND ASK A DOCTOR IF
symptoms persist for more than 3 days
If breast-feeding, ask a health professional before use.
Keep out of reach of children. If swallowed, get medical help or contact a Poison Control Center right away.

DIRECTIONS
- use only as directed
- to spray, squeeze bottle quickly and firmly

adults and children 12 years and older
- 2 or 3 sprays in each nostril not more often than every 4 hours

children under 12 years
- ask a doctor

OTHER INFORMATION
- store at room temperature
- protect from light

INACTIVE INGREDIENTS
anhydrous citric acid, benzalkonium chloride, purified water, sodium chloride, sodium citrate

QUESTIONS OR COMMENTS?
1-800-986-0369 (Mon-Fri 9AM-5PM EST) or www.bayercare.com

NEO-SYNEPHRINE SEVERE SINUS CONGESTION SPRAY (oxymetazoline hydrochloride)

Bayer HealthCare

DRUG FACTS

Active Ingredient(s)	Purpose(s)
Oxymetazoline HCl 0.05%	Nasal decongestant

USES
- temporarily relieves nasal congestion:
  - due to common cold
  - due to hay fever or other upper respiratory allergies (allergic rhinitis)
- temporarily relieves stuffy nose
- helps clear nasal passages; shrinks swollen membranes
- temporarily restores freer breathing through the nose
- helps decongest sinus openings and passages; temporarily relieves sinus congestion and pressure

ASK A DOCTOR BEFORE USE IF YOU HAVE
- heart disease
- high blood pressure
- thyroid disease
- diabetes
- difficulty in urination due to enlargement of the prostate gland

WHEN USING THIS PRODUCT
- **do not exceed recommended dosage**
- do not use more than 3 days. Use only as directed. Frequent or prolonged use may cause nasal congestion to recur or worsen.
- temporary discomfort may occur such as burning, stinging, sneezing, and an increase in nasal discharge
- use of this container by more than one person may spread infection

STOP USE AND ASK A DOCTOR IF
- symptoms persist for more than 3 days

If pregnant or breast-feeding, ask a health professional before use.
Keep out of reach of children. If swallowed, get medical help or contact a Poison Control Center right away.

DIRECTIONS
- use only as directed
- to spray, squeeze bottle quickly and firmly

adults and children 6 to under 12 years (with adult supervision)	2 or 3 sprays in each nostril not more often than every 10 to 12 hours. Do not exceed 2 doses in 24 hours.
children under 6 years	ask a doctor

OTHER INFORMATION
- store at room temperature
- protect from light

INACTIVE INGREDIENTS
benzalkonium chloride, dibasic sodium phosphate, edetate disodium, glycerin, monobasic sodium phosphate, purified water, sodium chloride

QUESTIONS OR COMMENTS?
1-800-986-0369 (Mon – Fri 9AM – 5PM EST) or
www.bayercare.com

NICODERM CQ (nicotine)

GlaxoSmithKline Consumer Healthcare LP

Active Ingredient(s) (in each patch)(clear)
Nicotine, 21 mg delivered over 24 hours

Active Ingredient(s) (in each patch)(clear)
Nicotine, 14 mg delivered over 24 hours

Active Ingredient(s) (in each patch)(clear)
Nicotine, 7 mg delivered over 24 hours

Active Ingredient(s) (in each patch)(opaque)
Nicotine, 21 mg delivered over 24 hours

Purpose(s)
Stop smoking aid

USES
reduces withdrawal symptoms, including nicotine craving,
associated with quitting smoking

WARNINGS
**If you are pregnant or breast-feeding, only use this medicine
on the advice of your health care provider.**
Smoking can seriously harm your child. Try to stop smoking
without using any nicotine replacement medicine. This medicine
is believed to be safer than smoking. However, the risks to your
child from this medicine are not fully known.

DO NOT USE
- if you continue to smoke, chew tobacco, use snuff, or use a
  nicotine gum or other nicotine containing products

ASK A DOCTOR BEFORE USE IF YOU HAVE
- heart disease, recent heart attack, or irregular heartbeat.
  Nicotine can increase your heart rate.
- high blood pressure not controlled with medication. Nicotine
  can increase your blood pressure.
- an allergy to adhesive tape or have skin problems because you
  are more likely to get rashes

ASK A DOCTOR OR PHARMACIST BEFORE USE IF YOU ARE
- using a non-nicotine stop smoking drug
- taking a prescription medicine for depression or asthma. Your
  prescription dose may need to be adjusted.

WHEN USING THIS PRODUCT
- don not smoke even when not wearing the patch. The nicotine
  in your skin will still be entering your blood stream for
  several hours after you take off the patch.
- if you have vivid dreams or other sleep disturbances remove
  this patch at bedtime

STOP USE AND ASK A DOCTOR IF
- skin redness caused by the patch does not go away after four
  days, or if your skin swells, or you get a rash
- irregular heartbeat or palpitations occur
- you get symptoms of nicotine overdose such as nausea,
  vomiting, dizziness, weakness and rapid heartbeat

Keep out of reach of children and pets.
Used patches have enough nicotine to poison children and pets.
If swallowed, get medical help or contact a Posion Control
Center right away. Dispose of the used patches by folding sticky
ends together. Replace in pouch and discard.

DIRECTIONS (CLEAR)
- **if you are under 18 years of age, ask a doctor before use**
- before using this product, read the enclosed User's Guide for
  complete directions and other information
- stop smoking completely when you begin using the patch
- **if you smoke more than 10 cigarettes per day,** use
  according to the following 10-week schedule:

STEP 1	STEP 2	STEP 3
Use one 21 mg patch/day	Use one 14 mg patch/day	Use one 7 mg patch/day
Weeks 1-6	Week 7-8	Week 9-10

- if you smoke **10 or less cigarettes per day,** do not use
  STEP 1 (21mg). Start with **STEP 2 (14mg)** for 6 weeks, then
  STEP 3 (7mg) for 2 weeks and then stop.
- steps 2 and 3 allow you to gradually reduce your level of
  nicotine. Completing the full program will increase your
  chances of quitting successfully.
- apply one new patch every 24 hours on skin that is dry, clean
  and hairless. Save pouch for disposing of the patch after use.
- remove backing from patch and immediately press onto skin.
  Hold for 10 seconds.
- wash hands after applying or removing patch. Throw away
  the patch by folding sticky ends together. Replace in its pouch
  and discard. See enclosed User's Guide for safety and
  handling.
- you may wear the patch for 16 or 24 hours
- if you crave cigarettes when you wake up, wear the patch for
  24 hours
- if you have vivid dreams or other sleep disturbances, you may
  remove the patch at bedtime and apply a new one in the
  morning
- the used patch should be removed and a new one applied to a
  different skin site at the same time each day
- do not wear more than one patch at a time
- do not cut patch in half or into smaller pieces
- do not leave patch on for more than 24 hours because it may
  irritate your skin and loses strength after 24 hours
- stop using the patch at the end of 10 weeks. If you started
  with **STEP 2,** stop using the patch at the end of 8 weeks. If
  you still feel the need to use the patch, talk to your doctor.

DIRECTIONS (OPAQUE)
- **if you are under 18 years of age, ask a doctor before use**
- before using this product, read the enclosed User's Guide for
  complete directions and other information
- stop smoking completely when you begin using the patch
- **if you smoke more than 10 cigarettes per day,** use
  according to the follow 10 week schedule:

STEP 1	STEP 2	STEP 3
Use one 21 mg patch/day	Use one 14 mg patch/day	Use one 7 mg patch/day
Weeks 1-6	Week 7-8	Week 9-10

- if you smoke **10 or less cigarettes per day,** do not use
  STEP 1 (21mg). Start with **STEP 2 (14mg)** for 6 weeks, then
  STEP 3 (7mg) for 2 weeks and then stop.
- steps 2 and 3 allow you to gradually reduce your level of
  nicotine. Completing the full program will increase your
  chances of quitting successfully.
- apply one new patch every 24 hours on skin that is dry, clean
  and hairless. Save pouch for disposing of the patch after use.
- remove backing from patch and immediately press onto skin.
  Hold for 10 seconds.
- wash hands after applying or removing patch. Throw away
  the patch by folding sticky ends together. Replace in its pouch
  and discard. See enclosed User's Guide for safety and
  handling.
- you may wear the patch for 16 or 24 hours
- if you crave cigarettes when you wake up, wear the patch for
  24 hours

- if you have vivid dreams or other sleep disturbances, you may remove the patch at bedtime and apply a new one in the morning
- to avoid possible burns, remove patch before undergoing any MRI (magnetic resonance imaging) procedures
- the used patch should be removed and a new one applied to a different skin site at the same time each day
- do not wear more than one patch at a time
- do not cut patch in half or into smaller pieces
- do not leave patch on for more than 24 hours because it may irritate your skin and loses strength after 24 hours
- stop using the patch at the end of 10 weeks. If you started with **STEP 2**, stop using the patch at the end of 8 weeks. If you still feel the need to use the patch, talk to your doctor

OTHER INFORMATION
store at 20-25°C (68-77°F)

INACTIVE INGREDIENTS (CLEAR)
ethylene vinyl acetate-copolymer, polyisobutylene and high density polyethylene between clear polyester backings

INACTIVE INGREDIENTS (OPAQUE)
ethylene vinyl acetate-copolymer, polyisobutylene and high density polyethylene between pigmented and clear polyester backings

QUESTIONS OR COMMENTS?
call toll-free **1-800-834-5895** (English/Spanish) weekdays (9:00 a.m.-4:30 p.m. ET)

NICORETTE GUM (nicotine polacrilex)
GlaxoSmithKline Consumer Healthcare LP

Active Ingredient(s) (in each chewing piece)
Nicotine polacrilex (equal to 2mg nicotine)
Nicotine polacrilex (equal to 4mg nicotine)

Purpose(s)
Stop smoking aid

USE
- reduces withdrawal symptoms, including nicotine craving, associated with quitting smoking

WARNINGS
If you are pregnant or breast-feeding, only use this medicine on the advice of your health care provider.
Smoking can seriously harm your child. Try to stop smoking without using any nicotine replacement medicine. This medicine is believed to be safer than smoking. However, the risks to your child from this medicine are not fully known.

DO NOT USE
- if you continue to smoke, chew tobacco, use snuff, or use a nicotine patch or other nicotine containing products

ASK A DOCTOR BEFORE USE IF YOU HAVE
- a sodium-restricted diet
- heart disease, recent heart attack, or irregular heartbeat. Nicotine can increase your heart rate.
- high blood pressure not controlled with medication. Nicotine can increase blood pressure.
- stomach ulcer or diabetes

ASK A DOCTOR OR A PHARMACIST BEFORE USE IF YOU ARE
- using a non-nicotine stop smoking drug
- taking prescription medicine for depression or asthma. Your prescription dose may need to be adjusted.

STOP USE AND ASK A DOCTOR IF
- mouth, teeth or jaw problems occur
- irregular heartbeat or palpitations occur
- you get symptoms of nicotine overdose such as nausea, vomiting, dizziness, diarrhea, weakness and rapid heartbeat
- **(For Cinnamon Surge)** oral blistering occurs
-

Keep out of reach of children and pets.
Pieces of nicotine gum may have enough nicotine to make children and pets sick. Wrap used pieces of gum in paper and throw away in the trash. In case of overdose, get medical help or contact a Poison Control Center right away.

DIRECTIONS (2MG)
- **if you are under 18 years of age, ask a doctor before use**
- before using this product, read the enclosed User's Guide for complete directions and other important information
- stop smoking completely when you begin using the gum
- **if you smoke your first cigarette within 30 minutes of waking up**, use 4mg nicotine gum
- **if you smoke your first cigarette more than 30 minutes after waking up**, use 2mg nicotine gum according to the following 12 week schedule:

Weeks 1 to 6	Weeks 7 to 9	Weeks 10 to 12
1 piece every 1 to 2 hours	1 piece every 2 to 4 hours	1 piece every 4 to 8 hours

- nicotine gum is a medicine and must be used a certain way to get the best results
- chew the gum slowly until it tingles. Then park it between your cheek and gum. When the tingle is gone, begin chewing again, until the tingle returns.
- repeat this process until most of the tingle is gone (about 30 minutes)
- do not eat or drink for 15 minutes before chewing the nicotine gum, or while chewing a piece
- to improve your chances of quitting, use at least 9 pieces per day for the first 6 weeks
- if you experience strong or frequent cravings, you may use a second piece within the hour. However, do not continuously use one piece after another since this may cause you hiccups, heartburn, nausea or other side effects.
- do not use more than 24 pieces a day
- it is important to complete treatment. Stop using the nicotine gum at the end of 12 weeks. If you still feel the need to use nicotine gum, talk to your doctor.

DIRECTIONS (4 MG)
- **if you are under 18 years of age, ask a doctor before use**
- before using this product, read the enclosed User's Guide for complete directions and other important information
- stop smoking completely when you begin using the gum
- **if you smoke your first cigarette more than 30 minutes after waking up**, use 2mg nicotine gum
- **if you smoke your first cigarette within 30 minutes of waking up**, use 4mg nicotine gum according to the following 12 week schedule:

Weeks 1 to 6	Weeks 7 to 9	Weeks 10 to 12
1 piece every 1 to 2 hours	1 piece every 2 to 4 hours	1 piece every 4 to 8 hours

- nicotine gum is a medicine and must be used a certain way to get the best results
- chew the gum slowly until it tingles. Then park it between your cheek and gum. When the tingle is gone, begin chewing again, until the tingle returns.
- repeat this process until most of the tingle is gone (about 30 minutes)
- do not eat or drink for 15 minutes before chewing the nicotine gum, or while chewing a piece
- to improve your chances of quitting, use at least 9 pieces per day for the first 6 weeks

- if you experience strong or frequent cravings, you may use a second piece within the hour. However, do not continuously use one piece after another since this may cause you hiccups, heartburn, nausea or other side effects.
- do not use more than 24 pieces a day
- it is important to complete treatment. Stop using the nicotine gum at the end of 12 weeks. If you still feel the need to use nicotine gum, talk to your doctor.

OTHER INFORMATION (WHITE ICE MINT)
- **(2 mg) each piece contains:** calcium 94 mg, sodium 11 mg
- **(4 mg) each piece contains:** calcium 94 mg, sodium 13 mg
- store at 20-25°C (68-77°F)
- protect from light

OTHER INFORMATION (ORIGINAL)
- **each piece contains:** calcium 117 mg, sodium 13 mg
- store at 20-25°C (68-77°F)
- protect from light

OTHER INFORMATION (CINNAMON SURGE)
- **(2 mg) each piece contains:** calcium 94 mg, sodium 11 mg
- **(4 mg) each piece contains:** calcium 94 mg, sodium 13 mg
- store at 20-25°C (68-77°F)
- protect from light

OTHER INFORMATION (FRESH MINT)
- **(2 mg) each piece contains:** calcium 94 mg, sodium 11 mg
- **(4 mg) each piece contains:** calcium 94 mg, sodium 13 mg
- store at 20-25°C (68-77°F)
- protect from light

OTHER INFORMATION (MINT)
- **(2 mg) each piece contains:** calcium 94 mg, sodium 13 mg
- **(4 mg) each piece contains:** calcium 94 mg, sodium 14 mg
- store at 20-25°C (68-77°F)
- protect from light

OTHER INFORMATION (SPEARMINT BURST)
- **(2 mg) each piece contains:** calcium 94mg, sodium 11mg
- **(4 mg) each piece contains:** calcium 94mg, sodium 13mg
- store at 20-25°C (68-77°F)
- protect from light

INACTIVE INGREDIENTS WHITE ICE MINT
each 2 mg piece contains: acesulfame potassium, carnauba wax, edible ink, flavor, gum base, hypromellose, magnesium oxide, menthol, peppermint oil, polysorbate 80, sodium bicarbonate, sodium carbonate, starch, sucralose, titanium dioxide, xylitol
each 4 mg piece contains: acesulfame potassium, carnauba wax, D&C yellow #10 Al. lake, edible ink, flavor, gum base, hypromellose, magnesium oxide, menthol, peppermint oil, polysorbate 80, sodium carbonate, starch, sucralose, titanium dioxide, xylitol

INACTIVE INGREDIENTS ORIGINAL
each 2 mg piece contains: flavors, glycerin, gum base, sodium bicarbonate, sodium carbonate, sorbitol
each 4 mg piece contains: D&C yellow #10, flavors, glycerin, gum base, sodium carbonate, sorbitol

INACTIVE INGREDIENTS CINNAMON SURGE
each 2 mg piece contains: acacia, acesulfame potassium, carnauba wax, edible ink, gum base, hypromellose, magnesium oxide, menthol, natural and artificial cinnamon flavors, peppermint oil, polysorbate 80, sodium bicarbonate, sodium carbonate, sucralose, titanium dioxide, xylitol
each 4 mg piece contains: acacia, acesulfame potassium, carnauba wax, D&C yellow #10 Al. lake, edible ink, gum base, hypromellose, magnesium oxide, menthol, natural and artificial cinnamon flavors, peppermint oil, polysorbate 80, sodium carbonate, sucralose, titanium dioxide, xylitol

INACTIVE INGREDIENTS FRESH MINT
each 2 mg piece contains: acacia, acesulfame potassium, carnauba wax, edible ink, gum base, magnesium oxide, menthol, peppermint oil, sodium bicarbonate, sodium carbonate, titanium dioxide, xylitol
each 4 mg piece contains: acacia, acesulfame potassium, carnauba wax, D&C yellow #10 Al. lake, edible ink, gum base, magnesium oxide, menthol, peppermint oil, sodium carbonate, titanium dioxide, xylitol

INACTIVE INGREDIENTS MINT
each 2 mg piece contains: acesulfame potassium, gum base, magnesium oxide, menthol, peppermint oil, sodium bicarbonate, sodium carbonate, xylitol
each 4 mg piece contains: acesulfame potassium, D&C yellow #10 Al. lake, gum base, magnesium oxide, menthol, peppermint oil, sodium carbonate, xylitol

INACTIVE INGREDIENTS SPEARMINT BURST
each 2 mg piece contains: acesulfame potassium, carnauba wax, chamomile flavor, edible ink, gum base, gum arabica, hypromellose, levomenthol, magnesium oxide, peppermint flavor, polysorbate 80, spearmint flavor, sodium carbonate, sodium hydrogen carbonate, sucralose, titanium dioxide, xylitol
each 4 mg piece contains: acesulfame potassium, carnauba wax, chamomile flavor, D&C yllow #10 Al. lake, edible ink, gum base, gum arabica, hypromellose, levomenthol, magnesium oxide, peppermint flavor, polysorbate 80, spearmint flavor, sodium carbonate, sucralose, titanium dioxide, xylitol

QUESTIONS OR COMMENTS?
call toll-free **1-800-419-4766** (English/Spanish) weekdays (9:00 am-4:30 pm ET)
TO INCREASE YOUR SUCCESS IN QUITTING:
- You must be motivated to quit.
- **Use Enough**-Chew **at least 9 pieces** of Nicorette per day during the first six weeks.
- **Use Long Enough** - Use Nicorette for the full 12 weeks.
- **Use with a support program** as directed in the enclosed User's Guide.

To remove the gum, tear off single unit.
Peel off backing, starting at corner with loose edge.
Push gum through foil.
- not for sale to those under 18 years of age
- proof of age required
- not for sale in vending machines or from any source where proof of age cannot be verified

This product is protected in sealed blisters. **Do not use if individual blisters or printed backings are broken, open, or torn.**
Distributed by
GlaxoSmithKline Consumer Healthcare, L.P.
Moon Township, PA 15108
Made in Sweden
For more information and for a FREE individualized stop smoking program, please visit www.Nicorette.com or see inside for more details.
Free Audio CD upon request. See inside.

NICORETTE LOZENGES (nicotine polacrilex)
GlaxoSmithKline Consumer Healthcare LP

Active Ingredient(s) (in each lozenge) (2mg)
Nicotine polacrilex, 2mg

Active Ingredient(s) (in each lozenge) (4mg)
Nicotine polacrilex, 4mg

Purpose(s)
Stop smoking aid

USE
- reduces withdrawal symptoms, including nicotine craving, associated with quitting smoking

WARNINGS
If you are pregnant or breast-feeding, only use this medicine on the advice of your health care provider.
Smoking can seriously harm your child. Try to stop smoking without using any nicotine replacement medicine. This medicine is believed to be safer than smoking. However, the risks to your child from this medicine are not fully known.

DO NOT USE
- if you continue to smoke, chew tobacco, use snuff, or use a nicotine patch or other nicotine containing products

ASK A DOCTOR BEFORE USE IF YOU HAVE
- a sodium-restricted diet
- heart disease, recent heart attack, or irregular heartbeat. Nicotine can increase your heart rate.
- high blood pressure not controlled with medication. Nicotine can increase your blood pressure.
- stomach ulcer or diabetes

ASK A DOCTOR OR PHARMACIST BEFORE USE IF YOU ARE
- using a non-nicotine stop smoking drug
- taking prescription medicine for depression or asthma. Your prescription dose may need to be adjusted.

STOP USE AND ASK A DOCTOR IF
- mouth problems occur
- persistent indigestion or severe sore throat occurs
- irregular heartbeat or palpitations occur
- you get symptoms of nicotine overdose such as nausea, vomiting, dizziness, diarrhea, weakness and rapid heartbeat

Keep out of reach of children and pets.
Nicotine lozenges may have enough nicotine to make children and pets sick. If you need to remove the lozenge, wrap it in paper and throw away in the trash. In case of overdose, get medical help or contact a Poison Control Center right away.

DIRECTIONS (2MG)
- **if you are under 18 years of age, ask a doctor before use**
- before using this product, read the enclosed User's Guide for complete directions and other important information
- stop smoking completely when you begin using the lozenge
- **if you smoke your first cigarette within 30 minutes of waking up,** use 4mg nicotine lozenge
- **if you smoke your first cigarette more than 30 minutes after waking up,** use 2mg nicotine lozenge according to the following 12 week schedule:

Weeks 1 to 6	Weeks 7 to 9	Weeks 10 to 12
1 lozenge every 1 to 2 hours	1 lozenge every 2 to 4 hours	1 lozenge every 4 to 8 hours

- **nicotine lozenge is a medicine and must be used a certain way to get the best results**
- place the lozenge in your mouth and allow the lozenge to slowly dissolve (about 20-30 minutes). Minimize swallowing. **Do not chew or swallow lozenge.**
- you may feel a warm or tingling sensation
- occasionally move the lozenge from one side of your mouth to the other until completely dissolved (about 20-30 minutes)
- do not eat or drink 15 minutes before using or while the lozenge is in your mouth
- to improve your chances of quitting, use at least 9 lozenges per day for the first 6 weeks

- do not use more than one lozenge at a time or continuously use one lozenge after another since this may cause you hiccups, heartburn, nausea or other side effects
- **do not use more than 5 lozenges in 6 hours. Do not use more than 20 lozenges per day.**
- stop using the nicotine lozenge at the end of 12 weeks. If you still feel the need to use nicotine lozenges, talk to your doctor.

DIRECTIONS (4MG)
- **if you are under 18 years of age, ask a doctor before use**
- before using this product, read the enclosed User's Guide for complete directions and other important information
- stop smoking completely when you begin using the lozenge
- **if you smoke your first cigarette more than 30 minutes after waking up,** use 2mg nicotine lozenge
- **if you smoke your first cigarette within 30 minutes of waking up,** use 4mg nicotine lozenge according to the following 12 week schedule:

Weeks 1 to 6	Weeks 7 to 9	Weeks 10 to 12
1 lozenge every 1 to 2 hours	1 lozenge every 2 to 4 hours	1 lozenge every 4 to 8 hours

- **nicotine lozenge is a medicine and must be used a certain way to get the best results**
- place the lozenge in your mouth and allow the lozenge to slowly dissolve (about 20-30 minutes). Minimize swallowing. **Do not chew or swallow lozenge.**
- you may feel a warm or tingling sensation
- occasionally move the lozenge from one side of your mouth to the other until completely dissolved (about 20-30 minutes)
- do not eat or drink 15 minutes before using or while the lozenge is in your mouth
- to improve your chances of quitting, use at least 9 lozenges per day for the first 6 weeks
- do not use more than one lozenge at a time or continuously use one lozenge after another since this may cause you hiccups, heartburn, nausea or other side effects
- **do not use more than 5 lozenges in 6 hours. Do not use more than 20 lozenges per day.**
- stop using the nicotine lozenge at the end of 12 weeks. If you still feel the need to use nicotine lozenges, talk to your doctor.

OTHER INFORMATION (ORIGINAL)
- **each lozenge contains:** sodium, 18mg
- Phenylketonurics: Contains Phenylalanine 3.4 mg per lozenge
- store at 20-25°C (68-77°F)
- protect from light

NICORETTE® and associated logo designs and overall trade dress designs are trademarks owned and/or licensed to the GlaxoSmithKline group of companies.
Distributed By:
GlaxoSmithKline Consumer Healthcare, L.P.
Moon Township, PA 15108, Made in the Switzerland
©2010 GlaxoSmithKline
- not for sale to those under 18 years of age
- proof of age required
- not for sale in vending machines or from any source where proof of age cannot be verified

This product is protected in sealed blisters.
Do not use if individual blisters or printed backings are broken, open, or torn.
TO INCREASE YOUR SUCCESS IN QUITTING:
- You must be motivated to quit.
- **Use Enough-**Use **at least 9 lozenges** of Nicorette per day during the first six weeks.
- **Use Long Enough-**Use Nicorette for the full 12 weeks.
- **Use With a Support Program** as directed in the enclosed User's Guide.

For more information and for a FREE individualized stop smoking program, please visit www.Nicorette.com or see inside for more details.

OTHER INFORMATION (MINT)
- **each lozenge contains:** sodium, 18mg
- Phenylketonurics: Contains Phenylalanine 3.4 mg per lozenge
- store at 20-25°C (68-77°F)
- keep POPPAC tightly closed and protect from light

NICORETTE®, POPPAC ™ and associated logo designs and overall trade dress designs are trademarks owned and/or licensed to the GlaxoSmithKline group of companies.
Distributed By:
GlaxoSmithKline Consumer Healthcare, L.P.
Moon Township, PA 15108, Made in the Switzerland
©2010 GlaxoSmithKline
- not for sale to those under 18 years of age
- proof of age required
- not for sale in vending machines or from any source where proof of age cannot be verified

TAMPER EVIDENT FEATURE: Do not use if clear neckband printed "SEALED FOR SAFETY" is missing or broken.
Retain outer carton for full product uses, directions and warnings.

TO INCREASE YOUR SUCCESS IN QUITTING:
- You must be motivated to quit.
- **Use Enough**-Use **at least 9 lozenges** of Nicorette per day during the first six weeks.
- **Use Long Enough**-Use Nicorette for the full 12 weeks.
- **Use With a Support Program** as directed in the enclosed User's Guide.

Nicorette® POPPAC™
To open vial, push in child resistant band on the POPPAC with thumb.
Flip up the top of the POPPAC and remove lozenge. A small amount of powder on opening of the POPPAC is normal.
For more information and for a FREE individualized stop smoking program, please visit www.Nicorette.com or see inside for more details.

OTHER INFORMATION (CHERRY)
- **each lozenge contains:** sodium, 18mg
- store at 20-25°C (68-77°F)
- keep POPPAC tightly closed and protect from light

NICORETTE®, POPPAC ™ and associated logo designs and overall trade dress designs are trademarks owned and/or licensed to the GlaxoSmithKline group of companies.
Distributed By:
GlaxoSmithKline Consumer Healthcare, L.P.
Moon Township, PA 15108, Made in Switzerland.
©2010 GlaxoSmithKline
- not for sale to those under 18 years of age
- proof of age required
- not for sale in vending machines or from any source where proof of age cannot be verified

TAMPER EVIDENT FEATURE: Do not use if clear neckband printed "SEALED FOR SAFETY" is missing or broken.
Retain outer carton for full product uses, directions and warnings.

TO INCREASE YOUR SUCCESS IN QUITTING:
- You must be motivated to quit.
- **Use Enough**-Use **at least 9 lozenges** of Nicorette per day during the first six weeks.
- **Use Long Enough**-Use Nicorette for the full 12 weeks.
- **Use With a Support Program** as directed in the enclosed User's Guide.

Nicorette® POPPAC™
To open vial, push in child resistant band on the POPPAC with thumb.
Flip up the top of the POPPAC and remove lozenge. A small amount of powder on opening of the POPPAC is normal.
For more information and for a FREE individualized stop smoking program, please visit www.Nicorette.com or see inside for more details.

INACTIVE INGREDIENTS (ORIGINAL)
aspartame, calcium polycarbophil, flavor, magnesium stearate, mannitol, potassium bicarbonate, sodium alginate, sodium carbonate, xanthan gum

INACTIVE INGREDIENTS (MINT)
acacia, aspartame, calcium polycarbophil, corn syrup solids, flavors, lactose, magnesium stearate, maltodextrin, mannitol, potassium bicarbonate, sodium alginate, sodium carbonate, soy protein, triethyl citrate, xanthan gum

INACTIVE INGREDIENTS (CHERRY)
acesulfame potassium, benzyl alcohol, butylhydroxy toluene, calcium polycarbophil, coconut and/or palm kernel oil, eugenol, flavors, magnesium stearate, maltodextrin, mannitol, modified corn starch, potassium bicarbonate, sodium alginate, sodium carbonate, xanthan gum

QUESTIONS OR COMMENTS?
call toll-free **1-888-569-1743** (English/Spanish) weekdays (9:00 am-4:30 pm ET)

NIX (permethrin)
Insight Pharmaceuticals

DRUG FACTS
Active Ingredient(s) (in each fluid ounce) Purpose(s)
Permethrin 280 mg (1%).......................Lice treatment

USE
treats head lice

WARNINGS
For external use only

DO NOT USE
- on children under 2 months of age
- near the eyes
- inside the nose, ear, mouth, or vagina
- on lice in eyebrows or eyelashes. See your doctor.

ASK A DOCTOR BEFORE USE IF YOU ARE
- allergic to ragweed. May cause breathing difficulty or an asthmatic episode.

WHEN USING THIS PRODUCT
- keep eyes tightly closed and protect eyes with a washcloth or towel
- if product gets into the eyes, immediately flush with large amounts of water
- scalp itching or redness may occur

STOP USE AND SEE A DOCTOR IF
- breathing difficulty occurs
- eye irritation occurs
- skin or scalp irritation continues or infection occurs

If pregnant or breast-feeding, ask a health professional before use.
Keep out of reach of children. If swallowed, get medical help or contact a Poison Control Center right away.

DIRECTIONS
Inspect
- all household members should be checked by another person for lice and/or nits (eggs)
- use a magnifying glass in bright light to help you see the lice and nits (eggs)

- use a tool, such as a comb or two unsharpened pencils to lift and part the hair
- look for tiny nits near the scalp, beginning at the back of the neck and behind the ears
- small sections of hair (1-2 inches wide) should be examined at a time
- unlike dandruff, nits stick to the hair. Dandruff should move when lightly touched.
- if either lice or nits (eggs) are found, treat with Nix Creme Rinse

Treat
- wash hair with a shampoo without conditioner. Do not use a shampoo that contains a conditioner or a conditioner alone since this may decrease the activity of Nix. Rinse with water.
- towel dry hair so it is damp but not wet
- shake the bottle of Nix well
- completely saturate the hair and scalp with Nix. Begin to apply Nix behind the ears and at the back of the neck.
- keep Nix out of the eyes. Protect the eyes with a washcloth or towel.
- leave Nix on the hair for 10 minutes, but no longer
- rinse with warm water
- towel dry hair and comb out tangles
- if live lice are seen seven days or more after the first treatment, a second treatment should be given

Remove Lice/Nits
- remove nits by combing the hair with the special small tooth comb provided. Remaining nits may be removed by hand (using a throw-away glove), or cutting the nits out.
- use the nit comb provided and make sure the hair remains slightly damp while removing nits
- if the hair dries during combing, dampen it slightly with water
- part the hair into 4 sections. Work on one section at a time. Longer hair may take more time (1-2 hours).
- start at the top of the head on the section you have picked
- with one hand, lift a 1-2 inch wide strand of hair. Get the teeth of the comb as close to the scalp as possible and comb with a firm, even motion away from the scalp to the end of the hair.
- use clips to pin back each strand of hair after you have combed out the nits
- clean the comb completely as you go. Wipe the nits from the comb with a tissue and throw away the tissue in a sealed plastic bag to prevent the lice from coming back.
- after combing, recheck the entire head for nits and repeat combing if necessary
- check the affected head daily to remove any nits that you might have missed

OTHER INFORMATION
- read all the directions in the Consumer Information Insert and warnings before use. Keep the carton. It contains important information.
- store at 20° to 25°C (68° to 77°F)

INACTIVE INGREDIENTS
balsam canada, cetyl alcohol, citric acid, FD&C yellow no. 6, fragrance, hydrolyzed animal protein, hydroxyethylcellulose, polyoxyethylene 10 cetyl ether, propylene glycol, stearalkonium chloride, water, isopropyl alcohol 5.6 g (20%), methylparaben 56 mg (0.2%), and propylparaben 22 mg (0.08%)

QUESTIONS OR COMMENTS?
call **1-888-LICE LINE (1-888-542-3546),** Monday to Friday, 9 AM-5 PM EST

How do head lice spread?
- head lice spread easily from close head-to-head or hand-to-head contact with persons who have lice
- they may also spread by sharing hats, helmets, scarves, headphones, brushes, combs, bedding and clothing

How do you know if you have lice?
- itching is the most common symptom
- scratching behind the ears or the back of the neck is a sign that you should check for head lice
- scabs or blood spots may be seen

How do you prevent the spread of lice?
- do not share or borrow personal items like combs, brushes, or headbands
- do not share or borrow hats, sweaters, coats, scarves, helmets, headphones, pillows or stuffed animals
- store hats in coat sleeves and hang coats separately, so that they do not touch other people's hats and coats
- wash under fingernails when you first see lice or nits (eggs)
- check your child's head daily when you hear of a lice outbreak in day care or school

I. Inspect
If you suspect head lice-check. Head lice may be hard to locate because they avoid light. Nits are easier to see.
- all household members should be checked by another person for lice and/or nits (eggs)
- use a magnifying glass in bright light to help you see the lice and nits (eggs)
- use a tool, such as a comb or two unsharpened pencils to lift and part the hair
- look for tiny nits near the scalp, beginning at the back of the neck and behind the ears
- small sections of hair (1-2 inches wide) should be examined at a time
- unlike dandruff, nits stick to the hair. Dandruff should move when lightly touched.
- if either lice or nits (eggs) are found, treat with Nix Creme Rinse

II. Treat
- wash hair with a shampoo without conditioner. Do not use a shampoo that contains a conditioner or a conditioner alone since this may decrease the activity of Nix. Rinse with water.
- towel dry hair so it is damp but not wet
- shake the bottle of Nix well
- completely saturate the hair and scalp with Nix. Begin to apply Nix behind the ears and at the back of the neck.
- keep Nix out of the eyes. Protect the eyes with a washcloth or towel.
- leave Nix on the hair for 10 minutes, but no longer
- rinse with warm water
- towel dry hair and comb out tangles
- if live lice are seen seven days or more after the first treatment, a second treatment should be given

III. Remove Lice/Nits
Treatment kills lice but does not remove the nits.
- remove nits by combing the hair with the special small tooth comb provided. Remaining nits may be removed by hand (using a throw-away glove), or cutting the nits out.
- use the nit comb provided and make sure the hair remains slightly damp while removing nits
- if the hair dries during combing, dampen it slightly with water
- part the hair into 4 sections. Work on one section at a time. Longer hair may take more time (1-2 hours).
- start at the top of the head on the section you have picked
- with one hand, lift a 1-2 inch wide strand of hair. Get the teeth of the comb as close to the scalp as possible and comb with a firm, even motion away from the scalp to the end of the hair.
- use clips to pin back each strand of hair after you have combed out the nits
- clean the comb completely as you go. Wipe the nits from the comb with a tissue and throw away the tissue in a sealed plastic bag to prevent the lice from coming back.
- after combing, recheck the entire head for nits and repeat combing if necessary
- check the affected head daily to remove any nits that you might have missed

IV. Clean home and personal items

After using Nix Creme Rinse, it is very important to clean personal items and your home to prevent the spread of lice. Nits may live away from the human head for about 7-12 days. Lice may live away from the human head for about 1 day.

- all personal head gear (hats, hair ribbons, etc.), scarves, coats, towels and bed linens should be washed in hot water (above 130°F), then dried in the dryer using the hottest cycle for at least 20 minutes
- personal combs, including nit combs, and brushes should be soaked in hot water (above 130°F) for at least 10 minutes
- personal articles such as clothing, bedspreads, blankets, pillows or stuffed animals that cannot be washed should be dry-cleaned or sealed tightly in a plastic bag for a period of at least 4 weeks. Items should be taken out of the plastic bag outdoors and shaken out very hard before using again.
- for anything you cannot wash, dry-clean or store in a plastic bag, spray with Nix Lice Control Spray.
- vacuum everywhere. Vacuum all carpets, mattresses, upholstered furniture and car seats that may have been used by infested household members.

WARNINGS
For external use only

DO NOT USE
- on children under 2 months of age
- near the eyes
- inside the nose, ear, mouth, or vagina
- on lice in eyebrows or eyelashes. See your doctor.

ASK A DOCTOR BEFORE USE IF YOU ARE
- allergic to ragweed. May cause breathing difficulty or an asthmatic episode.

WHEN USING THIS PRODUCT
- keep eyes tightly closed and protect eyes with a washcloth or towel
- if product gets into the eyes, immediately flush with large amounts of water
- scalp itching or redness may occur

STOP USE AND SEE A DOCTOR IF
- breathing difficulty occurs
- eye irritation occurs
- skin or scalp irritation continues or infection occurs

If pregnant or breast-feeding, ask a health professional before use.
Keep out of reach of children. If swallowed, get medical help or contact a Poison Control Center right away.

QUESTIONS OR COMMENTS?
call **1-888-LICE LINE (1-888-542-3546),**
Monday to Friday, 9 AM-5 PM EST
www.insightpharma.com
Distributed by:
INSIGHT Pharmaceuticals Corp.
Langhorne, PA 19049-1749
66623A

NIX LICE CONTROL SPRAY (permethrin)
Insight Pharmaceuticals, LLC

DIRECTIONS FOR USE
It is a violation of Federal law to use this product in a manner inconsistent with its labeling.
FOR USE IN NON-FOOD AREAS OF HOMES
INDOOR APPLICATION
Surface Spraying: To kill lice and louse eggs, spray in an inconspicuous area to test for possible staining or discoloration.

Inspect again after drying, then proceed to spray entire area to be treated. Spray from a distance of 8 to 10 inches. Treat only those garments and parts of bedding, including mattresses and furniture that cannot be either laundered or dry cleaned. Allow all treated articles to dry thoroughly before use.
To control bedbugs: Spray mattresses lightly, particularly around tufts and seams. Take beds apart and spray in all joints. Allow all sprayed articles to dry thoroughly before use.
Do not use in food/feed areas of food/feed handling establishments, restaurants or other areas where food/feed is commercially prepared or processed. Do not use in serving areas while food is exposed or facility is in operation. Serving areas are areas where prepared foods are served such as dining rooms, but excluding areas where foods may be prepared or held.
In the home, cover all food handling surfaces, cover or remove all food and cooking utensils or wash thoroughly after treatment.
Do not apply to classrooms while in use.
Not for Use in Federally Inspected Meat and Poultry Plants. Application is prohibited directly into sewers or drains, or into any area like a gutter where drainage to sewers, storms drains, water bodies, or aquatic habitat can occur. Do not allow the product to enter any drain during or after application.

QUESTIONS OR COMMENTS?
1-888-542-3546

OCCUFRESH (purified water)
Optics Laboratory, Inc

Active Ingredient(s) (in each ml)
PURIFIED WATER 99.1%

Purpose(s) Section
EYE WASHING

INDICATIONS AND USE SECTION
FOR CLEANING THE EYE TO HELP RELIEVE IRRITATION, DISCOMFORT, BURNING, STINGING, SMARTING OR ITCHING BY REMOVING LOOSE FOREIGN MATERIAL, AIR POLLUTANTS (SMOG OR POLLEN) OR CHLORINATED WATER

WARNINGS SECTION
TO AVOID CONTAMINATION, DO NOT TOUCH TIP OF CONTAINER TO ANY SURFACE. DO NOT REUSE. ONCE OPENED, DISCARD.
IF YOU EXPERIENCE EYE PAIN, CHANGES IN VISION, CONTINUED REDNESS OR IRRITATION OF THE EYE, OR IF THE CONDITION WORSENS OR PERSISTS CONSULT A DOCTOR.
OBTAIN IMMEDIATE MEDICAL TREATMENT FOR ALL OPEN WOUNDS IN OR NEAR THE EYES.
IF SOLUTION CHANGES COLOR OR BECOMES CLOUDY DO NOT USE.

DOSAGE AND ADMINISTRATION SECTION

DIRECTIONS
DO NOT DILUTE SOLUTION OR REUSE BOTTLE.

WITHOUT CUP: HOLD CONTAINER A FEW INCHES ABOVE THE EYE. CONTROL RATE OF FLOW BY PRESSURE ON BOTTLE. FLUSH AFFECTED AREA AS NEEDED.

WITH CUP: RINSE CUP WITH CLEAN WATER IMMEDIATELY BEFORE EACH USE. AVOID CONTAMINATION OF RIM AND INSIDE SURFACE OF CUP. FILL CUP WITH HALF FULL AND APPLY THE CUP TO THE AFFECTED EYE, PRESSING TIGHTLY TO PREVENT THE ESCAPE OF THE LIQUID AND TILT THE HEAD

BACKWARD. OPEN EYELIDS WIDE AND ROTATE THE EYEBALL TO ENSURE THOROUGH BATHING WITH THE WASH. RINSE CUP WITH CLEAN WATER AFTER EACH USE.

OTHER INFORMATION
STORE AT ROOM TEMPERATURE 15-30 DEGREES C (59-86 DEGREES F)

KEEP OUT OF REACH OF CHILDREN
KEEP OUT OF REACH OF CHILDREN. IF SWALLOWED, GET MEDICAL HELP OR CONTACT A POISON CONTROL CENTER RIGHT AWAY.

INACTIVE INGREDIENTS SECTION
sodium chloride 0.65%, sodium borate 0.02%, boric acid 0.32%

QUESTIONS OR COMMENTS?
800-966-6788

OCEAN FOR KIDS SALINE NASAL SPRAY
Valeant Consumer

USES
- To help relieve congestion by thinning mucus
- To soothe dry irritated nasal passages due to allergies, cold and flu
- To help reduce nosebleeds due to nasal dryness
- To return moisture lost to drug-induced dryness
- To moisturize and irrigate membranes following nasal surgery

THREE DELIVERY OPTIONS IN ONE BOTTLE
- Upright, the OCEAN® Nasal Spray bottle delivers a fine mist.
- Held horizontally, the bottle produces a stream.
- When held upside down the spray bottle delivers saline drops with a gentle squeeze.

INGREDIENTS
0.65% sodium chloride, purified water (USP), glycerin, phenylcarbinol, sodium phosphate monobasic, sodium hydroxide, benzalkonium chloride

DIRECTIONS
When held upright, the bottle delivers a fine mist. Held horizontally, the bottle produces a stream, and when held upside down, the bottle delivers drops of saline with a gentle squeeze. Drops are recommended for infants.

WARNINGS
- Sealed with printed neckband for your protection: use only if intact.
- The use of this dispenser by more than one person may spread infection.

QUESTIONS OR COMMENTS?
Call the OCEAN Hotline: 1-800-343-9497

OCEAN SALINE NASAL SPRAY
Valeant Consumer

USES
- For nasal dryness due to allergies, cold, flu, rhinitis, and sinusitis
- To help relieve congestion by thinning mucus
- To return moisture caused by drug-induced dryness
- To help reduce nosebleeds from dryness

- To moisturize and irrigate membranes following nasal surgery
- To relieve dryness associated with oxygen treatments and CPAP machines for sleep apnea
- For general moisturizing in dry, cold climates
- To moisturize the nose while spending time in an encloses spaces such as during air travel

INGREDIENTS
0.65% sodium chloride saline solution made isotonic (0.9%) by the addition of preservative systems and buffers, which reduce nasal irritation. Contains benzyl alcohol and benzalkonium chloride as preservatives.

DIRECTIONS
For children and adults, squeeze bottle twice in each nostril as often as needed or as directed by physician. For infants, use drop application. Hold bottle upright for spray, horizontally for stream, upside down for drop.

WARNINGS
- Sealed with printed neckband for your protection: use only if intact.
- The use of this dispenser by more than one person may spread infection.

QUESTIONS OR COMMENTS?
Call the OCEAN Hotline: 1-800-343-9497

OCEAN GEL NASAL MOISTURIZER
Valeant Consumer

USES
- To soothe dry skin in and around the nose
- To relieve dryness associated with oxygen treatments and CPAP machines for sleep apnea
- For moisturizing the sensitive areas where dryness occurs more frequently (i.e., elbows, knuckles)
- To help retain moisture longer for enhanced nasal dryness relief
- For extra moisturizing in dry, cold climates

INGREDIENTS
purified water, glycerin, carbomer 940, trolamine, hyaluronan, methylparaben, propylparaben

DIRECTIONS
Apply to the affected areas in and around the nose. Re-apply as often as necessary.

WARNINGS
- Do not use if foil safety seal under cap is broken or missing.
- For topical use only.

QUESTIONS OR COMMENTS?
Call the OCEAN Hotline: 1-800-343-9497

OPCON-A (naphazoline hydrochloride and pheniramine maleate)
Bausch & Lomb Incorporated

Active Ingredient(s)
Naphazoline HCl (0.02675%)
Pheniramine maleate (0.315%)

Purpose(s)
Redness reliever
Antihistamine

USES
- temporarily relieves itching and redness caused by pollen, ragweed, grass, animal hair and dander.

WARNINGS

DO NOT USE
- if you are sensitive to any ingredient in this product
- if solution changes color or becomes cloudy

ASK A DOCTOR BEFORE USE IF YOU HAVE
- heart disease
- high blood pressure
- trouble urinating due to an enlarged prostate gland
- narrow angle glaucoma

WHEN USING THIS PRODUCT
- overuse may cause more eye redness
- pupils may become enlarged temporarily
- do not touch tip of container to any surface to avoid contamination
- you may feel a brief tingling after putting drops in eye
- replace cap after use
- remove contact lenses before using

STOP USE AND ASK A DOCTOR IF YOU EXPERIENCE
- eye pain
- changes in vision
- redness or irritation of the eye that worsens or lasts more than 72 hours.

Keep out of reach of children.
If swallowed, get medical help or contact a Poison Control Center right away. Accidental oral ingestion in infants and children may lead to coma and marked reduction in body temperature.

DIRECTIONS
- **Adults and children 6 years of age and older:** Instill 1 or 2 drops in the affected eye(s) up to 4 times daily.
- **Children under 6 years:** ask a doctor

OTHER INFORMATION
- store at 20°-25°C (68°-77°F)
- protect from light
- use before expiration date marked on the carton or bottle

INACTIVE INGREDIENTS
benzalkonium chloride, boric acid, edetate disodium, hypromellose, purified water, sodium borate, sodium chloride

QUESTIONS OR COMMENTS?
Call: 1-800-553-5340

COLGATE ORABASE (benzocaine)
Colgate Oral Pharmaceuticals, Inc.

DRUG FACTS

Active Ingredient(s)
Benzocaine 20%

Purpose(s)
Oral pain reliever

USE
for the temporary relief of pain associated with canker sores, due to minor irritation or injury of the mouth and gums, or due to minor irritation of the mouth and gums caused by dentures or orthodontic appliances

WARNINGS

DO NOT USE
- for more than 7 days unless directed by a dentist or physician
- if you have a history of allergy to local anesthetics such as procaine, butacaine, benzocaine, or other "caine" anesthetics

WHEN USING THIS PRODUCT
- do not exceed recommended dosage
- avoid contact with eyes
- localized allergic reactions may occur after prolonged or repeated use

STOP USE AND ASK A DOCTOR IF
- sore mouth symptoms do not improve in 7 days
- swelling, rash or fever develops
- irritation, pain or redness persists or worsens

Keep out of reach of children. If more than used for pain relief is accidentally swallowed, get medical help or contact a Poison Control Center immediately.

DIRECTIONS
- adults and children 2 years and older: gently dab paste on the site of irritation with a cotton swab or fingertip
- allow to remain in place at least 1 minute and then spit out
- use up to 4 times daily or as directed by a dentist or physician
- children under 12 years of age should be supervised in the use of the product
- children under 2 years of age: consult a dentist or physician

OTHER INFORMATION
store at controlled room temperature, 68-77°F (20-25°C)

INACTIVE INGREDIENTS
butylparaben, cellulose gum, ethylparaben, flavor, methylparaben, mineral oil, pectin, polyethylene, propylparaben, xanthan gum

QUESTIONS OR COMMENTS?
call toll free **1-800-962-2345**

ORAJEL ANTISEPTIC RINSE FOR MOUTH SORES (hydrogen peroxide)
Church & Dwight Co., Inc.

Active ingredient(s) Purpose(s)
hydrogen peroxide 1.5% Oral debriding agent

USES
for temporary use in cleansing minor wounds or minor gum inflammation resulting form:
minor dental procedures accidental injury
orthodontic appliances canker sores
dentures other irritations of the mouth and gumsAids in the removal of phlegm, mucus, other secretions associated with occasional sore mouth

WARNINGS

DO NOT USE
this product for more than 7 days unless directed by a dentist or doctor

WHEN USING THIS PRODUCT
do not swallow

STOP USE AND SEE YOUR DENTIST OR DOCTOR PROMPTLY IF
swelling, rash or fever develops; irritations, pain or redness persists or worsens; sore mouth symptoms do not improve in 7 days
Keep out of reach of children. in case of overdose or allergic reaction, get medical help or contact a Poison Control Center right away

DIRECTIONS
- remove imprinted safety seal from bottle cap; to remove child-resistant cap, squeeze smooth sides of cap while turning.
- Reclose tightly.
- Ready to use, no mixing needed
- Adults and children 2 years of age and older: Swish one-half capful (2 teaspoons-10mL) around the mouth over the affected area for at least 1 minute and then spit out.
- Use up to 4 times daily after meals and at bedtime or as directed by a dentist or doctor
- Children under 12 year of age: Should be supervised in the use of this product
- Children under 2 years of age: Consult a dentist or doctor

OTHER INFORMATION
cap tightly; keep away from heat or direct sunlight; do not use if safety seal is broken or missing

INACTIVE INGREDIENTS
alcohol (4.1% by volume), blue 1, disodium EDTA, methylparaben, methyl salicylate, phosphoric acid, poloxamer 338, purified water, sodium saccharin, sorbitol

QUESTIONS OR COMMENTS?
call us at **1-800-952-5080** M-F 9am-5pm ET or visit our website at www.orajel.com

ORAJEL FILM-FORMING CANKER SORE GEL
(benzocaine and menthol)
Church & Dwight Co. Inc.

DRUG FACTS

Active Ingredient(s)	Purpose(s)
Benzocaine 15%	Oral pain reliever
Menthol 2%	Oral pain reliever

USE
for the temporary relief of pain associated with • minor irritation or injury of the mouth and gums • canker sores

WARNINGS
Allergy alert: do not use this product if you have a history of allergy to local anesthetics such as procaine, butacaine, benzocaine, or other "caine" anesthetics
Flammable: keep away from fire or flame. Avoid smoking during the application and until product has dried.

DO NOT USE
• more than directed • for more than 7 days unless directed by a dentist or doctor

STOP USE AND ASK A DOCTOR IF
• sore mouth symptoms do not improve in 7 days • swelling, rash or fever develops • irritation, pain, or redness persists or worsens
Keep out of reach of children. In case of overdose or allergic reaction, get medical help or contact a Poison Control Center right away.

DIRECTIONS
• cut open tip of tube on score mark • do not use if tube tip is cut prior to opening
• do not peel off protective film • use up to 4 times daily or as directed by a dentist or doctor

Adults and children 2 years of age and over	Dry affected area. Apply with cotton swab or finger. Allow gel to dry for 30-60 seconds into protective film.
Children under 12 years of age	Should be supervised in the use of this product
Children under 2 years of age	Ask a dentist or doctor

INACTIVE INGREDIENTS
acesulfame potassium, alcohol (76.4% by volume), ethylcellulose, flavor, polycarbophil, water

QUESTIONS OR COMMENTS?
call us at **1-800-952-5080** M-F 9am-5pm ET or visit our website at www.orajel.com

ORAJEL FOR ALL MOUTH SORES MAXIMUM STRENGTH (benzocaine)
Church & Dwight Co., Inc.

Active Ingredient(s)
Benzocaine 20%

Purpose(s)
Oral Pain Reliever

USES
for the temporary relief of pain associated with canker sores, cold sores, fever blisters minor irritation or injury of the mouth and gums

WARNINGS
Allergy Alert
do not use this product if your have a history of allergy to local anesthetics such as procaine, butacaine, benzocaine or other "caine" anesthetics

DO NOT USE
more than directed, for more than 7 days unless told to do so by a dentist or doctor

STOP USE AND ASK A DENTIST OF DOCTOR IF
sore mouth symptoms do not get better in 7 days; swelling, rash or fever develops; irritation, pain or redness does not go away

Keep out of reach of children. in case of overdose or allergic reaction, get medical help or contact a Poison Control Center right away

DIRECTIONS
Adults and Children Hold swab with solid white tip down
2 years of age and older Bend and snap open swab tip with the colored rings
Apply product to affected area
Use up to 4 times daily or as directed by a dentist or doctor

OTHER INFORMATION
do not use if label seal is broken prior to purchase, or if colored rings on tip are not orange

INACTIVE INGREDIENTS
flavor, polyethylene glycol, purified water, red 40, sodium
saccharin, yellow 5

QUESTIONS OR COMMENTS?
call us at **1-800-952-5080** M-F 9am-5pm ET or visit our website
at www.orajel.com

ORAJEL MOUTH SORE GEL (benzalkonium
chloride, benzocaine, and zinc chloride)
Church & Dwight Co., Inc.

DRUG FACTS

Active Ingredient(s)	Purpose(s)
Benzalkonium chloride 0.02%	Oral antiseptic
Benzocaine 20%	Oral pain reliever
Zinc chloride 0.1%	Oral astringent

USES
for the temporary relief of pain associated with • canker sores •
cold sores • fever blisters • minor irritation or injury of the
mouth and gums. To help protect against infection in minor oral
irritation.

WARNINGS
Allergy alert: do not use this product if you have a history of
allergy to local anesthetics such as procaine, butacaine,
benzocaine or other "caine" anesthetics

DO NOT USE
• more than directed • for more than 7 days unless directed by
a dentist or doctor

STOP USE AND ASK A DOCTOR IF
• sore mouth symptoms do not improve in 7 days • swelling,
rash or fever develops • irritation, pain or redness persists or
worsens
Keep out of reach of children.
In case of overdose or allergic reaction, get medical help or
contact a Poison Control Center right away

DIRECTIONS
• cut open tip of tube on score mark • do not use if tube tip is
cut prior to opening

Adults and children 2 years of age and over	Apply to affected area up to 4 times daily or as directed by a dentist or doctor
Children under 12 years of age	Should be supervised in the use of this product
Children under 2 years of age	Ask a dentist or doctor

INACTIVE INGREDIENTS
allantoin, carbomer, edetate disodium, mentha piperota
(peppermint) oil, polyethylene glycol, polysorbate 60, propylene
glycol, propyl gallate, water, pvp, sodium saccharin, sorbic acid,
stearyl alcohol

QUESTIONS OR COMMENTS?
call us at **1-800-952-5080** M-F 9am-5pm ET or visit our website
at **www.orajel.com**

PAMPRIN MAX MENSTRUAL PAIN RELIEF
(acetaminophen, aspirin, and caffeine)
Chattem, Inc.

DRUG FACTS

Active Ingredient(s)
(in each caplet)
Acetaminophen 250 mg
Aspirin 250 mg (NSAID*)

Purpose(s)
Pain reliever

Active Ingredient(s)
(in each caplet)
Caffeine 65 mg

Purpose(s)
Diuretic
*nonsteroidal anti-inflammatory drug

USES
for the temporary relief of these symptoms associated with
menstrual periods:
• cramps
• headache
• backache
• fatigue
• bloating

WARNINGS
Reye's syndrome: Children and teenagers who have or are
recovering from chicken pox or flu-like symptoms should not use
this product. When using this product, if changes in behavior
with nausea and vomiting occur, consult a doctor because these
symptoms could be an early sign of Reye's syndrome, a rare but
serious illness.
Allergy alert: Aspirin may cause a severe allergic reaction
which may include:
• hives
• facial swelling
• asthma (wheezing)
• shock

Liver warning: This product contains acetaminophen. Severe
liver damage may occur if you take
• more than 8 caplets in 24 hours, which is the maximum daily
amount
• with other drugs containing acetaminophen
• 3 or more alcoholic drinks every day while using this product

Stomach bleeding warning: This product contains an NSAID,
which may cause severe stomach bleeding. The chance is higher
if you
• are age 60 or older
• have had stomach ulcers or bleeding problems
• take a blood thinning (anticoagulant) or steroid drug
• take other drugs containing prescription or nonprescription
NSAIDs [aspirin, ibuprofen, naproxen, or others]
• have 3 or more alcoholic drinks every day while using this
product
• take more or for a longer time than directed

Caffeine warning: The recommended dose of this product
contains about as much caffeine as a cup of coffee. Limit the use
of caffeine-containing medications, foods, or beverages while
taking this product because too much caffeine may cause
nervousness, irritability, sleeplessness, and occasionally, rapid
heartbeat.

DO NOT USE
• if you are allergic to aspirin or any other pain reliever/fever
reducer

- with any other drug containing acetaminophen (prescription or nonprescription). If you are not sure whether a drug contains acetaminophen, ask a doctor or pharmacist.

ASK A DOCTOR BEFORE USE IF
- you have liver disease
- the stomach bleeding warning applies to you
- you have a history of stomach problems, such as heartburn
- you have high blood pressure, heart disease, liver cirrhosis, or kidney disease
- you are taking a diuretic

ASK A DOCTOR OR PHARMACIST BEFORE USE
if you are taking a prescription drug for gout, diabetes or arthritis

STOP USE AND ASK A DOCTOR IF
- an allergic reaction occurs. Seek medical help right away.
- you experience any of the following signs of stomach bleeding:
  - feel faint
  - vomit blood
  - have bloody or black stools
  - have stomach pain that does not get better
- redness or swelling is present
- new symptoms occur
- pain gets worse or lasts more than 10 days
- fever gets worse or lasts more than 3 days
- ringing in the ears or loss of hearing occurs

If pregnant or breast-feeding,
ask a health professional before use. It is especially important not to use aspirin during the last 3 months of pregnancy unless definitely directed to do so by a doctor because it may cause problems in the unborn child or complications during delivery.

Keep out of reach of children.
In case of overdose, get medical help or contact a Poison Control Center right away. Quick medical attention is critical for adults as well as for children even if you do not notice any signs or symptoms.

DIRECTIONS
adults and children 12 years and over:
- take 2 caplets with water every 6 hours as needed
- do not exceed 8 caplets in a 24 hour period or as directed by a doctor
- do not use more than directed (see warnings)
children under 12 years: ask a doctor

INACTIVE INGREDIENTS
D&C red no. 27 lake, FD&C red no. 40 lake, fractionated coconut oil, hypromellose, maltodextrin, microcrystalline cellulose, polydextrose, polyvinylpyrrolidone, pregelatinized starch, silica, sodium starch glycolate, starch, stearic acid, talc, titanium dioxide (245-171)

PAMPRIN MULTISYMPTOM MENSTRUAL PAIN RELIEF (acetaminophen, pamabrom, and pyrilamine maleate)

Chattem, Inc.

DRUG FACTS

Active Ingredient(s)
(in each caplet)
Acetaminophen 500 mg

Purpose(s)
Pain reliever

Active Ingredient(s)
(in each caplet)
Pamabrom 25 mg

Purpose(s)
Diuretic

Active Ingredient(s)
(in each caplet)
Pyrilamine maleate 15 mg

Purpose(s)
Antihistamine

USES
for the temporary relief of these symptoms associated with menstrual periods:
- cramps
- headache
- bloating
- backache
- water-weight gain
- muscular aches
- irritability

WARNINGS
Liver warning: This product contains acetaminophen. Severe liver damage may occur if you take
- more than 8 caplets in 24 hours, which is the maximum daily amount
- with other drugs containing acetaminophen
- 3 or more alcoholic drinks every day while using this product

DO NOT USE
with any other drug containing acetaminophen (prescription or nonprescription). If you are not sure whether a drug contains acetaminophen, ask a doctor or pharmacist.

ASK A DOCTOR BEFORE USE IF
you have
- liver disease
- glaucoma
- a breathing problem such as emphysema or chronic bronchitis
- difficulty in urination due to enlargement of the prostate gland

ASK A DOCTOR OR PHARMACIST BEFORE USE
if you are
- taking the blood thinning drug warfarin
- taking sedatives or tranquilizers

WHEN USING THIS PRODUCT
- you may get drowsy, avoid alcoholic beverages
- alcohol, sedatives and tranquilizers may increase drowsiness
- use caution when driving or operating machinery
- excitability may occur, especially in children

STOP USE AND ASK A DOCTOR IF
- pain gets worse or lasts for more than 10 days
- fever gets worse or lasts for more than 3 days
- new symptoms occur
- redness or swelling is present

If pregnant or breast-feeding,
ask a health professional before use.

Keep out of reach of children.
In case of overdose, get medical help or contact a Poison Control Center right away. Quick medical attention is critical for adults as well as for children even if you do not notice any signs or symptoms.

DIRECTIONS
adults and children 12 years and over:
- take 2 caplets with water every 6 hours as needed
- do not exceed 8 caplets in a 24 hour period or as directed by a doctor
- do not use more than directed (see warnings)
children under 12 years: ask a doctor

INACTIVE INGREDIENTS
crospovidone, magnesium stearate, povidone, pregelatinized starch, sodium starch glycolate, stearic acid (224-186)

PEDIACARE CHILDREN 24 HOUR ALLERGY
(cetirizine hydrochloride)
Blacksmith Brands, Inc.

DRUG FACTS

Active Ingredient(s) (in each 5 mL)	Purpose(s)
Cetirizine hydrochloride 5 mg	Antihistamine

USES
Temporarily Relieves
- Sneezing
- Itchy, watery eyes
- Runny nose
- Itchy throat or nose

WARNINGS

DO NOT USE
- If you have ever had an allergic reaction to this product or any of its ingredients or to an antihistamine containing hydroxyzine

ASK A DOCTOR IF THE CHILD HAS
- **Liver or kidney disease. Your doctor should determine if you need a different dose.**

ASK A DOCTOR OR A PHARMACIST BEFORE USE
- If the child is taking sedatives or tranquilizers

WHEN USING THIS PRODUCT
- Drowsiness may occur
- Avoid alcoholic drinks
- Alcohol, sedatives, and tranquilizers may increase drowsiness
- Be careful when driving a motor vehicle or operating machinery

STOP USE AND ASK A DOCTOR IF
- An allergic reaction to this product occurs. Seek medical help right away.

If Pregnant or breast-feeding:
- If breast-feeding: not recommended
- If pregnant: ask a health professional before use

Keep this and all drugs out of reach of children.
In case of overdose, get medical help or contact a Poison Control Center (1-800-222-1222) right away.

DIRECTIONS
- Find right dosage on the chart. **Use age to dose.**
- **Use only enclosed dosing cup designed for use with this product.** Do not use any other dosing device.
- Take once daily.
- Do not take more than recommended dose on package.

Weight (lbs)	Age (yrs)	Dose (mL)
(n/a)	Children under 2 years of age	Ask a doctor
(n/a)	Children 2 to under 6 years of age	2.5 mL once daily. If needed, dose can be increased to a maximum of 5 mL once daily or 2.5 mL every 12 hours. Do not give more than 5 mL in 24 hours.
(n/a)	Adults and children 6 years and over	5 mL or 10 mL once daily depending on severity of symptoms; do not take more than 10 mL in 24 hours.
(n/a)	Adults 65 years and older	5 mL once daily; do not take more than 5 mL in 24 hours.
(n/a)	**Consumers with liver or kidney disease**	Ask a doctor.

INACTIVE INGREDIENTS
artificial grape flavor, glacial acetic acid, glycerin, methylparaben, natural and artificial banana flavor, propylene glycol, propylparaben, purified water, sodium acetate (anhydrous), sucrose

QUESTIONS OR COMMENTS?
Call **1-888-474-3099** or email customerService@pediacare.com

PEDIACARE CHILDREN'S ALLERGY
(diphenhydramine HCl)
Blacksmith Brands, Inc.

PediaCare Children's Allergy Cherry Flavor

DRUG FACTS
Active Ingredient(s)
(in each 5 mL)*
Diphenhydramine HCl 12.5 mg

Purpose(s)
Antihistamine/cough suppressant
*5 mL = one teaspoon

USES
- temporarily relieves these symptoms due to hay fever or other upper respiratory allergies:
- runny nose
- sneezing
- itchy, watery eyes
- temporarily relieves cough due to inhaled irritants

WARNINGS

DO NOT USE
- to make a child sleepy
- with any other product containing diphenhydramine, even one used on skin

ASK A DOCTOR BEFORE USE IF THE CHILD HAS
- persistent or chronic cough such as occurs with asthma
- cough accompanied by excessive phlegm (mucus)
- a breathing problem such as chronic bronchitis
- glaucoma

ASK A DOCTOR OR PHARMACIST BEFORE USE
if the child is taking sedatives or tranquilizers

WHEN USING THIS PRODUCT
- excitability may occur, especially in children
- marked drowsiness may occur
- sedatives and tranquilizers may increase drowsiness

STOP USE AND ASK A DOCTOR IF
- cough gets worse or lasts for more than 7 days
- cough tends to come back or occurs with fever, rash or headache that lasts

These could be signs of a serious condition.

Keep out of reach of children
In case of overdose, get medical help or contact a Poison Control Center right away. (1-800-222-1222)

DIRECTIONS
- find right dose on chart below
- use only enclosed dosing cup designed for use with this product. Do not use any other dosing device.
- if needed, repeat dose every 4 hours
- do not use more than 6 times in 24 hours

Age (yr)	Dose (tsp)
Under 4 years	Do not use
4 to 5 years	Do not use unless directed by a doctor
6 to 11 years	1 teaspoonful

Attention: use only enclosed dosing cup specifically designed for use with this product. Do not use any other dosing device.

OTHER INFORMATION
- each teaspoon contains: **sodium 14 mg**
- store between 20-25°C (68-77°F). Protect from light. Store in outer carton until contents used.
- **do not use if bottle wrap, or foil inner seal imprinted "Safety Seal®" is broken or missing**
- see bottom panel for lot number and expiration date

INACTIVE INGREDIENTS
anhydrous citric acid, D&C red #33, FD&C red #40, flavors, glycerin, monoammonium glycyrrhizinate, poloxamer 407, purified water, sodium benzoate, sodium chloride, sodium citrate, sucrose

QUESTIONS OR COMMENTS?
call **1-888-474-3099**

PediaCare Children's Allergy Bubblegum Flavor

DRUG FACTS

Active Ingredient(s)
(in each 5 mL, 1 teaspoon)
Diphenhydramine HCl 12.5 mg

Purpose(s)
Antihistamine

USES
temporarily relieves these symptoms due to hay fever or other upper respiratory allergies:
- runny nose
- sneezing
- itchy, watery eyes
- itching of the nose or throat

WARNINGS

DO NOT USE
- to make a child sleepy
- with any other product containing diphenhydramine, even one used on skin

ASK A DOCTOR BEFORE USE IF THE CHILD HAS
- glaucoma
- a breathing problem such as chronic bronchitis

ASK A DOCTOR OR PHARMACIST BEFORE USE
if the child is taking sedatives or tranquilizers

WHEN USING THIS PRODUCT
- marked drowsiness may occur
- sedatives and tranquilizers may increase drowsiness
- excitability may occur, especially in children

Keep out of reach of children
In case of overdose, seek professional assistance or contact a Poison Control Center (1-800-222-1222) immediately.

DIRECTIONS
- use only enclosed dosing cup designed for use with this product. Do not use any other dosing device.
- take every 4 to 6 hours
- do not take more than 6 doses in 24 hours
- tsp = teaspoon, mL = milliliter, mg = milligram

Age (yr)	Dose (tsp)
children 6 to 11 years	1 to 2 teaspoonfuls (5 mL to 10 mL)
children 4 to 5 years	Do not use unless directed by a doctor
children under 4 years	do not use

OTHER INFORMATION
- **each teaspoon contains:** sodium 6 mg
- store at room temperature

INACTIVE INGREDIENTS
citric acid, flavors, glycerin, poloxamer 407, purified water, red 33, red 40, sodium benzoate, sodium chloride, sodium citrate, sugar

QUESTIONS OR COMMENTS?
call **1-888-474-3099**

PEDIACARE CHILDREN'S COUGH & CONGESTION (NO ACETAMINOPHEN)
(dextromethorphan and guaifenesin)
Blacksmith Brands, Inc.

DRUG FACTS

Active Ingredient(s) (in each 5 mL)	Purpose(s)
Dextromethorphan HBr, USP 5 mg	Cough suppressant
Guaifenesin USP 100 mg	Expectorant

USES
Temporarily Relieves
- Cough
- Chest congestion
- Mucus

WARNINGS

DO NOT USE
- In a child who is taking a prescription monoamine oxidase inhibitor (MAOI) (certain drugs for depression, psychiatric or emotional conditions, or Parkinson's disease) or for 2 weeks after stopping the MAOI drug. If you do not know if your child's prescription drug contains an MAOI, ask a doctor or pharmacist before giving this product.

ASK A DOCTOR BEFORE USE IF YOUR CHILD HAS
- A cough accompanied by excessive phlegm (mucus)
- A persistent or chronic cough such as occurs with asthma or chronic bronchitis

WHEN USING THIS PRODUCT
Do not use more than directed.

STOP USE AND ASK A DOCTOR IF
- Cough gets worse or lasts more than 7 days
- Cough comes back or occurs with fever

These could be signs of a serious illness.
Keep this and all drugs out of reach of children.
In case of accidental overdose, seek professional assistance or contact a Poison Control Center immediately (1-800-222-1222)

DIRECTIONS
- Find right dosage on the chart. **If possible, use weight to dose; otherwise, use age.**
- Do not use more than 6 times in 24 hours.
- Use only enclosed dosing cup specifically designed for use with this product. Do not use any other dosing device.

Weight (lbs)	Age (yrs)	Dose (mL)
Under 36	Under 4	Do not use
36-47	4 - 6	2.5-5
48-95	6-11	5-10

INACTIVE INGREDIENTS
citric acid anhydrous, dextrose, flavors, glycerin, methyl paraben, potassium sorbate, propylene glycol, propyl paraben, purified water, red 33, red 40, saccharin sodium, sodium hydroxide, sucralose, xanthan gum

QUESTIONS OR COMMENTS?
Call **1-888-474-3099** or email CustomerService@pediacare.com

PEDIACARE CHILDREN'S FEVER REDUCER PLUS COUGH & RUNNY NOSE WITH ACETAMINOPHEN (acetaminophen, chlorpheniramine, and dextromethorphan)
Blacksmith Brands, Inc.

DRUG FACTS

Active Ingredient(s) (in each 5 mL)	Purpose(s)
Acetaminophen 160 mg	Pain reliever/fever reducer
Chlorpheniramine maleate 1 mg	Antihistamine
Dextromethorphan HBr 5 mg	Cough suppressant

USES
Temporarily Relieves
- Minor aches and pains
- Cough
- Headache
- Sore throat
- Sneezing and runny nose
- Fever

WARNINGS
Liver warning
This product contains acetaminophen. Severe liver damage may occur if your child takes:
- More than 5 doses in 24 hours, which is the maximum daily amount.

Sore throat warning
- If sore throat is severe, persists for more than 2 days, or is accompanied or followed by fever, headache, rash, nausea or vomiting, consult a doctor promptly.

DO NOT USE
- To make a child sleepy.
- In a child who is taking a prescription monoamine oxidase inhibitor (MAOI) (certain drugs for depression, psychiatric or emotional conditions, or Parkinson's disease) or for 2 weeks after stopping the MAOI drug. If you do not know if your child's prescription drug contains an MAOI, ask a doctor or pharmacist before giving this product.
- With any other drug containing acetaminophen (prescription or nonprescription). If you are not sure whether a drug contains acetaminophen, ask a doctor or pharmacist.

ASK A DOCTOR BEFORE USE IF YOUR CHILD HAS
- Glaucoma
- A breathing problem such as chronic bronchitis
- Cough that occurs with too much phlegm (mucus)
- Persistent or chronic cough such as occurs with asthma
- Liver disease

ASK A DOCTOR OR A PHARMACIST BEFORE USE IF YOUR CHILD IS TAKING
- Sedatives or tranquilizers
- The blood-thinning drug warfarin

WHEN USING THIS PRODUCT
- **Do not exceed recommended dose (see overdose warning)**
- May cause excitability, especially in children
- Marked drowsiness may occur
- Sedatives and tranquilizers may increase drowsiness

STOP USE AND ASK A DOCTOR IF
- New symptoms occur
- Fever gets worse or lasts for more than 3 days
- Redness or swelling is present
- Pain, nasal congestion or cough gets worse or lasts for more than 5 days
- Cough comes back or occurs with rash or headache that lasts

These could be signs of a serious condition.
Keep this and all drugs out of reach of children.

OVERDOSE WARNING
Taking more than the recommended dose (overdose) could cause major health problems, including liver damage. In case of accidental overdose, seek professional assistance or contact a Poison Control Center immediately (1-800-222-1222). Quick medical attention is critical even if you do not notice any signs or symptoms.

DIRECTIONS
- Find right dosage on the chart. **If possible, use weight to dose; otherwise, use age.**
- Shake well before using.
- If needed, repeat dose every 4 hours while symptoms last.
- Do not use more than 5 times in 24 hours.

Weight (lbs)	Age (yrs)	Dose (mL)
Under 36	Under 4	Do not use
36-47	4 - 5	Do not use unless directed by a doctor
48-95	6-11	10

INACTIVE INGREDIENTS
acesulfame potassium, carboxymethylcellulose sodium, cellulose, citric acid, flavors, glycerin, high-fructose corn syrup, purified water, red 33, red 40, sodium benzoate, sorbitol, xanthan gum

QUESTIONS OR COMMENTS?
Call **1-888-474-3099** or email CustomerService@pediacare.com

PEDIACARE CHILDREN'S FEVER REDUCER PLUS COUGH & SORE THROAT WITH ACETAMINOPHEN (acetaminophen and dextromethorphan)

Blacksmith Brands, Inc.

DRUG FACTS

Active Ingredient(s) (in each 5 mL)	Purpose(s)
Acetaminophen 160 mg	Pain reliever/fever reducer
Dextromethorphan HBr 5 mg	Cough suppressant

USES
Temporarily Relieves
- Minor aches and pains
- Cough
- Headache
- Sore throat
- Fever

WARNINGS
Liver warning
This product contains acetaminophen. Severe liver damage may occur if your child takes:
- More than 5 doses in 24 hours, which is the maximum daily amount.

Sore throat warning
- If sore throat is severe, persists for more than 2 days, or is accompanied or followed by fever, headache, rash, nausea or vomiting, consult a doctor promptly.

DO NOT USE
- To make a child sleepy.
- In a child who is taking a prescription monoamine oxidase inhibitor (MAOI) (certain drugs for depression, psychiatric or emotional conditions, or Parkinson's disease) or for 2 weeks after stopping the MAOI drug. If you do not know if your child's prescription drug contains an MAOI, ask a doctor or pharmacist before giving this product.
- With any other drug containing acetaminophen (prescription or nonprescription). If you are not sure whether a drug contains acetaminophen, ask a doctor or pharmacist.

ASK A DOCTOR BEFORE USE IF YOUR CHILD HAS
- Glaucoma
- Cough that occurs with too much phlegm (mucus)
- Persistent or chronic cough such as occurs with asthma
- Liver disease

ASK A DOCTOR OR A PHARMACIST BEFORE USE IF YOUR CHILD IS TAKING
- The blood-thinning drug warfarin

WHEN USING THIS PRODUCT
- **Do not exceed recommended dose (see overdose warning)**
- May cause excitability, especially in children
- Marked drowsiness may occur
- Sedatives and tranquilizers may increase drowsiness

STOP USE AND ASK A DOCTOR IF
- New symptoms occur
- Fever gets worse or lasts for more than 3 days
- Redness or swelling is present
- Pain, nasal congestion or cough gets worse or lasts for more than 5 days
- Cough comes back or occurs with rash or headache that lasts

These could be signs of a serious condition.
Keep this and all drugs out of reach of children.

OVERDOSE WARNING
Taking more than the recommended dose (overdose) could cause major health problems, including liver damage. In case of accidental overdose, seek professional assistance or contact a Poison Control Center immediately (1-800-222-1222). Quick medical attention is critical even if you do not notice any signs or symptoms.

DIRECTIONS
- Find right dosage on the chart. **If possible, use weight to dose; otherwise, use age.**
- Shake well before using
- If needed, repeat dose every 4 hours while symptoms last.
- Do not use more than 5 times in 24 hours.

Weight (lbs)	Age (yrs)	Dose (mL)
Under 36	Under 4	Do not use
36-47	4 - 5	Do not use unless directed by a doctor
48-95	6-11	10

INACTIVE INGREDIENTS
acesulfame potassium, carboxymethylcellulose sodium, cellulose, citric acid, flavors, glycerin, high-fructose corn syrup, purified water, red 33, red 40, sodium benzoate, sorbitol, xanthan gum

QUESTIONS OR COMMENTS?
Call 1-888-474-3099 or email CustomerService@pediacare.com

PEDIACARE CHILDREN'S FEVER REDUCER PLUS FLU WITH ACETAMINOPHEN

(acetaminophen, chlorpheniramine, dextromethorphan, and phenylephrine)

Blacksmith Brands, Inc.

DRUG FACTS

Active Ingredient(s) (in each 5 mL)	Purpose(s)
Acetaminophen 160 mg	Pain reliever/Fever reducer
Chlorpheniramine maleate 1 mg	Antihistamine
Dextromethorphan HBr 5 mg	Cough suppressant
Phenylephrine HCl 2.5 mg	Nasal decongestant

USES

Temporarily Relieves
- Minor aches and pains
- Cough
- Headache
- Sore throat
- Sneezing and runny nose
- Stuffy nose
- Fever

WARNINGS

Liver warning

This product contains acetaminophen. Severe liver damage may occur if your child takes:
- More than 5 doses in 24 hours, which is the maximum daily amount.

Sore throat warning
- If sore throat is severe, persists for more than 2 days, or is accompanied or followed by fever, headache, rash, nausea or vomiting, consult a doctor promptly.

DO NOT USE
- To make a child sleepy.
- In a child who is taking a prescription monoamine oxidase inhibitor (MAOI) (certain drugs for depression, psychiatric or emotional conditions, or Parkinson's disease) or for 2 weeks after stopping the MAOI drug. If you do not know if your child's prescription drug contains an MAOI, ask a doctor or pharmacist before giving this product.
- With any other drug containing acetaminophen (prescription or nonprescription). If you are not sure whether a drug contains acetaminophen, ask a doctor or pharmacist.

ASK A DOCTOR BEFORE USE IF YOUR CHILD HAS
- Glaucoma
- Thyroid disease
- Diabetes
- High blood pressure
- Heart disease
- A breathing problem such as chronic bronchitis
- Cough that occurs with too much phlegm (mucus)
- Persistent or chronic cough such as occurs with asthma
- Liver disease

ASK A DOCTOR OR A PHARMACIST BEFORE USE IF YOUR CHILD IS TAKING
- Sedatives or tranquilizers
- The blood-thinning drug warfarin

WHEN USING THIS PRODUCT
- May cause excitability, especially in children
- Marked drowsiness may occur
- Sedatives and tranquilizers may increase drowsiness

STOP USE AND ASK A DOCTOR IF
- New symptoms occur
- Nervousness, dizziness or sleeplessness occur
- Fever gets worse or lasts for more than 3 days
- Redness or swelling is present
- Pain, nasal congestion or cough gets worse or lasts for more than 5 days
- Cough comes back or occurs with rash or headache that lasts

These could be signs of a serious condition.
Keep this and all drugs out of reach of children.

OVERDOSE WARNING

Taking more than the recommended dose (overdose) could cause major health problems, including liver damage. In case of accidental overdose, seek professional assistance or contact a Poison Control Center immediately (1-800-222-1222). Quick medical attention is critical even if you do not notice any signs or symptoms.

DIRECTIONS
- Find right dosage on the chart. **If possible, use weight to dose; otherwise, use age.**
- Shake well before using.
- If needed, repeat dose every 4 hours while symptoms last.
- Do not use more than 5 times in 24 hours.

Weight (lbs)	Age (yrs)	Dose (mL)
Under 36	Under 4	Do not use
36-47	4 - 5	Do not use unless directed by a doctor
48-95	6-11	10

INACTIVE INGREDIENTS

carboxymethylcellulose sodium, cellulose, citric acid, flavors, glycerin, purified water, red 33, red 40, sodium benzoate, sorbitol, sucrose, xanthan gum

QUESTIONS OR COMMENTS?

Call **1-888-474-3099** or email CustomerService@pediacare.com

PEDIACARE CHILDREN'S FEVER REDUCER PLUS MULTI-SYMPTOM COLD WITH ACETAMINOPHEN (acetaminophen, chlorpheniramine, dextromethorphan, and phenylephrine)

Blacksmith Brands, Inc.

DRUG FACTS

Active Ingredient(s) (in each 5 mL)	Purpose(s)
Acetaminophen 160 mg	Pain reliever/Fever reducer
Chlorpheniramine maleate 1 mg	Antihistamine
Dextromethorphan HBr 5 mg	Cough suppressant
Phenylephrine HCl 2.5 mg	Nasal decongestant

USES

Temporarily Relieves
- Minor aches and pains
- Cough

- Headache
- Sore throat
- Sneezing and runny nose
- Stuffy nose
- Fever

WARNINGS
Liver warning
This product contains acetaminophen. Severe liver damage may occur if your child takes:
- More than 5 doses in 24 hours, which is the maximum daily amount.

Sore throat warning
- If sore throat is severe, persists for more than 2 days, or is accompanied or followed by fever, headache, rash, nausea or vomiting, consult a doctor promptly.

DO NOT USE
- To make a child sleepy.
- In a child who is taking a prescription monoamine oxidase inhibitor (MAOI) (certain drugs for depression, psychiatric or emotional conditions, or Parkinson's disease) or for 2 weeks after stopping the MAOI drug. If you do not know if your child's prescription drug contains an MAOI, ask a doctor or pharmacist before giving this product.
- With any other drug containing acetaminophen (prescription or nonprescription). If you are not sure whether a drug contains acetaminophen, ask a doctor or pharmacist.

ASK A DOCTOR BEFORE USE IF YOUR CHILD HAS
- Glaucoma
- Thyroid disease
- Diabetes
- High blood pressure
- Heart disease
- A breathing problem such as chronic bronchitis
- Cough that occurs with too much phlegm (mucus)
- Persistent or chronic cough such as occurs with asthma
- Liver disease

ASK A DOCTOR OR A PHARMACIST BEFORE USE IF YOUR CHILD IS TAKING
- Sedatives or tranquilizers
- The blood-thinning drug warfarin

WHEN USING THIS PRODUCT
- **Do not exceed recommended dose (see overdose warning)**
- May cause excitability, especially in children
- Marked drowsiness may occur
- Sedatives and tranquilizers may increase drowsiness

STOP USE AND ASK A DOCTOR IF
- New symptoms occur
- Nervousness, dizziness or sleeplessness occur
- Fever gets worse or lasts for more than 3 days
- Redness or swelling is present
- Pain, nasal congestion or cough gets worse or lasts for more than 5 days
- Cough comes back or occurs with rash or headache that lasts

These could be signs of a serious condition.
Keep this and all drugs out of reach of children.

OVERDOSE WARNING
Taking more than the recommended dose (overdose) could cause major health problems, including liver damage. In case of accidental overdose, seek professional assistance or contact a Poison Control Center immediately (1-800-222-1222). Quick medical attention is critical even if you do not notice any signs or symptoms.

DIRECTIONS
- Find right dosage on the chart. **If possible, use weight to dose; otherwise, use age.**
- Shake well before using.
- If needed, repeat dose every 4 hours while symptoms last.
- Do not use more than 5 times in 24 hours.

Weight (lbs)	Age (yrs)	Dose (mL)
Under 36	Under 4	Do not use
36-47	4 - 5	Do not use unless directed by a doctor
48-95	6-11	10

INACTIVE INGREDIENTS
blue 1, carboxymethylcellulose sodium, cellulose, citric acid, flavors, glycerin, purified water, red 33, red 40, sodium benzoate, sorbitol, sucrose, xanthan gum

QUESTIONS OR COMMENTS?
Call **1-888-474-3099** or email CustomerService@pediacare.com

---

PEDIACARE CHILDREN'S DAYTIME MULTI-SYMPTOM COLD (NO ACETAMINOPHEN) (dextromethorphan and phenylephrine)

Blacksmith Brands, Inc.

DRUG FACTS

Active Ingredient(s) (in each 5 mL)	Purpose(s)
Dextromethorphan HBr 5 mg	Cough suppressant
Phenylephrine HCl 2.5 mg	Nasal decongestant

USES
Temporarily Relieves
- Cough
- Nasal congestion

WARNINGS

DO NOT USE
- In a child under 4 years of age
- In a child who is taking a prescription monoamine oxidase inhibitor (MAOI) (certain drugs for depression, psychiatric or emotional conditions, or Parkinson's disease) or for 2 weeks after stopping the MAOI drug. If you do not know if your child's prescription drug contains an MAOI, ask a doctor or pharmacist before giving this product.

ASK A DOCTOR BEFORE USE IF YOUR CHILD HAS
- Heart disease
- High blood pressure
- Thyroid disease
- Diabetes
- A persistent or chronic cough such as occurs with asthma
- A cough accompanied by excessive phlegm (mucus)
- A sodium-restricted diet

WHEN USING THIS PRODUCT
- Do not exceed recommended dosage.

STOP USE AND ASK A DOCTOR IF
- Nervousness, dizziness or sleeplessness occur
- Symptoms do not improve within 7 days, or occur with a fever

- Cough persists for more than 7 days, comes back or occurs with a fever, rash or persistent headache. These could be signs of a serious condition.

Keep out of reach of children

In case of overdose, get medical help or contact a Poison Control Center right away (1-800-222-1222).

DIRECTIONS

- Find right dosage on the chart. **If possible, use weight to dose; otherwise, use age.**
- Use only enclosed dosing cup designed for use with this product. Do not use any other dosing device.
- If needed, repeat dose every 4 hours while symptoms last.
- Do not use more than 6 times in 24 hours.

Weight (lbs)	Age (yrs)	Dose (mL)
Under 36	Under 4	Do not use
36-43	4-5	5
48-95	6-11	10

INACTIVE INGREDIENTS

acesulfame potassium, alcohol, benzoic acid, citric acid, edetate disodium, FD&C red 40, flavors, maltitol solution, propylene glycol, purified water, sodium citrate

QUESTIONS OR COMMENTS?

Call **1-888-474-3099** or email CustomerService@pediacare.com

---

PEDIACARE CHILDREN'S NIGHTTIME MULTI-SYMPTOM COLD (NO ACETAMINOPHEN) (diphenhydramine HCl and phenylephrine HCl)

Blacksmith Brands, Inc.

DRUG FACTS

Active Ingredient(s) (in each 5 mL)	Purpose(s)
Diphenhydramine HCl 6.25 mg	Cough suppressant
Phenylephrine HCl 2.5 mg	Nasal decongestant

USES

Temporarily Relieves
- Sneezing
- Runny nose
- Itchy nose or throat
- Itchy or watery eyes
- Nasal and sinus congestion
- Cough

WARNINGS

DO NOT USE
- To make child sleepy.
- In a child under 4 years of age
- In a child who is taking prescription monoamine oxidase inhibitor (MAOI)(certain drugs for depression, psychiatric or emotional conditions, or Parkinson's disease), or for 2 weeks after stopping the MAOI drug. If you do not know if your child's prescription drug contains an MAOI, ask a doctor or pharmacist before giving this product.
- With any other product containing diphenhydramine, even one used on skin

ASK A DOCTOR BEFORE USE IF YOUR CHILD HAS
- Heart disease
- Glaucoma
- High blood pressure
- Diabetes
- Thyroid disease
- A breathing problem such as chronic bronchitis
- Chronic cough that lasts, or occurs with asthma
- Cough that occurs with too much phlegm (mucus)

ASK A DOCTOR OR A PHARMACIST BEFORE USE IF YOUR CHILD IS TAKING
- sedatives or tranquilizers

WHEN USING THIS PRODUCT
- Do not exceed recommended dose
- Marked drowsiness may occur
- Sedatives and tranquilizers may increase drowsiness
- Excitability may occur, especially in children

STOP USE AND ASK A DOCTOR IF
- Nervousness, dizziness or sleeplessness occurs
- Symptoms do not improve within 7 days, or occur with a fever
- Cough persists for more than 7 days, comes back or occurs with a fever, rash or persistent headache. These could be signs of a serious condition.

Keep out of reach of children.

In case of accidental overdose, get medical help or contact a Poison Control Center (1-800-222-1222) right away.

DIRECTIONS

- Find right dosage on the chart. **If possible, use weight to dose; otherwise, use age.**
- Use only enclosed dosing cup designed for use with this product. Do not use any other dosing device.
- If needed, repeat dose every 4 hours while symptoms last.
- Do not use more than 6 times in 24 hours.

Weight (lbs)	Age (yrs)	Dose (mL)
Under 36	Under 4	Do not use
36-47	4 - 5	Do not use unless directed by a doctor
48-95	6-11	10

INACTIVE INGREDIENTS

acesulfame potassium, benzoic acid, citric acid, edetate disodium, FD&C blue 1, FD&C red 40, flavor, maltitol solution, propylene glycol, purified water, sodium citrate

QUESTIONS OR COMMENTS?

Call **1-888-474-3099** or email CustomerService@pediacare.com

---

PEDIACARE CHILDREN'S FEVER REDUCER/ PAIN RELIEVER ACETAMINOPHEN ORAL SUSPENSION (acetaminophen)

Blacksmith Brands, Inc.

DRUG FACTS

Active Ingredient(s) (in each 5 mL)	Purpose(s)
Acetaminophen 160 mg	Pain reliever/Fever reducer

USES

temporarily relieves
- Fever
- minor aches and pains

WARNINGS
Liver warning
This product contains acetaminophen. Severe liver damage may occur if your child takes:
- more than 5 doses in 24 hours, which is the maximum daily amount

Sore throat warning
- If sore throat is severe, persists for more than 2 days, or is accompanied or followed by fever, headache, rash, nausea or vomiting, consult a doctor promptly.

DO NOT USE
- With any other drug containing acetaminophen (prescription or nonprescription). If you are not sure whether a drug contains acetaminophen, ask a doctor or pharmacist.

ASK A DOCTOR BEFORE USE IF YOUR CHILD
- Has liver disease.
- Is taking the blood-thinning drug warfarin.

WHEN USING THIS PRODUCT
- **do not exceed recommended dose**
- Taking more than the recommended dose (overdose) may not provide more relief and may cause liver damage

STOP USE AND ASK A DOCTOR IF
- Pain gets worse or lasts for more than 5 days
- Fever gets worse or lasts for more than 3 days
- New symptoms occur
- Redness or swelling is present

These could be signs of a serious condition.
Keep out of the reach of children.

OVERDOSE WARNING
Taking more than the recommended dose (overdose) could cause major health problems, including liver damage. In case of accidental overdose, seek professional assistance or contact a Poison Control Center (1-800-222-1222) right away. Quick medical attention is critical even if you do not notice any signs or symptoms.

DIRECTIONS
- **this product does not contain directions or complete warnings for adult use.**
- **shake well before using.**
- find right dosage on the chart. If possible, use weight to dose; otherwise, use age.
- use only enclosed dosing cup designed for use with this product. Do not use any other dosing device.
- if needed, repeat dose every 4 hours while symptoms last
- do not give more than 5 times in 24 hours.
- do not give for more than 5 days unless directed by a doctor

Weight (lbs)	Age (yrs)	Dose (mL)
6-23	0-23	Use PediaCare® Infants Acetaminophen Oral Suspension
24-35	2-3	5
36-47	4-5	7.5
48-59	6-8	10
60-71	9-10	12.5
72-95	11	15

INACTIVE INGREDIENTS
Cherry Flavor: acesulfame potassium, butylparaben, carboxymethylcellulose sodium, cellulose, citric acid, flavors, glycerin, high-fructose corn syrup, propylene glycol, purified water, red 40, sodium benzoate, sorbitol, xanthan gum

Non-Staining Cherry Flavor: butylparaben, carboxymethylcellulose sodium, cellulose, citric acid, flavors, glycerin, high-fructose corn syrup, propylene glycol, purified water, sodium benzoate, sorbitol, sucralose, xanthan gum
Grape Flavor: blue 1, butylparaben, carboxymethylcellulose sodium, cellulose, citric acid, flavors, glycerin, high - fructose corn syrup, propylene glycol, purified water, Red 33, sodium benzoate, sorbitol, sucralose, xanthan gum

QUESTIONS OR COMMENTS?
Call **1-888-474-3099** or email CustomerService@pediacare.com

PEDIACARE CHILDRENS (ibuprofen)
Medtech Products Inc.

DRUG FACTS

Active Ingredient(s)
(in each 5 mL = 1 teaspoon)
Ibuprofen, USP 100 mg (NSAID)*

Purpose(s)
Pain reliever/ fever reducer
*nonsteroidal anti-inflammatory drug

USES
temporarily:
- relieves minor aches and pains due to the common cold, flu, sore throat, headache and toothache
- reduces fever

WARNINGS
Allergy alert: Ibuprofen may cause a severe allergic reaction, especially in people allergic to aspirin. Symptoms may include:
- hives
- asthma (wheezing)
- skin reddening
- facial swelling
- shock
- rash
- blisters

If an allergic reaction occurs, stop use and seek medical help right away.
Stomach bleeding warning: This product contains a nonsteroidal anti-inflammatory drug (NSAID), which may cause severe stomach bleeding.
The chances are higher if your child:
- has had stomach ulcers or bleeding problems
- takes a blood thinning (anticoagulant) or steroid drug
- takes other drugs containing prescription or nonprescription NSAIDs (aspirin, ibuprofen, naproxen, or others)
- takes more or for a longer time than directed

Sore throat warning: Severe or persistent sore throat or sore throat accompanied by high fever, headache, nausea, and vomiting may be serious. Consult doctor promptly. Do not use more than 2 days to administer to children under 3 years of age unless directed by doctor.

DO NOT USE
- if the child has ever had an allergic reaction to any other pain reliever/fever reducer
- right before or after heart surgery

ASK A DOCTOR BEFORE USE IF
- stomach bleeding warning applies to your child
- child has a history of stomach problems, such as heartburn
- child has not been drinking fluids
- child has lost a lot of fluid due to vomiting or diarrhea
- child has high blood pressure, heart disease, liver cirrhosis, or kidney disease
- child is taking a diuretic

ASK A DOCTOR OR PHARMACIST BEFORE USE IF THE CHILD IS
- under a doctor's care for any serious condition
- taking any other drug

WHEN USING THIS PRODUCT
- take with food or milk if stomach upset occurs
- the risk of heart attack or stroke may increase if you use more than directed or for longer than directed

STOP USE AND ASK A DOCTOR IF
- child experiences any of the following signs of stomach bleeding
  - feels faint
  - vomits blood
  - has bloody or black stools
- has stomach pain that does not get better
- the child does not get any relief within the first day (24 hours) of treatment
- fever or pain gets worse or lasts more than 3 days
- redness or swelling is present in the painful area
- any new symptoms appear

Keep out of reach of children.
In case of overdose, get medical help or contact a Poison Control Center (1-800-222-1222) right away.

DIRECTIONS
- **This product does not contain directions or complete warnings for adult use**
- **Do not give more than directed**
- Shake well before using
- Find right does on chart below. If possible, use weight to dose; otherwise use age.
- Use only enclosed measuring cup
- If needed, repeat dose every **6-8 hours**
- Do not use more than **4 times a day**
- Replace original bottle cap to maintain child resistance

Dosing Chart		
Weight (lb)	**Age (yr)**	**Dose (tsp or mL)**
	Under 2 years	ask a doctor
24-35 lbs	2-3 years	1 tsp or 5 mL
36-47 lbs	4-5 years	1 ½ tsp or 7.5 mL
48-59 lbs	6-8 years	2 tsp or 10 mL
60-71 lbs	9-10 years	2 ½ tsp or 12.5 mL
72-95 lbs	11 years	3 tsp or 15 mL

OTHER INFORMATION
- **do not use if printed neckband is broken or missing**
- store between 20-25°C (68-77°F)
- see bottom panel for lot number and expiration date

INACTIVE INGREDIENTS
citric acid, flavors, glycerin, hypromellose, polysorbate-80, purified water, sodium benzoate, sucrose, xanthan gum

QUESTIONS OR COMMENTS?
1-888-474-3099 Mon.-Fri. 8:00am to 8:00pm EST or visit us at www.PediaCare.com

PEDIACARE INFANTS FEVER REDUCER/ PAIN RELIEVER WITH ACETAMINOPHEN
(acetaminophen)

Blacksmith Brands, Inc.

DRUG FACTS

Active Ingredient(s) (in each 5 mL)	Purpose(s)
Acetaminophen 160 mg	Pain reliever/Fever reducer

USES
Temporarily Relieves
- Fever
- Minor aches and pains

WARNINGS
Liver warning
This product contains acetaminophen. Severe liver damage may occur if your child takes:
- More than 5 doses in 24 hours, which is the maximum daily amount.
- With other drugs containing acetaminophen

Sore throat warning
- If sore throat is severe, persists for more than 2 days, or is accompanied or followed by fever, headache, rash, nausea or vomiting, consult a doctor promptly.

DO NOT USE
- With any other drug containing acetaminophen (prescription or nonprescription). If you are not sure whether a drug contains acetaminophen, ask a doctor or pharmacist.
- If your child is allergic to acetaminophen or any of the inactive ingredients in this product.

ASK A DOCTOR BEFORE USE IF YOUR CHILD
- Has liver disease
- Is taking the blood-thinning drug warfarin

WHEN USING THIS PRODUCT
- **Do not exceed recommended dose (see overdose warning)**

STOP USE AND ASK A DOCTOR IF
- Pain gets worse or lasts for more than 5 days
- Fever gets worse or lasts for more than 3 days
- New symptoms occur
- Redness or swelling is present

These could be signs of a serious condition.
Keep this and all drugs out of reach of children.

OVERDOSE WARNING
Taking more than the recommended dose (overdose) could cause major health problems, including liver damage. In case of accidental overdose, seek professional assistance or contact a Poison Control Center (1-800-222-1222) right away. Quick medical attention is critical even if you do not notice any signs or symptoms.

DIRECTIONS
- **This product does not contain directions or complete warnings for adult use.**
- **Shake well before using.**
- Find right dosage on the chart. If possible, use weight to dose; otherwise, use age.
- Use only enclosed dosing cup designed for use with this product. Do not use any other dosing device.
- If needed, repeat dose every 4 hours while symptoms last.

- Do not give more than 5 times in 24 hours.
- Do not give for more than 5 days unless directed by a doctor.

Weight (lbs)	Age (yrs)	Dose (mL)
Under 24	Under 2	Ask a doctor
24-35	2-3	5
36 and over	4-11	Use PediaCare® Children Acetaminophen Oral Suspension

INACTIVE INGREDIENTS
Cherry: acesulfame potassium, butylparaben, carboxymethylcellulose sodium, cellulose, citric acid, flavors, glycerin, high-fructose corn syrup, propylene glycol, purified water, red 40, sodium benzoate, sorbitol, sucralose, xanthan gum
Non-Staining Cherry: butylparaben, carboxymethylcellulose sodium, cellulose, citric acid, flavors, glycerin, high-fructose corn syrup, propylene glycol, purified water, sodium benzoate, sorbitol, sucralose, xanthan gum
Bubble Gum: butylparaben, carboxymethylcellulose sodium, cellulose, citric acid, flavors, glycerin, high-fructose corn syrup, propylene glycol, purified water, red 33, red 40, sodium benzoate, sorbitol, sucralose, xanthan gum
Grape: blue 1, butylparaben, carboxymethylcellulose sodium, cellulose, citric acid, flavors, glycerin, high-fructose corn syrup, propylene glycol, purified water, red 33, sodium benzoate, sorbitol, sucralose, xanthan gum

QUESTIONS OR COMMENTS?
Call **1-888-474-3099** or email CustomerService@pediacare.com

PEDIACARE INFANTS GAS RELIEF DROPS
(simethicone)

Blacksmith Brands, Inc.

DRUG FACTS

Active Ingredient(s) (in each 0.3 mL)	Purpose(s)
Simethicone 20 mg	Anti-Gas

USES
Temporarily Relieves
- Symptoms of gas frequently caused by air swallowing or certain formulas or foods

WHEN USING THIS PRODUCT
- Do not exceed 12 doses per day
Keep out of reach of children.
- In case of overdose, get medical help or contact a Poison Control Center (1-800-222-1222) right away.

DIRECTIONS
- Shake well before using.
- All dosages may be repeated as needed, after meals and at bedtime.
- Fill enclosed dropper to recommended dosage level.
- Dispense liquid slowly into baby's mouth, toward inner cheek.
- May mix with 1 fl. oz. of cool water, infant formula or other suitable liquids.
- Clean dropper after each use and replace original cap.

Weight (lbs)	Age (yrs)	Dose (mL)
Under 24	Infants under 2	0.3
24 and over	Children 2 and over	0.6

INACTIVE INGREDIENTS
benzoic acid, D&C red 22, D&C red 28, magnesium aluminum silicate, natural flavor, purified water, sorbitol, xanthan gum

QUESTIONS OR COMMENTS?
Call **1-888-474-3099** or email CustomerService@pediacare.com

PEPCID AC MAXIMUM STRENGTH
(famotidine)

McNeil Consumer Pharmaceuticals Co.

DRUG FACTS

Active Ingredient(s) (in each tablet)
Famotidine 20 mg

Purpose(s)
Acid reducer

USES
- relieves heartburn associated with acid indigestion and sour stomach
- prevents heartburn associated with acid indigestion and sour stomach brought on by eating or drinking certain food and beverages

WARNINGS
Allergy alert
Do not use if you are allergic to famotidine or other acid reducers

DO NOT USE
- if you have trouble or pain swallowing food, vomiting with blood, or bloody or black stools. These may be signs of a serious condition. See your doctor.
- if you have kidney disease, except under the advice and supervision of a doctor
- with other acid reducers

ASK A DOCTOR BEFORE USE IF YOU HAVE
- had heartburn over 3 months. This may be a sign of a more serious condition.
- heartburn with **lightheadedness, sweating, or dizziness**
- chest pain or shoulder pain with shortness of breath; sweating; pain spreading to arms, neck or shoulders; or lightheadedness
- frequent **chest pain**
- frequent wheezing, particularly with heartburn
- unexplained weight loss
- nausea or vomiting
- stomach pain

STOP USE AND ASK A DOCTOR IF
- your heartburn continues or worsens
- you need to take this product for more than 14 days
If pregnant or breast-feeding, ask a health professional before use.
Keep out of reach of children. In case of overdose, get medical help or contact a Poison Control Center right away.

DIRECTIONS
- adults and children 12 years and over:
- to **relieve** symptoms, swallow 1 tablet with a glass of water. Do not chew.

- to **prevent** symptoms, swallow 1 tablet with a glass of water at any time from **10 to 60 minutes before** eating food or drinking beverages that cause heartburn
- do not use more than 2 tablets in 24 hours
- children under 12 years: ask a doctor

OTHER INFORMATION
- read the directions and warnings before use
- keep the carton. It contains important information.
- store at 20°-25°C (68°-77°F)
- protect from moisture

INACTIVE INGREDIENTS
carnauba wax, hydroxypropyl cellulose, hypromellose, magnesium stearate, microcrystalline cellulose, pregelatinized starch, talc, titanium dioxide

QUESTIONS OR COMMENTS?
1-800-755-4008 toll-free or 215-273-8755 (collect)

PEPCID AC ORIGINAL STRENGTH (famotidine)
Johnson & Johnson Merck Consumer Pharmaceuticals

DRUG FACTS

Active Ingredient(s) (in each tablet)
Famotidine 10 mg

Purpose(s)
Acid reducer

USES
- relieves heartburn associated with acid indigestion and sour stomach
- prevents heartburn associated with acid indigestion and sour stomach brought on by eating or drinking certain food and beverages

WARNINGS
Allergy alert
Do not use if you are allergic to famotidine or other acid reducers

DO NOT USE
- if you have trouble or pain swallowing food, vomiting with blood, or bloody or black stools. These may be signs of a serious condition. See your doctor.
- with other acid reducers
- **Ask a doctor before use if you have**
- had heartburn over 3 months. This may be a sign of a more serious condition.
- heartburn with **lightheadedness, sweating, or dizziness**
- chest pain or shoulder pain with shortness of breath; sweating; pain spreading to arms, neck or shoulders; or lightheadedness
- frequent **chest pain**
- frequent wheezing, particularly with heartburn
- unexplained weight loss
- nausea or vomiting
- stomach pain

STOP USE AND ASK A DOCTOR IF
- your heartburn continues or worsens
- you need to take this product for more than 14 days

If pregnant or breast-feeding, ask a health professional before use.
Keep out of reach of children. In case of overdose, get medical help or contact a Poison Control Center right away.

DIRECTIONS
- adults and children 12 years and over:
- to **relieve** symptoms, swallow 1 tablet with a glass of water. Do not chew.
- to **prevent** symptoms, swallow 1 tablet with a glass of water at any time from **15 to 60 minutes before** eating food or drinking beverages that cause heartburn
- do not use more than 2 tablets in 24 hours
- children under 12 years: ask a doctor

OTHER INFORMATION
- read the directions and warnings before use
- keep the carton. It contains important information.
- store at 20°-30°C (68°-86°F)
- protect from moisture

INACTIVE INGREDIENTS
hydroxypropyl cellulose, hypromellose, magnesium stearate, microcrystalline cellulose, red iron oxide, starch, talc, titanium dioxide ·

QUESTIONS OR COMMENTS?
1-800-755-4008 (English) or 1-888-466-8746 (Spanish)

PEPCID COMPLETE BERRY
PEPCID COMPLETE COOL MINT
PEPCIL COMPLETE TROPICAL FRUIT
(famotidine, calcium carbonate, and magnesium hydroxide)
McNeil Consumer Pharmaceuticals Co.

DRUG FACTS

Active Ingredient(s) (in each chewable tablet)	Purpose(s)
Famotidine 10 mg	Acid reducer
Calcium carbonate 800 mg	Antacid
Magnesium hydroxide 165 mg	Antacid

USES
Relieves heartburn associated with acid indigestion and sour stomach.

WARNINGS
Allergy Alert: Do not use if you are allergic to famotidine or other acid reducers

DO NOT USE
- if you have trouble or pain swallowing food, vomiting with blood, or bloody or black stools. These may be signs of a serious condition. See your doctor.
- With other acid reducers

ASK A DOCTOR BEFORE USE IF YOU HAVE
- had heartburn over 3 months. This may be a sign of a more serious condition.
- heartburn with **lightheadedness, sweating or dizziness**
- chest pain or shoulder pain with shortness of breath; sweating; pain spreading to arms, neck or shoulders; or lightheadedness
- frequent **chest pain**
- frequent wheezing, particularly with heartburn
- unexplained weight loss
- nausea or vomiting
- stomach pain

ASK A DOCTOR OR A PHARMACIST BEFORE USE IF YOU ARE

- presently taking a prescription drug. Antacids may interact with certain prescription drugs.

STOP USE AND ASK A DOCTOR IF

- your heartburn continues or worsens
- you need to take this product for more than 14 days

If pregnant or breast-feeding, ask a health professional before use.

Keep out of reach of children. In case of overdose, get medical help or contact a Poison Control Center right away.

DIRECTIONS

adults and children 12 years and over:
- do not swallow tablet whole: chew completely
- to relieve symptoms, **chew** 1tablet before swallowing
- do not use more than 2 chewable tablets in 24 hours

children under 12 years: ask a doctor

OTHER INFORMATION

- each tablet contains: **calcium 320 mg; magnesium 70 mg**
- read the directions and warnings before use
- keep the carton. It contains important information.
- store at 20°-30°C (68°-86°F)
- protect from moisture

INACTIVE INGREDIENTS

Tropical Fruit Flavor: cellulose acetate, corn starch, corn syrup solids, crospovidone, dextrose, FD&C yellow #5 aluminum lake (tartrazine), FD&C yellow aluminum lake #6, flavors, gum arabic, hydroxypropyl cellulose, hypromellose, lactose, magnesium stearate, maltodextrin, mineral oil, sucralose, triacetin
Berry Flavor: cellulose acetate, corn starch, crospovidone, D&C red #7 calcium lake, dextrose, FD&C blue #1 aluminum lake, FD&C red #40 aluminum lake, flavors, gum arabic, hydroxypropyl cellulose, hypromellose, lactose, magnesium stearate, maltodextrin, mineral oil, sucralose
Cool Mint Flavor: cellulose acetate, corn starch, crospovidone, D&C yellow #10 aluminum lake, dextrose, FD&C blue #1 aluminum lake, flavors, gum arabic, hydroxypropyl cellulose, hypromellose, lactose, magnesium stearate, maltodextrin, mineral oil, sucralose

---

PEPTO BISMOL ORIGINAL (bismuth subsalicylate)

Procter & Gamble

DRUGS FACTS

Active Ingredient(s) (in each 30 mL Dose Cup or 2 Tablespoons)	Purpose(s)
Bismuth subsalicylate 525 mg	upset stomach reliever and antidiarrheal

USES

Relieves
- travelers' diarrhea
- diarrhea
- upset stomach due to overindulgence in food and drink, including:
  - heartburn
  - indigestion
  - nausea
  - gas
  - belching
  - fullness

WARNINGS

Reye's syndrome: Children and teenagers who have or are recovering from chicken pox or flu-like symptoms should not use this product. When using this product, if changes in behavior with nausea or vomiting occur, consult a doctor because these symptoms could be an early sign of Reye's syndrome, a rare but serious illness.

Allergy alert: Contains salicylate. Do not take if you are:
- allergic to salicylates (including aspirin)
- taking other salicylate products

DO NOT USE

if you have:
- an ulcer
- a bleeding problem
- bloody or black stool

ASK A DOCTOR BEFORE USE

if you have:
- fever
- mucus in the stool

ASK A DOCTOR OR PHARMACIST BEFORE USE IF YOU ARE

taking any drug for:
- anticoagulation (thinning the blood)
- diabetes
- gout
- arthritis

If pregnant or breast-feeding, ask a health professional before use.

Keep out of reach of children. In case of overdose, get medical help or contact a Poison Control Center right away

DIRECTIONS

- Shake well before use.
- For accurate dosing, use dose cup or tablespoon (TBSP).
- Adults and children 12 years and over:
  - 1 dose (30 mL or 2 TBSP) every ½ to 1 hour as needed.
  - Do not exceed 8 doses (240 mL or 16 TBSP) in 24 hours.
  - Use until diarrhea stops, but not more than 2 days.
- Not for children under 12 years of age.
- Drink plenty of clear fluids to help prevent dehydration caused by diarrhea.

OTHER INFORMATION

- When using this product a temporary, but harmless, darkening of the stool and/or tongue may occur.
- Each 30 mL dose cup contains:
  - Magnesium 25 mg
  - Sodium 8 mg.
  - Salicylate 261 mg.
- Low sodium
- Protect from freezing.
- Avoid excessive heat (over 104° F or 40° C).
- TAMPER EVIDENT: Do not use if printed shrinkband is missing or broken.

INACTIVE INGREDIENTS

benzoic acid, D&C red No. 22, D&C red No. 28, flavor, magnesium aluminum silicate, methylcellulose, saccharin sodium, salicylic acid, sodium salicylate, sorbic acid, water

QUESTIONS OR COMMENTS?

1-800-717-3786

CHILDREN'S PEPTO ANTACID (calcium carbonate)

Procter & Gamble

Children's Pepto Antacid Chewable Tablets

DRUG FACTS

Active Ingredient(s) (in each caplet)	Calcium carbonate 400 mg
Purpose(s)	Antacid

USES

Relieves:
• Heartburn
• Sour stomach
• Acid indigestion
• Upset stomach due to these symptoms or overindulgence in food and drink

WARNINGS

ASK A DOCTOR OR PHARMACIST BEFORE USE IF
the child is presently taking a prescription drug.
Antacids may interact with certain prescription drugs.

STOP USE AND ASK A DOCTOR IF
symptoms last more than two weeks.
Keep this and all drugs out of the reach of children.

DIRECTIONS
• Find the right dose on the chart below based on weight (preferred). Otherwise, use age.
• Repeat dose as needed.
• Do not take more than 3 tablets (ages 2-5) or 6 tablets (ages 6-11) in a 24-hour period, or use the maximum dosage for more than two weeks, except under the advice and supervision of a doctor.

DOSING CHART

Weight (lbs.)	Under 24	24 to 47	48 to 95
Age	Under 2 yrs	2 to 5 yrs	6 to 11 yrs
Dose	Ask a doctor	1 tablet	2 tablets

OTHER INFORMATION
• Each tablet contains: calcium 161 mg
• Sodium free
• Store at room temperature; avoid excessive humidity.

INACTIVE INGREDIENTS
flavor, magnesium stearate, mannitol, povidone, red 27 aluminum lake, sorbitol, sugar, talc

QUESTIONS OR COMMENTS?
1-800-944-9606

PEPTO-BISMOL MAX STRENGTH LIQUID
(bismuth subsalicylate)

Procter & Gamble

DRUG FACTS

Active Ingredient(s) (in each 30 ML Dose Cup or 2 Tablespoons)
Bismuth subsalicylate 1050 mg

Purpose(s)
Upset stomach reliever and antidiarrheal

USES
relieves
• travelers' diarrhea
• diarrhea
• upset stomach
• due to overindulgence in food and drink, including
• heartburn
• indigestion
• nausea
• gas
• belching
• fullness

WARNINGS
Reye's syndrome
Children and teenagers who have or are recovering from chicken pox or flu-like symptoms should not use this product. When using this product, if changes in behavior with nausea and vomiting occur, consult a doctor because these symptoms could be an early sign of Reye's syndrome, a rare but serious illness.

Allergy alert
Contains salicylate. Do not take if you are
• allergic to salicylates (including aspirin)
• taking other salicylate products

DO NOT USE IF
you have
• an ulcer
• a bleeding problem
• bloody or black stool

ASK A DOCTOR BEFORE USE IF YOU HAVE
• fever
• mucus in the stool

ASK A DOCTOR OR PHARMACIST BEFORE USE IF YOU ARE
taking any drug for
• anticoagulation (thinning the blood)
• diabetes
• gout
• arthritis

WHEN USING THIS PRODUCT
a temporary, but harmless, darkening of the stool and/or tongue may occur

STOP USE AND ASK A DOCTOR IF
• symptoms get worse or last more than 2 days
• ringing in the ears or loss of hearing occurs
• diarrhea lasts more than 2 days

If pregnant or breast feeding, ask a health professional before use.
Keep out of reach of children. In case of overdose, get medical help or contact a Poison Control Center right away.

DIRECTIONS
• shake well before use
• for accurate dosing, use dose cup or tablespoon (TBSP)
• adults and children 12 years and over: 1 dose (2 Tbsp or 30 ml) every hour as needed
• not for use until diarrhea stops but not more than 2 days
• children under 12 years of age
• drink plenty of clear fluids to help prevent dehydration caused by diarrhea

OTHER INFORMATION
- **each 30 mL dose cup contains:** magnesium 25 mg - sodium 8 mg
- salicylate 236 mg
- low sodium
- protect from freezing
- avoid excessive heat (over 104°F or 40°C)
- TAMPER EVIDENT: Do not use if printed shrinkband is missing or broken.

INACTIVE INGREDIENTS
benzoic acid, D&C red No. 22, D&C red No. 28, flavor, magnesium aluminum silicate, methylcellulose, saccharin sodium, salicylic acid, sodium salicylate, sorbic acid, water

QUESTIONS?
1-800-717-3786
Dist. by Procter & Gamble,
Cincinnati OH 45202

PEPTO-BISMOL TO GO (bismuth subsalicylate)
Procter & Gamble

DRUG FACTS

Active Ingredient(s) (in each tablet)
Bismuth subsalicylate 262 mg

Purpose(s)
Upset stomach reliever and antidiarrheal

USES
relieves
- travelers' diarrhea
- diarrhea
- upset stomach due to overindulgence in food and drink, including:
  - heartburn
  - indigestion
  - nausea
  - gas
  - belching
  - fullness

WARNINGS
Reye's syndrome
Children and teenagers who have or are recovering from chicken pox or flu-like symptoms should not use this product. When using this product, if changes in behavior with nausea and vomiting occur, consult a doctor because these symptoms could be an early sign of Reye's syndrome, a rare but serious illness.

Allergy alert: Contains salicylate.

Do not take if you are
- allergic to salicylates (including aspirin)
- taking other salicylate products

DO NOT USE
if you have
- an ulcer
- a bleeding problem
- bloody or black stool

ASK A DOCTOR BEFORE USE IF YOU HAVE
- fever
- mucus in the stool

ASK A DOCTOR OR PHARMACIST BEFORE USE IF YOU ARE
taking any drug for
- anticoagulation (thinning the blood)
- diabetes
- gout
- arthritis

WHEN USING THIS PRODUCT
a temporary, but harmless, darkening of the stool and/or tongue may occur

STOP USE AND ASK A DOCTOR IF
- symptoms get worse or last more than 2 days
- ringing in the ears or loss of hearing occurs
- diarrhea lasts more than 2 days

If pregnant or breast feeding, ask a health professional before use.
Keep out of reach of children. In case of overdose, get medical help or contact a Poison Control Center right away.

DIRECTIONS
- chew or dissolve in mouth
- adults and children 12 years and over: 2 tablets every 1/2 to 1 hour as needed
- do not exceed 8 doses (16 tablets) in 24 hours
- use until diarrhea stops but not more than 2 days
- children under 12 years: ask a doctor
- drink plenty of clear fluids to help prevent dehydration caused by diarrhea

OTHER INFORMATION
- **each tablet contains:** calcium 140 mg
- sodium less than 1 mg
- salicylate 99 mg
- very low sodium
- sugar free
- avoid excessive heat (over 104°F or 40°C)

INACTIVE INGREDIENTS
adipic acid, calcium carbonate, flavor, magnesium stearate, mannitol, povidone, red 27 aluminum lake, red 40 aluminum lake, saccharin sodium, talc

QUESTIONS OR COMMENTS?
1-800-717-3786
Dist. by Procter & Gamble, Cincinnati OH 45202

PEPTO-BISMOL INSTACOOL (bismuth subsalicylate)
The Procter & Gamble

DRUG FACTS

Active Ingredient(s) (in each tablet)
Bismuth subsalicylate 262 mg

Purpose(s)
Upset stomach reliever and antidiarrheal

USES
relieves
- travelers' diarrhea
- diarrhea
- upset stomach due to overindulgence in food and drink, including:
  - heartburn
  - indigestion
  - nausea
  - gas

- belching
- fullness

WARNINGS
Reye's syndrome
Children and teenagers who have or are recovering from chicken pox or flu-like symptoms should not use this product. When using this product, if changes in behavior with nausea and vomiting occur, consult a doctor because these symptoms could be an early sign of Reye's syndrome, a rare but serious illness.

Allergy alert
Contains salicylate. Do not take if you are
- allergic to salicylates (including aspirin)
- taking other salicylate products

DO NOT USE IF
you have
- an ulcer
- a bleeding problem
- bloody or black stool

ASK A DOCTOR BEFORE USE IF YOU HAVE
- fever
- mucus in the stool

ASK A DOCTOR OR PHARMACIST BEFORE USE IF YOU ARE
taking any drug for
- anticoagulation (thinning the blood)
- diabetes
- gout
- arthritis

WHEN USING THIS PRODUCT
a temporary, but harmless, darkening of the stool and/or tongue may occur

STOP USE AND ASK A DOCTOR IF
- symptoms get worse or last more than 2 days
- ringing in the ears or loss of hearing occurs
- diarrhea lasts more than 2 days

If pregnant or breast feeding, ask a health professional before use.
Keep out of reach of children. In case of overdose, get medical help or contact a Poison Control Center right away.

DIRECTIONS
- chew or dissolve in mouth
- adults and children 12 years and over: 2 tablets every 1/2 to 1 hour as needed
- do not exceed 8 doses (16 tablets) in 24 hours
- use until diarrhea stops but not more than 2 days
- children under 12 years: ask a doctor
- drink plenty of clear fluids to help prevent dehydration caused by diarrhea

OTHER INFORMATION
- **each tablet contains:** calcium 85 mg
- sodium less than 1 mg
- salicylate 100 mg
- very low sodium
- sugar free
- avoid excessive heat (over 104°F or 40°C)

INACTIVE INGREDIENTS
calcium carbonate, flavor, magnesium stearate, mannitol, povidone, red 27 aluminum lake, saccharin sodium, talc

QUESTIONS OR COMMENTS?
1-800-717-3786

Made in Mexico by Procter & Gamble
Manufactura S. de R. L. de C.V.
Dist. by Procter & Gamble, Cincinnati OH 45202

PERI-COLACE TABLETS (docusate sodium and sennosides)
Purdue Products L.P.

HOW THEY ARE SUPPLIED
- Each tablet contains 50 mg docusate sodium and 8.6 mg sennosides
- Tablets: 10s, 30s, 60s

MECHANISM OF ACTION
The active ingredients in Peri-Colace Tablets are docusate sodium and standardized senna concentrate. These ingredients are used together to help relieve occasional constipation. Docusate sodium works to soften the stool. Standardized senna concentrate is a laxative that helps to gently stimulate motility of the intestines.

RECOMMENDED DOSES
Take only by mouth. Doses may be taken as a single daily dose, preferable in the evening, or in divided doses.
Usual daily dose:
- Adults and children 12 years of age and older: take 2-4 tablets daily
- Children 6 to under 12 years: take 1-2 tablets daily
- Children 2 to under 6 years of age: take up to 1 tablet daily
- Children under 2: ask a doctor

WARNINGS
- Use laxatives for no longer than seven (7) days, unless directed otherwise by a doctor.
- Do not use if you are presently taking mineral oil unless told to do so by a doctor.
- Ask a doctor before use if you have:
  - Stomach pain
  - Nausea
  - Vomiting
  - Noticed a sudden change in bowel habits that lasts over two weeks
- Stop use and ask a doctor if you have rectal bleeding or fail to have a bowel movement after use of a laxative. These could be signs of a serious condition.
- If pregnant or breast-feeding, ask a health professional before use.
- Keep out of reach of children. In case of overdose, get medical help or contact a Poison Control Center right away.

PHAZYME (simethicone)
GlaxoSmithKline Consumer Healthcare LP

Active Ingredient(s) (in each softgel)
Simethicone 180 mg

Purpose(s)
Anti-gas

USE
- relieves bloating, pressure or fullness commonly referred to as gas

WARNINGS

STOP USE AND ASK A DOCTOR
if condition persists

Keep out of reach of children.

DIRECTIONS
- swallow one or two softgels as needed after a meal
- do not exceed two softgels per day except under the advice and supervision of a physician

OTHER INFORMATION
- store at room temperature 59°-86° F (15°- 30°C)

INACTIVE INGREDIENTS
FD&C yellow no. 6, gelatin, glycerin, white edible ink

QUESTIONS OR COMMENTS?
call toll-free **1-866-255-5204** (English/Spanish) weekdays

POLYSPORIN (polymyxin B and bacitracin zinc)
Johnson & Johnson Consumer Products Company, Division of Johnson & Johnson Consumer Companies, Inc.

DRUG FACTS

Active Ingredient(s) (in each gram)	Purpose(s)
Bacitracin 500 units	First aid antibiotic
Polymyxin B 10,000 units	First aid antibiotic

USE
first aid to help prevent infection in minor:
- cuts
- scrapes
- burns

WARNINGS
For external use only.

DO NOT USE
- if you are allergic to any of the ingredients
- in the eyes
- over large areas of the body

ASK A DOCTOR BEFORE USE IF YOU HAVE
- deep or puncture wounds
- animal bites
- serious burns

STOP USE AND ASK A DOCTOR IF
- you need to use longer than 1 week
- condition persists or gets worse
- rash or other allergic reaction develops

Keep out of reach of children. If swallowed, get medical help or contact a Poison Control Center right away.

DIRECTIONS
- clean the affected area
- apply a light dusting of the powder on the area 1 to 3 times daily
- may be covered with a sterile bandage

OTHER INFORMATION
- store at 20° to 25°C (68° to 77° F)
- do not refrigerate

INACTIVE INGREDIENT
lactose base

QUESTIONS OR COMMENTS?
call **1-800-223-0182**

PREPARATION H HYDROCORTISONE
(hydrocortisone)

Pfizer Consumer Healthcare

DRUG FACTS

Active Ingredient(s)
Hydrocortisone 1%

Purpose(s)
Anti-itch

USES
- temporary relief of external anal itching
- temporary relief of itching associated with minor skin irritations and rashes
- other uses of this product should be only under the advice and supervision of a doctor

WARNINGS
For external use only

DO NOT USE
for the treatment of diaper rash. Consult a doctor.

WHEN USING THIS PRODUCT
- avoid contact with the eyes
- do not exceed the recommended daily dosage unless directed by a doctor
- do not put into the rectum by using fingers or any mechanical device or applicator

STOP USE AND ASK A DOCTOR IF
- bleeding occurs
- condition worsens
- symptoms persist for more than 7 days or clear up and occur again within a few days. Do not begin use of any other hydrocortisone product unless you have consulted a doctor.

Keep out of reach of children.
If swallowed, get medical help or contact a Poison Control Center right away.

DIRECTIONS
- adults: when practical, cleanse the affected area by patting or blotting with an appropriate cleansing wipe. Gently dry by patting or blotting with a tissue or soft cloth before application of this product.
- when first opening the tube, puncture foil seal with top end of cap
- adults and children 12 years of age and older: apply to the affected area not more than 3 to 4 times daily
- children under 12 years of age: do not use, consult a doctor

OTHER INFORMATION
store at 20-25°C (68-77°F)

INACTIVE INGREDIENTS
anhydrous citric acid, butylated hydroxyanisole, carboxymethylcellulose sodium, cetyl alcohol, citric acid monohydrate, edetate disodium, glycerin, glyceryl oleate, glyceryl stearate, lanolin, methylparaben, propyl gallate, propylene glycol, propylparaben, purified water, simethicone emulsion, sodium benzoate, sodium lauryl sulfate, stearyl alcohol, white petrolatum, xanthan gum

QUESTIONS OR COMMENTS?
Call weekdays 9 AM to 5 PM EST at **1-800-99PrepH** or **1-800-997-7374**.

PREPARATION H COOLING GEL (phenylephrine HCl and witch hazel)

Wyeth Consumer Healthcare

DRUG FACTS

Active Ingredient(s)
Phenylephrine HCl 0.25%
Witch hazel 50.0%

Purpose(s)
Vasoconstrictor
Astringent

USES
- helps relieve the local itching and discomfort associated with hemorrhoids
- temporary relief of irritation and burning
- temporarily shrinks hemorrhoidal tissue
- aids in protecting irritated anorectal areas

WARNINGS
For external use only

ASK A DOCTOR BEFORE USE IF YOU HAVE
- heart disease
- high blood pressure
- thyroid disease
- diabetes
- difficulty in urination due to enlargement of the prostate gland

ASK A DOCTOR OR PHARMACIST BEFORE USE IF YOU ARE
presently taking a prescription drug for high blood pressure or depression.

WHEN USING THIS PRODUCT
- do not exceed the recommended daily dosage unless directed by a doctor
- do not put this product into the rectum by using fingers or any mechanical device or applicator

STOP USE AND ASK A DOCTOR IF
- bleeding occurs
- condition worsens or does not improve within 7 days

If pregnant or breast-feeding,
ask a health professional before use.

Keep out of reach of children.
If swallowed, get medical help or contact a Poison Control Center right away.

DIRECTIONS
- adults: when practical, cleanse the affected area by patting or blotting with an appropriate cleansing wipe. Gently dry by patting or blotting with a tissue or a soft cloth before applying gel.
- when first opening the tube, puncture foil seal with top end of cap
- apply externally to the affected area up to 4 times daily, especially at night, in the morning or after each bowel movement
- children under 12 years of age: ask a doctor

OTHER INFORMATION
store at 20-25°C (68-77°F)

INACTIVE INGREDIENTS
aloe barbadensis leaf juice, edetate disodium, hydroxyethyl cellulose, methylparaben, polysorbate 80, propylene glycol, propylparaben, purified water, sodium citrate, sulisobenzone, vitamin E acetate

QUESTIONS OR COMMENTS?
Call weekdays 9 AM to 5 PM EST at **1-800-99PrepH** or **1-800-997-7374.**

PREPARATION H CREAM MAX STRENGTH (glycerin, petrolatum, phenylephrine HCl, and pramoxine HCl)

Pfizer Consumer Healthcare

DRUG FACTS

Active Ingredient(s)
Glycerin 14.4%
Phenylephrine HCl 0.25%
Pramoxine HCl 1%
White petrolatum 15%

Purpose(s)
Protectant
Vasoconstrictor
Local anesthetic
Protectant

USES
- for temporary relief of pain, soreness and burning
- helps relieve the local itching and discomfort associated with hemorrhoids
- temporarily shrinks hemorrhoidal tissue
- temporarily provides a coating for relief of anorectal discomforts
- temporarily protects the inflamed, irritated anorectal surface to help make bowel movements less painful

WARNINGS
For external use only

ASK A DOCTOR BEFORE USE IF YOU HAVE
- heart disease
- high blood pressure
- thyroid disease
- diabetes
- difficulty in urination due to enlargement of the prostate gland

ASK A DOCTOR OR PHARMACIST BEFORE USE IF YOU ARE
presently taking a prescription drug for high blood pressure or depression.

WHEN USING THIS PRODUCT
- do not exceed the recommended daily dosage unless directed by a doctor
- do not put into the rectum by using fingers or any mechanical device or applicator

STOP USE AND ASK A DOCTOR IF
- bleeding occurs
- condition worsens or does not improve within 7 days
- an allergic reaction develops
- the symptom being treated does not subside or if redness, irritation, swelling, pain, or other symptoms develop or increase

If pregnant or breast-feeding,
ask a health professional before use.

Keep out of reach of children.
If swallowed, get medical help or contact a Poison Control Center right away.

DIRECTIONS
- adults: when practical, cleanse the affected area by patting or blotting with an appropriate cleansing wipe. Gently dry by patting or blotting with a tissue or a soft cloth before applying cream.
- when first opening the tube, puncture foil seal with top end of cap
- apply externally or in the lower portion of the anal canal only
- apply externally to the affected area up to 4 times daily, especially at night, in the morning or after each bowel movement
- for application in the lower anal canal: remove cover from dispensing cap. Attach dispensing cap to tube. Lubricate dispensing cap well, then gently insert dispensing cap partway into the anus.
- thoroughly cleanse dispensing cap after each use and replace cover
- children under 12 years of age: ask a doctor

OTHER INFORMATION
store at 20-25°C (68-77°F)

INACTIVE INGREDIENTS
aloe barbadensis leaf extract, anhydrous citric acid, butylated hydroxyanisole, carboxymethylcellulose sodium, cetyl alcohol, citric acid monohydrate, dexpanthenol, edetate disodium, glyceryl monostearate, methylparaben, mineral oil, polyoxyl lauryl ether, polyoxyl stearyl ether, propyl gallate, propylene glycol, propylparaben, purified water, sodium benzoate, stearyl alcohol, tocopherols excipient, vitamin E acetate, xanthan gum

QUESTIONS OR COMMENTS?
Call weekdays 9 AM to 5 PM EST at **1-800-99PrepH** or **1-800-997-7374.**

PREPARATION H HEMORRHOIDAL OINTMENT (mineral oil, petrolatum, and phenylephrine HCl)
Pfizer Consumer Healthcare

DRUG FACTS

Active Ingredient(s)
Mineral oil 14%
Petrolatum 74.9%
Phenylephrine HCl 0.25%

Purpose(s)
Protectant
Protectant
Vasoconstrictor

USES
- helps relieve the local itching and discomfort associated with hemorrhoids
- temporarily shrinks hemorrhoidal tissue and relieves burning
- temporarily provides a coating for relief of anorectal discomforts
- temporarily protects the inflamed, irritated anorectal surface to help make bowel movements less painful

WARNINGS
For external and/or intrarectal use only

ASK A DOCTOR BEFORE USE IF YOU HAVE
- heart disease
- high blood pressure
- thyroid disease
- diabetes
- difficulty in urination due to enlargement of the prostate gland

ASK A DOCTOR OR PHARMACIST BEFORE USE IF YOU ARE
presently taking a prescription drug for high blood pressure or depression.

WHEN USING THIS PRODUCT
do not exceed the recommended daily dosage unless directed by a doctor.

STOP USE AND ASK A DOCTOR IF
- bleeding occurs
- condition worsens or does not improve within 7 days
- introduction of applicator into the rectum causes additional pain

If pregnant or breast-feeding, ask a health professional before use.

Keep out of reach of children. If swallowed, get medical help or contact a Poison Control Center right away.

DIRECTIONS
- adults: when practical, cleanse the affected area by patting or blotting with an appropriate cleansing wipe. Gently dry by patting or blotting with a tissue or a soft cloth before applying ointment.
- when first opening the tube, puncture foil seal with top end of cap
- apply to the affected area up to 4 times daily, especially at night, in the morning or after each bowel movement
- intrarectal use:
  - remove cover from applicator, attach applicator to tube, lubricate applicator well and gently insert applicator into the rectum
  - thoroughly cleanse applicator after each use and replace cover
- also apply ointment to external area
- regular use provides continual therapy for relief of symptoms
- children under 12 years of age: ask a doctor

OTHER INFORMATION
store at 20-25°C (68-77°F)

INACTIVE INGREDIENTS
benzoic acid, butylated hydroxyanisole, corn oil, glycerin, lanolin, lanolin alcohols, methylparaben, mineral oil, paraffin, propylparaben, purified water, shark liver oil, thymus vulgaris (thyme) flower/leaf oil, tocopherols excipient, white wax

QUESTIONS OR COMMENTS?
Call weekdays 9 AM to 5 PM EST at **1-800-99PrepH** or **1-800-997-7374**

PREPARATION H SUPPOSITORIES (cocoa butter and phenylephrine HCl)
Pfizer Consumer Healthcare

DRUG FACTS

Active Ingredient(s)
Cocoa butter 85.39%
Phenylephrine HCl 0.25%

Purpose(s)
Protectant
Vasoconstrictor

USES
- helps relieve the local itching and discomfort associated with hemorrhoids
- temporarily relieves burning and shrinks hemorrhoidal tissue

- temporarily provides a coating for relief of anorectal discomforts
- temporarily protects the inflamed, irritated anorectal surface to help make bowel movements less painful

WARNINGS
For rectal use only

ASK A DOCTOR BEFORE USE IF YOU HAVE
- heart disease
- high blood pressure
- thyroid disease
- diabetes
- difficulty in urination due to enlargement of the prostate gland

ASK A DOCTOR OR PHARMACIST BEFORE USE IF YOU ARE
presently taking a prescription drug for high blood pressure or depression

WHEN USING THIS PRODUCT
do not exceed the recommended daily dosage unless directed by a doctor

STOP USE AND ASK A DOCTOR IF
- bleeding occurs
- condition worsens or does not improve within 7 days

If pregnant or breast-feeding,
ask a health professional before use.

Keep out of reach of children.
If swallowed, get medical help or contact a Poison Control Center right away.

DIRECTIONS
- adults: when practical, cleanse the affected area by patting or blotting with an appropriate cleansing wipe. Gently dry by patting or blotting with a tissue or a soft cloth before insertion of this product.
- detach one suppository from the strip; remove the foil wrapper before inserting into the rectum as follows:
  - hold suppository with rounded end up
  - as shown, carefully separate foil tabs by inserting tip of fingernail at end marked "peel down"
  - slowly and evenly peel apart (do not tear) foil by pulling tabs down both sides, to expose the suppository
  - remove exposed suppository from wrapper
  - insert one suppository into the rectum up to 4 times daily, especially at night, in the morning or after each bowel movement
- children under 12 years of age: ask a doctor

OTHER INFORMATION
store at 20-25°C (68-77°F)

INACTIVE INGREDIENTS
corn starch, methylparaben, propylparaben, shark liver oil

QUESTIONS OR COMMENTS?
Call weekdays 9 AM to 5 PM EST at **1-800-99PrepH** or **1-800-997-7374.**

PREPARATION H TOTABLES BURNING RELIEF GEL (phenylephrine hydrochloride and witch hazel)

Pfizer Consumer Healthcare

DRUG FACTS

Active Ingredient(s)	Purpose(s)
Phenylephrine HCl 0.25%	Vasoconstrictor
Witch hazel 50.0%	Astringent

USES
- helps relieve the local itching and discomfort associated with hemorrhoids
- temporary relief of irritation and burning
- temporarily shrinks hemorrhoidal tissue
- aids in protecting irritated anorectal areas

WARNINGS
For external use only

ASK A DOCTOR BEFORE USE IF YOU HAVE
- heart disease
- high blood pressure
- thyroid disease
- diabetes
- difficulty in urination due to enlargement of the prostate gland

ASK A DOCTOR OR PHARMACIST BEFORE USE IF YOU ARE
presently taking a prescription drug for high blood pressure or depression.

WHEN USING THIS PRODUCT
- do not exceed the recommended daily dosage unless directed by a doctor
- do not put this product into the rectum by using fingers or any mechanical device or applicator

STOP USE AND ASK A DOCTOR IF
- bleeding occurs
- condition worsens or does not improve within 7 days

If pregnant or breast-feeding, ask a health professional before use.
Keep out of reach of children. If swallowed, get medical help or contact a Poison Control Center right away.

DIRECTIONS
- adults: when practical, cleanse the affected area by patting or blotting with an appropriate cleansing wipe. Gently dry by patting or blotting with a tissue or a soft cloth before applying gel.
- when first opening the tube, puncture foil seal with top end of cap
- apply externally to the affected area up to 4 times daily, especially at night, in the morning or after each bowel movement
- children under 12 years of age: ask a doctor

OTHER INFORMATION
Store at 20°-25°C (68-77°F)

INACTIVE INGREDIENTS
aloe barbadensis leaf juice, edetate disodium, hydroxyethyl cellulose, methylparaben, polysorbate 80, propylene glycol, propylparaben, purified water, sodium citrate, sulisobenzone, vitamin E acetate

PREPARATION H TOTABLES IRRITATION RELIEF WIPES (witch hazel)

Pfizer Consumer Healthcare

DRUG FACTS

Active Ingredient(s)	Purpose(s)
Witch hazel 50.0%	Astringent

USES
- helps relieve the local itching and discomfort associated with hemorrhoids
- temporary relief of irritation and burning
- aids in protecting irritated anorectal areas

WARNINGS
For external use only

WHEN USING THIS PRODUCT
- do not exceed the recommended daily dosage unless directed by a doctor
- do not put this product into the rectum by using fingers or any mechanical device or applicator

STOP USE AND ASK A DOCTOR IF
- bleeding occurs
- condition worsens or does not improve within 7 days

If pregnant or breast-feeding, ask a health professional before use.
Keep out of reach of children. If swallowed, get medical help or contact a Poison Control Center right away.

DIRECTIONS
- adults: unfold wipe and cleanse the area by gently wiping, patting or blotting. If necessary, repeat until all matter is removed from the area.
- use up to 6 times daily or after each bowel movement and before applying topical hemorrhoidal treatments, and then discard
- children under 12 years of age: consult a doctor

OTHER INFORMATION
- store at 20°-25°C (68-77°F)
- for best results, flush only one or two wipes at a time

INACTIVE INGREDIENTS
aloe barbadensis leaf juice, anhydrous citric acid, capryl/capramidopropyl betaine, diazolidinyl urea, glycerin, methylparaben, propylene glycol, propylparaben, purified water, sodium citrate

QUESTIONS OR COMMENTS?
Call weekdays 9 AM to 5 PM EST at **1-800-99PrepH or 1-800-997-7374**

PREPARATION H TOTABLES PAIN RELIEF CREAM (glycerin, phenylephrine hydrochloride, pramoxine hydrochloride, and petrolatum)

Pfizer Consumer Healthcare

DRUG FACTS

Active Ingredient(s)	Purpose(s)
Glycerin 14.4%	Protectant
Phenylephrine HCl 0.25%	Vasoconstrictor
Pramoxine HCl 1%	Local anesthetic
White petrolatum 15%	Protectant

USES
- for temporary relief of pain, soreness and burning
- helps relieve the local itching and discomfort associated with hemorrhoids
- temporarily shrinks hemorrhoidal tissue
- temporarily provides a coating for relief of anorectal discomforts
- temporarily protects the inflamed, irritated anorectal surface to help make bowel movements less painful

WARNINGS
For external use only

ASK A DOCTOR BEFORE USE IF YOU HAVE
- heart disease
- high blood pressure
- thyroid disease
- diabetes
- difficulty in urination due to enlargement of the prostate gland

ASK A DOCTOR OR PHARMACIST BEFORE USE IF YOU ARE
presently taking a prescription drug for high blood pressure or depression.

WHEN USING THIS PRODUCT
- do not exceed the recommended daily dosage unless directed by a doctor
- do not put into the rectum by using fingers or any mechanical device or applicator

STOP USE AND ASK A DOCTOR IF
- bleeding occurs
- condition worsens or does not improve within 7 days
- an allergic reaction develops
- the symptom being treated does not subside or if redness, irritation, swelling, pain, or other symptoms develop or increase

If pregnant or breast-feeding, ask a health professional before use.
Keep out of reach of children. If swallowed, get medical help or contact a Poison Control Center right away.

DIRECTIONS
- adults: when practical, cleanse the affected area by patting or blotting with an appropriate cleansing wipe. Gently dry by patting or blotting with a tissue or a soft cloth before applying cream.
- when first opening the tube, puncture foil seal with top end of cap
- apply externally to the affected area up to 4 times daily, especially at night, in the morning or after each bowel movement
- children under 12 years of age: ask a doctor

OTHER INFORMATION
Store at 20°-25°C (68-77°F)

INACTIVE INGREDIENTS
aloe barbadensis leaf extract, anhydrous citric acid, butylated hydroxyanisole, carboxymethylcellulose sodium, cetyl alcohol, citric acid monohydrate, dexpanthenol, edetate disodium, glyceryl monostearate, methylparaben, mineral oil, polyoxyl lauryl ether, polyoxyl stearyl ether, propyl gallate, propylene glycol, propylparaben, purified water, sodium benzoate, stearyl alcohol, tocopherols excipient, vitamin E acetate, xanthan gum

QUESTIONS OR COMMENTS?
Call weekdays 9 AM to 5 PM EST at **1-800-99PrepH or 1-800-997-7374.**

PREVACID 24 HR (lansoprazole)

Novartis Consumer Health, Inc.

Active Ingredient(s)
Lansoprazole 15mg

Purpose(s)
Acid reducer

USES
- treats frequent heartburn (occurs **2 or more** days a week)
- not intended for immediate relief of heartburn; this drug may take 1 to 4 days for full effect

WARNINGS
Allergy alert: Do not use if you are allergic to lansoprazole

DO NOT USE
- if you have trouble or pain swallowing food, vomiting with blood, or bloody or black stools. These may be signs of a serious condition. See your doctor.

ASK DOCTOR
- warfarin (blood-thinning medicine)
- prescription antifungal or anti-yeast medicines
- digoxin (heart medicine)
- theophylline (asthma medicine)
- tacrolimus (immune system medicine)
- atazanavir (medicine for HIV infection)

STOP USE AND ASK A DOCTOR IF
- your heartburn continues or worsens
- you need to take this product for more than 14 days
- you need to take more than 1 course of treatment every 4 months

If pregnant or breast feeding
If pregnant or breast-feeding, ask a health professional before use.

Keep out of reach of children

In case of overdose
get medical help or contact a Poison Control Center right away.

DIRECTIONS
- adults 18 years of age and older
- this product is to be used once a day (every 24 hours), every day for 14 days
- it may take 1 to 4 days for full effect, although some people get complete relief of symptoms within 24 hours
- **14-Day Course of Treatment**
  - swallow 1 capsule with a glass of water before eating in the morning
  - take every day for 14 days
  - do not take more than 1 capsule a day
  - swallow whole. Do not crush or chew capsules.

- do not use for more than 14 days unless directed by your doctor
- **Repeated 14-Day Courses (if needed)**
  - you may repeat a 14-day course every 4 months
  - **do not take for more than 14 days or more often than every 4 months unless directed by a doctor**
- children under 18 years of age: ask a doctor before use. Heartburn in children may sometimes be caused by a serious condition.

OTHER INFORMATION
- read the directions, warnings and package insert before use
- keep the carton and package insert. They contain important information.
- store at 20-25° C (68-77 ° F)
- keep product out of high heat and humidity
- protect product from moisture

INACTIVE INGREDIENTS
colloidal silicon dioxide, D&C red no. 28, FD&C blue no. 1, FD&C green no. 3, FD&C red no. 40, gelatin, hydroxypropyl cellulose, low substituted hydroxypropyl cellulose, magnesium carbonate, methacrylic acid copolymer, polyethylene glycol, polysorbate 80, starch, sucrose, sugar sphere, talc, titanium dioxide

QUESTIONS OR COMMENTS?
1-800-452-0051
Distributed by: **Novartis Consumer Health, Inc.,** Parsippany, NJ 07054-0622 ©2009 U.S. Patent No. 4,628,098 PREVACID® is a registered trademark of Takeda Pharmaceuticals North America, Inc.

PRILOSEC OTC (omeprazole magnesium)

Procter & Gamble

DRUG FACTS

Active Ingredient(s) (in each tablet)
Omeprazole magnesium delayed-release tablet 20.6 mg (equivalent to 20 mg omeprazole).

Purpose(s)
Acid reducer

USE
- treats frequent heartburn (occurs **2 or more** days a week)
- not intended for immediate relief of heartburn; this drug may take 1 to 4 days for full effect

WARNINGS
Allergy alert
Do not use if you are allergic to omeprazole

DO NOT USE
if you have trouble or pain swallowing food, vomiting with blood, or bloody or black stools.
These may be signs of a serious condition. See your doctor.

ASK A DOCTOR BEFORE USE IF YOU HAVE
- had heartburn over 3 months.
  This may be a sign of a more serious condition.
- heartburn with **lightheadedness, sweating or dizziness**
- chest pain or shoulder pain with shortness of breath; sweating; pain spreading to arms, neck or shoulders; or lightheadedness
- frequent **chest pain**
- frequent wheezing, particularly with heartburn
- unexplained weight loss
- nausea or vomiting
- stomach pain

ASK A DOCTOR OR PHARMACIST BEFORE USE IF YOU ARE

taking
- warfarin, clopidogrel, or cilostazol (blood-thinning medicines)
- prescription antifungal or anti-yeast medicines
- diazepam (anxiety medicine)
- digoxin (heart medicine)
- tacrolimus (immune system medicine)
- prescription antiretrovirals (medicines for HIV infection)

STOP USE AND ASK A DOCTOR IF
- your heartburn continues or worsens
- you need to take this product for more than 14 days
- you need to take more than 1 course of treatment every 4 months

If pregnant or breast-feeding, ask a health professional before use.

Keep out of reach of children. In case of overdose, get medical help or contact a Poison Control Center right away.

DIRECTIONS
- for adults 18 years of age and older
- this product is to be used once a day (every 24 hours), every day for 14 days
- it may take 1 to 4 days for full effect; some people get complete relief of symptoms within 24 hours
  14-Day Course of Treatment
  - swallow 1 tablet with a glass of water before eating in the morning
  - take every day for 14 days
  - do not take more than 1 tablet a day
  - do not use for more than 14 days unless directed by your doctor
  - swallow whole. Do not chew or crush tablets.
  Repeated 14-Day Courses (if needed)
  - you may repeat a 14-day course every 4 months
  - **do not take for more than 14 days or more often than every 4 months unless directed by a doctor**
- children under 18 years of age: ask a doctor. Heartburn in children may sometimes be caused by a serious condition.

OTHER INFORMATION
- read the directions and warnings before use
- keep the carton. It contains important information.
- store at 20-25°C (68-77°F) and protect from moisture

INACTIVE INGREDIENTS
glyceryl monostearate, hydroxypropyl cellulose, hypromellose, iron oxide, magnesium stearate, methacrylic acid copolymer, microcrystalline cellulose, paraffin, polyethylene glycol 6000, polysorbate 80, polyvinylpyrrolidone, sodium stearyl fumarate, starch, sucrose, talc, titanium dioxide, triethyl citrate

QUESTIONS OR COMMENTS?
1-800-289-9181
Dist. by Procter & Gamble, Cincinnati, OH 45202
Product of Sweden

REFRESH CELLUVISC (carboxymethylcellulose sodium)
Allergan, Inc.

DRUG FACTS

Active Ingredient(s)
Carboxymethylcellulose sodium 1%

Purpose(s)
Eye lubricant

USES
- For the temporary relief of burning, irritation, and discomfort due to dryness of the eye or exposure to wind or sun.
- May be used as a protectant against further irritation.

WARNINGS
- **For external use only.**
- **To avoid contamination, do not touch tip of container to any surface. Do not reuse. Once opened, discard.**
- **Do not touch unit-dose tip to eye.**
- **If solution changes color or becomes cloudy, do not use.**

STOP USE AND ASK A DOCTOR IF
you experience eye pain, changes in vision, continued redness or irritation of the eye, or if the condition worsens or persists for more than 72 hours.
Keep out of reach of children. If swallowed, get medical help or contact a Poison Control Center right away.

DIRECTIONS
To open, **TWIST AND PULL TAB TO REMOVE.** Instill 1 or 2 drops in the affected eye(s) as needed and discard container.

OTHER INFORMATION
- Use only if single-use container is intact.
- **REFRESH® CELLUVISC® may cause temporary blurring due to its viscosity.**
- **Store at 59°-86°F (15°-30°C).**
- **Use before expiration date marked on container.**
- **RETAIN THIS CARTON FOR FUTURE REFERENCE.**

INACTIVE INGREDIENTS
calcium chloride, potassium chloride, purified water, sodium chloride, and sodium lactate.

QUESTIONS OR COMMENTS?
1.800.433.8871, M-F 6 AM-4:30 PM Pacific Time
refreshbrand.com

REFRESH CLASSIC (polyvinyl alcohol and povidone)
Allergan, Inc.

DRUG FACTS

Active Ingredient(s)
Polyvinyl Alcohol 1.4%
Povidone 0.6%

Purpose(s)
Eye lubricant
Eye lubricant

USES
- For the temporary relief of burning, irritation, and discomfort due to dryness of the eye or exposure to wind or sun.
- May be used as a protectant against further irritation.

WARNINGS
- **For external use only.**
- **To avoid contamination, do not touch tip of container to any surface. Do not reuse. Once opened, discard.**
- **Do not touch unit-dose tip to eye.**
- **If solution changes color or becomes cloudy, do not use.**

STOP USE AND ASK A DOCTOR IF
you experience eye pain, changes in vision, continued redness or irritation of the eye, or if the condition worsens or persists for more than 72 hours.

Keep out of reach of children. If swallowed, get medical help or contact a Poison Control Center right away.

DIRECTIONS
To open, **TWIST AND PULL TAB TO REMOVE.** Instill 1 or 2 drops in the affected eye(s) as needed and discard container.

OTHER INFORMATION
• **Use only if single-use container is intact.**
• **Use before expiration date marked on container.**
• **Store at 59°-86°F (15°-30°C).**
• **RETAIN THIS CARTON FOR FUTURE REFERENCE.**

INACTIVE INGREDIENTS
purified water and sodium chloride. May also contain hydrochloric acid and/or sodium hydroxide to adjust pH.

QUESTIONS OR COMMENTS?
1.800.433.8871, M-F 6 AM-4:30 PM Pacific Time
refreshbrand.com

REFRESH LACRI-LUBE (mineral oil and petrolatum)
Allergan, Inc.

DRUG FACTS

Active Ingredient(s)
Mineral Oil 42.5%
White Petrolatum 56.8%

Purpose(s)
Eye lubricant
Eye lubricant

USES
• For use as a protectant against further irritation or to relieve dryness of the eye.

WARNINGS
• **For external use only.**
• **To avoid contamination, do not touch tip of container to any surface.**
• **Replace cap after using.**

STOP USE AND ASK A DOCTOR IF
you experience eye pain, changes in vision, continued redness or irritation of the eye, or if the condition worsens or persists for more than 72 hours.
Keep out of reach of children. If swallowed, get medical help or contact a Poison Control Center right away.

DIRECTIONS
Pull down the lower lid of the affected eye and apply a small amount (one-fourth inch) of ointment to the inside of the eyelid.

OTHER INFORMATION
• **Use only if imprinted tape seals on top and bottom flaps are intact and clearly legible.**
• **Store away from heat. Protect from freezing.**
• **Use before expiration date marked on container.**
• **Store at 59°-86°F (15°-30°C)**
• **RETAIN THIS CARTON FOR FUTURE REFERENCE.**

INACTIVE INGREDIENTS
chlorobutanol and lanolin alcohols.

QUESTIONS OR COMMENTS?
1.800.433.8871
M-F 6 AM-4:30 PM
Pacific Time
refreshbrand.com

REFRESH LIQUIGEL (carboxymethylcellulose sodium)
Allergan, Inc.

DRUG FACTS

Active Ingredient(s)
Carboxymethylcellulose sodium 1%

Purpose(s)
Eye lubricant

USES
• For the temporary relief of burning, irritation, and discomfort due to dryness of the eye or exposure to wind or sun.
• May be used as a protectant against further irritation.

WARNINGS
• **For external use only.**
• **To avoid contamination, do not touch tip of container to any surface. Replace cap after using.**
• **If solution changes color or becomes cloudy, do not use.**

STOP USE AND ASK A DOCTOR IF
you experience eye pain, changes in vision, continued redness or irritation of the eye, or if the condition worsens or persists for more than 72 hours.
Keep out of reach of children. If swallowed, get medical help or contact a Poison Control Center right away.

DIRECTIONS
Instill 1 or 2 drops in the affected eye(s) as needed.

OTHER INFORMATION
• **Use only if imprinted tape seals on top and bottom flaps are intact and clearly legible.**
• **Use before expiration date marked on container.**
• **Store at 59°-86° F (15°-30° C).**
• **RETAIN THIS CARTON FOR FUTURE REFERENCE.**

INACTIVE INGREDIENTS
boric acid, calcium chloride, magnesium chloride, potassium chloride, purified water, PURITE® (stabilized oxychloro complex), sodium borate, and sodium chloride.

QUESTIONS OR COMMENTS?
1.800.433.8871
M-F 6 AM-4:30 PM
Pacific Time
refreshbrand.com
Refresh®
Make your dry eyes feel better with the drops doctors recommend.
REFRESH LIQUIGEL® Lubricant Eye Drops provides extra strength moisturizing relief, plus protection, for dry, irritated eyes with our thick gel formula.
REFRESH LIQUIGEL® comes in a convenient multi-dose bottle and is safe to use as often as needed, so your eyes can feel good-anytime, anywhere.
refreshbrand.com
REFRESH LIQUIGEL® uses the safe and gentle preservative PURITE®.
Allergan, Inc.
2525 Dupont Drive
Irvine, CA 92612, U.S.A.
© 2010 Allergan, Inc.
® marks owned by Allergan, Inc.
U.S. Patent 5,424,078
Made in the U.S.A.

REFRESH OPTIVE (carboxymethylcellulose sodium and glycerin)

Allergan, Inc.

DRUG FACTS

Active Ingredient(s)
Carboxymethylcellulose sodium 0.5%
Glycerin 0.9%

Purpose(s)
Eye lubricant
Eye lubricant

USES
• For the temporary relief of burning, irritation, and discomfort due to dryness of the eye or exposure to wind or sun.
• May be used as a protectant against further irritation.

WARNINGS
• **For external use only.**
• **To avoid contamination, do not touch tip of container to any surface. Replace cap after using.**
• **If solution changes color or becomes cloudy, do not use.**

STOP USE AND ASK A DOCTOR IF
you experience eye pain, changes in vision, continued redness, or irritation of the eye, or if the condition worsens or persists for more than 72 hours.
Keep out of reach of children. If swallowed, get medical help or contact a Poison Control Center right away.

DIRECTIONS
Instill 1 or 2 drops in the affected eye(s) as needed.

OTHER INFORMATION
• **Use only if imprinted tape seals on top and bottom flaps are intact and clearly legible.**
• **Use before expiration date marked on container.**
• **Store at 59°-86°F (15°-30°C).**
• **RETAIN THIS CARTON FOR FUTURE REFERENCE.**

INACTIVE INGREDIENTS
boric acid; calcium chloride dihydrate; erythritol; levocarnitine; magnesium chloride hexahydrate; potassium chloride; purified water; PURITE® (stabilized oxychloro complex); sodium borate decahydrate; and sodium citrate dihydrate.

QUESTIONS OR COMMENTS?
1.800.433.8871
M-F 6 AM-4:30 PM
Pacific Time
refreshbrand.com

REFRESH OPTIVE ADVANCED

(carboxymethylcellulose sodium, glycerin, and polysorbate 80)

Allergan, Inc.

DRUG FACTS

Active Ingredient(s)
Carboxymethylcellulose sodium 0.5%
Glycerin 1%
Polysorbate 80 0.5%

Purpose(s)
Eye lubricant
Eye lubricant
Eye lubricant

USES
• For the temporary relief of burning, irritation, and discomfort due to dryness of the eye or exposure to wind or sun.
• May be used as a protectant against further irritation.

WARNINGS
• **For external use only.**
• **To avoid contamination, do not touch tip of container to any surface. Replace cap after using.**
• **If solution changes color, do not use.**

STOP USE AND ASK A DOCTOR IF
you experience eye pain, changes in vision, continued redness, or irritation of the eye, or if the condition worsens or persists for more than 72 hours.
Keep out of reach of children. If swallowed, get medical help or contact a Poison Control Center right away.

DIRECTIONS
Instill 1 or 2 drops in the affected eye(s) as needed.

OTHER INFORMATION
• **Use only if imprinted tape seals on top and bottom flaps are intact and clearly legible.**
• **Use before expiration date marked on container.**
• **Store at 59°-86°F (15°-30°C).**
• **RETAIN THIS CARTON FOR FUTURE REFERENCE.**

INACTIVE INGREDIENTS
boric acid; castor oil; erythritol; levocarnitine; carbomer copolymer type A; purified water; and PURITE® (stabilized oxychloro complex). May also contain hydrochloric acid and/or sodium hydroxide to adjust pH.

QUESTIONS OR COMMENTS?
1.800.433.8871
M-F 6 AM-4:30 PM Pacific Time
refreshbrand.com

REFRESH OPTIVE SENSITIVE

(carboxymethylcellulose sodium and glycerin)

Allergan, Inc.

DRUG FACTS

Active Ingredient(s)
Carboxymethylcellulose sodium 0.5%
Glycerin 0.9%

Purpose(s)
Eye lubricant
Eye lubricant

USES
• For the temporary relief of burning, irritation, and discomfort due to dryness of the eye or exposure to wind or sun.
• May be used as a protectant against further irritation.

WARNINGS
• **For external use only.**
• **To avoid contamination, do not touch tip of container to any surface. Do not reuse. Once opened, discard.**
• **Do not touch unit-dose tip to eye.**
• **If solution changes color, do not use.**

STOP USE AND ASK A DOCTOR IF

you experience eye pain, changes in vision, continued redness or irritation of the eye, or if the condition worsens or persists for more than 72 hours.

Keep out of reach of children. If swallowed, get medical help or contact a Poison Control Center right away.

DIRECTIONS

To open, **TWIST AND PULL TAB TO REMOVE.** Instill 1 or 2 drops in the affected eye(s) as needed and discard container.
*lf used for post-operative (e.g., LASIK) dryness and discomfort, follow your eye doctor's instructions.

OTHER INFORMATION

- **Use only if single-use container is intact.**
- **Use before expiration date marked on container.**
- **Store at 59°-86°F (15°-30°C).**
- **RETAIN THIS CARTON FOR FUTURE REFERENCE.**

INACTIVE INGREDIENTS

boric acid, calcium chloride dihydrate, erythritol, levocarnitine, magnesium chloride hexahydrate, potassium chloride, purified water, sodium borate decahydrate, and sodium citrate dihydrate.

QUESTIONS OR COMMENTS?

1.800.433.8871 M-F 6 AM-4:30 PM Pacific Time
refreshbrand.com
Refresh Optive Sensitive
Lubricant Eye Drops
Allergan, Inc.

REFRESH PLUS (carboxymethylcellulose sodium)

Allergan, Inc.

DRUG FACTS

Active Ingredient(s)
Carboxymethylcellulose sodium 0.5%

Purpose(s)
Eye lubricant

USES

- For the temporary relief of burning, irritation, and discomfort due to dryness of the eye or exposure to wind or sun.
- May be used as a protectant against further irritation.

WARNINGS

- **For external use only.**
- **To avoid contamination, do not touch tip of container to any surface. Do not reuse. Once opened, discard.**
- **Do not touch unit-dose tip to eye.**
- **If solution changes color or becomes cloudy, do not use.**

STOP USE AND ASK A DOCTOR IF

you experience eye pain, changes in vision, continued redness or irritation of the eye, or if the condition worsens or persists for more than 72 hours.

Keep out of reach of children. If swallowed, get medical help or contact a Poison Control Center right away.

DIRECTIONS

To open, **TWIST AND PULL TAB TO REMOVE.** Instill 1 or 2 drops in the affected eye(s) as needed and discard container.
*lf used for post-operative (e.g., LASIK) dryness and discomfort, follow your eye doctor's instructions.

OTHER INFORMATION

- **Use only if single-use container is intact.**
- **Use before expiration date marked on container.**
- **Store at 59°-86°F (15°-30°C)**
- **RETAIN THIS CARTON FOR FUTURE REFERENCE.**

INACTIVE INGREDIENTS

calcium chloride, magnesium chloride, potassium chloride, purified water, sodium chloride, and sodium lactate.
May also contain hydrochloric acid and/or sodium hydroxide to adjust pH.

QUESTIONS OR COMMENTS?

1.800.433.8871, M-F 6 AM-4:30 PM Pacific Time
refreshbrand.com

REFRESH P.M. (mineral oil and petrolatum)

Allergan, Inc.

DRUG FACTS

Active Ingredient(s)
Mineral Oil 42.5% and White Petrolatum 57.3%

Purpose(s)
Eye lubricant

USES

- For the temporary relief of burning, irritation, and discomfort due to dryness of the eye or exposure to wind or sun.
- May be used as a protectant against further irritation.

WARNINGS

- **For external use only.**
- **To avoid contamination, do not touch tip of container to any surface. Replace cap after using.**

STOP USE AND ASK A DOCTOR IF

you experience eye pain, changes in vision, continued redness or irritation of the eye, or if the condition worsens or persists for more than 72 hours.

Keep out of reach of children. If swallowed, get medical help or contact a Poison Control Center right away.

DIRECTIONS

Pull down the lower lid of the affected eye and apply a small amount (one
fourth inch) of ointment to the inside of the eyelid.

OTHER INFORMATION

- **Store away from heat.**
- **Protect from freezing.**
- **Use only if imprinted tape seals on top and bottom flaps are intact and clearly legible.**
- **Use before expiration date marked on container.**
- **Store at 59°-86°F (15°-30°C).**
- **RETAIN THIS CARTON FOR FUTURE REFERENCE.**

INACTIVE INGREDIENTS

lanolin alcohols

QUESTIONS OR COMMENTS?

1.800.433.8871
M-F 6 AM-4:30 PM Pacific Time
refreshbrand.com

RHINARIS NASAL GEL (polyethylene glycol and propylene glycol)
Pendopharm

DRUGS FACTS

Active ingredient(s)
Mixture of polyethylene glycol 15% and propylene glycol 20% in a gel adjusted to pH 5.5

USES
- To help moisturize and lubricate dry nasal passages caused by low humidity in homes, office buildings, hotels and airplanes.
- Provides long-lasting relief

WARNINGS
- For nasal use only.
- Keep out of reach of children.

DIRECTIONS
Adults: Apply a small amount of gel into each nostril every four (4) hours or as needed

OTHER INFORMATION
- Protect from freezing.

INACTIVE INGREDIENTS
purified water, carbomer 934P, sodium carboxymethylcellulose, sodium hydroxide, sodium chloride, potassium chloride, benzalkonium chloride

RHINARIS NASAL MIST
Pendopharm

DRUGS FACTS

Active ingredient(s)
Mixture of polyethylene glycol 15% and propylene glycol 5% in a solution adjusted to pH 6.0.

USES
- Helps moisturize and lubricate dry nasal passages caused by low humidity in homes, office buildings, hotels and airplanes.
- Provides long-lasting relief.

WARNINGS
- For nasal use only.
- Keep out of reach of children.

DIRECTIONS
- Adults: One (1) or two (2) sprays into each nostril every four (4) hours or as needed.
- Please refer to the package insert included with the product for detailed directions of use.

INACTIVE INGREDIENTS
purified water, sodium chloride, potassium chloride, potassium phosphate monobasic, benzalkonium chloride, dibasic sodium phosphate anhydrous

RHINARIS SALINE NASAL DROPS (KIDS)
(sodium chloride)
Pharmascience Inc.

DRUG FACTS

Active Ingredient(s)
Sodium Chloride 0.9%

USES
- gently moisturizes dry nasal passages, helping your child breathe easier

WARNINGS
- For nasal use only.
- Keep out of reach of children.

DIRECTIONS
- Infants and children: Gently tilt your child's head backwards and squeeze one (1) drop into each nostril, one (1) to three (3) times daily.

OTHER INFORMATION
- Protect from freezing.

INGREDIENTS
purified water, sodium chloride (0.9%), benzalkonium chloride

RHINARIS SINUS SALINE NASAL RINSE
Pendopharm

DRUGS FACTS

Active ingredient(s)
Purified water, sodium chloride, sodium biphosphate, sodium bicarbonate, trisodium EDTA, benzethonium chloride (as a preservative). May contain phosphoric acid to adjust pH.

USES
- Rinses away excess mucus in heavily blocked nasal passages to ease breathing.
- Helps to remove inhaled pollen, dust and pollutants that can cause allergies and sinus problems.

WARNINGS
- For nasal use only.
- Keep out of reach of children.
- For children under 8 years of age, please consult your physician before using.
- If nasal irritation, ear pressure or ear pain occurs, discontinue use and contact your physician.

DIRECTIONS
- Adults and children (8 years and older): One (1) spray (approx. 15–30 mL) per nostril, once daily as needed, or as directed by a health professional.
- Please refer to the product label for detailed directions of use.

OTHER INFORMATION
- Non-medicated. No rebound effect.
- Unique delivery system with no-spill cap.
- Refillable bottle (840 mL refill available).
- Protect from freezing.

RID HOME LICE, BEDBUG, & DUST MITE SPRAY (permethrin)

Bayer HealthCare LLC.

Active Ingredient(s)
Permethrin†. 0.50%
OTHER INGREDIENTS†† 99.50%
Total: 100.00%
†Cis/trans ratio: Max 55% (±) cis and Min 45% (±) trans
††Contains petroleum distillate

PRECAUTIONARY STATEMENT HAZARDS TO HUMANS CAUTION

Harmful if swallowed or absorbed through skin. Avoid inhalation of spray mist. Causes eye irritation. Avoid contact with skin, eyes or clothing. Wash thoroughly with soap and water after handling. Avoid contamination of feed and foodstuffs. Remove pets and birds and cover fish aquaria before space spraying or surface applications. **This product is not for use on humans.** Vacate room after treatment and ventilate before reoccupying. Do not allow children or pets to contact treated areas until surfaces are dry.
PHYSICAL OR CHEMICAL HAZARDS Contents under pressure. Do not use or store near heat or open flame. Do not puncture or incinerate container. Exposure to temperatures above 130°F (54°C) may cause bursting.

FIRST AID

Call poison control center or doctor immediately for treatment advice. Have the product container or label with you when calling a poison control center or doctor, or going for treatment. For MEDICAL Emergencies or other information call 1-800-RID-LICE (1-800-743-5423). For TRANSPORT Emergencies only call 1-800-424-9300.

If swallowed
- Immediately call a poison control center or doctor.
- Do not induce vomiting unless told to do so by a poison control center or doctor.
- Do not give any liquid to the person.
- Do not give anything by mouth to an unconscious person.

If in eyes
- Hold eye open and rinse slowly and gently with water for 15-20 minutes.
- Remove contact lenses, if present, after the first 5 minutes, then continue rinsing eye.

If inhaled
- Move person to fresh air.
- If person is not breathing, call 911 or an ambulance, then give artificial respiration, preferably by mouth-to mouth, if possible.

If on skin or clothing
- Take off contaminated clothing.
- Rinse skin immediately with plenty of water for 15-20 minutes.

NOTE TO PHYSICIAN

Contains petroleum distillate-vomiting may cause aspiration pneumonia.

DIRECTIONS FOR USE

It is a violation of Federal law to use this product in a manner inconsistent with its labeling. See can label for complete directions.
SHAKE WELL BEFORE USING
Remove protective cap; hold container upright and spray from a distance of 8-10 inches. We recommend that those with asthma or severe allergies consult their doctor before using this product and have someone else apply this product.
*Spray only those garments and parts of bedding including mattresses and furniture, that cannot be either laundered or dry-cleaned. Do not use on sheets or pillowcases.

STORAGE AND DISPOSAL

Storage: Store in a cool, dry area away from children and pets and away from heat, sparks and open flame. Do not transport or store below 32°F (0°C).
Container Disposal: Do Not Puncture or Incinerate.
If empty: Place in trash or offer for recycling if available.
If partly filled: Call your local solid waste agency or 1-800-CLEANUP for disposal instructions.

KEEP OUT OF REACH OF CHILDREN

RID LICE & EGG COMB-OUT GEL

Bayer HealthCare LLC.

USE

To make egg and nit removal from the hair faster and easier.

WARNINGS

For external use only. Keep out of reach of children.

DIRECTIONS FOR USE

- **Before using, read Consumer Information Insert for complete directions.**
- Use AFTER shampooing with **RID® Lice Killing Shampoo** or other similar product to kill lice and eggs.
- Towel dry hair and comb out tangles with regular comb.
- Apply RID® Lice & Egg Comb-Out Gel to one section of damp hair at a time.
- Massage well to ensure that the product covers the entire section.
- Pay special attention to the areas behind the ears and at the nape of the neck where nits and eggs are more likely to be found.
- Comb out the dead lice, eggs, and nits with the enclosed RID® comb. (See insert for additional combing instructions). **This step is very important.**
- If hair dries during combing, dampen slightly with water and re-apply gel as needed.
- Rinse thoroughly with warm water, after you have combed entire head. Disinfect combs with hot water (130°F).

OTHER INFORMATION

- Protect from freezing and excessive heat.
- It is important to wash in hot water (130°F) all clothing, bedding, towels, and hair products (combs, brushes) used by infested persons.
- Dry clean non-washable fabrics.
- To eliminate infestation of furniture and bedding that cannot be washed or dry cleaned, a multi-use lice spray may be used.
- **This product does not kill lice or their eggs.** Use this product only after treating with RID® Lice Killing Shampoo or other similar product.

INGREDIENTS

Purified Water, Glycerin, Hydroxyethylcellulose, PG-Hydroxyethylcellulose Cocodimonium Chloride, Polysorbate 20, DMDM Hydantoin, Fragrance, Iodopropynyl Butylcarbamate.

QUESTIONS OR COMMENTS?

1-800-RID-LICE (1-800-743-5423) (Mon-Fri 9AM-5PM EST) or www.ridlice.com

RID LICE KILLING SHAMPOO (piperonyl butoxide and pyrethrum extract)
Bayer HealthCare LLC.

Active Ingredient(s)
Piperonyl butoxide (4%). Lice treatment
Pyrethrum extract (equivalent to 0.33% pyrethrins). Lice treatment

USES
treats head, pubic (crab), and body lice

WARNINGS
For external use only

DO NOT USE
• near the eyes
• inside the nose, mouth, or vagina
• on lice in eyebrows or eyelashes. See a doctor if lice are present in these areas.

ASK A DOCTOR OR PHARMACIST BEFORE USE IF YOU ARE
allergic to ragweed. May cause breathing difficulty or an asthmatic attack.

WHEN USING THIS PRODUCT
• keep eyes tightly closed and protect eyes with a washcloth or towel
• if product gets into the eyes, flush with water right away
• scalp itching or redness may occur

STOP USE AND ASK A DOCTOR IF
• breathing difficulty occurs
• eye irritation occurs
• skin or scalp irritation continues or infection occurs

Keep out of reach of children. If swallowed, get medical help or contact a Poison Control Center right away.

DIRECTIONS
Important: Read warnings before use
Adults and children 2 years and over:
Inspect
• check each household member with a magnifying glass in bright light for lice/nits (eggs)
• look for tiny nits near scalp, beginning at back of neck and behind ears
• examine small sections of hair at a time
• unlike dandruff which moves when touched, nits stick to the hair
• if either lice or nits are found, treat with this product
Treat
• apply thoroughly to DRY HAIR or other affected area. For head lice, first apply behind ears and to back of neck.
• allow product to remain for 10 minutes, but no longer
• use warm water to form a lather, shampoo, then thoroughly rinse
• for head lice, towel dry hair and comb out tangles
Remove lice and their eggs (nits)
• use a fine-tooth or special lice/nit comb. Remove any remaining nits by hand (using a throw-away glove).
• hair should remain slightly damp while removing nits
• if hair dries during combing, dampen slightly with water
• for head lice, part hair into sections. Do one section at a time starting on top of head. Longer hair may take 1 to 2 hours.
• lift a 1- to 2-inch wide strand of hair. Place comb as close to scalp as possible and comb with a firm, even motion away from scalp.
• pin back each strand of hair after combing
• clean comb often. Wipe nits away with tissue and discard in a plastic bag. Seal bag and discard to prevent lice from coming back.
• after combing, thoroughly recheck for lice/nits. Repeat combing if necessary.
• check daily for any lice/nits that you missed
• a second treatment must be done in 7 to 10 days to kill any newly hatched lice
• if infestation continues, see a doctor for other treatments
Children under 2 years: ask a doctor

OTHER INFORMATION
• keep carton for important product information
• see Consumer Information Insert for additional information
• protect from excessive heat

INACTIVE INGREDIENTS
ammonium laureth sulfate, fragrance, PEG-25 hydrogenated castor oil, polyquaternium-10, purified water, SD alcohol

QUESTIONS OR COMMENTS?
1-800-RID-LICE (1-800-743-5423) (Mon-Fri 9AM-5PM EST) or www.ridlice.com

CHILDREN'S ROBITUSSIN COUGH AND COLD CF (dextromethorphan HBr, guaifenesin, and phenylephrine HCl)
Pfizer Consumer

DRUG FACTS
Active Ingredient(s) (in each 5 mL tsp)
Dextromethorphan HBr, USP 5 mg
Guaifenesin, USP 50 mg
Phenylephrine HCl, USP 2.5 mg

Purpose(s)
Cough suppressant
Expectorant
Nasal decongestant

USES
• helps loosen phlegm (mucus) and thin bronchial secretions to drain bronchial tubes
• temporarily relieves these symptoms occurring with a cold:
  • nasal congestion
  • cough due to minor throat and bronchial irritation

WARNINGS

DO NOT USE
• if you are now taking a prescription monoamine oxidase inhibitor (MAOI) (certain drugs for depression, psychiatric, or emotional conditions, or Parkinson's disease), or for 2 weeks after stopping the MAOI drug. If you do not know if your prescription drug contains an MAOI, ask a doctor or pharmacist before taking this product.

ASK A DOCTOR BEFORE USE IF YOU HAVE
• heart disease
• high blood pressure
• thyroid disease
• diabetes
• trouble urinating due to an enlarged prostate gland
• cough that occurs with too much phlegm (mucus)
• cough that lasts or is chronic such as occurs with smoking, asthma, chronic bronchitis or emphysema

Ask a doctor or pharmacist before use if you are taking any other oral nasal decongestant or stimulant.

WHEN USING THIS PRODUCT
do not use more than directed

STOP USE AND ASK A DOCTOR IF
- you get nervous, dizzy, or sleepless
- symptoms do not get better within 7 days or are accompanied by a fever
- cough lasts more than 7 days, comes back, or is accompanied by fever, rash, or persistent headache. These could be signs of a serious condition.

If pregnant or breast-feeding,
ask a health professional before use.

Keep out of the reach of children.
In case of overdose, get medical help or contact a Poison Control Center right away.

DIRECTIONS
- do not take more than 6 doses in any 24-hour period

age	dose
children under 6 years	do not use
children 6 to under 12 years	2 teaspoons every 4 hours
adults and children 12 years and over	4 teaspoons every 4 hours

OTHER INFORMATION
- **each teaspoon contains:** sodium 3 mg
- store at 20-25°C (68-77°F. Do not refrigerate.)
- dosage cup provided

INACTIVE INGREDIENTS
anhydrous citric acid, artificial flavor, FD&C red no. 40, glycerin, propylene glycol, purified water, sodium benzoate, sodium citrate, sorbitol solution, sucralose

QUESTIONS OR COMMENTS?
call weekdays from 9 AM to 5 PM EST at **1-800-762-4675**

CHILDREN'S ROBITUSSIN COUGH AND COLD LONG-ACTING (chlorpheniramine maleate and dextrometrorphan HBr)

Pfizer Consumer

DRUG FACTS

Active Ingredient(s) (in each 5 mL tsp)
Chlorpheniramine maleate, USP 1 mg
Dextromethorphan HBr, USP 7.5 mg

Purpose(s)
Antihistamine
Cough suppressant

USES
- temporarily relieves cough due to minor throat and bronchial irritation as may occur with a cold
- temporarily relieves these symptoms due to hay fever or other upper respiratory allergies:
  - runny nose
  - sneezing
  - itchy, watery eyes
  - itching of the nose or throat

WARNINGS
DO NOT USE
- to sedate a child or to make a child sleepy
- if you are now taking a prescription monoamine oxidase inhibitor (MAOI) (certain drugs for depression, psychiatric, or emotional conditions, or Parkinson's disease), or for 2 weeks after stopping the MAOI drug. If you do not know if your prescription drug contains an MAOI, ask a doctor or pharmacist before taking this product.

ASK A DOCTOR BEFORE USE IF YOU HAVE
- trouble urinating due to an enlarged prostate gland
- glaucoma
- a cough that occurs with too much phlegm (mucus)
- a breathing problem or chronic cough that lasts or as occurs with smoking, asthma, chronic bronchitis or emphysema

ASK A DOCTOR OR PHARMACIST BEFORE USE IF YOU ARE
taking sedatives or tranquilizers

WHEN USING THIS PRODUCT
- **do not use more than directed**
- marked drowsiness may occur
- avoid alcoholic drinks
- alcohol, sedatives, and tranquilizers may increase drowsiness
- be careful when driving a motor vehicle or operating machinery
- excitability may occur, especially in children

STOP USE AND ASK A DOCTOR IF
cough lasts more than 7 days, comes back, or is accompanied by fever, rash, or persistent headache. These could be signs of a serious condition.

If pregnant or breast-feeding,
ask a health professional before use.

Keep out of reach of children.
In case of overdose, get medical help or contact a Poison Control Center right away.

DIRECTIONS
- do not take more than 4 doses in any 24-hour period

age	dose
under 6 years	do not use
6 to under 12 years	2 teaspoons every 6 hours
12 years and older	4 teaspoons every 6 hours

OTHER INFORMATION
- **each teaspoon contains:** sodium 3 mg
- store at 20-25°C (68-77°F)
- dosage cup provided

INACTIVE INGREDIENTS
anhydrous citric acid, artificial & natural flavors, FD&C red no. 40, glycerin, lactic acid, propylene glycol, purified water, sodium benzoate, sodium citrate, sorbitol solution, sucralose

QUESTIONS OR COMMENTS?
Call weekdays from 9 AM to 5 PM EST at **1-800-762-4675**

CHILDREN'S ROBITUSSIN COUGH LONG-ACTING (dextromethorphan HBr)

Pfizer Consumer

DRUG FACTS

Active Ingredient(s) (in each 5 mL tsp)
Dextromethorphan HBr, USP 7.5 mg

Purpose(s)
Cough suppressant

USE
temporarily relieves cough due to minor throat and bronchial irritation as may occur with a cold

WARNINGS

DO NOT USE
• if you are now taking a prescription monoamine oxidase inhibitor (MAOI) (certain drugs for depression, psychiatric, or emotional conditions, or Parkinson's disease), or for 2 weeks after stopping the MAOI drug. If you do not know if your prescription drug contains an MAOI, ask a doctor or pharmacist before taking this product.

ASK A DOCTOR BEFORE USE IF YOU HAVE
• cough that occurs with too much phlegm (mucus)
• cough that lasts or is chronic such as occurs with smoking, asthma, or emphysema

STOP USE AND ASK A DOCTOR IF
cough lasts more than 7 days, comes back, or is accompanied by fever, rash, or persistent headache. These could be signs of a serious condition.

If pregnant or breast-feeding,
ask a health professional before use.

Keep out of reach of children.
In case of overdose, get medical help or contact a Poison Control Center right away.

DIRECTIONS
• do not take more than 4 doses in any 24-hour period

age	dose
children under 6 years	do not use
children 6 to under 12 years	2 teaspoons every 6 to 8 hours
adults and children 12 years and older	4 teaspoons every 6 to 8 hours

OTHER INFORMATION
• **each teaspoon contains:** sodium 5 mg
• store at 20-25°C (68-77°F)
• dosage cup provided

INACTIVE INGREDIENTS
anhydrous citric acid, artificial flavor, FD&C red no. 40, glycerin, high fructose corn syrup, propylene glycol, purified water, saccharin sodium, sodium benzoate, sodium chloride, sodium citrate

QUESTIONS OR COMMENTS?
Call weekdays from 9 AM to 5 PM EST at **1-800-762-4675**

ROBITUSSIN COUGH AND CHEST CONGESTION DM (dextromethorphan HBr and guaifenesin)

Pfizer Consumer

DRUG FACTS

Active Ingredient(s) (in each 5 mL tsp)
Dextromethorphan HBr, USP 10 mg
Guaifenesin, USP 100 mg

Purpose(s)
Cough suppressant
Expectorant

USES
• temporarily relieves cough due to minor throat and bronchial irritation as may occur with a cold
• helps loosen phlegm (mucus) and thin bronchial secretions to drain bronchial tubes

WARNINGS

DO NOT USE
• if you are now taking a prescription monoamine oxidase inhibitor (MAOI) (certain drugs for depression, psychiatric, or emotional conditions, or Parkinson's disease), or for 2 weeks after stopping the MAOI drug. If you do not know if your prescription drug contains an MAOI, ask a doctor or pharmacist before taking this product.

ASK A DOCTOR BEFORE USE IF YOU HAVE
• cough that occurs with too much phlegm (mucus)
• cough that lasts or is chronic such as occurs with smoking, asthma, chronic bronchitis, or emphysema

STOP USE AND ASK A DOCTOR IF
cough lasts more than 7 days, comes back, or is accompanied by fever, rash, or persistent headache. These could be signs of a serious condition.

If pregnant or breast-feeding,
ask a health professional before use.

Keep out of reach of children.
In case of overdose, get medical help or contact a Poison Control Center right away.

DIRECTIONS
• do not take more than 6 doses in any 24-hour period
• this adult product is not intended for use in children under 12 years of age

age	dose
adults and children 12 years and over	2 teaspoons every 4 hours
children under 12 years	do not use

OTHER INFORMATION
Robitussin Cough & Chest Congestion DM
• **each teaspoon contains:** sodium 7 mg
• store at 20-25°C (68-77°F)
• dosage cup provided

Robitussin Cough & Chest Congestion Sugar Free DM
• **each teaspoon contains:** sodium 4 mg
• store at 20-25°C (68-77°F)
• alcohol-free
• dosage cup provided

INACTIVE INGREDIENTS

Robitussin Cough & Chest Congestion DM
anhydrous citric acid, FD&C red no. 40, glycerin, high fructose corn syrup, menthol, natural flavor, propylene glycol, purified water, sodium benzoate, sodium citrate, sucralose

Robitussin Cough & Chest Congestion Sugar Free DM
acesulfame potassium, artificial & natural flavor, citric acid monohydrate, glycerin, methylparaben, polyethylene glycol, povidone, propylene glycol, purified water, saccharin sodium, sodium benzoate

QUESTIONS OR COMMENTS?

call weekdays from 9 AM to 5 PM EST at **1-800-762-4675**

ROBITUSSIN MAXIMUM STRENGTH COUGH + CHEST CONGESTION DM

(dextromethorphan hydrobromide and guaifenesin)

Pfizer Consumer

DRUG FACTS

Active Ingredient(s) (in each 5 mL tsp)	Purpose(s)
Dextromethorphan HBr, USP 10 mg	Cough suppressant
Guaifenesin, USP 200 mg	Expectorant

USES

- temporarily relieves cough due to minor throat and bronchial irritation as may occur with a cold
- helps loosen phlegm (mucus) and thin bronchial secretions to drain bronchial tubes

WARNINGS

DO NOT USE
if you are now taking a prescription monoamine oxidase inhibitor (MAOI) (certain drugs for depression, psychiatric, or emotional conditions, or Parkinson's disease), or for 2 weeks after stopping the MAOI drug. If you do not know if your prescription drug contains an MAOI, ask a doctor or pharmacist before taking this product.

ASK A DOCTOR BEFORE USE IF YOU HAVE
- cough that occurs with too much phlegm (mucus)
- cough that lasts or is chronic such as occurs with smoking, asthma, chronic bronchitis, or emphysema

STOP USE AND ASK A DOCTOR IF
cough lasts more than 7 days, comes back, or is accompanied by fever, rash, or persistent headache. These could be signs of a serious condition.
If pregnant or breast-feeding, ask a health professional before use.
Keep out of reach of children. In case of overdose, get medical help or contact a Poison Control Center right away.

DIRECTIONS

- shake well before using
- do not take more than 6 doses in any 24-hour period
- this adult product is not intended for use in children under 12 years of age

age	dose
adults and children 12 years and over	2 teaspoons every 4 hours
children under 12 years	do not use

OTHER INFORMATION

- **each teaspoon contains:** sodium 5 mg
- store at 20-25°C (68-77°F).
- alcohol-free
- dosage cup provided

INACTIVE INGREDIENTS

anhydrous citric acid, artificial & natural flavors, carboxymethylcellulose sodium, D&C red no. 33, FD&C red no. 40, glycerin, high fructose corn syrup, menthol, microcrystalline cellulose, polyethylene glycol, povidone, propylene glycol, purified water, saccharin sodium, sodium benzoate, sorbitol solution, xanthan gum

QUESTIONS OR COMMENTS?

Call weekdays from 9 AM to 5 PM EST at **1-800-762-4675**

ROBITUSSIN PEAK COLD COUGH PLUS CHEST CONGESTION DM (dextromethorphan HBr and guaifenesin)

Pfizer Consumer

DRUG FACTS

Active Ingredient(s) (in each 10 mL)
Dextromethorphan HBr, USP 20 mg
Guaifenesin, USP 200 mg

Purpose(s)
Cough suppressant
Expectorant

USES

- temporarily relieves cough due to minor throat and bronchial irritation as may occur with a cold
- helps loosen phlegm (mucus) and thin bronchial secretions to drain bronchial tubes

WARNINGS

DO NOT USE
if you are now taking a prescription monoamine oxidase inhibitor (MAOI) (certain drugs for depression, psychiatric, or emotional conditions, or Parkinson's disease), or for 2 weeks after stopping the MAOI drug. If you do not know if your prescription drug contains an MAOI, ask a doctor or pharmacist before taking this product.

ASK A DOCTOR BEFORE USE IF YOU HAVE
- cough that occurs with too much phlegm (mucus)
- cough that lasts or is chronic such as occurs with smoking, asthma, chronic bronchitis or emphysema

STOP USE AND ASK A DOCTOR IF
cough lasts more than 7 days, comes back, or is accompanied by fever, rash, or persistent headache. These could be signs of a serious condition.

If pregnant or breast-feeding,
ask a health professional before use.

Keep out of reach of children.
In case of overdose, get medical help or contact a Poison Control Center right away.

DIRECTIONS

- do not take more than 6 doses in any 24-hour period
- measure only with dosing cup provided
- keep dosing cup with product
- ml = milliliter
- this adult product is not intended for use in children under 12 years of age

age	dose
adults and children 12 years and over	10 mL every 4 hours
children under 12 years	do not use

OTHER INFORMATION
Robitussin Peak Cold Cough+Chest Congestion DM
• **each 10 mL contains:** sodium 7 mg
• store at 20-25°C (68-77°F). Do not refrigerate.

Robitussin Peak Cold Sugar-Free Cough+Chest Congestion DM
• **each 10 mL contains:** sodium 5 mg
• store at 20-25°C (68-77°F). Do not refrigerate.
• alcohol-free

INACTIVE INGREDIENTS
Robitussin Peak Cold Cough+Chest Congestion DM
anhydrous citric acid, FD&C red no. 40, glycerin, high fructose corn syrup, menthol, natural flavor, propylene glycol, purified water, sodium benzoate, sodium citrate, sucralose

Robitussin Peak Cold Sugar-Free Cough+Chest Congestion DM
acesulfame potassium, artificial & natural flavor, citric acid monohydrate, glycerin, methylparaben, polyethylene glycol, povidone, propylene glycol, purified water, saccharin sodium, sodium benzoate

QUESTIONS OR COMMENTS?
call weekdays from 9 AM to 5 PM EST at **1-800-762-4675**
For most recent product information, **visit www.robitussin.com**

ROBITUSSIN PEAK COLD MULTI-SYMPTOM COLD CF (dextromethorphan hydrobromide, guaifenesin, and phenylephrine hydrochloride)
Pfizer Consumer

DRUG FACTS

Active Ingredient(s) (in each 10 mL)	Purpose(s)
Dextromethorphan HBr, USP 20 mg	Cough suppressant
Guaifenesin, USP 200 mg	Expectorant
Phenylephrine HCl, USP 10 mg	Nasal decongestant

USES
• helps loosen phlegm (mucus) and thin bronchial secretions to drain bronchial tubes
• temporarily relieves these symptoms occurring with a cold:
  • nasal congestion
  • cough due to minor throat and bronchial irritation

WARNINGS

DO NOT USE
if you are now taking a prescription monoamine oxidase inhibitor (MAOI) (certain drugs for depression, psychiatric, or emotional conditions, or Parkinson's disease), or for 2 weeks after stopping the MAOI drug. If you do not know if your prescription drug contains an MAOI, ask a doctor or pharmacist before taking this product.

ASK A DOCTOR BEFORE USE IF YOU HAVE
• heart disease
• high blood pressure
• thyroid disease
• diabetes
• trouble urinating due to an enlarged prostate gland
• cough that occurs with too much phlegm (mucus)
• cough that lasts or is chronic such as occurs with smoking, asthma, chronic bronchitis or emphysema

ASK A DOCTOR OR PHARMACIST BEFORE USE IF YOU ARE
taking any other oral nasal decongestant or stimulant.

WHEN USING THIS PRODUCT
do not use more than directed.

STOP USE AND ASK A DOCTOR IF
• you get nervous, dizzy, or sleepless
• symptoms do not get better within 7 days or are accompanied by fever
• cough lasts more than 7 days, comes back, or is accompanied by fever, rash, or persistent headache. These could be signs of a serious condition.

If pregnant or breast-feeding, ask a health professional before use.
Keep out of reach of children. In case of overdose, get medical help or contact a Poison Control Center right away.

DIRECTIONS
• do not take more than 6 doses in any 24-hour period
• measure only with dosing cup provided
• keep dosing cup with product
• ml = milliliter
• this adult product is not intended for use in children under 12 years of age

age	dose
adults and children 12 years and over	10 mL every 4 hours
children under 12 years	Do not use

OTHER INFORMATION
• **each 10 mL contains:** sodium 6 mg
• store at 20-25°C (68-77°F). Do not refrigerate.

INACTIVE INGREDIENTS
anhydrous citric acid, FD&C red no. 40, glycerin, menthol, natural & artificial flavor, propylene glycol, purified water, sodium benzoate, sodium citrate, sorbitol solution, sucralose

QUESTIONS OR COMMENTS?
call weekdays from 9 AM to 5 PM EST at **1-800-762-4675**
For most recent product information, **visit www.robitussin.com**

ROBITUSSIN PEAK COLD NASAL RELIEF
(acetaminophen and phenylephrine HCl)
Pfizer Consumer

DRUG FACTS

Active Ingredient(s) (in each tablet)
Acetaminophen, USP 325 mg
Phenylephrine HCl, USP 5 mg

Purpose(s)
Pain reliever/Fever reducer
Nasal decongestant

USES
- temporarily relieves these symptoms associated with a cold or flu, hay fever or other upper respiratory allergies:
  - nasal congestion
  - sinus congestion and pressure
  - reduces swelling of nasal passages
  - restores freer breathing through the nose
  - headache
  - sore throat
  - minor aches and pains
- temporarily reduces fever

WARNINGS
Liver warning:
This product contains acetaminophen. Severe liver damage may occur if you take
- more than 12 tablets in any 24-hour period, which is the maximum daily amount
- with other drugs containing acetaminophen
- 3 or more alcoholic drinks every day while using this product

Sore throat warning:
If sore throat is severe, persists for more than 2 days, is accompanied or followed by fever, headache, rash, nausea, or vomiting, consult a doctor promptly.

DO NOT USE
- if you are now taking a prescription monoamine oxidase inhibitor (MAOI) (certain drugs for depression, psychiatric, or emotional conditions, or Parkinson's disease), or for 2 weeks after stopping the MAOI drug. If you do not know if your prescription drug contains an MAOI, ask a doctor or pharmacist before taking this product.
- with any other drug containing acetaminophen (prescription or nonprescription). If you are not sure whether a drug contains acetaminophen ask a doctor or pharmacist.

ASK A DOCTOR BEFORE USE IF YOU HAVE
- liver disease
- heart disease
- high blood pressure
- thyroid disease
- diabetes
- trouble urinating due to an enlarged prostate gland

ASK A DOCTOR OR PHARMACIST BEFORE USE IF YOU ARE
- taking the blood thinning drug warfarin
- taking any other oral nasal decongestant or stimulant
- taking any other pain reliever/fever reducer

WHEN USING THIS PRODUCT
do not use more than directed

STOP USE AND ASK A DOCTOR IF
- you get nervous, dizzy, or sleepless
- pain or nasal congestion gets worse or lasts more than 7 days
- fever gets worse or lasts more than 3 days
- redness or swelling is present
- new symptoms occur

If pregnant or breast-feeding,
ask a health professional before use.

Keep out of reach of children.
In case of overdose, get medical help or contact a Poison Control Center right away. Prompt medical attention is critical for adults as well as for children, even if you do not notice any signs or symptoms.

DIRECTIONS
- do not use more than 12 tablets in any 24-hour period
- do not exceed recommended dosage. Taking more than the recommended dose (overdose) may cause serious liver damage

- this adult product is not intended for use in children under 12 years of age

age	dose
adults and children 12 years and over	2 tablets every 4 hours
children under 12 years	do not use

OTHER INFORMATION
- store at 20-25°C (68-77°F)
- tamper-evident individual blisters

INACTIVE INGREDIENTS
calcium stearate, croscarmellose sodium, crospovidone, hypromellose, microcrystalline cellulose, polyethylene glycol, povidone, pregelatinized starch, stearic acid

QUESTIONS OR COMMENTS?
Call weekdays from 9 AM to 5 PM EST at **1-800-762-4675**

ROBITUSSIN PEAK COLD NIGHTTIME MULTI-SYMPTOM COLD (acetaminophen, diphenhydramine HCl, and phenylephrine HCl)

Pfizer Consumer

DRUG FACTS

Active Ingredient(s) (in each 5 mL tsp)
Acetaminophen, USP 640 mg
Diphenhydramine HCl, USP 25 mg
Phenylephrine HCl, USP 10 mg

Purpose(s)
Pain reliever/Fever reducer
Antihistamine/Cough suppressant
Nasal decongestant

USES
- temporarily relieves these symptoms occurring with a cold or flu, hay fever, or other upper respiratory allergies:
  - headache
  - nasal congestion
  - sore throat
  - cough
  - minor aches and pains
  - runny nose
  - sneezing
  - itchy, watery eyes
  - itching of the nose or throat
- temporarily reduces fever

WARNINGS
Liver warning:
This product contains acetaminophen. Severe liver damage may occur if user takes
- more than 24 teaspoons in any 24-hour period, which is the maximum daily amount
- with other drugs containing acetaminophen
- 3 or more alcoholic drinks every day while using this product

Sore throat warning:
If sore throat is severe, persists for more than 2 days, is accompanied or followed by fever, headache, rash, nausea, or vomiting, consult a doctor promptly.

DO NOT USE
- to sedate a child or to make a child sleepy
- if you are now taking a prescription monoamine oxidase inhibitor (MAOI) (certain drugs for depression, psychiatric, or emotional conditions, or Parkinson's disease), or for 2 weeks

after stopping the MAOI drug. If you do not know if your prescription drug contains an MAOI, ask a doctor or pharmacist before taking this product.
- with any other drug containing acetaminophen (prescription or nonprescription). If you are not sure whether a drug contains acetaminophen ask a doctor or pharmacist.
- with any other product containing diphenhydramine, even one used on skin

ASK A DOCTOR BEFORE USE IF USER HAS
- liver disease
- heart disease
- high blood pressure
- thyroid disease
- diabetes
- trouble urinating due to an enlarged prostate gland
- glaucoma
- cough that occurs with too much phlegm (mucus)
- a breathing problem or chronic cough that lasts or as occurs with smoking, asthma, chronic bronchitis, or emphysema

ASK A DOCTOR OR PHARMACIST BEFORE USE IF USER IS
- taking the blood thinning drug warfarin
- taking any other oral nasal decongestant or stimulant
- taking any other pain reliever/fever reducer
- taking sedatives or tranquilizers

WHEN USING THIS PRODUCT
- **do not use more than directed**
- marked drowsiness may occur
- avoid alcoholic drinks
- alcohol, sedatives, and tranquilizers may increase drowsiness
- be careful when driving a motor vehicle or operating machinery
- excitability may occur, especially in children

STOP USE AND ASK A DOCTOR IF
- user gets nervous, dizzy, or sleepless
- pain, cough, or nasal congestion gets worse or lasts more than 5 days (children) or 7 days (adults)
- fever gets worse or lasts more than 3 days
- redness or swelling is present
- cough comes back or occurs with rash or headache that lasts. These could be signs of a serious condition.
- new symptoms occur

If pregnant or breast-feeding,
ask a health professional before use.

Keep out of reach of children.
In case of overdose, get medical help or contact a Poison Control Center right away. Prompt medical attention is critical for adults as well as for children, even if you do not notice any signs or symptoms.

DIRECTIONS
- do not take more than 6 doses in any 24-hour period
- do not exceed recommended dosage. Taking more than the recommended dose (overdose) may cause serious liver damage.
- this adult product is not intended for use in children under 12 years of age

age	dose
adults and children 12 years and over	20 mL every 4 hours
children under 12 years	do not use

OTHER INFORMATION
- **each 20 mL contains:** sodium 15 mg
- store at 20-25°C (68-77°F)

INACTIVE INGREDIENTS
anhydrous citric acid, artificial flavor, edetate disodium, FD&C red no. 40, glycerin, menthol, polyethylene glycol, propyl gallate, propylene glycol, purified water, sodium benzoate, sodium citrate, sorbitol solution, sucralose

QUESTIONS OR COMMENTS?
call weekdays from 9 AM to 5 PM EST at **1-800-762-4675**

ROBITUSSIN PEAK COLD NIGHTTIME NASAL RELIEF (acetaminophen, chlorpheniramine maleate, and phenylephrine HCl)

Pfizer Consumer

DRUG FACTS

Active Ingredient(s) (in each tablet)
Acetaminophen, USP 325 mg
Chlorpheniramine maleate, USP 2 mg
Phenylephrine HCl, USP 5 mg

Purpose(s)
Pain reliever/Fever reducer
Antihistamine
Nasal decongestant

USES
- temporarily relieves these symptoms associated with a cold, or flu:
  - headache
  - nasal congestion
  - sore throat
  - fever
  - minor aches and pains
- temporarily relieves minor aches, pains and headache as well as these symptoms of hay fever or other upper respiratory allergies:
  - runny nose
  - sneezing
  - nasal congestion
  - itching of the nose or throat
  - itchy, watery eyes
- temporarily relieves minor aches, pains, headache and nasal congestion as well as sinus congestion and pressure, and reduces swelling of nasal passages

WARNINGS
Liver warning:
This product contains acetaminophen. Severe liver damage may occur if you take
- more than 12 tablets in any 24-hour period, which is the maximum daily amount
- with other drugs containing acetaminophen
- 3 or more alcoholic drinks every day while using this product

Sore throat warning:
If sore throat is severe, persists for more than 2 days, is accompanied or followed by fever, headache, rash, nausea, or vomiting, consult a doctor promptly.

DO NOT USE
- to sedate a child or to make a child sleepy
- if you are now taking a prescription monoamine oxidase inhibitor (MAOI) (certain drugs for depression, psychiatric, or emotional conditions, or Parkinson's disease), or for 2 weeks after stopping the MAOI drug. If you do not know if your prescription drug contains an MAOI, ask a doctor or pharmacist before taking this product.
- with any other drug containing acetaminophen (prescription or nonprescription). If you are not sure whether a drug contains acetaminophen ask a doctor or pharmacist.

ASK A DOCTOR BEFORE USE IF YOU HAVE
- liver disease
- heart disease
- high blood pressure
- thyroid disease
- diabetes
- trouble urinating due to an enlarged prostate gland
- glaucoma
- a breathing problem such as emphysema, asthma, or chronic bronchitis

ASK A DOCTOR OR PHARMACIST BEFORE USE IF YOU ARE
- taking the blood thinning drug warfarin
- taking any other oral nasal decongestant or stimulant
- taking any other pain reliever/fever reducer
- taking sedatives or tranquilizers

WHEN USING THIS PRODUCT
- **do not use more than directed**
- drowsiness may occur
- avoid alcoholic drinks
- alcohol, sedatives, and tranquilizers may increase drowsiness
- be careful when driving a motor vehicle or operating machinery
- excitability may occur, especially in children

STOP USE AND ASK A DOCTOR IF
- you get nervous, dizzy, or sleepless
- pain or nasal congestion gets worse or lasts more than 7 days
- fever gets worse or lasts more than 3 days
- redness or swelling is present
- new symptoms occur

If pregnant or breast-feeding,
ask a health professional before use.

Keep out of reach of children.
In case of overdose, get medical help or contact a Poison Control Center right away. Prompt medical attention is critical for adults as well as for children, even if you do not notice any signs or symptoms.

DIRECTIONS
- do not use more than 12 tablets in any 24-hour period
- do not exceed recommended dosage. Taking more than the recommended dose (overdose) may cause serious liver damage
- this adult product is not intended for use in children under 12 years of age

age	dose
adults and children 12 years and over	2 tablets every 4 hours
children under 12 years	do not use

OTHER INFORMATION
- store at 20-25°C (68-77°F)
- tamper-evident individual blisters

INACTIVE INGREDIENTS
calcium stearate, croscarmellose sodium, crospovidone, D&C yellow no. 10 aluminum lake, FD&C yellow no. 6 aluminum lake, hypromellose, microcrystalline cellulose, polyethylene glycol, povidone, pregelatinized starch, stearic acid

QUESTIONS OR COMMENTS?
Call weekdays from 9 AM to 5 PM EST at **1-800-762-4675**

SARNA (camphor and menthol)
Stiefel Laboratories, Inc

Active Ingredient(s)
Camphor 0.5%
Menthol 0.5%

Purpose(s)
external analgesic

USES
for the temporary relief of pain and itching associated with minor skin irritations such as poison ivy/oak/sumac, sunburn, insect bites, and minor cuts and scrapes

WARNINGS
For external use only

WHEN USING THIS PRODUCT
- avoid contact with the eyes.

STOP USE AND ASK A DOCTOR IF
- condition worsens
- symptoms persist for more than 7 days or clear up and occur again within a few days.

Keep out of reach of children.
If swallowed, get medical help or contact a Poison Control Center right away.

DIRECTIONS
- To open, squeeze cap tightly and turn pump counter-clockwise.

Adults and children 2 years of age and older:
- apply to affected area not more than 3 to 4 times daily.

Children under 2 years of age: consult a doctor.

OTHER INFORMATION
Side effects may be reported to 1-888-438-7426.

INACTIVE INGREDIENTS
carbomer 940, cetyl alcohol, DMDM hydantoin, fragrance, glyceryl stearate, isopropyl myristate, PEG-8 stearate, PEG-100 stearate, petrolatum, purified water, sodium hydroxide, stearic acid.
Find more about Sarna!
Stiefel Laboratories, Inc.
Research Triangle Park, NC 27709
www.sarna-skincare.com
Made in Canada

SARNA (pramoxine hydrochloride)
Stiefel Laboratories, Inc

Active Ingredient(s)
Pramoxine hydrochloride 1%

Purpose(s)
external analgesic

USE
for the temporary relief of itching associated with minor skin irritations

WARNINGS
For external use only

WHEN USING THIS PRODUCT
- avoid contact with the eyes.

STOP USE AND ASK A DOCTOR IF
• condition worsens
• symptoms persist for more than 7 days or clear up and occur again within a few days.

Caution -- Do not use in the eyes or nose. Not for prolonged use. Do not apply to large areas of the body. If redness, irritation, swelling, or pain persists or increases, discontinue use unless directed by a physician.

Keep out of reach of children.
If swallowed, get medical help or contact a Poison Control Center right away.

DIRECTIONS
• To open, squeeze cap tightly and turn pump counter-clockwise.
Adults and children 2 years of age and older:
• apply to affected area not more than 3 to 4 times daily.
Children under 2 years of age: consult a doctor.

OTHER INFORMATION
Side effects may be reported to 1-888-438-7426

INACTIVE INGREDIENTS
benzyl alcohol, carbomer 940, cetyl alcohol, dimethicone, glyceryl stearate, isopropyl myristate, PEG-8 stearate, PEG-100 stearate, petrolatum, purified water, sodium hydroxide, stearic acid
Find more about Sarna!
Stiefel Laboratories, Inc.
Research Triangle Park, NC 27709
www.sarna-skincare.com
Made in Canada
A099718

SENOKOT (sennosides)
Purdue Products LP

DRUG FACTS

Active Ingredient(s) (in each tablet)
Sennosides 8.6 mg

Purpose(s)
Laxative

USES
• relieves occasional constipation (irregularity)
• generally produces a bowel movement in 6-12 hours

WARNINGS

DO NOT USE
• laxative products for longer than 1 week unless directed by a doctor

ASK A DOCTOR BEFORE USE IF YOU HAVE
• stomach pain
• nausea
• vomiting
• noticed a sudden change in bowel habits that continues over a period of 2 weeks

STOP USE AND ASK A DOCTOR IF
you have rectal bleeding or fail to have a bowel movement after use of a laxative. These may indicate a serious condition.
If pregnant or breast-feeding, ask a health professional before use.

Keep out of reach of children. In case of overdose, get medical help or contact a Poison Control Center right away.

DIRECTIONS
• take preferably at bedtime or as directed by a doctor

age	starting dosage	maximum dosage
adults and children 12 years of age and over	2 tablets once a day	4 tablets twice a day
children 6 to under 12 years	1 tablet once a day	2 tablets twice a day
children 2 to under 6 years	1/2 tablet once a day	1 tablet twice a day
children under 2 years	ask a doctor	ask a doctor

OTHER INFORMATION
• each tablet contains: **calcium 10 mg**
• store at 25°C (77°F); excursions permitted between 15°-30°C (59°-86°F)

INACTIVE INGREDIENTS
dicalcium phosphate, magnesium stearate, microcrystalline cellulose, pregelatinized starch

SENOKOT-S (docusate sodium and sennosides)
Purdue Products LP

DRUG FACTS

Active Ingredient(s) (in each tablet)
Docusate sodium 50 mg
Sennosides 8.6 mg

Purpose(s)
Stool softener
Laxative

USES
• relieves occasional constipation (irregularity)
• generally produces a bowel movement in 6-12 hours

WARNINGS

DO NOT USE
• if you are now taking mineral oil, unless directed by a doctor
• laxative products for longer than 1 week unless directed by a doctor

ASK A DOCTOR BEFORE USE IF YOU HAVE
• stomach pain
• nausea
• vomiting
• noticed a sudden change in bowel habits that continues over a period of 2 weeks

STOP USE AND ASK A DOCTOR IF
you have rectal bleeding or fail to have a bowel movement after use of a laxative. These may indicate a serious condition.
If pregnant or breast-feeding, ask a health professional before use.
Keep out of reach of children.
In case of overdose, get medical help or contact a Poison Control Center right away.

DIRECTIONS
• take preferably at bedtime or as directed by a doctor

age	starting dosage	maximum dosage
adults and children 12 years of age and over	2 tablets once a day	4 tablets twice a day
children 6 to under 12 years	1 tablet once a day	2 tablets twice a day
children 2 to under 6 years	1/2 tablet once a day	1 tablet twice a day
children under 2 years	ask a doctor	ask a doctor

OTHER INFORMATION
• each tablet contains: **sodium 4 mg VERY LOW SODIUM**
• store at 25°C (77°F); excursions permitted between 15°-30°C (59°-86°F)

INACTIVE INGREDIENTS
corn starch, D&C yellow #10 aluminum lake, FD&C yellow #6 aluminum lake, guar gum, lecithin, magnesium stearate, microcrystalline cellulose, polyethylene glycol, polyvinyl alcohol, silicon dioxide, sodium benzoate, talc, and titanium dioxide
©2009 Purdue Products L.P.
Made in Canada
Dist. by: **Purdue Products L.P.**
Stamford, CT 06901-3431
302205-0A

SENOKOTXTRA (sennosides)
Purdue Products LP

DRUG FACTS

Active Ingredient(s) (in each tablet)
Sennosides 17.2 mg

Purpose(s)
Laxative

USES
• relieves occasional constipation (irregularity)
• generally produces a bowel movement in 6-12 hours

WARNINGS

DO NOT USE
• laxative products for longer than 1 week unless directed by a doctor

ASK A DOCTOR BEFORE USE IF YOU HAVE
• stomach pain
• nausea
• vomiting
• noticed a sudden change in bowel movements that continues over a period of 2 weeks

STOP USE AND ASK A DOCTOR IF
you have rectal bleeding or fail to have a bowel movement after use of a laxative. These may indicate a serious condition.
If pregnant or breast-feeding, ask a health professional before use.
Keep out of reach of children. In case of overdose, get medical help or contact a Poison Control Center right away.

DIRECTIONS
• take preferably at bedtime or as directed by a doctor

age	starting dosage	maximum dosage
adults and children 12 years of age and over	1 tablet once a day	2 tablets twice a day
children 6 to under 12 years	1/2 tablet once a day	1 tablet twice a day
children under 6	ask a doctor	ask a doctor

OTHER INFORMATION
• each tablet contains: **calcium 25 mg**
• store at 25°C (77°F); excursions permitted between 15°-30°C (59°-86°F)

INACTIVE INGREDIENTS
croscarmellose sodium, dicalcium phosphate, hypromellose, lactose anhydrous, magnesium stearate, microcrystalline cellulose, mineral oil, stearic acid, tartaric acid
©2009 Purdue Products L.P.
Dist. by: **Purdue Products L.P.**
Stamford, CT 06901-3431
302105-0B

SIMPLY SALINE ALLERGY AND SINUS RELIEF (purified water and sodium chloride)
Church & Dwight Co., Inc.

INGREDIENTS
Purified water, and 3% sodium chloride.)

USES
Comforting mist helps dry congestion as gentle misting flushes dust, dirt, pollen and congestion from nasal and sinus passages.

WARNINGS
• The use of this dispenser by more than one person may spread infection.
• **KEEP OUT OF REACH OF CHILDREN.**
• Contents under pressure.
• Do not puncture or incinerate.
• Store between 59° and 86°F (15° and 30°C).
• Avoid spraying in eyes.

DIRECTIONS
To flush & irrigate, tilt head to the side over sink or use in shower. Insert nozzle into one nostril depressing as a gentle mist fills sinus passages and flows out nostrils. Repeat in other nostril.

SIMPLY SALINE BABY NASAL MOISTURIZER PLUS ALOE VERA
Church & Dwight Co., Inc.

INGREDIENTS
Water, propylene glycol, hydroxyethylcellulose, sodium chloride, aloe barbadensis leaf extract (aloe vera), allantoin, methylparaben, propylparaben.)

WARNINGS
If irritation develops or condition worsens, discontinue use and consult your physician. Do not insert into the nose.
KEEP OUT OF REACH OF CHILDREN.

DIRECTIONS

Apply around the nose to relieve dryness and soreness. Use as often as needed.

For best results, use after a saline nasal spray, like **Simply Saline®** Baby Nasal Relief.

SIMPLY SALINE BABY NASAL RELIEF

(purified water and sodium chloride)

Church & Dwight Co., Inc.

INGREDIENTS

Purified water, 0.9% sodium chloride.

USES

Comforting mist helps relieve symptoms of dry, irritated nose as gentle misting flushes dust, dirt, pollen and congestion from nasal and sinus passages.)

WARNINGS

- The use of this dispenser by more than one person may spread infection.
- **KEEP OUT OF REACH OF CHILDREN. EXCEPT UNDER ADULT SUPERVISION.**
- Contents under pressure.
- Do not puncture or incinerate.
- Store between 59° and 86°F (15° and 30°C).
- Avoid spraying in eyes.

DIRECTIONS

To flush & irrigate, tilt head to the side over sink or use in shower. Insert nozzle into one nostril depressing as a gentle mist fills sinus passages and flows out nostrils. Repeat in other nostril.

To moisturize, insert nozzle into each nostril and press as moisture is restored to dry nasal passages. **USE AS OFTEN AS NEEDED (NON-HABIT FORMING, NON-ADDICTING).**

SIMPLY SALINE BABY SWABS (water, glycerin, sodium chloride, and methylparaben)

Church & Dwight Co., Inc.

- Remove one swab from the sheet. Tear wrapper as indicated on the wrapper.
- Hold the swab with colored ring pointing upward, bend the colored ring tip gently until it snaps.
- Hold the swab with the colored ring upward for 1-2 seconds to allow the liquid to flow down to the solid white tip.
- Gently insert saturated solid white tip just past the nasal opening. Clean/Moisturize nostril by using a circular motion as long as needed.
  DO NOT PUT THE SWAB TOO FAR INTO THE NOSE. IMPROPER USE CAN CAUSE INJURY.
  Discard swab after use. Reusing of swab may cause infection.

WARNINGS

If irritation develops or condition worsens, discontinue use and consult your physician. Do Not Swallow.

The use of one swab by more than one person may spread infection.

KEEP OUT OF REACH OF CHILDREN.

INGREDIENTS

Water, Glycerin, Sodium Chloride, Methylparaben.

SIMPLY SALINE CHILDREN'S COLD FORMULA PLUS MOISTURIZERS (*Luffa operculata* and *sabadilla*)

Church & Dwight Co., Inc.

DRUG FACTS

Active Ingredient(s)	Purpose(s)
Luffa operculata 6X HPUS	Runny nose, nasal dryness, sinus congestion, post-nasal drip
Sabadilla 6X HPUS	Sneezing, runny nose, itching

USES

according to homeopathic principles, the active ingredients in this medication temporarily relieve symptoms of:
- nasal congestion
- runny nose due to colds and flu
- post-nasal drip
- dry, irritated nasal passages
- sinus congestion and pressure

WARNINGS

ASK A DOCTOR BEFORE USE IF YOU
- are prone to ear, nose or throat sensitivity
- are susceptible to nose bleeds

WHEN USING THIS PRODUCT
- contents under pressure
- do not puncture or incinerate
- store between 59° and 86°F (15° and 30°C)
- avoid spraying in eyes

STOP USE AND CONSULT A DOCTOR IF
symptoms persist beyond 7 days or worsen
- initial exacerbation of symptoms may occur
- the use of this container by more than one person may spread infection

If pregnant or breast-feeding, ask a health professional before use

KEEP OUT OF REACH OF CHILDREN.

DIRECTIONS

for adults and children 2 years and older. Simply Saline® Nasal Mist can be used as often as necessary. Non-habit forming.
- to flush and irrigate, tilt head to the side over sink. Insert nozzle into one nostril, depressing as a gentle mist fills sinus passages and flows out nostrils. **OR,**
- to moisturize and relieve congestion, insert nozzle into each nostril and press shortly as moisture is restored to dry nasal passages.

OTHER INFORMATION

active ingredients are microdiluted in accordance with the Homeopathic Pharmacopoeia of the United States and are therefore non-toxic and have no known side effects

INACTIVE INGREDIENTS

benzalkonium chloride, glycerin, phenylcarbinol, purified water, sodium bicarbonate, sodium chloride

The letters "HPUS" indicate that the components in this product are officially monographed in the Homeopathic Pharmacopoeia of the United States.

SIMPLY SALINE COLD FORMULA PLUS MENTHOL (*Luffa operculata* and *sabadilla*)
Church & Dwight Co., Inc.

DRUG FACTS

Active Ingredient(s)	Purpose(s)
Luffa operculata 6X HPUS	Runny nose, nasal dryness, sinus congestion, post-nasal drip
Sabadilla 6X HPUS	Sneezing, runny nose, itching

USES
according to homeopathic principles, the active ingredients in this medication temporarily relieve symptoms of:
• nasal congestion
• runny nose due to colds and flu
• post-nasal drip
• dry, irritated nasal passages
• sinus congestion and pressure

WARNINGS

ASK A DOCTOR BEFORE USE IF YOU
• are prone to ear, nose or throat sensitivity
• are susceptible to nose bleeds

WHEN USING THIS PRODUCT
• contents under pressure
• do not puncture or incinerate
• store between 59° and 86°F (15° and 30°C)
• avoid spraying in eyes

STOP USE AND CONSULT A DOCTOR IF
symptoms persist beyond 7 days or worsen
• initial exacerbation of symptoms may occur
• the use of this container by more than one person may spread infection
If pregnant or breast-feeding, ask a health professional before use
KEEP OUT OF REACH OF CHILDREN.

DIRECTIONS
for adults and children 2 years and older. **Simply Saline®** Nasal Mist can be used as often as necessary. Non-habit forming.
• to flush and irrigate, tilt head to the side over sink. Insert nozzle into one nostril, depressing as a gentle mist fills sinus passages and flows out nostrils. **OR,**
• to moisturize and relieve congestion, insert nozzle into each nostril and press shortly as moisture is restored to dry nasal passages.

OTHER INFORMATION
active ingredients are microdiluted in accordance with the Homeopathic Pharmacopoeia of the United States and are therefore non-toxic and have no known side effects

INACTIVE INGREDIENTS
benzalkonium chloride, glycerin, menthol, phenylcarbinol, purified water, sodium bicarbonate, sodium chloride

SIMPLY SALINE NASAL RELIEF (purified water and sodium chloride)
Church & Dwight Co., Inc.

INGREDIENTS
Purified water, 0.9% sodium chloride.

USES
Comforting mist helps relieve symptoms of dry, irritated nose as gentle misting flushes dust and dirt and pollen and congestion from nasal and sinus passages.)

WARNINGS
• The use of this dispenser by more than one person may spread infection.
• **KEEP OUT OF REACH OF CHILDREN.**
• Contents under pressure.
• Do not puncture or incinerate.
• Store between 59° and 86°F (15° and 30°C).
• Avoid spraying in eyes.

DIRECTIONS
To flush & irrigate, tilt head to the side over sink or use in shower. Insert nozzle into one nostril depressing as a gentle mist fills sinus passages and flows out nostrils. Repeat in other nostril.
To moisturize, insert nozzle into each nostril and press as moisture is restored to dry nasal passages. **USE AS OFTEN AS NEEDED (NON-HABIT FORMING, NON-ADDICTING).**

SINEX 12 HOUR DECONGESTANT NASAL SPRAY (oxymetazoline hydrochloride)
The Procter & Gamble

DRUG FACTS

Active Ingredient(s)	Purpose(s)
Oxymetazoline HCl 0.05%	Nasal decongestant

USES
Temporarily relieves
• Nasal Congestion due to colds
• Hay Fever
• Upper Respiratory Allergies

WARNINGS
Failure to follow these warnings could result in serious consequences.

ASK A DOCTOR BEFORE USE IF YOU HAVE
• Heart disease
• Thyroid disease
• Diabetes
• High blood pressure
• Trouble urinating due to enlarged prostate gland

WHEN USING THIS PRODUCT
• **Do not exceed recommended dosage.**
• Use of this container by more than one person may spread infection.
• Temporary burning, stinging, sneezing, or increased nasal discharge may occur.
• Frequent or prolonged use may cause nasal congestion to recur or worsen.

STOP USE AND ASK A DOCTOR IF
• Symptoms persist for more than 3 days

If pregnant or breast-feeding, ask a health professional before use.
Keep out of reach of children. In case of accidental ingestion, get medical help or contact a Poison Control Center right away.
Tamper evident: End flaps sealed with a sticker for your protection.

DIRECTIONS
• Adults and children 6 years and older (with adult supervision): 2 or 3 sprays in each nostril without tilting your head, not more often than every 10 to 12 hours. Do not exceed 2 doses in 24 hours.
• Children 2 to under 6 years: Ask a doctor.
• Children under 2 years: Do not use.

OTHER INFORMATION
• Store at room temperature.

INACTIVE INGREDIENTS
benzalkonium chloride, chlorhexidine gluconate, citric acid, disodium EDTA, fragrance, purified water, sodium citrate, sodium hydroxide, tyloxapol

QUESTIONS OR COMMENTS?
Call **1-800-873-8276**

SINEX 12 HOUR DECONGESTANT ULTRAFINE MIST MOISTURIZING NASAL SPRAY (oxymetazoline HCl)

The Procter & Gamble

DRUG FACTS

Active Ingredient(s)	Purpose(s)
Oxymetazoline HCl 0.05%	Nasal decongestant

USES
Temporarily relieves
• Nasal Congestion due to colds
• Hay Fever
• Upper Respiratory Allergies

WARNINGS
Failure to follow these warnings could result in serious consequences.

ASK A DOCTOR BEFORE USE IF YOU HAVE
• Heart disease
• Thyroid disease
• Diabetes
• High blood pressure
• Trouble urinating due to enlarged prostate gland

WHEN USING THIS PRODUCT
• **Do not exceed recommended dosage.**
• Use of this container by more than one person may spread infection.
• Temporary burning, stinging, sneezing, or increased nasal discharge may occur.
• Frequent or prolonged use may cause nasal congestion to recur or worsen.

STOP USE AND ASK A DOCTOR IF
• Symptoms persist for more than 3 days

If pregnant or breast-feeding, ask a health professional before use.
Keep out of reach of children. In case of accidental ingestion, get medical help or contact a Poison Control Center right away.
Tamper evident: Carton sealed for your protection.

DIRECTIONS
Remove protective cap. Before using for the first time, prime the pump by firmly depressing its rim several times. Hold container with thumb at base and nozzle between first and second fingers. Without tilting your head, insert nozzle into nostril. Fully depress rim with a firm, even stroke and inhale deeply.
• Adults and children 6 years and older (with adult supervision): 2 or 3 sprays in each nostril, not more often than every 10 - 12 hours. Do not exceed 2 doses in 24 hours.
• Children 2 to under 6 years: Ask a doctor.
• Children under 2 years: Do not use.

OTHER INFORMATION
• Store at room temperature.

INACTIVE INGREDIENTS
benzalkonium chloride, chlorhexidine gluconate, citric acid, disodium EDTA, purified water, sodium citrate, sodium hydroxide, tyloxapol

QUESTIONS OR COMMENTS?
Call **1-800-873-8276**.

SINEX 12 HOUR DECONGESTANT ULTRAFINE MIST NASAL SPRAY

(oxymetazoline HCl)

The Procter & Gamble

DRUG FACTS

Active Ingredient(s)	Purpose(s)
Oxymetazoline HCl 0.05%	Nasal decongestant

USES
Temporarily relieves
• Nasal Congestion due to colds
• Hay Fever
• Upper Respiratory Allergies

WARNINGS
Failure to follow these warnings could result in serious consequences.

ASK A DOCTOR BEFORE USE IF YOU HAVE
• Heart disease
• High blood pressure
• Thyroid disease
• Diabetes
• Trouble urinating due to enlarged prostate gland

WHEN USING THIS PRODUCT
• **Do not exceed recommended dosage.**
• Use of this container by more than one person may spread infection.
• Temporary burning, stinging, sneezing, or increased nasal discharge may occur.
• Frequent or prolonged use may cause nasal congestion to recur or worsen.

STOP USE AND ASK A DOCTOR IF
• Symptoms persist for more than 3 days

If pregnant or breast-feeding, ask a health professional before use.

Keep out of reach of children. In case of accidental ingestion, get medical help or contact a Poison Control Center right away.

Tamper evident: Carton sealed for your protection.

DIRECTIONS
Remove protective cap. Before using for the first time, prime the pump by firmly depressing its rim several times. Hold container with thumb at base and nozzle between first and second fingers. Without tilting your head, insert nozzle into nostril. Fully depress rim with a firm, even stroke and inhale deeply.
• Adults and children 6 years and older (with adult supervision): 2 or 3 sprays in each nostril, not more often than every 10 to 12 hours. Do not exceed 2 doses in 24 hours.
• Children 2 to under 6 years: Ask a doctor.
• Children under 2 years: Do not use.

OTHER INFORMATION
• Store at room temperature.

INACTIVE INGREDIENTS
acesulfame potassium, aloe vera, benzalkonium chloride, chlorhexidine gluconate, citric acid, disodium EDTA, fragrance, purified water, sodium citrate, sodium hydroxide, sorbitol, tyloxapol

QUESTIONS OR COMMENTS?
Call **1-800-873-8276.**

SOLARCAINE COOL ALOE (lidocaine hydrochloride)
MSD Consumer Care, Inc.

DRUG FACTS

Active Ingredient(s)
Lidocaine hydrochloride 0.5%

Purpose(s)
External analgesic

USES
temporarily relieves pain and itching due to:
• minor skin irritations
• minor burns
• sunburn
• scrapes
• minor cuts
• insect bites

WARNINGS
For external use only

DO NOT USE
in large quantities, particularly over raw surfaces or blistered areas

WHEN USING THIS PRODUCT
keep out of eyes

STOP USE AND ASK A DOCTOR IF
• condition gets worse
• symptoms last more than 7 days
• symptoms clear up and occur again in a few days

Keep out of reach of children. If swallowed, get medical help or contact a Poison Control Center right away.

DIRECTIONS
• adults and children 2 years of age and older: apply to affected area not more than 3 to 4 times daily
• children under 2 years of age: ask a doctor

INACTIVE INGREDIENTS
aloe barbadensis leaf juice, water, propylene glycol, glycerin, triethanolamine, isopropyl alcohol (0.06% v/v), polysorbate 80, carbomer, diazolidinyl urea, menthol, disodium EDTA, yellow 5, blue 1
© Copyright & Distributed by MSD
Consumer Care, Inc., PO Box 377,
Memphis, TN 38151 USA, a subsidiary
of Merck & Co., Inc.,
Whitehouse Station, NJ USA

SOLARCAINE COOL ALOE SPRAY (lidocaine)
MSD Consumer Care, Inc.

DRUG FACTS

Active Ingredient(s)
Lidocaine 0.5%

Purpose(s)
External analgesic

USES
temporarily relieves pain and itching due to:
• sunburn
• minor burns
• minor cuts
• scrapes
• insect bites
• minor skin irritations

WARNINGS
For external use only
Flammable: Do not use while smoking or near heat or flame

WHEN USING THIS PRODUCT

DO NOT USE
in large quantities, particularly over raw surfaces or blistered areas

WHEN USING THIS PRODUCT
• keep out of eyes
• use only as directed. Intentional misuse by deliberately concentrating and inhaling the contents can be harmful or fatal.
• do not puncture or incinerate. Contents under pressure. Do not store at temperatures above 120°F.

STOP USE AND ASK A DOCTOR IF
• condition gets worse
• symptoms last more than 7 days
• symptoms clear up and occur again in a few days

Keep out of reach of children. If swallowed, get medical help or contact a Poison Control Center right away.

DIRECTIONS
• shake well
• adults and children 2 years of age and older: apply to affected area not more than 3 to 4 times daily
• children under 2 years of age: ask a doctor
• to apply to face, spray in palm of hand and gently apply

INACTIVE INGREDIENTS
aloe barbadensis leaf juice, isobutane, propane, propylene glycol, glycerin, simethicone, tocopheryl acetate (vitamin E acetate),

triethanolamine, carbomer, diazolidinyl urea, methylparaben, propylparaben, disodium cocoamphodipropionate, disodium EDTA
© Copyright & Distributed by MSD Consumer Care, Inc., PO Box 377 Memphis, TN 38151 USA, a subsidiary of Merck & Co., Inc., Whitehouse Station, NJ USA

SOMINEX MAX (diphenhydramine HCl)
Medtech Products Inc.

DRUG FACTS

Active Ingredient(s)
(in each caplet)
Diphenhydramine HCl 50mg

Purpose(s)
Nighttime sleep-aid

USE
helps reduce difficultly falling asleep

WARNINGS

DO NOT USE
- in children under 12 years of age
- with any other product containing diphenhydramine, even one used on skin
- with other antihistamines

ASK A DOCTOR BEFORE USE IF YOU HAVE
- a breathing problem such as emphysema or chronic bronchitis
- glaucoma
- trouble urinating due to an enlarged prostate gland

ASK A DOCTOR OR PHARMACIST BEFORE USE IF YOU ARE
taking sedatives or tranquilizers

WHEN USING THIS PRODUCT
avoid alcoholic beverages
- be careful when driving a motor vehicle or operating machinery

STOP USE AND ASK A DOCTOR IF
sleeplessness persists continuously for more than 2 weeks. Insomnia may be a symptom of serious underlying medical illness.

If pregnant or breast-feeding,
ask a health professional before use.

Keep out of reach of children.

OVERDOSE WARNING
In case of accidental overdose get medical help or contact a Poison Control Center right away.

DIRECTIONS
- adults and children 12 years and over: take 1 caplet at bedtime if needed, or as directed by your doctor

OTHER INFORMATION
- each caplet contains: **calcium 50 mg**
- store below 25ºC (77ºF)

INACTIVE INGREDIENTS
carnauba wax, crospovidone, dibasic calcium phosphate, FD&C blue #1 aluminum lake, hydroxypropyl methylcellulose, magnesium stearate, microcrystalline cellulose, polyethylene glycol, polysorbate 80, silicon dioxide, starch, titanium dioxide

QUESTIONS OR COMMENTS?
1-866-255-5202 (English/Spanish)

SOMINEX (diphenhydramine HCl)
GlaxoSmithKline Consumer Healthcare LP

Active Ingredient(s) (in each tablet)
Diphenhydramine HCl 25 mg

Active Ingredient(s) (in each caplet)
Diphenhydramine HCl 50 mg

Purpose(s)
Nighttime sleep-aid

USE
helps reduce difficulty falling asleep

WARNINGS

DO NOT USE
- in children under 12 years of age
- with any other product containing diphenhydramine, even one used on skin
- with other antihistamines

ASK A DOCTOR BEFORE USE IF YOU HAVE
- a breathing problem such as emphysema or chronic bronchitis
- glaucoma
- trouble urinating due to an enlarged prostate gland

ASK A DOCTOR OR PHARMACIST BEFORE USE IF YOU ARE
taking sedatives or tranquilizers

WHEN USING THIS PRODUCT
- avoid alcoholic beverages
- be careful when driving a motor vehicle or operating machinery

STOP USE AND ASK A DOCTOR IF
- sleeplessness persists continuously for more than 2 weeks. Insomnia may be a symptom of serious underlying medical illness.

If pregnant or breast-feeding,
ask a health professional before use.

Keep out of reach of children.
(Original Formula)
In case of accidental overdose, get medical help or contact a Poison Control Center right away.

OVERDOSE WARNING: (MAXIMUM STRENGTH)
In case of overdose, get medical help or contact a Poison Control Center right away.

DIRECTIONS (ORIGINAL FORMULA)
- adults and children 12 years and older: take 2 tablets at bedtime if needed, or as directed by a doctor

DIRECTIONS (MAXIMUM STRENGTH)
- adults and children 12 years and older: take 1 caplet at bedtime if needed or as directed by your doctor

OTHER INFORMATION (ORIGINAL FORMULA)
- **each tablet contains:** calcium 70 mg
- store below 25°C (77°F)

OTHER INFORMATION (MAXIMUM STRENGTH)
- **each caplet contains:** calcium 50 mg
- store below 25°C (77°F)

INACTIVE INGREDIENTS (ORIGINAL FORMULA)
dibasic calcium phosphate, FD&C blue #1 aluminum lake, magnesium stearate, microcrystalline cellulose, silicon dioxide, starch

INACTIVE INGREDIENTS (MAXIMUM STRENGTH)
carnauba wax, crospovidone, dibasic calcium phosphate, FD&C blue #1 aluminum lake, hydroxypropyl methylcellulose, magnesium stearate, microcrystalline cellulose, polyethylene glycol, polysorbate 80, silicon dioxide, starch, titanium dioxide

QUESTIONS OR COMMENTS?
1-800-245-1040 (English/Spanish) weekdays or visit essentialsforlivingwell.com

---

CHILDREN'S SUDAFED PE COLD AND COUGH (dextromethorphan hydrobromide and phenylephrine hydrochloride)
McNeil Consumer Healthcare Div. McNeil-PPC, Inc

DRUG FACTS

Active Ingredient(s) (in each 5 mL)*	Purpose(s)
Dextromethorphan HBr 5 mg	Cough suppressant
Phenylephrine HCl 2.5 mg	Nasal decongestant
*5 mL = one teaspoon	

USE
- temporarily relieves these symptoms due to the common cold, hay fever, or other upper respiratory allergies:
  - cough
  - nasal congestion

WARNINGS

DO NOT USE
- in a child who is taking a prescription monoamine oxidase inhibitor (MAOI) (certain drugs for depression, psychiatric or emotional conditions, or Parkinson's disease), or for 2 weeks after stopping the MAOI drug. If you do not know if your child's prescription drug contains an MAOI, ask a doctor or pharmacist before giving this product.

ASK A DOCTOR BEFORE USE IF THE CHILD HAS
- heart disease
- high blood pressure
- thyroid disease
- diabetes
- persistent or chronic cough such as occurs with asthma
- cough that occurs with too much phlegm (mucus)
- a sodium-restricted diet

WHEN USING THIS PRODUCT
do not exceed recommended dose

STOP USE AND ASK A DOCTOR IF
- nervousness, dizziness, or sleeplessness occur
- symptoms do not improve within 7 days or occur with a fever
- cough gets worse or lasts for more than 7 days
- cough tends to come back or occurs with fever, rash or headache that lasts

These could be signs of a serious condition.
Keep out of reach of children. In case of overdose, get medical help or contact a Poison Control Center right away. (1-800-222-1222)

DIRECTIONS
- find right dose on chart below
- use only enclosed dosing cup designed for use with this product. Do not use any other dosing device.
- if needed, repeat dose every 4 hours
- do not give more than 6 times in 24 hours.

Age (yr)	Dose (tsp)
under 4 years	do not use
4 to 5 years	1 teaspoonful (5 mL)
6 to 11 years	2 teaspoonfuls (10 mL)

Attention: use only enclosed dosing cup specifically designed for use with this product. Do not use any other dosing device.

OTHER INFORMATION
- each teaspoon contains: **sodium 15 mg**
- store between 20-25°C (68-77°F). Protect from light. Store in outer carton until contents are used.
- **do not use if bottle wrap, or foil inner seal imprinted "SAFETY SEAL®" is broken or missing**
- see bottom panel for lot number and expiration date

INACTIVE INGREDIENTS
anhydrous citric acid, carboxymethylcellulose sodium, edetate disodium, FD&C blue #1, FD&C red #40, flavors, glycerin, purified water, sodium benzoate, sodium citrate, sorbitol solution, sucralose

QUESTIONS OR COMMENTS?
call **1-888-217-2117**

CHILDREN'S SUDAFED NASAL DECONGESTANT (pseudoephedrine hydrochloride)
McNeil Consumer Healthcare Div. McNeil-PPC, Inc

DRUG FACTS

Active Ingredient(s) (in each 5 mL = 1 teaspoonful)
Pseudoephedrine HCl 15 mg

Purpose(s)
Nasal decongestant

USES
- temporarily relieves nasal congestion due to the common cold, hay fever or other upper respiratory allergies
- temporarily relieves sinus congestion and pressure
- promotes nasal and/or sinus drainage

WARNINGS

DO NOT USE
in a child who is taking a prescription monoamine oxidase inhibitor (MAOI) (certain drugs for depression, psychiatric or emotional conditions, or Parkinson's disease), or for 2 weeks after stopping the MAOI drug. If you do not know if your child's prescription drug contains an MAOI, ask a doctor or pharmacist before giving this product.

ASK A DOCTOR BEFORE USE IF THE CHILD HAS
- heart disease
- high blood pressure
- thyroid disease
- diabetes

WHEN USING THIS PRODUCT
do not exceed recommended dose

STOP USE AND ASK A DOCTOR IF
• nervousness, dizziness, or sleeplessness occur
• symptoms do not improve within 7 days or occur with a fever

Keep out of reach of children. In case of overdose, get medical help or contact a Poison Control Center right away. (1-800-222-1222)

DIRECTIONS
• find right dose on chart below
• mL = milliliter; tsp = teaspoonful
• repeat dose every 4 to 6 hours
• do not use more than 4 times in 24 hours

Age (yr)	Dose (mL or tsp)
under 4 years	do not use
4 to 5 years	5 mL (1 tsp)
6 to 11 years	10 mL (2 tsp)

Attention: use only enclosed dosing cup designed for use with this product. Do not use any other dosing device.

OTHER INFORMATION
• **each 5 mL (1 tsp) contains:** sodium 5 mg
• store between 20-25°C (68-77°F)
• **do not use if bottle wrap, or foil inner seal imprinted "SAFETY SEAL®" is broken or missing**
• see bottom panel for lot number and expiration date

INACTIVE INGREDIENTS
anhydrous citric acid, edetate disodium, FD&C blue no. 1, FD&C red no. 40, flavor, glycerin, menthol, poloxamer 407, polyethylene glycol, povidone K-90, purified water, saccharin sodium, sodium benzoate, sodium citrate, sorbitol solution

QUESTIONS OR COMMENTS?
call **1-888-217-2117**

CHILDREN'S SUDAFED PE NASAL DECONGESTANT (phenylephrine hydrochloride)
McNeil Consumer Healthcare Div. McNeil-PPC, Inc

DRUG FACTS

Active Ingredient(s) (in each 5 mL = 1 teaspoonful)
Phenylephrine HCl 2.5 mg

Purpose(s)
Nasal decongestant

USE
temporarily relieves nasal congestion due to the common cold, hay fever or other upper respiratory allergies

WARNINGS

DO NOT USE
in a child who is taking a prescription monoamine oxidase inhibitor (MAOI) (certain drugs for depression, psychiatric or emotional conditions, or Parkinson's disease), or for 2 weeks after stopping the MAOI drug. If you do not know if your child's prescription drug contains an MAOI, ask a doctor or pharmacist before giving this product.

ASK A DOCTOR BEFORE USE IF THE CHILD HAS
• heart disease
• high blood pressure
• thyroid disease
• diabetes
• a sodium-restricted diet

WHEN USING THIS PRODUCT
do not exceed recommended dose

STOP USE AND ASK A DOCTOR IF
• nervousness, dizziness, or sleeplessness occur
• symptoms do not improve within 7 days or occur with a fever

Keep out of reach of children. In case of overdose, get medical help or contact a Poison Control Center right away. (1-800-222-1222)

DIRECTIONS
• find right dose on chart below
• mL = milliliter; tsp = teaspoonful
• repeat dose every 4 hours
• do not use more than 6 times in 24 hours

Age (yr)	Dose (mL or tsp)
under 4 years	do not use
4 to 5 years	5 mL (1 tsp)
6 to 11 years	10 mL (2 tsp)

Attention: use only enclosed dosing cup designed for use with this product. Do not use any other dosing device.

OTHER INFORMATION
• **each 5 mL (1 tsp) contains:** sodium 14 mg
• store between 20-25°C (68-77°F). Protect from light. Store in outer carton until contents are used.
• **do not use if bottle wrap, or foil inner seal imprinted "Safety Seal®" is broken or missing**
• see bottom panel for lot number and expiration date

INACTIVE INGREDIENTS
anhydrous citric acid, carboxymethylcellulose sodium, edetate disodium, FD&C red #40, flavors, glycerin, purified water, sodium benzoate, sodium citrate, sorbitol solution, sucralose

QUESTIONS OR COMMENTS?
call **1-888-217-2117**

SUDAFED 12 HOUR (pseudoephedrine hydrochloride)
McNeil Consumer Healthcare Div. McNeil-PPC, Inc

DRUG FACTS

Active Ingredient(s) (in each tablet)
Pseudoephedrine HCl 120 mg

Purpose(s)
Nasal decongestant

USES
• temporarily relieves nasal congestion due to the common cold, hay fever or other upper respiratory allergies
• temporarily relieves sinus congestion and pressure

WARNINGS

DO NOT USE
if you are now taking a prescription monoamine oxidase inhibitor (MAOI) (certain drugs for depression, psychiatric or emotional conditions, or Parkinson's disease), or for 2 weeks after stopping the MAOI drug. If you do not know if your prescription drug contains an MAOI, ask a doctor or pharmacist before taking this product.

ASK A DOCTOR BEFORE USE IF YOU HAVE
• heart disease
• high blood pressure

- thyroid disease
- diabetes
- trouble urinating due to an enlarged prostate gland

WHEN USING THIS PRODUCT
do not exceed recommended dosage

STOP USE AND ASK A DOCTOR IF
- nervousness, dizziness, or sleeplessness occur
- symptoms do not improve within 7 days or occur with a fever

If pregnant or breast-feeding, ask a health professional before use.
Keep out of reach of children. In case of overdose, get medical help or contact a Poison Control Center right away. (1-800-222-1222)

DIRECTIONS

adults and children 12 years and over	take 1 tablet every 12 hours do not take more than 2 tablets in 24 hours
children under 12 years	do not use this product in children under 12 years of age

OTHER INFORMATION
- store at 59° to 77°F in a dry place. Protect from light
- **do not use if carton is opened or if blister unit is broken**
- see side panel for lot number and expiration date

INACTIVE INGREDIENTS
candelilla wax, FD&C blue no. 1 aluminum lake, hypromellose, magnesium stearate, microcrystalline cellulose, polyethylene glycol, povidone, propylene glycol, shellac, talc, and titanium dioxide.

QUESTIONS OR COMMENTS?
call **1-888-217-2117** (toll-free) or **215-273-8755** (collect)

SUDAFED 12 HOUR PRESSURE AND PAIN
(naproxen sodium and pseudoephedrine hydrochloride)
McNeil Consumer Healthcare Div. McNeil-PPC, Inc

DRUG FACTS

Active Ingredient(s) (in each caplet)	Purpose(s)
Naproxen sodium 220 mg (naproxen 200 mg) (NSAID)*	Pain reliever/fever reducer
Pseudoephedrine HCl 120 mg, extended-release	Nasal decongestant
*nonsteroidal anti-inflammatory drug	

USES
temporarily relieves these cold, sinus, and flu symptoms:
- sinus pressure
- minor body aches and pains
- headache
- nasal and sinus congestion (promotes sinus drainage and restores freer breathing through the nose)
- fever

WARNINGS
Allergy alert
Naproxen sodium may cause a severe allergic reaction, especially in people allergic to aspirin. Symptoms may include:

- hives
- facial swelling
- asthma (wheezing)
- shock
- skin reddening
- rash
- blisters

If an allergic reaction occurs, stop use and seek medical help right away.

Stomach bleeding warning
This product contains an NSAID, which may cause severe stomach bleeding. The chance is higher if you:
- are age 60 or older
- have had stomach ulcers or bleeding problems
- take a blood thinning (anticoagulant) or steroid drug
- take other drugs containing prescription or nonprescription NSAIDs (aspirin, ibuprofen, naproxen, or others)
- have 3 or more alcoholic drinks every day while using this product
- take more or for a longer time than directed

DO NOT USE
- if you have ever had an allergic reaction to any other pain reliever/fever reducer
- right before or after heart surgery
- if you are now taking a prescription monoamine oxidase inhibitor (MAOI) (certain drugs for depression, psychiatric, or emotional conditions, or Parkinson's disease), or for 2 weeks after stopping the MAOI drug. If you do not know if your prescription drug contains an MAOI, ask a doctor or pharmacist before taking this product.
- in children under 12 years of age

ASK A DOCTOR BEFORE USE IF
- the stomach bleeding warning applies to you
- you have a history of stomach problems, such as heartburn
- you have high blood pressure, heart disease, liver cirrhosis, or kidney disease
- you are taking a diuretic
- you have problems or serious side effects from taking pain relievers or fever reducers
- you have
  - asthma
  - diabetes
  - thyroid disease
  - trouble urinating due to an enlarged prostate gland

ASK A DOCTOR OR PHARMACIST BEFORE USE IF YOU ARE
- under a doctor's care for any serious condition
- taking any other drug

WHEN USING THIS PRODUCT
- take with food or milk if stomach upset occurs
- the risk of heart attack or stroke may increase if you use more than directed or for longer than directed

STOP USE AND ASK A DOCTOR IF
- you experience any of the following signs of stomach bleeding:
  - feel faint
  - vomit blood
  - have bloody or black stools
  - have stomach pain that does not get better
- redness or swelling is present in the painful area
- any new symptoms appear
- fever gets worse or lasts more than 3 days
- you have difficulty swallowing or the caplet feels stuck in your throat
- you get nervous, dizzy, or sleepless
- nasal congestion lasts more than 7 days

If pregnant or breast-feeding, ask a health professional before use. It is especially important not to use naproxen sodium during the last 3 months of pregnancy unless definitely

directed to do so by a doctor because it may cause problems in the unborn child or complications during delivery.
Keep out of reach of children. In case of overdose, get medical help or contact a Poison Control Center right away. (1-800-222-1222)

DIRECTIONS
- **do not take more than directed**
- **the smallest effective dose should be used**
- **swallow whole;** do not crush or chew
- **drink a full glass of water with each dose**

adults and children 12 years and older	**1 caplet every 12 hours** do not take more than 2 caplets in 24 hours
children under 12 years	do not use

OTHER INFORMATION
- **each caplet contains:** sodium 20 mg
- **do not use if carton is opened or if blister unit is broken**
- store at 20-25°C (68-77°F)
- store in a dry place

INACTIVE INGREDIENTS
colloidal silicon dioxide, hypromellose, lactose monohydrate, magnesium stearate, microcrystalline cellulose, polyethylene glycol, polysorbate 80, povidone, talc, titanium dioxide

QUESTIONS OR COMMENTS?
1-888-217-2117

SUDAFED 24 HOUR (pseudoephedrine hydrochloride)

McNeil Consumer Healthcare Div McNeil-PPC, Inc

DRUG FACTS

Active Ingredient(s) (in each tablet)
Pseudoephedrine HCl 240 mg

Purpose(s)
Nasal decongestant

USES
- temporarily relieves nasal congestion due to the common cold, hay fever or other upper respiratory allergies
- reduces swelling of nasal passages
- relieves sinus pressure

WARNINGS

DO NOT USE
if you are now taking a prescription monoamine oxidase inhibitor (MAOI) (certain drugs for depression, psychiatric or emotional conditions, or Parkinson's disease), or for 2 weeks after stopping the MAOI drug. If you do not know if your prescription drug contains an MAOI, ask a doctor or pharmacist before taking this product.

ASK A DOCTOR BEFORE USE IF YOU HAVE
- heart disease
- high blood pressure
- thyroid disease
- diabetes
- trouble urinating due to an enlarged prostate gland
- had obstruction or narrowing of the bowel. Rarely, tablets of this kind may cause bowel obstruction (blockage), usually in people with severe narrowing of the bowel (esophagus, stomach or intestine).

WHEN USING THIS PRODUCT
do not exceed recommended dosage

STOP USE AND ASK A DOCTOR IF
- nervousness, dizziness, or sleeplessness occur
- symptoms do not improve within 7 days or occur with a fever
- you experience persistent abdominal pain or vomiting

If pregnant or breast-feeding, ask a health professional before use.
Keep out of reach of children. In case of overdose, get medical help or contact a Poison Control Center right away. (1-800-222-1222)

DIRECTIONS

adults and children 12 years and over	**swallow one** whole tablet with water every 24 hours **do not exceed one tablet in 24 hours** **do not divide, crush, chew or dissolve the tablet** the tablet does not completely dissolve and may be seen in the stool (this is normal)
children under 12 years	do not use this product in children under 12 years of age

OTHER INFORMATION
- each tablet contains: **sodium 10 mg**
- store at 15° to 25°C (59° to 77°F) in a dry place
- **do not use if carton is opened or if individual blister seals are broken or opened**
- see side panel for lot number and expiration date

INACTIVE INGREDIENTS
cellulose, cellulose acetate, hydroxypropyl cellulose, hypromellose, magnesium stearate, polyethylene glycol, polysorbate 80, povidone, sodium chloride, and titanium dioxide

QUESTIONS OR COMMENTS?
call **1-888-217-2117**

SUDAFED CONGESTION (pseudoephedrine hydrochloride)

McNeil Consumer Healthcare Div. McNeil-PPC, Inc

USES
- temporarily relieves sinus congestion and pressure
- temporarily relieves nasal congestion due to the common cold, hay fever, or other upper-respiratory allergies

DIRECTIONS
adults and children 12 years and over
- take 2 tablets every 4 to 6 hours
- do not take more than 8 tablets in 24 hours

children ages 6 to 11 years
- take 1 tablet every 4 to 6 hours
- do not take more than 4 tablets in 24 hours

children under 6 years
- do not use this product for children under 6 years of age

WARNINGS

DO NOT USE
if you are now taking a prescription monoamine oxidase inhibitor (MAOI) (certain drugs for depression, psychiatric or emotional conditions or Parkinson's disease), or for 2 weeks after stopping the MAOI drug. If you do not know if your

prescription drug contains an MAOI, ask a doctor or pharmacist before taking this product.

ASK A DOCTOR BEFORE USE IF YOU HAVE
- heart disease
- high blood pressure
- thyroid disease
- diabetes
- trouble urinating due to an enlarged prostate gland

WHEN USING THIS PRODUCT
do not exceed recommended dose

STOP USE AND ASK A DOCTOR IF
- nervousness, dizziness, or sleeplessness occurs
- symptoms do not improve within 7 days or occur with a fever

If pregnant or breast-feeding, ask a health professional before use.
Keep out of reach of children. In case of overdose, get medical help or contact a Poison Control Center right away (1-800-222-1222).

INGREDIENTS

Active Ingredient(s) (in each tablet)	Purpose(s)
Pseudoephedrine HCl 30 mg	Nasal decongestant

INACTIVE INGREDIENTS
carnauba wax, colloidal silicon dioxide, D&C yellow #10 aluminum lake, FD&C red #40 aluminum lake, FD&C yellow #6 aluminum lake, iron oxide, magnesium stearate, microcrystalline cellulose, polyethylene glycol, polyvinyl alcohol, pregelatinized starch, shellac, sodium starch glycolate, talc, titanium dioxide

SUDAFED PE COLD+COUGH (acetaminophen, dextromethorphan HBr, guaifenesin, and phenylephrine HCl)

McNeil Consumer Healthcare Div. McNeil-PPC, Inc

DRUG FACTS

Active Ingredient(s) (in each caplet)	Purpose(s)
Acetaminophen 325 mg	Pain reliever/fever reducer
Dextromethorphan HBr 10 mg	Cough suppressant
Guaifenesin 100 mg	Expectorant
Phenylephrine HCl 5 mg	Nasal decongestant

USES
- temporarily relieves these symptoms due to the common cold:
  - nasal congestion
  - headache
  - minor aches and pains
  - cough
  - sore throat
- helps loosen phlegm (mucus) and thin bronchial secretions to drain bronchial tubes and make coughs more productive
- temporarily reduces fever

WARNINGS
Liver warning: This product contains acetaminophen. Severe liver damage may occur if you take
- more than 12 caplets in 24 hours, which is the maximum daily amount

- with other drugs containing acetaminophen
- 3 or more alcoholic drinks every day while using this product

Sore throat warning: If sore throat is severe, persists for more than 2 days, is accompanied or followed by fever, headache, rash, nausea, or vomiting, consult a doctor promptly.

DO NOT USE
- with any other drug containing acetaminophen (prescription or nonprescription). If you are not sure whether a drug contains acetaminophen, ask a doctor or pharmacist.
- if you are now taking a prescription monoamine oxidase inhibitor (MAOI) (certain drugs for depression, psychiatric or emotional conditions or Parkinson's disease), or for 2 weeks after stopping the MAOI drug. If you do not know if your prescription drug contains an MAOI, ask a doctor or pharmacist before taking this product.
- if you have ever had an allergic reaction to this product or any of its ingredients.

ASK A DOCTOR BEFORE USE IF YOU HAVE
- liver disease
- heart disease
- high blood pressure
- thyroid disease
- diabetes
- trouble urinating due to an enlarged prostate gland
- persistent or chronic cough such as occurs with smoking, asthma, chronic bronchitis, or emphysema
- cough that occurs with too much phlegm (mucus)

ASK A DOCTOR OR PHARMACIST BEFORE USE IF YOU ARE
- taking the blood-thinning drug warfarin

WHEN USING THIS PRODUCT
- **do not exceed recommended dose**

STOP USE AND ASK A DOCTOR IF
- nervousness, dizziness, or sleeplessness occur
- pain, cough, or nasal congestion gets worse or lasts more than 7 days
- fever gets worse or lasts more than 3 days
- redness or swelling is present
- new symptoms occur
- cough comes back or occurs with rash or headache that lasts

These could be signs of a serious condition.
If pregnant or breast-feeding, ask a health professional before use.
Keep out of reach of children.

OVERDOSE WARNING
Taking more than the recommended dose (overdose) may cause liver damage. In case of overdose, get medical help or contact a Poison Control Center right away (1-800-222-1222). Quick medical attention is critical for adults as well as for children even if you do not notice any signs or symptoms.

DIRECTIONS
do not use more than directed (see overdose warning)
adults and children 12 years and over
- take 2 caplets every 4 hours
- do not take more than 12 tablets in 24 hours

children under 12 years
- do not use this adult product for children under 12 years of age; this will provide more than the recommended dose (overdose) and may cause liver damage

OTHER INFORMATION
- contains FD&C yellow #5 aluminum lake (tartrazine) as a color additive
- each caplet contains: **sodium 3 mg**
- store between 20-25°C (68-77°F)

INACTIVE INGREDIENTS
carnauba wax, croscarmellose sodium, FD&C yellow #5
aluminum lake (tartrazine), FD&C yellow #6 aluminum lake,
hydroxypropyl cellulose, hypromellose, magnesium stearate,
microcrystalline cellulose, polyethylene glycol, polysorbate 80,
pregelatinized starch, titanium dioxide

QUESTIONS OR COMMENTS?
Call **1-888-217-2117**

SUDAFED PE CONGESTION (phenylephrine HCl)
McNeil Consumer Healthcare Div. McNeil-PPC, Inc

DRUG FACTS

Active Ingredient(s) (in each tablet)	Purpose(s)
Phenylephrine HCl 10 mg	Nasal decongestant

USES
- temporarily relieves sinus congestion and pressure
- temporarily relieves nasal congestion due to the common cold, hay fever, or other upper-respiratory allergies

DO NOT USE
If you are now taking a prescription monoamine oxidase
inhibitor (MAOI) (certain drugs for depression, psychiatric or
emotional conditions or Parkinson's disease), or for 2 weeks
after stopping the MAOI drug. If you do not know if your
prescription drug contains an MAOI, ask a doctor or pharmacist
before taking this product.

ASK A DOCTOR BEFORE USE IF YOU HAVE
- heart disease
- high blood pressure
- thyroid disease
- diabetes
- trouble urinating due to an enlarged prostate gland

WHEN USING THIS PRODUCT
- **do not exceed recommended dose**

STOP USE AND ASK A DOCTOR IF
- nervousness, dizziness, or sleeplessness occurs
- symptoms do not improve within 7 days or occur with a fever

If pregnant or breast-feeding, ask a health professional
before use.
Keep out of reach of children. In case of overdose, get
medical help or contact a Poison Control Center right away
(1-800-222-1222).

DIRECTIONS
adults and children 12 years and over
- take 1 tablet every 4 hours
- do not take more than 6 tablets in 24 hours

children under 12 years
- do not use this product for children under 12 years of age

OTHER INFORMATION
- store between 20-25°C (68-77°&F)

INACTIVE INGREDIENTS
carnauba wax, corn starch, D&C yellow #10 aluminum lake,
FD&C red #40 aluminum lake, FD&C yellow #6 aluminum lake,
magnesium stearate, microcrystalline cellulose, polyethylene
glycol, polyvinyl alcohol, powdered cellulose, pregelatinized
starch, sodium starch glycolate, talc, titanium dioxide

QUESTIONS OR COMMENTS?
Call **1-888-217-2117**

SUDAFED PE DAY & NIGHT COLD
(acetaminophen, dextromethorphan hydrobromide,
guaifenesin, and phenylephrine hydrochloride)
McNeil Consumer Healthcare Div. McNeil-PPC, Inc

OVERVIEW
Daytime - SUDAFED PE® Cold+Cough
Get relief from coughing, congestion, and sore throat—plus, help
loosen mucus to make coughs more productive.
- New look, same effective relief you trust

Nighttime - SUDAFED PE® Nighttime Cold
Relieves your cold symptoms, so you can get the rest you need.

USES
Daytime - SUDAFED PE® Cold+Cough
- temporarily relieves these symptoms due to the common cold:
  - nasal congestion
  - headache
  - minor aches and pains
  - cough
  - sore throat
- helps loosen phlegm (mucus) and thin bronchial secretions to drain bronchial tubes and make coughs more productive
- temporarily reduces fever

Nighttime - SUDAFED PE® Nighttime Cold
- temporarily relieves these symptoms of hay fever and the common cold
  - runny nose
  - sneezing
  - headache
  - minor aches and pains
  - nasal congestion
  - sore throat
- temporarily relieves these additional symptoms of hay fever:
  - itching of the nose or throat
  - itchy, watery eyes
- temporarily reduces fever

DIRECTIONS
do not use more than directed (see overdose warning)
adults and children 12 years and over
- take 2 caplets every 4 hours
- do not take more than 12 caplets in 24 hours

children under 12 years
- do not use this adult product for children under 12 years of age; this will provide more than the recommended dose (overdose) and may cause liver damage

WARNINGS
Daytime - SUDAFED PE® Cold+Cough
Liver warning: This product contains acetaminophen. Severe
liver damage may occur if you take
- more than 12 caplets in 24 hours, which is the maximum daily amount
- with other drugs containing acetaminophen
- 3 or more alcoholic drinks every day while using this product

Sore throat warning: If sore throat is severe, persists for
more than 2 days, is accompanied or followed by fever,
headache, rash, nausea, or vomiting, consult a doctor promptly.

DO NOT USE
- with any other drug containing acetaminophen (prescription or nonprescription). If you are not sure whether a drug contains acetaminophen, ask a doctor or pharmacist.
- if you are now taking a prescription monoamine oxidase inhibitor (MAOI) (certain drugs for depression, psychiatric or

emotional conditions or Parkinson's disease), or for 2 weeks after stopping the MAOI drug. If you do not know if your prescription drug contains an MAOI, ask a doctor or pharmacist before taking this product.
- if you have ever had an allergic reaction to this product or any of its ingredients

ASK A DOCTOR BEFORE USE IF YOU HAVE
- liver disease
- heart disease
- high blood pressure
- thyroid disease
- diabetes
- trouble urinating due to an enlarged prostate
- persistent or chronic cough such as occurs with smoking, asthma, chronic bronchitis, or emphysema
- cough that occurs with too much phlegm (mucus)

ASK A DOCTOR OR PHARMACIST BEFORE USE IF
you are taking the blood-thinning drug warfarin

WHEN USING THIS PRODUCT
do not exceed recommended dose

STOP USE AND ASK A DOCTOR IF
- nervousness, dizziness, or sleeplessness occur
- pain, cough or nasal congestion gets worse or lasts more than 7 days
- fever gets worse or lasts more than 3 days
- redness or swelling is present
- new symptoms occur
- cough comes back or occurs with rash or headache that lasts

These could be signs of a serious condition.
If pregnant or breast-feeding, ask a health professional before use.
Keep out of reach of children.

OVERDOSE WARNING
Taking more than the recommended dose (overdose) may cause liver damage. In case of overdose, get medical help or contact a Poison Control Center right away (1-800-222-1222). Quick medical attention is critical for adults as well as for children even if you do not notice any signs or symptoms.

Nighttime — SUDAFED PE® Nighttime Cold
Liver warning: This product contains acetaminophen. Severe liver damage may occur if you take
- more than 12 caplets in 24 hours, which is the maximum daily amount
- with other drugs containing acetaminophen
- 3 or more alcoholic drinks every day while using this product

Sore throat warning: If sore throat is severe, persists for more than 2 days, is accompanied or followed by fever, headache, rash, nausea, or vomiting, consult a doctor promptly.

DO NOT USE
- with any other drug containing acetaminophen (prescription or nonprescription). If you are not sure whether a drug contains acetaminophen, ask a doctor or pharmacist.
- with any other product containing diphenhydramine, even one used on skin
- if you are now taking a prescription monoamine oxidase inhibitor (MAOI) (certain drugs for depression, psychiatric or emotional conditions or Parkinson's disease), or for 2 weeks after stopping the MAOI drug. If you do not know if your prescription drug contains an MAOI, ask a doctor or pharmacist before taking this product.
- if you have ever had an allergic reaction to this product or any of its ingredients.

ASK A DOCTOR BEFORE USE IF YOU HAVE
- liver disease
- heart disease

- high blood pressure
- thyroid disease
- diabetes
- trouble urinating due to an enlarged prostate gland
- a breathing problem such as emphysema or chronic bronchitis
- glaucoma

ASK A DOCTOR OR PHARMACIST BEFORE USE IF YOU ARE
- taking the blood-thinning drug warfarin
- taking sedatives or tranquilizers

WHEN USING THIS PRODUCT
- **do not exceed recommended dose**
- excitability may occur, especially in children
- marked drowsiness may occur
- alcohol, sedatives, and tranquilizers may increases drowsiness
- avoid alcoholic drinks
- be careful when driving a motor vehicle or operating machinery

STOP USE AND ASK A DOCTOR IF
- nervousness, dizziness, or sleeplessness occur
- pain or nasal congestion gets worse or lasts more than 7 days
- fever gets worse or lasts more than 3 days
- redness or swelling is present
- new symptoms occur

These could be signs of a serious condition.
If pregnant or breast-feeding, ask a health professional before use.
Keep out of reach of children.

OVERDOSE WARNING
Taking more than the recommended dose (overdose) may cause liver damage. In case of overdose, get medical help or contact a Poison Control Center right away (1-800-222-1222). Quick medical attention is critical for adults as well as for children even if you do not notice any signs or symptoms.

INGREDIENTS
Daytime - SUDAFED PE® Cold+Cough

Active Ingredient(s) (in each caplet)	Purpose(s)
Acetaminophen 325 mg	Pain reliever/fever reducer
Dextromethorphan HBr 10 mg	Cough suppressant
Guaifenesin 100 mg	Expectorant
Phenylephrine HCl 5 mg	Nasal decongestant

INACTIVE INGREDIENTS
carnauba wax, croscarmellose sodium, FD&C yellow #5 aluminum lake (tartrazine), FD&C yellow #6 aluminum lake, hydroxypropyl cellulose, hypromellose, magnesium stearate, microcrystalline cellulose, polyethylene glycol, polysorbate 80, pregelatinized starch, titanium dioxide
Nighttime - SUDAFED PE® Nighttime Cold

Active Ingredient(s) (in each caplet)	Purpose(s)
Acetaminophen 325 mg	Pain reliever/fever reducer
Diphenhydramine HCl 25 mg	Antihistamine
Phenylephrine HCl 5 mg	Nasal decongestant

INACTIVE INGREDIENTS
carnauba wax, corn starch, FD&C blue #1 aluminum lake, hypromellose, magnesium stearate, microcrystalline cellulose, polyethylene glycol, polyvinyl alcohol, sodium citrate, sodium starch glycolate, talc, titanium dioxide

OTHER INFO
Daytime - SUDAFED PE® Cold+Cough
- contains FD&C yellow #5 aluminum lake (tartrazine) as a color additive
- each caplet contains: **sodium 3 mg**
- store between 20-25°C (68-77°F)

Nighttime - SUDAFED PE® Nighttime Cold
- store between 20-25°C (68-77°F)

QUESTIONS OR COMMENTS?
Call **1-888-217-2117**

SUDAFED PE NON-DRYING SINUS
(phenylephrine HCl and guaifenesin)
McNeil Consumer Healthcare Div. McNeil-PPC, Inc

OVERVIEW
Get relief from sinus pressure and congestion, and in a non-drying formula.)
- Non-drowsy formula
- Available in a box of 24
- New look, same effective relief you trust

USES
- temporarily relieves nasal congestion
- promotes nasal and/or sinus drainage
- temporarily relieves sinus congestion and pressure
- helps loosen phlegm (mucus) and thin bronchial secretions to rid the bronchial passageways of bothersome mucus and make coughs more productive

DIRECTIONS
adults and children 12 years and over
- take 2 caplets every 4 hours
- do not take more than 12 tablets in 24 hours

children under 12 years
- do not use this product for children under 12 years of age

WARNINGS

DO NOT USE
if you are now taking a prescription monoamine oxidase inhibitor (MAOI) (certain drugs for depression, psychiatric or emotional conditions or Parkinson's disease), or for 2 weeks after stopping the MAOI drug. If you do not know if your prescription drug contains an MAOI, ask a doctor or pharmacist before taking this product.

ASK A DOCTOR BEFORE USE IF YOU HAVE
- heart disease
- high blood pressure
- thyroid disease
- diabetes
- trouble urinating due to an enlarged prostate gland
- persistent or chronic cough such as occurs with smoking, asthma, chronic bronchitis, or emphysema
- cough that occurs with too much phlegm (mucus)

WHEN USING THIS PRODUCT
do not exceed recommended dose

STOP USE AND ASK A DOCTOR IF
- nervousness, dizziness, or sleeplessness occurs
- symptoms do not improve within 7 days or occur with a fever
- cough gets worse or lasts more than 7 days
- cough tends to come back or occurs with fever, rash or headache that lasts

These could be signs of a serious condition

If pregnant or breast-feeding, ask a health professional before use.
Keep out of reach of children. In case of overdose, get medical help or contact a Poison Control Center right away (1-800-222-1222).

INGREDIENTS

Active Ingredient(s) (in each caplet)	Purpose(s)
Guaifenesin 200 mg	Expectorant
Phenylephrine HCl 5 mg	Nasal decongestant

INACTIVE INGREDIENTS
carnauba wax, croscarmellose sodium, D&C yellow #10 aluminum lake, FD&C blue #1 aluminum lake, FD&C blue #2 aluminum lake, hydroxypropyl cellulose, magnesium stearate, microcrystalline cellulose, polyethylene glycol, polyvinyl alcohol, powdered cellulose, pregelatinized starch, talc, titanium dioxide

OTHER INFO
- each caplet contains: **sodium 3 mg**
- store between 20-25°C (68-77°F)

QUESTIONS OR COMMENTS?
Call **1-888-217-2117**

SUDAFED PE PRESSURE PLUS PAIN
(acetaminophen and phenylephrine hydrochloride)
McNeil Consumer Healthcare Div. McNeil-PPC, Inc

DRUG FACTS

Active Ingredient(s) (in each caplet)	Purpose(s)
Acetaminophen 325 mg	Pain reliever/fever reducer
Phenylephrine HCl 5 mg	Nasal decongestant

USES
- temporarily relieves these symptoms associated with hay fever or other respiratory allergies, and the common cold:
  - sinus congestion and pressure
  - headache
  - minor aches and pains
  - nasal congestion
- promotes sinus drainage
- temporarily reduces fever

WARNINGS
Liver warning
This product contains acetaminophen. The maximum daily dose of this product is 10 caplets (3,250 mg acetaminophen) in 24 hours. Severe liver damage may occur if you take
- more than 4,000 mg of acetaminophen in 24 hours
- with other drugs containing acetaminophen
- 3 or more alcoholic drinks every day while using this product

DO NOT USE
- with any other drug containing acetaminophen (prescription or nonprescription). If you are not sure whether a drug contains acetaminophen, ask a doctor or pharmacist.
- if you are now taking a prescription monoamine oxidase inhibitor (MAOI) (certain drugs for depression, psychiatric or emotional conditions, or Parkinson's disease), or for 2 weeks after stopping the MAOI drug. If you do not know if your prescription drug contains an MAOI, ask a doctor or pharmacist before taking this product.

- if you have ever had an allergic reaction to this product or any of its ingredients

ASK A DOCTOR BEFORE USE IF YOU HAVE
- liver disease
- heart disease
- high blood pressure
- thyroid disease
- diabetes
- trouble urinating due to an enlarged prostate gland

ASK A DOCTOR OR PHARMACIST BEFORE USE IF YOU ARE
taking the blood thinning drug warfarin

WHEN USING THIS PRODUCT
do not exceed recommended dose

STOP USE AND ASK A DOCTOR IF
- nervousness, dizziness, or sleeplessness occur
- pain or nasal congestion gets worse or lasts more than 7 days
- fever gets worse or lasts more than 3 days
- redness or swelling is present
- new symptoms occur

These could be signs of a serious condition.
If pregnant or breast-feeding, ask a health professional before use.
Keep out of reach of children.

OVERDOSE WARNING
In case of overdose, get medical help or contact a Poison Control Center right away. (1-800-222-1222) Quick medical attention is critical for adults as well as for children even if you do not notice any signs or symptoms.

DIRECTIONS
- **do not use more than directed (see overdose warning)**

adults and children 12 years and over	take 2 caplets every 4 hours do not take more than 10 caplets in 24 hours
children under 12 years	ask a doctor

OTHER INFORMATION
- store between 20-25°C (68-77°F)
- **do not use if carton is opened or if blister unit is broken**

INACTIVE INGREDIENTS
carnauba wax, corn starch, FD&C yellow no. 6 aluminum lake, hypromellose, magnesium stearate, microcrystalline cellulose, polyethylene glycol, polysorbate 80, powdered cellulose, pregelatinized starch, sodium starch glycolate, titanium dioxide

QUESTIONS OR COMMENTS?
call **1-888-217-2117** (toll-free) or **215-273-8755** (collect)

SUDAFED PE SEVERE COLD (acetaminophen, diphenhydramine HCl, and phenylephrine HCl)
McNeil Consumer Healthcare Div. McNeil-PPC, Inc

DRUG FACTS

Active Ingredient(s) (in each caplet)	Purpose(s)
Acetaminophen 325 mg	Pain reliever
Diphenhydramine HCl 12.5 mg	Antihistamine/cough suppressant
Phenylephrine HCl 5 mg	Nasal decongestant

USES
temporarily relieves these symptoms due to the common cold:
- runny nose
- sneezing
- headache
- minor aches and pains
- nasal congestion
- cough
- sore throat

temporarily relieves sinus congestion and pressure

WARNINGS
Liver warning: This product contains acetaminophen. Severe liver damage may occur if you take
- more than 12 caplets in 24 hours, which is the maximum daily amount
- with other drugs containing acetaminophen
- 3 or more alcoholic drinks every day while using this product

Sore throat warning: If sore throat is severe, persists for more than 2 days, is accompanied or followed by fever, headache, rash, nausea, or vomiting, consult a doctor promptly.

DO NOT USE
- with any other drug containing acetaminophen (prescription or nonprescription). If you are not sure whether a drug contains acetaminophen, ask a doctor or pharmacist.
- with any other product containing diphenhydramine, even one used on skin
- if you are now taking a prescription monoamine oxidase inhibitor (MAOI) (certain drugs for depression, psychiatric or emotional conditions or Parkinson's disease), or for 2 weeks after stopping the MAOI drug. If you do not know if your prescription drug contains an MAOI, ask a doctor or pharmacist before taking this product.
- if you have ever had an allergic reaction to this product or any of its ingredients

ASK A DOCTOR BEFORE USE IF YOU HAVE
- liver disease
- heart disease
- high blood pressure
- thyroid disease
- diabetes
- trouble urinating due to an enlarged prostate gland
- cough accompanied by too much phlegm (mucus)
- persistent or chronic cough such as occurs with smoking, asthma, chronic bronchitis, or emphysema
- breathing problem such as emphysema or chronic bronchitis
- glaucoma

ASK A DOCTOR OR PHARMACIST BEFORE USE IF YOU ARE
- taking the blood-thinning drug warfarin
- taking sedatives or tranquilizers

WHEN USING THIS PRODUCT
- **do not exceed recommended dose**
- excitability may occur, especially in children
- marked drowsiness may occur
- alcohol, sedatives, and tranquilizers may increase drowsiness
- avoid alcoholic drinks
- be careful when driving a motor vehicle or operating machinery

STOP USE AND ASK A DOCTOR IF
- nervousness, dizziness, or sleeplessness occur
- pain, cough or nasal congestion gets worse or lasts more than 7 days
- fever gets worse or lasts more than 3 days
- redness or swelling is present
- new symptoms occur
- cough comes back or occurs with rash or headache that lasts

These could be signs of a serious condition.

If pregnant or breast-feeding, ask a health professional before use.

Keep out of reach of children.

OVERDOSE WARNING
Taking more than the recommended dose (overdose) may cause liver damage. In case of overdose, get medical help or contact a Poison Control Center right away (1-800-222-1222). Quick medical attention is critical for adults as well as for children even if you do not notice any signs or symptoms.

DIRECTIONS
do not use more than directed (see overdose warning)

adults and children 12 years and over
- take 2 caplets every 4 hours
- do not take more than 12 caplets in 24 hours

children under 12 years
- do not use this adult product for children under 12 years of age; this will provide more than the recommended dose (overdose) and may cause liver damage

OTHER INFORMATION
- store between 20-25°C (68-77°F)

INACTIVE INGREDIENTS
carnauba wax, corn starch, hypromellose, magnesium stearate, microcrystalline cellulose, polyethylene glycol, polyvinyl alcohol, sodium citrate, sodium starch glycolate, talc, titanium dioxide

QUESTIONS OR COMMENTS?
Call **1-888-217-2117**

SUDAFED PE SINUS+ALLERGY

(chlorpheniramine maleate and phenylephrine HCl)

McNeil Consumer Healthcare Div. McNeil-PPC, Inc

DRUG FACTS

Active Ingredient(s) (in each tablet)	Purpose(s)
Chlorpheniramine maleate 4 mg	Antihistamine
Phenylephrine HCl 10 mg	Nasal decongestant

USES
temporarily relieves these symptoms due to hay fever (allergic rhinitis) or other upper-respiratory allergies:
- runny nose
- sneezing
- itchy, watery eyes
- nasal congestion
- itching of the nose or throat
- sinus congestion and pressure

DO NOT USE
if you are now taking a prescription monoamine oxidase inhibitor (MAOI) (certain drugs for depression, psychiatric or emotional conditions or Parkinson's disease), or for 2 weeks after stopping the MAOI drug. If you do not know if your prescription drug contains an MAOI, ask a doctor or pharmacist before taking this product.

ASK A DOCTOR BEFORE USE IF YOU HAVE
- heart disease
- high blood pressure
- thyroid disease
- diabetes
- trouble urinating due to an enlarged prostate gland
- a breathing problem such as emphysema or chronic bronchitis
- glaucoma

ASK A DOCTOR OR PHARMACIST BEFORE USE IF YOU ARE
- taking sedatives or tranquilizers

WHEN USING THIS PRODUCT
- do not exceed recommended dose
- excitability may occur, especially in children
- drowsiness may occur
- alcohol, sedatives, and tranquilizers may increase drowsiness
- avoid alcoholic drinks
- be careful when driving a motor vehicle or operating machinery

STOP USE AND ASK A DOCTOR IF
- nervousness, dizziness, or sleeplessness occurs
- symptoms do not improve within 7 days or occur with a fever

If pregnant or breast-feeding, ask a health professional before use.

Keep out of reach of children. In case of overdose, get medical help or contact a Poison Control Center right away (1-800-222-1222).

DIRECTIONS
adults and children 12 years and over
- take 1 tablet every 4 hours
- do not take more than 6 tablets in 24 hours

children under 12 years
- do not use this product for children under 12 years of age

OTHER INFORMATION
- store between 20-25°C (68-77°F)

INACTIVE INGREDIENTS
carnauba wax, corn starch, magnesium stearate, microcrystalline cellulose, polyethylene glycol, polyvinyl alcohol, powdered cellulose, pregelatinized starch, sodium starch glycolate, talc, titanium dioxide

QUESTIONS OR COMMENTS?
Call **1-888-217-2117**

SUDAFED PE TRIPLE ACTION (acetaminophen, guaifenesin, and phenylephrine HCl)

McNeil Consumer Healthcare Div. McNeil-PPC, Inc

DRUG FACTS

Active Ingredient(s) (in each caplet)	Purpose(s)
Acetaminophen 325 mg	Pain reliever
Guaifenesin 200 mg	Expectorant
Phenylephrine HCl 5 mg	Nasal decongestant

USES

for the temporary relief of:
- sinus congestion and pressure
- headache
- minor aches and pains
- nasal congestion

helps loosen phlegm (mucus) and thin bronchial secretions, to rid the bronchial passageways of bothersome mucus and makes coughs more productive

WARNINGS

Liver warning: This product contains acetaminophen. Severe liver damage may occur if you take
- more than 12 caplets in 24 hours, which is the maximum daily amount
- with other drugs containing acetaminophen
- 3 or more alcoholic drinks every day while using this product

DO NOT USE

- with any other product containing acetaminophen (prescription or nonprescription). If you are not sure whether a drug contains acetaminophen, ask a doctor or pharmacist.
- if you are now taking a prescription monoamine oxidase inhibitor (MAOI) (certain drugs for depression, psychiatric or emotional conditions or Parkinson's disease), or for 2 weeks after stopping the MAOI drug. If you do not know if your prescription drug contains an MAOI, ask a doctor or pharmacist before taking this product.
- if you have ever had an allergic reaction to this product or any of its ingredients

ASK A DOCTOR BEFORE USE IF YOU HAVE

- liver disease
- heart disease
- high blood pressure
- thyroid disease
- diabetes
- trouble urinating due to an enlarged prostate gland
- persistent or chronic cough such as occurs with smoking, asthma, chronic bronchitis, or emphysema
- cough that occurs with too much phlegm (mucus)

ASK A DOCTOR OR PHARMACIST BEFORE USE IF YOU ARE

- taking the blood-thinning drug warfarin

WHEN USING THIS PRODUCT

- **do not exceed recommended dose**

STOP USE AND ASK A DOCTOR IF

- nervousness, dizziness, or sleeplessness occur
- pain, nasal congestion or cough gets worse or lasts more than 7 days
- fever gets worse or lasts more than 3 days
- redness or swelling is present
- new symptoms occur
- cough comes back or occurs with rash or headache that lasts

These could be signs of a serious condition.
If pregnant or breast-feeding, ask a health professional before use.
Keep out of reach of children.

OVERDOSE WARNING

Taking more than the recommended dose (overdose) may cause liver damage. In case of overdose, get medical help or contact a Poison Control Center right away (1-800-222-1222). Quick medical attention is critical for adults as well as for children even if you do not notice any signs or symptoms.

DIRECTIONS

do not use more than directed (see overdose warning)
adults and children 12 years and over
- take 2 caplets every 4 hours
- do not take more than 12 caplets in 24 hours

children under 12 years
- do not use this adult product for children under 12 years of age; this will provide more than the recommended dose (overdose) and may cause liver damage

OTHER INFORMATION

- each caplet contains: **sodium 3 mg**
- store between 20-25°C (68-77°F)

INACTIVE INGREDIENTS

carnauba wax, croscarmellose sodium, hydroxypropyl cellulose, hypromellose, magnesium stearate, microcrystalline cellulose, pregelatinized starch, titanium dioxide, triacetin

QUESTIONS OR COMMENTS?

Call **1-888-217-2117**

SUDAFED TRIPLE ACTION (acetaminophen, guaifenesin, and pseudoephedrine HCl)

McNeil Consumer Healthcare Div. McNeil-PPC, Inc

DRUG FACTS

Active Ingredient(s) (in each caplet)	Purpose(s)
Acetaminophen 325 mg	Pain reliever
Guaifenesin 200 mg	Expectorant
Pseudoephedrine HCl 30 mg	Nasal decongestant

USES

for the temporary relief of:
- sinus congestion and pressure
- headache
- minor aches and pains
- nasal congestion

helps loosen phlegm (mucus) and thin bronchial secretions to rid the bronchial passageways of bothersome mucus and makes coughs more productive

WARNINGS

Liver warning: This product contains acetaminophen. Severe liver damage may occur if you take
- more than 8 caplets in 24 hours, which is the maximum daily amount for this product
- with other drugs containing acetaminophen
- 3 or more alcoholic drinks every day while using this product

DO NOT USE
- with any other product containing acetaminophen (prescription or nonprescription). If you are not sure whether a drug contains acetaminophen, ask a doctor or pharmacist.
- if you are now taking a prescription monoamine oxidase inhibitor (MAOI) (certain drugs for depression, psychiatric or emotional conditions or Parkinson's disease), or for 2 weeks after stopping the MAOI drug. If you do not know if your prescription drug contains an MAOI, ask a doctor or pharmacist before taking this product.
- if you have ever had an allergic reaction to this product or any of its ingredients

ASK A DOCTOR BEFORE USE IF YOU HAVE
- liver disease
- heart disease
- high blood pressure
- thyroid disease
- diabetes
- trouble urinating due to an enlarged prostate gland
- persistent or chronic cough such as occurs with smoking, asthma, chronic bronchitis, or emphysema
- cough that occurs with too much phlegm (mucus)

ASK A DOCTOR OR PHARMACIST BEFORE USE IF YOU ARE
- taking the blood-thinning drug warfarin

WHEN USING THIS PRODUCT
- **do not exceed recommended dose**

STOP USE AND ASK A DOCTOR IF
- nervousness, dizziness, or sleeplessness occur
- pain, nasal congestion or cough gets worse or lasts more than 7 days
- fever gets worse or lasts more than 3 days
- redness or swelling is present
- new symptoms occur
- cough comes back or occurs with rash or headache that lasts

These could be signs of a serious condition.
If pregnant or breast-feeding, ask a health professional before use.
Keep out of reach of children.

OVERDOSE WARNING
Taking more than the recommended dose (overdose) may cause liver damage. In case of overdose, get medical help or contact a Poison Control Center right away (1-800-222-1222). Quick medical attention is critical for adults as well as for children even if you do not notice any signs or symptoms.

DIRECTIONS
do not use more than directed (see overdose warning)
adults and children 12 years and over
- take 2 caplets every 4 to 6 hours
- do not take more than 8 caplets in 24 hours

children under 12 years
- do not use this adult product for children under 12 years of age; this will provide more than the recommended dose (overdose) and may cause liver damage

OTHER INFORMATION
- each caplet contains: **sodium 3 mg**
- store between 20-25°C (68-77°F)

INACTIVE INGREDIENTS
colloidal silicon dioxide, croscarmellose sodium, microcrystalline cellulose, polyethylene glycol, polyvinyl alcohol, povidone, pregelatinized starch, stearic acid, talc, titanium dioxide

QUESTIONS OR COMMENTS?
Call **1-888-217-2117**

SURFAK STOOL SOFTENER (docusate calcium)
Chattem, Inc.

DRUG FACTS

Active Ingredient(s) (in each softgel)
Docusate calcium 240 mg

Purpose(s)
Stool softener laxative

USES
- relieves occasional constipation (irregularity)
- generally produces a bowel movement in 12 to 72 hours

WARNINGS

DO NOT USE
- when stomach pain, nausea or vomiting are present unless directed by a doctor

ASK A DOCTOR BEFORE USE IF YOU HAVE
- stomach pain, nausea or vomiting
- a sudden change in bowel habits that lasts over 2 weeks

ASK A DOCTOR OR PHARMACIST BEFORE USE IF YOU ARE
presently taking mineral oil

STOP USE AND ASK A DOCTOR IF
- you have rectal bleeding or failure to have a bowel movement after use. These could be signs of a serious condition.
- you need to use a laxative for more than 1 week

If pregnant or breast-feeding, ask a health professional before use.

Keep out of reach of children.
In case of overdose, get medical help or contact a Poison Control Center right away.

DIRECTIONS
- adults and children 12 years of age or over: one softgel daily
- children under 12 years of age: ask a doctor

OTHER INFORMATION
- protect from heat, humidity and light

INACTIVE INGREDIENTS
corn oil, gelatin, glycerin, hypromellose, isopropyl alcohol, mannitol, propylene glycol, red 33, red 40, sorbitol, titanium dioxide, water (283-042)

SYSTANE (polyethylene glycol and propylene glycol)
Alcon Research, Ltd

Active Ingredient(s)
Polyethylene Glycol 400 0.4%. . . . . Lubricant
Propylene Glycol 0.3%. . . . . Lubricant

WARNINGS
For external use only.

DO NOT USE
- if this product changes color or becomes cloudy
- if you are sensitive to any ingredient in this product

WHEN USING THIS PRODUCT
- do not touch tip of container to any surface to avoid contamination
- do not reuse
- once opened, discard

STOP USE AND ASK A DOCTOR IF
• you feel eye pain
• changes in vision occur
• redness or irritation of the eye(s) gets worse, persists or lasts more than 72 hours

Keep out of reach of children.
If swallowed, get medical help or contact a Poison Control Center right away.

USES
For the temporary relief of burning and irritation due to dryness of the eye

DIRECTIONS
• Instill 1 or 2 drops in the affected eye(s) as needed.

OTHER INFORMATION
• Store at room temperature.
• Protect from light.

INACTIVE INGREDIENTS
boric acid, calcium chloride, hydroxypropyl guar, magnesium chloride, potassium chloride, purified water, sodium chloride, zinc chloride. May contain hydrochloric acid and/or sodium hydroxide to adjust pH.

QUESTIONS OR COMMENTS?
In the U.S. call 1-800-757-9195
www.systane.com MedInfo@AlconLabs.com

SYSTANE BALANCE (propylene glycol)

Alcon Laboratories, Inc.

Restorative Formula
Clinical Strength
Intensive Therapy
Alcon®
Sterile
10 mL (1/3 FL OZ)

DRUG FACTS

Active Ingredient(s)
Propylene Glycol 0.6%

Purpose(s)
Lubricant

USES
• For the temporary relief of burning and irritation due to dryness of the eye

WARNINGS
For external use only.

DO NOT USE
• if this product changes color
• if you are sensitive to any ingredient in this product

WHEN USING THIS PRODUCT
• do not touch tip of container to any surface to avoid contamination
• replace cap after each use

STOP USE AND ASK A DOCTOR IF
• you feel eye pain
• changes in vision occur
• redness or irritation of the eye(s) gets worse, persists or lasts more than 72 hours

Keep out of reach of children.
If swallowed, get medical help or contact a Poison Control Center right away.

DIRECTIONS
• Shake well before using.
• Instill 1 or 2 drops in the affected eye(s) as needed.

OTHER INFORMATION
• Store at room temperature

INACTIVE INGREDIENTS:
boric acid, dimyristoyl phosphatidylglycerol, edetate disodium, hydroxypropyl guar, mineral oil, polyoxyl 40 stearate, POLYQUAD® (polyquaternium-1) 0.001% preservative, sorbitan tristearate, sorbitol and purified water. May contain hydrochloric acid and/or sodium hydroxide to adjust pH.

QUESTIONS OR COMMENTS?
In the U.S. call **1-800-757-9195**
www.systane.com
MedInfo@AlconLabs.com
TAMPER EVIDENT: For your protection, this bottle has an imprinted seal around the neck. Do not use if seal is damaged or missing at time of purchase.
Upgrade to a higher standard of relief. SYSTANE® BALANCE Lubricant Eye Drops has the proven power to restore the natural tear's lipid layer to treat dryness and provide long lasting relief.
U.S. Patent Nos. 5,278,151; 5,294,607; 5,578,586; 6,583,124; 6,838,449; 6,849,253
© 2010 Alcon, Inc.
Alcon®
Alcon Laboratories, Inc.
6201 South Freeway
Fort Worth, TX 76134 USA
Printed in USA

SYSTANE GEL DROPS (polyethylene glycol and propylene glycol)

Alcon Laboratories, Inc.

SYSTANE Gel Drops

DRUG FACTS

Active Ingredient(s)	Purpose(s)
Polyethylene Glycol 400 0.4%	Lubricant
Propylene Glycol 0.3%	Lubricant

USES
• For the temporary relief of burning and irritation due to dryness of the eye

WARNINGS
For external use only.

DO NOT USE
• if this product changes color or becomes cloudy
• if you are sensitive to any ingredient in this product

WHEN USING THIS PRODUCT
• do not touch tip of container to any surface to avoid contamination
• replace cap after each use

STOP USE AND ASK A DOCTOR IF
- you feel eye pain
- changes in vision occur
- redness or irritation of the eye(s) gets worse, persists or lasts more than 72 hours

Keep out of reach of children.
If swallowed, get medical help or contact a Poison Control Center right away.

DIRECTIONS
- Shake well before using.
- Instill 1 or 2 drops in the affected eye(s) as needed.

OTHER INFORMATION
- Store at room temperature.

INACTIVE INGREDIENTS
aminomethylpropanol, boric acid, edetate disodium, hydroxypropyl guar, POLYQUAD (polyquaternium-1) 0.001% preservative, potassium chloride, sodium chloride, sorbitol and purified water. May contain hydrochloric acid and/or sodium hydroxide to adjust pH.

QUESTIONS OR COMMENTS?
In the U.S., call 1-800-757-9195
www.systane.com

SYSTANE NIGHTTIME (mineral oil and white petrolatum)
Alcon Laboratories, Inc.

OTC - ACTIVE INGREDIENT SECTION
Mineral Oil 3%
White Petrolatum 94%

OTC - PURPOSE SECTION
Lubricant

INDICATIONS & USAGE SECTION
- For use as a lubricant to prevent further irritation or to relieve dryness of the eye.

WARNINGS SECTION
For external use only

OTC - DO NOT USE SECTION
- if you are sensitive to any ingredient in this product

OTC - WHEN USING SECTION
- remove contact lenses before using
- to avoid contamination, do not touch tip of container to any surface
- replace cap after using

OTC - STOP USE SECTION AND ASK A DOCTOR IF
- you feel eye pain
- changes in vision occur
- redness or irritation of the eye(s) gets worse, persists or lasts more than 72 hours

OTC - KEEP OUT OF REACH OF CHILDREN SECTION
If swallowed, get medical help or contact a Poison Control Center right away.

DOSAGE & ADMINISTRATION SECTION
Pull down the lower lid of the affected eye and apply a small amount (one-fourth inch) of ointment to the inside of the eyelid.

OTHER INFORMATION
- Store at 8°-27°C (46°-80°F).

INACTIVE INGREDIENT SECTION
anhydrous liquid lanolin 3%.

QUESTIONS OR COMMENTS?
In the U.S., call 1-800-757-9195 or visit www.systane.com

SYSTANE PRESERVATIVE-FREE FORMULA
(polyethylene glycol and propylene glycol)
Alcon Laboratories, Inc.

Active Ingredient(s)	Purpose(s)
Polyethylene Glycol 400 0.4%	Lubricant
Propylene Glycol 0.3%	Lubricant

USES
- For the temporary relief of burning and irritation due to dryness of the eye.

WARNINGS
For external use only.

DO NOT USE
- if this product changes color or becomes cloudy
- if you are sensitive to any ingredient in this product

WHEN USING THIS PRODUCT
- do not touch tip of container to any surface to avoid contamination
- do not reuse
- once opened, discard

STOP USE AND ASK A DOCTOR IF
- you feel eye pain
- changes in vision occur
- redness or irritation of the eye(s) gets worse or lasts more than 72 hours

Keep out of reach of children.
If swallowed, get medical help or contact a Poison Control Center right away.

DIRECTIONS
- Instill 1 or 2 drops in the affected eye(s) as needed.

OTHER INFORMATION
- Store at room temperature.
- Protect from light.

INACTIVE INGREDIENTS
boric acid, calcium chloride, hydroxypropyl guar, magnesium chloride, potassium chloride, purified water, sodium chloride, zinc chloride. May contain hydrochloric acid and/or sodium hydroxide to adjust pH.

QUESTIONS OR COMMENTS?
In the U.S., call 1-800-757-9195

SYSTANE ULTRA (polyethylene glycol and propylene glycol)

Alcon Research Ltd

Active Ingredient(s)
Polyethylene Glycol 400 0.4% . . . . Lubricant
Propylene Glycol 0.3%. . . . . Lubricant

USES
For the temporary relief of burning and irritation due to dryness of the eye

WARNINGS
For external use only.

DO NOT USE
• if this product changes color or becomes cloudy
• if you are sensitive to any ingredient in this product

WHEN USING THIS PRODUCT
• do not touch tip of container to any surface to avoid contamination
• do not reuse
• once opened, discard

STOP USE AND ASK A DOCTOR IF
• you feel eye pain
• changes in vision occur
• redness or irritation of the eye(s) gets worse, persists or lasts more than 72 hours

Keep out of reach of children.
If swallowed, get medical help or contact a Poison Control Center right away.

DIRECTIONS
• Instill 1 or 2 drops in the affected eye(s) as needed.

OTHER INFORMATION
• Store at room temperature

INACTIVE INGREDIENTS
aminomethylpropanol, boric acid, hydroxypropyl guar, potassium chloride, purified water, sodium chloride, sorbitol. May contain hydrochloric acid and/or sodium hydroxide to adjust pH.

QUESTIONS OR COMMENTS?
In the U.S. call 1-800-757-9195
www.systane.com

SYSTANE ULTRA LUBRICANT EYE DROPS PRESERVATIVE-FREE FORMULA (polyethylene glycol and propylene glycol)

Alcon Laboratories, Inc.

SYSTANE ULTRA Preservative-Free Formula

DRUG FACTS

Active Ingredient(s)	Purpose(s)
Polyethylene Glycol 400 0.4%	Lubricant
Propylene Glycol 0.3%	Lubricant

USES
• For the temporary relief of burning and irritation due to dryness of the eye

WARNINGS
For external use only.

DO NOT USE
• if this product changes color or becomes cloudy
• if you are sensitive to any ingredient in this product

WHEN USING THIS PRODUCT
• do not touch tip of container to any surface to avoid contamination
• do not reuse
• once opened, discard

STOP USE AND ASK A DOCTOR IF
• you feel eye pain
• changes in vision occur
• redness or irritation of the eye(s) gets worse, persists or lasts more than 72 hours

Keep out of reach of children.
If swallowed, get medical help or contact a Poison Control Center right away.

DIRECTIONS
• Instill 1 or 2 drops in the affected eye(s) as needed.

OTHER INFORMATION
• Store at room temperature.

INACTIVE INGREDIENTS
aminomethylpropanol, boric acid, hydroxypropyl guar, potassium chloride, purified water, sodium chloride, sorbitol. May contain hydrochloric acid and/or sodium hydroxide to adjust pH.

QUESTIONS OR COMMENTS?
In the U.S., call 1-800-757-9195

TEARS NATURALE FORTE (dextran 70, glycerin, and hypromellose)

Alcon Laboratories, Inc.

OTC - ACTIVE INGREDIENT SECTION

Active Ingredient(s)
Dextran 70 0.1%
Glycerin 0.2%
Hypromellose 0.3%

OTC - PURPOSE SECTION

Purpose(s)
Lubricant

INDICATIONS & USAGE SECTION

USES
For the temporary relief of burning and irritation due to dryness of the eye and for use as a protectant against further irritation. For the temporary relief of discomfort due to minor irritations of the eye or to exposure to wind or sun.

WARNINGS SECTION

WARNINGS
For external use only

OTC - DO NOT USE SECTION

DO NOT USE
• if this solution changes color or becomes cloudy
• if you are sensitive to any ingredient in this product

OTC - WHEN USING SECTION

WHEN USING THIS PRODUCT
- remove contact lenses before using
- do not touch tip of container to any surface to avoid contamination
- replace cap after each use

OTC - STOP USE SECTION

STOP USE AND ASK A DOCTOR IF
- you feel eye pain
- changes in vision occur
- redness or irritation of the eye(s) gets worse or lasts more than 72 hours

OTC - KEEP OUT OF REACH OF CHILDREN SECTION
Keep out of reach of children.

If swallowed, get medical help or contact a Poison Control Center right away.

DOSAGE & ADMINISTRATION SECTION

DIRECTIONS
- Instill 1 or 2 drops in the affected eye(s) as needed.

OTHER SAFETY INFORMATION

OTHER INFORMATION
- store at room temperature.

INACTIVE INGREDIENT SECTION

INACTIVE INGREDIENTS
boric acid, calcium chloride, glycine, hydrochloric acid and/or sodium hydroxide (to adjust pH), magnesium chloride, POLYQUAD® (polyquaternium-1) 0.001% preservative, polysorbate 80, potassium chloride, purified water, sodium chloride, zinc chloride.

OTC - QUESTIONS SECTION

QUESTIONS OR COMMENTS?
In the U.S. call 1-800-757-9195
www.tearsnaturale.com

THERAFLU COLD & SORE THROAT
(acetaminophen, pheniramine maleate, and phenylephrine hydrochloride)

Novartis Consumer Health, Inc.

DRUG FACTS

Active Ingredient(s) (in each packet)	Purpose(s)
Acetaminophen 325 mg	Pain reliever/fever reducer
Pheniramine maleate 20 mg	Antihistamine
Phenylephrine hydrochloride 10 mg	Nasal decongestant

USES
- temporarily relieves these symptoms due to a cold:
  - minor aches and pains
  - headache
  - minor sore throat pain
  - nasal congestion
- temporarily reduces fever
- temporarily relieves these symptoms due to hay fever or other upper respiratory allergies:
  - runny nose
  - sneezing
  - itchy nose and throat
  - itchy, watery eyes

WARNINGS
Liver warning
This product contains acetaminophen. Severe liver damage may occur if you take
- more than 6 packets in 24 hours, which is the maximum daily amount
- with other drugs containing acetaminophen
- 3 or more alcoholic drinks every day while using this product

Sore throat warning
If sore throat is severe, persists for more than 2 days, is accompanied or followed by fever, headache, rash, nausea, or vomiting consult a doctor promptly.

DO NOT USE
- in a child under 4 years of age
- if you are allergic to acetaminophen
- with any other drug containing acetaminophen (prescription or nonprescription). If you are not sure whether a drug contains acetaminophen, ask a doctor or pharmacist.
- if you are now taking a prescription monoamine oxidase inhibitor (MAOI) (certain drugs for depression, psychiatric, or emotional conditions, or Parkinson's disease), or for 2 weeks after stopping the MAOI drug. If you do not know if your prescription drug contains an MAOI, ask a doctor or pharmacist before taking this product.

ASK A DOCTOR BEFORE USE IF YOU HAVE
- liver disease
- heart disease
- thyroid disease
- high blood pressure
- glaucoma
- diabetes
- a breathing problem such as emphysema, asthma or chronic bronchitis
- trouble urinating due to an enlarged prostate gland
- a sodium-restricted diet

ASK A DOCTOR OR PHARMACIST BEFORE USE IF YOU ARE
- taking the blood thinning drug warfarin
- taking sedatives or tranquilizers

WHEN USING THIS PRODUCT
- **do not exceed recommended dosage**
- avoid alcoholic drinks
- may cause drowsiness
- alcohol, sedatives, and tranquilizers may increase drowsiness
- be careful when driving a motor vehicle or operating machinery
- excitability may occur, especially in children

STOP USE AND ASK A DOCTOR IF
- nervousness, dizziness, or sleeplessness occurs
- pain, cough or nasal congestion gets worse or lasts more than 7 days
- fever gets worse or lasts more than 3 days
- redness or swelling is present
- new symptoms occur

If pregnant or breast-feeding, ask a health care professional before use.

Keep out of reach of children.
In case of overdose, get medical help or contact a Poison Control Center right away. Prompt medical attention is critical for adults as well as for children even if you do not notice any signs or symptoms.

DIRECTIONS
- **do not use more than directed**
- take every 4 hours; do not take more than 6 packets in 24 hours unless directed by a doctor

Age	Dose
children under 4 years of age	**do not use**
children 4 to under 12 years of age	do not use unless directed by a doctor
adults and children 12 years of age and over	one packet

- dissolve contents of one packet into 8 oz. hot water: sip while hot. Consume entire drink within 10-15 minutes.
- if using a microwave, add contents of one packet to 8 oz. of cool water: stir briskly before and after heating. Do not overheat.

OTHER INFORMATION
- **each packet contains:** sodium 44 mg
- store at controlled room temperature 20-25°C (68-77°F).

INACTIVE INGREDIENTS
acesulfame K, citric acid, D&C yellow #10, FD&C yellow #6, flavors, magnesium stearate, maltodextrin, silicon dioxide, sodium citrate, soy lecithin, sucrose, tribasic calcium phosphate

QUESTIONS OR COMMENTS?
Call **1-800-452-0051**

THERAFLU DAYTIME SEVERE COLD & COUGH (acetaminophen, dextromethorphan, hydrobromide, and phenylephrine hydrochloride)
Novartis Consumer Health, Inc.

DRUG FACTS

Active Ingredient(s)	Purpose(s)
Acetaminophen 650 mg	Pain reliever/fever reducer
Dextromethorphan hydrobromide 20 mg	cough suppressant
Phenylephrine hydrochloride 10 mg	Nasal decongestant

USES
- temporarily relieves these symptoms due to a cold:
  - minor aches and pains
  - minor sore throat pain
  - headache
  - nasal and sinus congestions
  - cough due to minor throat and bronchial irritation
- temporarily reduces fever

WARNINGS
Liver warning
This product contains acetaminophen. Severe liver damage may occur if you take
- more than 6 packets in 24 hours, which is the maximum daily amount
- with other drugs containing acetaminophen
- 3 or more alcoholic drinks every day while using this product

Sore throat warning
If sore throat is severe, persists for more than 2 days, is accompanied or followed by fever, headache, rash, nausea, or vomiting consult a doctor promptly.

DO NOT USE
- in a child under 4 years of age
- if you are allergic to acetaminophen
- with any other drug containing acetaminophen (prescription or nonprescription). If you are not sure whether a drug contains acetaminophen, ask a doctor or pharmacist.
- if you are now taking a prescription monoamine oxidase inhibitor (MAOI) (certain drugs for depression, psychiatric, or emotional conditions, or Parkinson's disease), or for 2 weeks after stopping the MAOI drug. If you do not know if your prescription drug contains an MAOI, ask a doctor or pharmacist before taking this product.

ASK A DOCTOR BEFORE USE IF YOU HAVE
- liver disease
- heart disease
- high blood pressure
- thyroid disease
- diabetes
- trouble urinating due to an enlarged prostate gland
- cough that occurs with too much phlegm (mucus)
- cough that lasts or is chronic such as occurs with smoking, asthma or emphysema

ASK A DOCTOR OR PHARMACIST BEFORE USE IF YOU ARE
- taking the blood thinning drug warfarin

WHEN USING THIS PRODUCT
- **do not exceed recommended dosage**

STOP USE AND ASK A DOCTOR IF
- nervousness, dizziness, or sleeplessness occurs
- fever gets worse or lasts more than 3 days
- redness or swelling is present
- new symptoms occur
- symptoms do not get better or worsen
- pain, cough or nasal congestion gets worse or lasts more than 7 days
- cough comes back or occurs with fever, rash or headache that lasts. These could be signs of a serious condition.

If pregnant or breast-feeding, ask a health care professional before use.

Keep out of reach of children.
In case of overdose, get medical help or contact a Poison Control Center right away. Prompt medical attention is critical for adults as well as for children even if you do not notice any signs or symptoms.

DIRECTIONS
- **do not use more than directed**
- take every 4 hours; do not take more than 6 packets in 24 hours unless directed by a doctor

Age	Dose
children under 4 years of age	**do not use**
children 4 to under 12 years of age	do not use unless directed by a doctor
adults and children 12 years of age and over	one packet

- dissolve contents of one packet into 8 oz. hot water: sip while hot. Consume entire drink within 10-15 minutes.
- if using a microwave, add contents of one packet to 8 oz. of cool water: stir briskly before and after heating. Do not overheat.

OTHER INFORMATION
- **each packet contains:** potassium 10 mg, sodium 20 mg
- **phenylketonurics:** contains phenylalanine 14 mg per packet

- store at controlled room temperature 20-25°C (68-77°F). Protect from excessive heat and moisture.

INACTIVE INGREDIENTS
acesulfame K, aspartame, citric acid, FD&C blue #1, FD&C red #40, flavors, maltodextrin, silicon dioxide, sodium citrate, sucrose, tribasic calcium phosphate

QUESTIONS OR COMMENTS?
Call 1-800-452-0051

THERAFLU FLU & CHEST CONGESTION
(acetaminophen and guaifenesin)

Novartis Consumer Health, Inc.

DRUG FACTS

Active Ingredient(s) (in each packet)	Purpose(s)
Acetaminophen 1000 mg	Pain reliever/fever reducer
Guaifenesin 400 mg	Expectorant

USES
- temporarily relieves these symptoms due to a cold:
  - minor aches and pains
  - headache
  - minor sore throat pain
- temporarily reduces fever
- helps loosen phlegm (mucus) and thin bronchial secretions to drain bronchial tubes and make coughs more productive

WARNINGS
Liver warning
This product contains acetaminophen. Severe liver damage may occur if you take
- more than 4 packets in 24 hours, which is the maximum daily amount
- with other drugs containing acetaminophen
- 3 or more alcoholic drinks every day while using this product

Sore throat warning
If sore throat is severe, persists for more than 2 days, is accompanied or followed by fever, headache, rash, nausea, or vomiting consult a doctor promptly.

DO NOT USE
- in a child under 4 years of age
- if you are allergic to acetaminophen
- with any other drug containing acetaminophen (prescription or nonprescription). If you are not sure whether a drug contains acetaminophen, ask a doctor or pharmacist.

ASK A DOCTOR BEFORE USE IF YOU HAVE
- liver disease
- cough that occurs with too much phlegm (mucus)
- cough that lasts or is chronic such as occurs with smoking, asthma, chronic bronchitis, or emphysema

ASK A DOCTOR OR PHARMACIST BEFORE USE IF YOU ARE
- taking the blood thinning drug warfarin

STOP USE AND ASK A DOCTOR IF
- pain or cough gets worse or lasts more than 7 days
- fever gets worse or lasts more than 3 days
- redness or swelling is present
- new symptoms occur
- cough comes back or occurs with fever, rash or headache that lasts. These could be signs of a serious condition.

If pregnant or breast-feeding, ask a health care professional before use.

Keep out of reach of children.
In case of overdose, get medical help or contact a Poison Control Center right away. Prompt medical attention is critical for adults as well as for children even if you do not notice any signs or symptoms.

DIRECTIONS
- **do not use more than directed**
- take every 6 hours; do not take more than 4 packets in 24 hours unless directed by a doctor

Age	Dose
children under 4 years of age	do not use
children 4 to under 12 years of age	do not use unless directed by a doctor
adults and children 12 years of age and over	one packet

- dissolve contents of one packet into 8 oz. hot water: sip while hot. Consume entire drink within 10-15 minutes.
- if using a microwave, add contents of one packet to 8 oz. of cool water: stir briskly before and after heating. Do not overheat.

OTHER INFORMATION
- **each packet contains:** potassium 10 mg, sodium 15 mg
- **phenylketonurics:** contains phenylalanine 24 mg per packet
- store at controlled room temperature 20-25°C (68-77°F).

INACTIVE INGREDIENTS
acesulfame K, aspartame, citric acid, D&C yellow #10, FD&C red #40, flavors, maltodextrin, silicon dioxide, sodium citrate, sucrose, tribasic calcium phosphate

QUESTIONS OR COMMENTS?
Call **1-800-452-0051**

THERAFLU FLU & SORE THROAT
(acetaminophen, pheniramine maleate, and phenylephrine hydrochloride)

Novartis Consumer Health, Inc.

DRUG FACTS

Active Ingredient(s) (in each packet)	Purpose(s)
Acetaminophen 650 mg	Pain reliever/fever reducer
Pheniramine maleate 20 mg	Antihistamine
Phenylephrine hydrochloride 10 mg	Nasal decongestant

USES
- temporarily relieves these symptoms due to a cold:
  - minor aches and pains
  - headache
  - minor sore throat pain
  - nasal congestions
- temporarily reduces fever
- temporarily relieves these symptoms due to hay fever or other upper respiratory allergies:
  - runny nose
  - sneezing
  - itchy nose and throat
  - itchy, watery eyes

WARNINGS

Liver warning

This product contains acetaminophen. Severe liver damage may occur if you take

- more than 6 packets in 24 hours, which is the maximum daily amount
- with other drugs containing acetaminophen
- 3 or more alcoholic drinks every day while using this product

Sore throat warning

If sore throat is severe, persists for more than 2 days, is accompanied or followed by fever, headache, rash, nausea, or vomiting consult a doctor promptly.

DO NOT USE

- in a child under 4 years of age
- if you are allergic to acetaminophen
- with any other drug containing acetaminophen (prescription or nonprescription). If you are not sure whether a drug contains acetaminophen, ask a doctor or pharmacist.
- if you are now taking a prescription monoamine oxidase inhibitor (MAOI) (certain drugs for depression, psychiatric, or emotional conditions, or Parkinson's disease), or for 2 weeks after stopping the MAOI drug. If you do not know if your prescription drug contains an MAOI, ask a doctor or pharmacist before taking this product.

ASK A DOCTOR BEFORE USE IF YOU HAVE

- liver disease
- heart disease
- high blood pressure
- thyroid disease
- diabetes
- glaucoma
- a breathing problem such as emphysema or chronic bronchitis
- trouble urinating due to an enlarged prostate gland
- a sodium-restricted diet

ASK A DOCTOR OR PHARMACIST BEFORE USE IF YOU ARE

- taking sedatives or tranquilizers
- taking the blood thinning drug warfarin

WHEN USING THIS PRODUCT

- **do not exceed recommended dosage**
- avoid alcoholic drinks
- may cause drowsiness
- alcohol, sedatives, and tranquilizers may increase drowsiness
- be careful when driving a motor vehicle or operating machinery
- excitability may occur, especially in children

STOP USE AND ASK A DOCTOR IF

- nervousness, dizziness, or sleeplessness occurs
- pain or nasal congestion gets worse or lasts more than 7 days
- fever gets worse or lasts more than 3 days
- redness or swelling is present
- new symptoms occur

If pregnant or breast-feeding, ask a health care professional before use.

Keep out of reach of children.

In case of overdose, get medical help or contact a Poison Control Center right away. Prompt medical attention is critical for adults as well as for children even if you do not notice any signs or symptoms.

DIRECTIONS

- **do not use more than directed**
- take every 4 hours; do not take more than 6 packets in 24 hours unless directed by a doctor

Age	Dose
children under 4 years of age	**do not use**
children 4 to under 12 years of age	do not use unless directed by a doctor
adults and children 12 years of age and over	one packet

- dissolve contents of one packet into 8 oz. hot water: sip while hot. Consume entire drink within 10-15 minutes.
- if using a microwave, add contents of one packet to 8 oz. of cool water: stir briskly before and after heating. Do not overheat.

OTHER INFORMATION

- **each packet contains:** potassium 10 mg, sodium 51 mg
- store at controlled room temperature 20-25°C (68-77°F).

INACTIVE INGREDIENTS

acacia, acesulfame K, aspartame, citric acid, D&C yellow #10, FD&C blue #1, FD&C red #40, flavors, lecithin, maltodextrin, medium chain triglycerides, mono & diglycerides, silicon dioxide, sodium chloride, sodium citrate, sucrose, triacetin, tribasic calcium phosphate

QUESTIONS OR COMMENTS?

Call **1-800-452-0051**

THERAFLU MAX-D SEVERE COLD & FLU

(acetaminophen, dextromethorphan hydrobromide, guaifenesin, and pseudoephedrine hydrochloride)

Novartis Consumer Health, Inc.

DRUG FACTS

Active Ingredient(s) (in each packet)	Purpose(s)
Acetaminophen 1000 mg	Pain reliever/fever reducer
Dextromethorphan HBr 30 mg	Cough suppressant
Guaifenesin 400 mg	Expectorant
Pseudoephedrine HCl 60 mg	Nasal decongestant

USES

- temporarily relieves these symptoms due to a cold:
  - minor aches and pains
  - headache
  - minor sore throat pain
  - cough
  - nasal congestion
  - helps decongest sinus openings and passages
- temporarily reduces fever
- helps loosen phlegm (mucus) and thin bronchial secretions to drain bronchial tubes and make coughs more productive

WARNINGS

Liver warning

This product contains acetaminophen. Severe liver damage may occur if you take

- more than 4 packets in 24 hours, which is the maximum daily amount
- with other drugs containing acetaminophen
- 3 or more alcoholic drinks every day while using this product

Sore throat warning

If sore throat is severe, persists for more than 2 days, is accompanied or followed by fever, headache, rash, nausea, or vomiting consult a doctor promptly.

DO NOT USE
- in a child under 4 years of age
- if you are allergic to acetaminophen
- with any other drug containing acetaminophen (prescription or nonprescription). If you are not sure whether a drug contains acetaminophen, ask a doctor or pharmacist
- if you are now taking a prescription monoamine oxidase inhibitor (MAOI) (certain drugs for depression, psychiatric, or emotional conditions, or Parkinson's disease), or for 2 weeks after stopping the MAOI drug. If you do not know if your prescription drug contains an MAOI, ask a doctor or pharmacist before taking this product.

ASK A DOCTOR BEFORE USE IF YOU HAVE
- liver disease
- heart disease
- diabetes
- thyroid disease
- high blood pressure
- trouble urinating due to an enlarged prostate gland
- cough that occurs with too much phlegm (mucus)
- cough that lasts or is chronic such as occurs with smoking, asthma, chronic bronchitis, or emphysema

ASK A DOCTOR OR PHARMACIST BEFORE USE IF YOU ARE
- taking the blood thinning drug warfarin

WHEN USING THIS PRODUCT
- **do not exceed recommended dosage**

STOP USE AND ASK A DOCTOR IF
- nervousness, dizziness, or sleeplessness occurs
- pain, nasal congestion or cough gets worse or lasts more than 7 days
- fever gets worse or lasts more than 3 days
- redness or swelling is present
- new symptoms occur
- cough comes back or occurs with fever, rash or headache that lasts. These could be signs of a serious condition.

If pregnant or breast-feeding, ask a health care professional before use.
Keep out of reach of children. In case of overdose, get medical help or contact a Poison Control Center right away. Prompt medical attention is critical for adults as well as for children even if you do not notice any signs or symptoms.

DIRECTIONS
- **do not use more than directed**
- **take every 6 hours; do not take more than 4 packets in 24 hours unless directed by a doctor**

children under 4 years of age	do not use
children 4 to under 12 years of age	do not use unless directed by a doctor
adults and children 12 years of age and over	one packet

- dissolve contents of one packet into 8 oz. hot water: sip while hot. Consume entire drink within 10-15 minutes.
- if using a microwave, add contents of one packet to 8 oz. of cool water: stir briskly before and after heating. Do not overheat.

OTHER INFORMATION
- **each packet contains:** calcium 10 mg, potassium 10 mg, sodium 15 mg
- **phenylketonurics:** contains phenylalanine 23.6 mg per packet
- store at controlled room temperature 20-25°C (68-77°F)

INACTIVE INGREDIENTS
acesulfame K, aspartame, citric acid, D&C yellow #10, FD&C red #40, flavors, maltodextrin, silicon dioxide, sodium citrate, sucrose, tribasic calcium phosphate

QUESTIONS OR COMMENTS?
Call 1-800-452-0051

THERAFLU MULTI SYMPTOM SEVERE COLD
(acetaminophen, dextromethorphan HBr, and phenylephrine HCl)
Novartis Consumer Health, Inc.

Active Ingredient(s)
Acetaminophen and 500 mg)
Dextromethorphan hydrobromide and 20 mg)
Phenylephrine hydrochloride, 10 mg

Purpose(s)
Pain reliever / fever reducer
Cough suppressant
Nasal decongestant

USES
- temporarily relieves these symptoms due to a cold:
- minor aches and pains • minor sore throat pain
- headache • nasal and sinus congestion
- cough due to minor throat and bronchial irritation
-
- temporarily reduces fever

WARNINGS
Liver warning: This product contains acetaminophen. Severe liver damage may occur if you take
- more than 6 packets in 24 hours, which is the maximum daily amount
- with other drugs containing acetaminophen
- 3 or more alcoholic drinks every day while using this product

Sore throat warning: If sore throat is severe, persists for more than 2 days, is accompanied or followed by fever, headache, rash. nausea, or vomiting consult a doctor promptly.

DO NOT USE
- in a child under 4 years of age
- if you are allergic to acetaminophen
- with any other drug containing acetaminophen (prescription or nonprescription). If you are not sure whether a drug contains acetaminophen, as a doctor or a pharmacist.
- if you are now taking a prescription monoamine oxidase inhibitor (MAOI) (certain drugs for depression, psychiatric, or emotional conditions, or Parkinson's disease), or for 2 weeks after stopping the MAOI drug. If you do not know if your prescription drug contains an MAOI, ask a doctor or pharmacist before taking this product.

ASK DOCTOR BEFORE USE IF YOU HAVE
- liver disease
- heart disease
- high blood pressure
- thyroid disease
- diabetes
- trouble urinating due to an enlarged prostate gland
- cough that occurs with too much phlegm (mucus)
- cough that lasts or is chronic such as occurs with smoking, asthma or emphysema

ASK A DOCTOR OR PHARMACIST BEFORE USE IF YOU ARE
- taking the blood thinning drug warfarin

WHEN USING THIS PRODUCT
- **do not exceed recommended dosage**

STOP USE AND ASK A DOCTOR IF
- nervousness, dizziness, or sleeplessness occurs
- fever gets worse or lasts more than 3 days
- redness or swelling is present
- new symptoms occur
- symptoms do not get better or worsen
- pain, cough or nasal congestion gets worse or lasts more than 7 days
- cough comes back or occurs with fever, rash or headache that lasts. These could be signs of a serious condition.

IF PREGNANT OR BREAST-FEEDING,
ask a health care professional before use.

KEEP OUT OF REACH OF CHILDREN
In case of overdose, get medical help or contact a Poison Control Center right away. Prompt medical attention is critical for adults as well as for children even if you do not notice any signs or symptoms.

DIRECTIONS
- **do not use more than directed**
- take every 4 hours; do not take more than 6 packets in 24 hours unless directed by a doctor

Age	Dose
children under 4 years of age	**do not use**
children 4 to under 12 years of age	do not use unless directed by a doctor
adults and children 12 years of age and over	one packet

- dissolve contents of one packet into 8 oz. hot water: sip while hot. Consume entire drink within 10 - 15 minutes.
- if using a microwave, add contents of one packet to 8 oz. of cool water: stir briskly before and after heating, Do not overheat.

OTHER INFORMATION
- **each packet contains**: potassium 10 mg, sodium 19 mg
- **phenylketonurics**: contains phenylalanine 20 mg per packet
- store at controlled room temperature 20-25°C (68-77°F). Protect from excessive heat and moisture.

INACTIVE INGREDIENTS
acesulfame K, aspartame, citric acid, D&C yellow #10, FD&C blue #1, FD&C red #40, flavors, maltodextrin, silicon dioxide, sodium citrate, sucrose, tribasic calcium phosphate

QUESTIONS OR COMMENTS?
call **1-800-452-0051**

THERAFLU NIGHTTIME SEVERE COLD & COUGH (acetaminophen, diphenhydramine hydrochloride, and phenylephrine hydrochloride)
Novartis Consumer Health, Inc.

DRUG FACTS

Active Ingredient(s) (in each packet)	Purpose(s)
Acetaminophen 650 mg	Pain reliever/fever reducer
Diphenhydramine hydrochloride 25 mg	Antihistamine/cough suppressant
Phenylephrine hydrochloride 10 mg	Nasal decongestant

USES
- temporarily relieves these symptoms due to a cold:
  - minor aches and pains
  - minor sore throat pain
  - headache
  - nasal and sinus congestions
  - runny nose
  - sneezing
  - itchy nose or throat
  - itchy, watery eyes due to hay fever
  - cough due to minor throat and bronchial irritation
- temporarily reduces fever

WARNINGS
Liver warning
This product contains acetaminophen. Severe liver damage may occur if you take
- more than 6 packets in 24 hours, which is the maximum daily amount
- with other drugs containing acetaminophen
- 3 or more alcoholic drinks every day while using this product

Sore throat warning
If sore throat is severe, persists for more than 2 days, is accompanied or followed by fever, headache, rash, nausea, or vomiting consult a doctor promptly.

DO NOT USE
- in a child under 4 years of age
- if you are allergic to acetaminophen
- with any other drug containing acetaminophen (prescription or nonprescription). If you are not sure whether a drug contains acetaminophen, ask a doctor or pharmacist.
- with any other product containing diphenhydramine, even one used on the skin
- if you are now taking a prescription monoamine oxidase inhibitor (MAOI) (certain drugs for depression, psychiatric, or emotional conditions, or Parkinson's disease), or for 2 weeks after stopping the MAOI drug. If you do not know if your prescription drug contains an MAOI, ask a doctor or pharmacist before taking this product.

ASK A DOCTOR BEFORE USE IF YOU HAVE
- liver disease
- heart disease
- high blood pressure
- thyroid disease
- diabetes
- glaucoma
- a sodium-restricted diet
- trouble urinating due to an enlarged prostate gland
- a breathing problem such as emphysema, asthma or chronic bronchitis
- cough that occurs with too much phlegm (mucus)

- cough that lasts or is chronic such as occurs with smoking, asthma or emphysema

ASK A DOCTOR OR PHARMACIST BEFORE USE IF YOU ARE
- taking sedatives or tranquilizers
- taking the blood thinning drug warfarin

WHEN USING THIS PRODUCT
- **do not exceed recommended dosage**
- avoid alcoholic drinks
- marked drowsiness may occur
- alcohol, sedatives and tranquilizers may increase drowsiness
- be careful when driving a motor vehicle or operating machinery
- excitability may occur, especially in children

STOP USE AND ASK A DOCTOR IF
- nervousness, dizziness, or sleeplessness occurs
- fever gets worse or lasts more than 3 days
- redness or swelling is present
- new symptoms occur
- symptoms do not get better or worsen
- pain, cough or nasal congestion gets worse or lasts more than 7 days
- cough comes back or occurs with fever, rash or headache that lasts. These could be signs of a serious condition.

If pregnant or breast-feeding, ask a health care professional before use.

Keep out of reach of children.
In case of overdose, get medical help or contact a Poison Control Center right away. Prompt medical attention is critical for adults as well as for children even if you do not notice any signs or symptoms.

DIRECTIONS
- **do not use more than directed**
- take every 4 hours; do not take more than 6 packets in 24 hours unless directed by a doctor

Age	Dose
children under 4 years of age	**do not use**
children 4 to under 12 years of age	do not use unless directed by a doctor
adults and children 12 years of age and over	one packet

- dissolve contents of one packet into 8 oz. hot water: sip while hot. Consume entire drink within 10-15 minutes.
- if using a microwave, add contents of one packet to 8 oz. of cool water: stir briskly before and after heating. Do not overheat.

OTHER INFORMATION
- **each packet contains:** potassium 10 mg, sodium 23 mg
- **phenylketonurics:** contains phenylalanine 13 mg per packet
- store at controlled room temperature 20-25°C (68-77°F). Protect from excessive heat and moisture.

INACTIVE INGREDIENTS
acesulfame K, aspartame, citric acid, D&C yellow #10, FD&C blue #1, FD&C red #40, flavors, maltodextrin, silicon dioxide, sodium citrate, sucrose, tribasic calcium phosphate

QUESTIONS OR COMMENTS?
Call **1-800-452-0051**

THERAFLU SINUS & COLD (acetaminophen, pheniramine maleate, and phenylephrine hydrochloride)
Novartis Consumer Health, Inc.

DRUG FACTS

Active Ingredient(s) (in each packet)	Purpose(s)
Acetaminophen 325 mg	Pain reliever/fever reducer
Pheniramine maleate 20 mg	Antihistamine
Phenylephrine hydrochloride 10 mg	Nasal decongestant

USES
- temporarily relieves these symptoms due to a cold:
  - nasal congestion
  - sinus congestion and pressure
  - minor aches and pains
  - headache
  - minor sore throat pain
- temporarily restores freer breathing through the nose
- helps clear nasal passages; shrinks swollen membranes
- temporarily reduces fever
- temporarily relieves these symptoms due to hay fever or other upper respiratory allergies:
  - runny nose
  - sneezing
  - itchy nose and throat
  - itchy, watery eyes

WARNINGS
Liver warning
This product contains acetaminophen. Severe liver damage may occur if you take
- more than 6 packets in 24 hours, which is the maximum daily amount
- with other drugs containing acetaminophen
- 3 or more alcoholic drinks every day while using this product

Sore throat warning
If sore throat is severe, persists for more than 2 days, is accompanied or followed by fever, headache, rash, nausea, or vomiting consult a doctor promptly.

DO NOT USE
- in a child under 4 years of age
- if you are allergic to acetaminophen
- with any other drug containing acetaminophen (prescription or nonprescription). If you are not sure whether a drug contains acetaminophen, ask a doctor or pharmacist.
- if you are now taking a prescription monoamine oxidase inhibitor (MAOI) (certain drugs for depression, psychiatric, or emotional conditions, or Parkinson's disease), or for 2 weeks after stopping the MAOI drug. If you do not know if your prescription drug contains an MAOI, ask a doctor or pharmacist before taking this product.

ASK A DOCTOR BEFORE USE IF YOU HAVE
- liver disease
- heart disease
- high blood pressure
- thyroid disease
- diabetes
- glaucoma
- a sodium-restricted diet
- trouble urinating due to an enlarged prostate gland
- a breathing problem such as emphysema, or chronic bronchitis
- cough that occurs with too much phlegm (mucus)

ASK A DOCTOR OR PHARMACIST BEFORE USE IF YOU ARE

- taking the blood thinning drug warfarin
- taking sedatives or tranquilizers

WHEN USING THIS PRODUCT

- **do not exceed recommended dosage**
- avoid alcoholic drinks
- may cause drowsiness
- alcohol, sedatives and tranquilizers may increase drowsiness
- be careful when driving a motor vehicle or operating machinery
- excitability may occur, especially in children

STOP USE AND ASK A DOCTOR IF

- nervousness, dizziness, or sleeplessness occurs
- fever gets worse or lasts more than 3 days
- redness or swelling is present
- new symptoms occur
- pain or nasal congestion gets worse or lasts more than 7 days

If pregnant or breast-feeding, ask a health care professional before use.

Keep out of reach of children.
In case of overdose, get medical help or contact a Poison Control Center right away. Prompt medical attention is critical for adults as well as for children even if you do not notice any signs or symptoms.

DIRECTIONS

- **do not use more than directed**
- take every 4 hours; do not take more than 6 packets in 24 hours unless directed by a doctor

Age	Dose
children under 4 years of age	**do not use**
children 4 to under 12 years of age	do not use unless directed by a doctor
adults and children 12 years of age and over	one packet

- dissolve contents of one packet into 8 oz. hot water: sip while hot. Consume entire drink within 10-15 minutes.
- if using a microwave, add contents of one packet to 8 oz. of cool water: stir briskly before and after heating. Do not overheat.

OTHER INFORMATION

- **each packet contains:** sodium 44 mg
- store at controlled room temperature 20-25°C (68-77°F).

INACTIVE INGREDIENTS

acesulfame K, citric acid, D&C yellow #10, FD&C yellow #6, flavors, magnesium stearate, maltodextrin, silicon dioxide, sodium citrate, soy lecithin, tribasic calcium phosphate

QUESTIONS OR COMMENTS?

Call **1-800-452-0051**

THERAFLU NIGHTTIME SEVERE COLD & COUGH (acetaminophen, diphenhydramine hydrochloride, and phenylephrine hydrochloride)

Novartis Consumer Health, Inc.

DRUG FACTS

Active Ingredient(s)	Purpose(s)
Acetaminophen 650 mg	Pain reliever/fever reducer
Diphenhydramine hydrochloride 25 mg	Antihistamine/cough suppressant
Phenylephrine hydrochloride 10 mg	Nasal decongestant

USES

- temporarily relieves these symptoms due to a cold:
  - minor aches and pains
  - minor sore throat pain
  - headache
  - nasal and sinus congestions
  - runny nose
  - sneezing
  - itchy nose or throat
  - itchy, watery eyes due to hay fever
  - cough due to minor throat and bronchial irritation
- temporarily reduces fever

WARNINGS

Liver warning: This product contains acetaminophen. Severe liver damage may occur if you take
- more than 6 packets in 24 hours, which is the maximum daily amount
- with other drugs containing acetaminophen
- 3 or more alcoholic drinks every day while using this product

Sore throat warning: If sore throat is severe, persists for more than 2 days, is accompanied or followed by fever, headache, rash, nausea, or vomiting consult a doctor promptly.

DO NOT USE

- in a child under 4 years of age
- if you are allergic to acetaminophen
- with any other drug containing acetaminophen (prescription or nonprescription). If you are not sure whether a drug contains acetaminophen, ask a doctor or pharmacist.
- with any other product containing diphenhydramine, even one used on the skin
- if you are now taking a prescription monoamine oxidase inhibitor (MAOI) (certain drugs for depression, psychiatric, or emotional conditions, or Parkinson's disease), or for 2 weeks after stopping the MAOI drug. If you do not know if your prescription drug contains an MAOI, ask a doctor or pharmacist before taking this product.

ASK A DOCTOR BEFORE USE IF YOU HAVE

- liver disease
- heart disease
- high blood pressure
- thyroid disease
- diabetes
- glaucoma
- a sodium-restricted diet
- trouble urinating due to an enlarged prostate gland
- a breathing problem such as emphysema, asthma or chronic bronchitis
- cough that occurs with too much phlegm (mucus)
- cough that lasts or is chronic such as occurs with smoking, asthma or emphysema

ASK A DOCTOR OR PHARMACIST BEFORE USE IF YOU ARE
- sedatives or tranquilizers
- taking the blood thinning drug warfarin

WHEN USING THIS PRODUCT
- **do not exceed recommended dosage**
- avoid alcoholic drinks
- marked drowsiness may occur
- alcohol, sedatives and tranquilizers may increase drowsiness
- be careful when driving a motor vehicle or operating machinery
- excitability may occur, especially in children

STOP USE AND ASK A DOCTOR IF
- nervousness, dizziness, or sleeplessness occurs
- fever gets worse or lasts more than 3 days
- redness or swelling is present
- new symptoms occur
- symptoms do not get better or worsen
- pain, cough or nasal congestion gets worse or lasts more than 7 days
- cough comes back or occurs with fever, rash or headache that lasts. These could be signs of a serious condition.

If pregnant or breast-feeding, ask a health care professional before use.

Keep out of reach of children.
In case of overdose, get medical help or contact a Poison Control Center right away. Prompt medical attention is critical for adults as well as for children even if you do not notice any signs or symptoms.

DIRECTIONS
- **do not use more than directed**
- take every 4 hours; do not take more than 6 packets in 24 hours unless directed by a doctor

Age	Dose
children under 4 years of age	do not use
children 4 to under 12 years of age	do not use unless directed by a doctor
adults and children 12 years of age and over	one packet

- dissolve contents of one packet into 8 oz. hot water: sip while hot. Consume entire drink within 10-15 minutes.
- if using a microwave, add contents of one packet to 8 oz. of cool water: stir briskly before and after heating. Do not overheat.

OTHER INFORMATION
- **each packet contains:** potassium 10 mg, sodium 23 mg
- **phenylketonurics:** contains phenylalanine 13 mg per packet
- store at controlled room temperature 20-25°C (68-77°F). Protect from excessive heat and moisture.

INACTIVE INGREDIENTS
acesulfame K, aspartame, citric acid, D&C yellow #10, FD&C blue #1, FD&C red #40, flavors, maltodextrin, silicon dioxide, sodium citrate, sucrose, tribasic calcium phosphate

QUESTIONS OR COMMENTS?
Call 1-800-452-0051

THERAFLU WARMING RELIEF COLD & CHEST CONGESTION (acetaminophen, guaifenesin, and phenylephrine hydrochloride)
Novartis Consumer Health, Inc.

DRUG FACTS

Active Ingredient(s) (in each tablespoonful, 15 mL)	Purpose(s)
Acetaminophen 325 mg	Pain reliever/fever reducer
Guaifenesin 200 mg	Expectorant
Phenylephrine HCl 5 mg	Nasal decongestant

USES
- temporarily relieves:
  - minor aches and pains
  - headache
  - minor sore throat pain
  - nasal and sinus congestion
- temporarily reduces fever
- helps loosen phlegm (mucus) and thin bronchial secretions to drain bronchial tubes and make cough more productive

WARNINGS
Liver warning
This product contains acetaminophen. Severe liver damage may occur if you take
- more than 6 doses (12 tablespoonfuls or 180 mL) in 24 hours, which is the maximum daily amount
- with other drugs containing acetaminophen
- 3 or more alcoholic drinks every day while using this product

Sore throat warning
If sore throat is severe, persists for more than 2 days, is accompanied or followed by fever, headache, rash, nausea, or vomiting consult a doctor promptly.

DO NOT USE
- in a child under 4 years of age
- if you are allergic to acetaminophen
- with any other drug containing acetaminophen (prescription or nonprescription). If you are not sure whether a drug contains acetaminophen, ask a doctor or pharmacist.
- if you are now taking a prescription monoamine oxidase inhibitor (MAOI) (certain drugs for depression, psychiatric, or emotional conditions, or Parkinson's disease), or for 2 weeks after stopping the MAOI drug. If you do not know if your prescription drug contains an MAOI, ask a doctor or pharmacist before taking this product.

ASK A DOCTOR BEFORE USE IF YOU HAVE
- liver disease
- heart disease
- high blood pressure
- thyroid disease
- diabetes
- cough that occurs with too much phlegm (mucus)
- trouble urinating due to an enlarged prostate gland
- cough that lasts or is chronic such as occurs with smoking, asthma, chronic bronchitis or emphysema

ASK A DOCTOR OR PHARMACIST BEFORE USE IF YOU ARE
- taking the blood thinning drug warfarin

WHEN USING THIS PRODUCT
- **do not exceed recommended dosage**

STOP USE AND ASK A DOCTOR IF
- nervousness, dizziness, or sleeplessness occurs
- pain, cough or nasal congestion gets worse or lasts more than 7 days
- fever gets worse or lasts more than 3 days
- redness or swelling is present
- symptoms do not improve within 7 days or are accompanied by fever
- new symptoms occur
- cough comes back or occurs with fever, rash or headache that lasts. These could be signs of a serious condition

If pregnant or breast-feeding, ask a health care professional before use.

Keep out of reach of children.
In case of overdose, get medical help or contact a Poison Control Center right away. Prompt medical attention is critical for adults as well as for children even if you do not notice any signs or symptoms.

DIRECTIONS
- **do not use more than directed**
- take every 4 hours, in dose cup provided, while symptoms persist
- do not take more than 6 doses (12 tablespoonfuls or 180 mL) in 24 hours

Age	Dose
children under 4 years of age	**do not use**
children 4 to under 12 years of age	do not use unless directed by a doctor
adults and children 12 years of age and over	2 tablespoonfuls (30 mL)

OTHER INFORMATION
- **each tablespoonful (15 mL) contains:** potassium 5 mg, sodium 9 mg
- store at controlled room temperature 20-25°C (68-77°F).

Do not refrigerate.

INACTIVE INGREDIENTS
acesulfame K, benzyl alcohol, citric acid, edetate disodium, FD&C yellow #6, maltitol solution, natural and artificial flavors, propylene glycol, purified water, sodium benzoate, sodium citrate

QUESTIONS OR COMMENTS?
Call 1-800-452-0051

THERAFLU WARMING RELIEF FLU & SORE THROAT (acetaminophen, diphenhydramine hydrochloride, and phenylephrine hydrochloride)

Novartis Consumer Health, Inc.

DRUG FACTS

Active Ingredient(s) (in each tablespoonful, 15 mL)	Purpose(s)
Acetaminophen 325 mg	Pain reliever/fever reducer
Diphenhydramine HCl 12.5 mg	Cough suppressant/antihistamine
Phenylephrine HCl 5 mg	Nasal decongestant

USES
- temporarily relieves:
  - minor aches and pains
  - headache
  - runny nose
  - sneezing
  - itchy nose or throat
  - itchy, watery eyes
  - minor sore throat pain
  - nasal and sinus congestion
  - cough due to minor throat and bronchial irritationas may occur with a cold
- temporarily reduces fever

WARNINGS
Liver warning
This product contains acetaminophen. Severe liver damage may occur if you take
- more than 6 doses (12 tablespoonfuls or 180 mL) in 24 hours, which is the maximum daily amount
- with other drugs containing acetaminophen
- 3 or more alcoholic drinks every day while using this product

Sore throat warning
If sore throat is severe, persists for more than 2 days, is accompanied or followed by fever, headache, rash, nausea, or vomiting consult a doctor promptly.

DO NOT USE
- in a child under 4 years of age
- if you are allergic to acetaminophen
- with any other drug containing acetaminophen (prescription or nonprescription). If you are not sure whether a drug contains acetaminophen, ask a doctor or pharmacist.
- if you are now taking a prescription monoamine oxidase inhibitor (MAOI) (certain drugs for depression, psychiatric, or emotional conditions, or Parkinson's disease), or for 2 weeks after stopping the MAOI drug. If you do not know if your prescription drug contains an MAOI, ask a doctor or pharmacist before taking this product.
- with any other product containing diphenhydramine, even one used on the skin

ASK A DOCTOR BEFORE USE IF YOU HAVE
- liver disease
- heart disease
- high blood pressure
- thyroid disease
- diabetes
- glaucoma
- a breathing problem such as emphysema, asthma or chronic bronchitis
- cough that occurs with too much phlegm (mucus)
- trouble urinating due to an enlarged prostate gland
- cough that lasts or is chronic such as occurs with smoking, asthma, chronic bronchitis or emphysema

ASK A DOCTOR OR PHARMACIST BEFORE USE IF YOU ARE
- taking sedatives or tranquilizers
- taking the blood thinning drug warfarin

WHEN USING THIS PRODUCT
- **do not exceed recommended dosage**
- avoid alcoholic drinks
- marked drowsiness may occur
- alcohol, sedatives and tranquilizers may increase drowsiness
- be careful when driving a motor vehicle or operating machinery
- excitability may occur, especially in children

STOP USE AND ASK A DOCTOR IF
- nervousness, dizziness, or sleeplessness occurs
- pain, cough or nasal congestion gets worse or lasts more than 7 days
- fever gets worse or lasts more than 3 days
- redness or swelling is present

- new symptoms occur
- cough comes back or occurs with fever, rash or headache that lasts. These could be signs of a serious condition.

If pregnant or breast-feeding, ask a health care professional before use.

Keep out of reach of children.
In case of overdose, get medical help or contact a Poison Control Center right away. Prompt medical attention is critical for adults as well as for children even if you do not notice any signs or symptoms.

DIRECTIONS
- **do not use more than directed**
- take every 4 hours, in dose cup provided, while symptoms persist
- do not take more than 6 doses (12 tablespoonfuls or 180 mL) in 24 hours

Age	Dose
children under 4 years of age	**do not use**
children 4 to under 12 years of age	do not use unless directed by a doctor
adults and children 12 years of age and over	2 tablespoonfuls (30 mL)

OTHER INFORMATION
- **each tablespoonful (15 mL) contains:** potassium 5 mg, sodium 7 mg
- store at controlled room temperature 20-25°C (68-77°F). Protect from excessive heat and moisture.

INACTIVE INGREDIENTS
acesulfame K, alcohol, citric acid, edetate disodium, FD&C blue #1, FD&C red #40, flavors, glycerin, maltitol solution, propylene glycol, purified water, sodium benzoate, sodium citrate

QUESTIONS OR COMMENTS?
Call **1-800-452-0051**

THERAFLU WARMING RELIEF DAYTIME SEVERE COLD & COUGH (acetaminophen, dextromethorphan hydrobromide, and phenylephrine hydrochloride)

Novartis Consumer Health, Inc.

DRUG FACTS

Active Ingredient(s) (in each tablespoonful, 15 mL)	Purpose(s)
Acetaminophen 325 mg	Pain reliever/fever reducer
Dextromethorphan HBr 10 mg	Cough suppressant
Phenylephrine HCl 5 mg	Nasal decongestant

USES
- temporarily relieves:
  - minor aches and pains
  - minor sore throat pain
  - headache
  - nasal congestion
  - cough due to minor throat and bronchial irritation as may occur with a cold
- temporarily reduces fever

WARNINGS
Liver warning
This product contains acetaminophen. Severe liver damage may occur if you take
- more than 6 doses (12 tablespoonfuls or 180 mL) in 24 hours, which is the maximum daily amount
- with other drugs containing acetaminophen
- 3 or more alcoholic drinks every day while using this product

Sore throat warning
If sore throat is severe, persists for more than 2 days, is accompanied or followed by fever, headache, rash, nausea, or vomiting consult a doctor promptly.

DO NOT USE
- in a child under 4 years of age
- if you are allergic to acetaminophen
- with any other drug containing acetaminophen (prescription or nonprescription). If you are not sure whether a drug contains acetaminophen, ask a doctor or pharmacist.
- if you are now taking a prescription monoamine oxidase inhibitor (MAOI) (certain drugs for depression, psychiatric, or emotional conditions, or Parkinson's disease), or for 2 weeks after stopping the MAOI drug. If you do not know if your prescription drug contains an MAOI, ask a doctor or pharmacist before taking this product.

ASK A DOCTOR BEFORE USE IF YOU HAVE
- liver disease
- heart disease
- high blood pressure
- thyroid disease
- diabetes
- cough that occurs with too much phlegm (mucus)
- trouble urinating due to an enlarged prostate gland
- cough that lasts or is chronic such as occurs with smoking, asthma, chronic bronchitis or emphysema

ASK A DOCTOR OR PHARMACIST BEFORE USE IF YOU ARE
- taking the blood thinning drug warfarin

WHEN USING THIS PRODUCT
- **do not exceed recommended dosage**

STOP USE AND ASK A DOCTOR IF
- nervousness, dizziness, or sleeplessness occurs
- pain, cough or nasal congestion gets worse or lasts more than 7 days
- fever gets worse or lasts more than 3 days
- redness or swelling is present
- new symptoms occur
- cough comes back or occurs with fever, rash or headache that lasts. These could be signs of a serious condition.

If pregnant or breast-feeding, ask a health care professional before use.

Keep out of reach of children.
In case of overdose, get medical help or contact a Poison Control Center right away. Prompt medical attention is critical for adults as well as for children even if you do not notice any signs or symptoms.

DIRECTIONS
- **do not use more than directed**
- take every 4 hours, in dose cup provided, while symptoms persist
- do not take more than 6 doses (12 tablespoonfuls or 180 mL) in 24 hours

Age	Dose
children under 4 years of age	**do not use**
children 4 to under 12 years of age	do not use unless directed by a doctor
adults and children 12 years of age and over	2 tablespoonfuls (30 mL)

OTHER INFORMATION
- **each tablespoonful (15 mL) contains:** sodium 8 mg
- store at controlled room temperature 20-25°C (68-77°F).

INACTIVE INGREDIENTS
acesulfame K, alcohol, citric acid, edetate disodium, FD&C blue #1, FD&C red #40, flavors, glycerin, maltitol solution, propylene glycol, purified water, sodium benzoate, sodium citrate

QUESTIONS OR COMMENTS?
Call **1-800-452-0051**

THERAFLU WARMING RELIEF NIGHTTIME SEVERE COLD & COUGH (acetaminophen, dextromethorphan hydrobromide, and phenylephrine hydrochloride)

Novartis Consumer Health, Inc.

DRUG FACTS

Active Ingredient(s) (in each tablespoon, 15 mL)	Purpose(s)
Acetaminophen 325 mg	Pain reliever/fever reducer
Dextromethorphan HBr 12.5 mg	Cough suppressant
Phenylephrine HCl 5 mg	Nasal decongestant

USES
- temporarily relieves:
  - minor aches and pains
  - headache
  - runny nose
  - sneezing
  - itchy nose or throat
  - itchy, watery eyes
  - minor sore throat pain
  - nasal and sinus congestion
  - cough due to minor throat and bronchial irritation as may occur with a cold
- temporarily reduces fever

WARNINGS
Liver warning
This product contains acetaminophen. Severe liver damage may occur if you take
- more than 6 doses (12 tablespoonfuls or 180 mL) in 24 hours, which is the maximum daily amount
- with other drugs containing acetaminophen
- 3 or more alcoholic drinks every day while using this product

Sore throat warning
If sore throat is severe, persists for more than 2 days, is accompanied or followed by fever, headache, rash, nausea, or vomiting consult a doctor promptly.

DO NOT USE
- in a child under 4 years of age
- if you are allergic to acetaminophen

- with any other drug containing acetaminophen (prescription or nonprescription). If you are not sure whether a drug contains acetaminophen, ask a doctor or pharmacist.
- if you are now taking a prescription monoamine oxidase inhibitor (MAOI) (certain drugs for depression, psychiatric, or emotional conditions, or Parkinson's disease), or for 2 weeks after stopping the MAOI drug. If you do not know if your prescription drug contains an MAOI, ask a doctor or pharmacist before taking this product.
- with any other product containing diphenhydramine, even one used on the skin

ASK A DOCTOR BEFORE USE IF YOU HAVE
- liver disease
- heart disease
- high blood pressure
- thyroid disease
- diabetes
- glaucoma
- a breathing problem such as emphysema, or chronic bronchitis
- cough that occurs with too much phlegm (mucus)
- trouble urinating due to an enlarged prostate gland
- cough that lasts or is chronic such as occurs with smoking, asthma, chronic bronchitis or emphysema

ASK A DOCTOR OR PHARMACIST BEFORE USE IF YOU ARE
- taking sedatives or tranquilizers
- taking the blood thinning drug warfarin

WHEN USING THIS PRODUCT
- **do not exceed recommended dosage**
- avoid alcoholic drinks
- marked drowsiness may occur
- alcohol, sedatives, and tranquilizers may increase drowsiness
- be careful when driving a motor vehicle or operating machinery
- excitability may occur, especially in children

STOP USE AND ASK A DOCTOR IF
- nervousness, dizziness, or sleeplessness occurs
- pain, cough or nasal congestion gets worse or lasts more than 7 days
- fever gets worse or lasts more than 3 days
- redness or swelling is present
- new symptoms occur
- symptoms do not get better or worsen
- cough comes back or occurs with fever, rash or headache that lasts. These could be signs of a serious condition.

If pregnant or breast-feeding, ask a health care professional before use.

Keep out of reach of children.
In case of overdose, get medical help or contact a Poison Control Center right away. Prompt medical attention is critical for adults as well as for children even if you do not notice any signs or symptoms.

DIRECTIONS
- **do not use more than directed**
- take every 4 hours, in dose cup provided, while symptoms persist
- do not take more than 6 doses (12 tablespoonfuls or 180 mL) in 24 hours

Age	Dose
children under 4 years of age	**do not use**
children 4 to under 12 years of age	do not use unless directed by a doctor
adults and children 12 years of age and over	2 tablespoonfuls (30 mL)

OTHER INFORMATION
- **each tablespoonful (15 mL) contains:** potassium 5 mg, sodium 7 mg
- store at controlled room temperature 20-25°C (68-77°F). Protect from excessive heat and moisture.

INACTIVE INGREDIENTS
acesulfame K, alcohol, citric acid, edetate disodium, FD&C blue #1, FD&C red #40, flavors, glycerin, maltitol solution, propylene glycol, purified water, sodium benzoate, sodium citrate

QUESTIONS OR COMMENTS?
Call **1-800-452-0051**

THERAFLU WARMING RELIEF SINUS & COLD (acetaminophen, diphenhydramine hydrochloride, and phenylephrine hydrochloride)

Novartis Consumer Health, Inc.

DRUG FACTS

Active Ingredient(s) (in each tablespoonful, 15 mL)	Purpose(s)
Acetaminophen 325 mg	Pain reliever/fever reducer
Diphenhydramine HCl 12.5 mg	Cough suppressant/antihistamine
Phenylephrine HCl 5 mg	Nasal decongestant

USES
- temporarily relieves:
  - minor aches and pains
  - headache
  - runny nose
  - sneezing
  - itchy nose or throat
  - itchy, watery eyes
  - minor sore throat pain
  - nasal and sinus congestion
  - cough due to minor throat and bronchial irritation as may occur with a cold
- temporarily reduces fever

WARNINGS
Liver warning
This product contains acetaminophen. Severe liver damage may occur if you take
- more than 6 doses (12 tablespoonfuls or 180 mL) in 24 hours, which is the maximum daily amount
- with other drugs containing acetaminophen
- 3 or more alcoholic drinks every day while using this product

Sore throat warning
If sore throat is severe, persists for more than 2 days, is accompanied or followed by fever, headache, rash, nausea, or vomiting consult a doctor promptly.

DO NOT USE
- in a child under 4 years of age
- if you are allergic to acetaminophen
- with any other drug containing acetaminophen (prescription or nonprescription). If you are not sure whether a drug contains acetaminophen, ask a doctor or pharmacist.
- if you are now taking a prescription monoamine oxidase inhibitor (MAOI) (certain drugs for depression, psychiatric, or emotional conditions, or Parkinson's disease), or for 2 weeks after stopping the MAOI drug. If you do not know if your prescription drug contains an MAOI, ask a doctor or pharmacist before taking this product.
- with any other product containing diphenhydramine, even one used on the skin

ASK A DOCTOR BEFORE USE IF YOU HAVE
- liver disease
- heart disease
- high blood pressure
- thyroid disease
- diabetes
- glaucoma
- a breathing problem such as emphysema, or chronic bronchitis
- cough that occurs with too much phlegm (mucus)
- trouble urinating due to an enlarged prostate gland
- cough that lasts or is chronic such as occurs with smoking, asthma, chronic bronchitis or emphysema

ASK A DOCTOR OR PHARMACIST BEFORE USE IF YOU ARE
- taking sedatives or tranquilizers
- taking the blood thinning drug warfarin

WHEN USING THIS PRODUCT
- **do not exceed recommended dosage**
- avoid alcoholic drinks
- marked drowsiness may occur
- alcohol, sedatives, and tranquilizers may increase drowsiness
- be careful when driving a motor vehicle or operating machinery
- excitability may occur, especially in children

STOP USE AND ASK A DOCTOR IF
- nervousness, dizziness, or sleeplessness occurs
- pain, cough or nasal congestion gets worse or lasts more than 7 days
- fever gets worse or lasts more than 3 days
- redness or swelling is present
- new symptoms occur
- cough comes back or occurs with fever, rash or headache that lasts. These could be signs of a serious condition.

If pregnant or breast-feeding, ask a health care professional before use.

Keep out of reach of children.
In case of overdose, get medical help or contact a Poison Control Center right away. Prompt medical attention is critical for adults as well as for children even if you do not notice any signs or symptoms.

DIRECTIONS
- **do not use more than directed**
- take every 4 hours, in dose cup provided, while symptoms persist
- do not take more than 6 doses (12 tablespoonfuls or 180 mL) in 24 hours

Age	Dose
children under 4 years of age	**do not use**
children 4 to under 12 years of age	do not use unless directed by a doctor
adults and children 12 years of age and over	2 tablespoonfuls (30 mL)

OTHER INFORMATION
- **each tablespoonful (15 mL) contains:** potassium 5 mg, sodium 7 mg
- store at controlled room temperature 20-25°C (68-77°F). Protect from excessive heat and moisture.

INACTIVE INGREDIENTS
acesulfame K, alcohol, citric acid, edetate disodium, FD&C blue #1, FD&C red #40, flavors, glycerin, maltitol solution, propylene glycol, purified water, sodium benzoate, sodium citrate

QUESTIONS OR COMMENTS?
Call **1-800-452-0051**

TINACTIN CREAM (tolnaftate)

MSD Consumer Care, Inc.

DRUG FACTS

Active Ingredient(s)
Tolnaftate 1%

Purpose(s)
Antifungal

USES
- cures most jock itch (tinea cruris)
- for effective relief of itching, chafing and burning

WARNINGS
For external use only

WHEN USING THIS PRODUCT
avoid contact with the eyes

STOP USE AND ASK A DOCTOR IF
- irritation occurs
- there is no improvement within 2 weeks

Do not use on children under 2 years of age except under the advice and supervision of a doctor.
Keep out of reach of children. If swallowed, get medical help or contact a Poison Control Center right away.

DIRECTIONS
- wash affected area and dry thoroughly
- apply a thin layer over affected area twice daily (morning and night)
- supervise children in the use of this product
- use daily for 2 weeks; if condition persists longer, ask a doctor
- this product is not effective on the scalp or nails

OTHER INFORMATION
store between 20° to 25°C (68° to 77°F)

INACTIVE INGREDIENTS
ceteth-20, cetostearyl alcohol, chlorocresol, mineral oil, propylene glycol, purified water, sodium phosphate monobasic, white petrolatum

QUESTIONS OR COMMENTS?
1-866-360-3266
Distributed by MSD Consumer Care, Inc., PO Box 377, Memphis, TN 38151 USA, a subsidiary of Merck & Co., Inc., Whitehouse Station, NJ USA.

TINACTIN POWDER SPRAY (tolnaftate)

MSD Consumer Care, Inc.

DRUG FACTS

Active Ingredient(s)
Tolnaftate 1%

Purpose(s)
Antifungal

USES
- cures most jock itch
- for effective relief of itching, chafing and burning

WARNINGS
For external use only
Flammable: Do not use while smoking or near heat or flame

WHEN USING THIS PRODUCT
- avoid contact with the eyes
- use only as directed. Intentional misuse by deliberately concentrating and inhaling contents can be harmful or fatal
- contents under pressure. Do not puncture or incinerate. Do not store at temperature above 120°F.

STOP USE AND ASK A DOCTOR IF
- irritation occurs
- there is no improvement within 2 weeks

Do not use on children under 2 years of age unless directed by a doctor.
Keep out of reach of children. If swallowed, get medical help or contact a Poison Control Center right away.

DIRECTIONS
- wash affected area and dry thoroughly
- shake can well and spray a thin layer over affected area twice daily (morning and night)
- supervise children in the use of this product
- use daily for 2 weeks; if condition persists longer, ask a doctor
- this product is not effective on the scalp or nails
- in case of clogging, clean nozzle with a pin

OTHER INFORMATION
store between 20° to 25°C (68° to 77°F)

INACTIVE INGREDIENTS
alcohol denat. (11% v/v), butylated hydroxytoluene, isobutane, PPG-12-buteth-16, talc

QUESTIONS OR COMMENTS?
1-866-360-3266
© Copyright & Distributed by
MSD Consumer Care, Inc.,
PO Box 377, Memphis,
TN 38151 USA,
a subsidiary of Merck & Co., Inc.,
Whitehouse Station, NJ USA.

TINACTIN SUPER ABSORBENT POWDER
(tolnaftate)

MSD Consumer Care, Inc.

DRUG FACTS

Active Ingredient(s)
Tolnaftate 1%

Purpose(s)
Antifungal

USES
- proven clinically effective in the treatment of most athlete's foot (tinea pedis) and ringworm (tinea corporis)
- helps prevent most athlete's foot with daily use
- for effective relief of itching, burning and cracking

WARNINGS
For external use only
Avoid contact with the eyes

STOP USE AND ASK A DOCTOR IF
- irritation occurs
- there is no improvement within 4 weeks

DO NOT USE
on children under 2 years of age except under the advice and supervision of a doctor.

Keep out of reach of children. If swallowed, get medical help or contact a Poison Control Center right away.

DIRECTIONS
- wash affected area and dry thoroughly
- apply a thin layer over affected area twice daily (morning and night)
- supervise children in the use of this product
- for athlete's foot: pay special attention to spaces between the toes; wear well-fitting, ventilated shoes and change shoes and socks at least once daily
- use daily for 4 weeks; if condition persists longer, ask a doctor
- to prevent athlete's foot, apply once or twice daily (morning and/or night)
- this product is not effective on the scalp or nails

OTHER INFORMATION
store between 20° to 25°C (68° to 77°F)

INACTIVE INGREDIENTS
benzethonium chloride, corn starch, kaolin, sodium bicarbonate

QUESTIONS OR COMMENTS?
1-866-360-3266

TINEACIDE PHYSICIAN FORMULA
(undecylenic acid)

Blaine Labs Inc.

Active Ingredient(s)
Undecylenic acid

INACTIVE INGREDIENTS
aloe vera, cetyl alcohol, clotrimazole, coco-caprylate caprate, disodium EDTA, glyceryl stearate, hydroxyethylcellulose, lavender oil, methylparaben, PEG-100, stearate, polysorbate 60, propylparaben, stearic acid, tea tree oil, triethanolamine, urea, water

USES
Cures Athlete's Foot (tinea pedis) jock itch (tinea cruris) and ringworm (tinea corporis).

USES FOR EFFECTIVE RELIEF OF ITCHING, CRACKING, BURNING AND DISCOMFORT WHICH CAN ACCOMPANY THESE CONDITIONS.

ASK YOUR PHYSICIANDO NOT USE ON CHILDREN UNDER 2 YEARS OF AGE UNLESS DIRECTED BY A PHYSICIAN

WHEN USING THIS PRODUCT
Wash the affected area with soap and water and dry thoroughly. Apply sparingly over affected area twice daily (morning and night) or as directed by a physician. For athlete's foot pay special attention to spaces between the toes. wear well-fitting ventilated shoes and change shoes and socks at least once daily. For athlete's foot and ringworm use daily for 4 weeks. for jock itch use daily for 2 weeks. If condition persists longer, consult a physician.

WARNINGS
For external use only. Avoid contact with eyes. If irritation occurs or if there is no improvement within 4 weeks (for athlete's foot or ringworm) or within 2 weeks (for jock itch) discontinue use and consult a physician. Keep this and all drugs out of the reach of children. In case of accidental ingestion seek professional assistance or contact a poison control center immediately.

TRIAMINIC THIN STRIPS ALLERGY
(diphenhydramine hydrochloride)

Novartis Consumer Health, Inc.

DRUG FACTS

Active Ingredient(s) (in each strip)	Purpose(s)
Diphenhydramine HCl 12.5 mg	Antihistamine

USES
- temporarily relieves
  - sneezing
  - runny nose
  - itchy nose or throat
  - itchy, watery eyes due to hay fever or other upper respiratory allergies

WARNINGS

DO NOT USE
- in a child under 4 years of age
- with any other product containing diphenhydramine, even one used on the skin
- for the purpose of making your child sleepy

ASK A DOCTOR BEFORE USE IF THE CHILD HAS
- glaucoma
- a breathing problem such as chronic bronchitis

ASK A DOCTOR OR PHARMACIST BEFORE USE IF THE CHILD IS
taking sedatives or tranquilizers

WHEN USING THIS PRODUCT
- marked drowsiness may occur
- sedatives and tranquilizers may increase the drowsiness effect
- excitability may occur, especially in children

Keep out of reach of children. In case of overdose, get medical help or contact a Poison Control Center right away.

DIRECTIONS
- may be given every 4 to 6 hours. Do not give more than 6 doses in 24 hours unless directed by a doctor.

Age	Dose
children 4 years of age	do not use
children 4 to under 6 years of age	do not use unless direccted by a doctor
children 6 to under 12 years of age	allow 1 or 2 strips to dissolve on tongue

OTHER INFORMATION
- store at controlled room temperature 20-25°C (68-77°F).

INACTIVE INGREDIENTS
acetone, alcohol, FD&C blue #1, FD&C red #40, flavors, hydroxypropyl cellulose, hypromellose, isopropyl alcohol, maltodextrin, microcrystalline cellulose, polyethylene glycol, pregelatinized starch, propylene glycol, purified water, sodium polystyrene sulfonate, sorbitol, sucralose, titanium dioxide

QUESTIONS OR COMMENTS?
Call **1-800-452-0051**

TRIAMINIC LONG ACTING COUGH
(dextromethorphan HBr)

Novartis Consumer Health, Inc.

DRUG FACTS

Active Ingredient(s) (in each 5 mL, 1 teaspoonful)	Purpose(s)
Dextromethorphan HBr 7.5 mg	Cough suppressant

USES
- temporarily relieves cough due to minor throat and bronchial irritation as may occur with a cold

WARNINGS

DO NOT USE
- in a child under 4 years of age
- in a child who is taking a prescription monoamine oxidase inhibitor (MAOI) (certain drugs for depression, psychiatric or emotional conditions, or Parkinson's disease), or for 2 weeks after stopping the MAOI drug. If you do not know if the child's prescription drug contains an MAOI, ask a doctor or pharmacist before giving this product.

ASK A DOCTOR BEFORE USE IF THE CHILD HAS
- cough that occurs with too much phlegm (mucus)
- cough that lasts or is chronic such as occurs with asthma

STOP USE AND ASK A DOCTOR IF
- cough persists for more than 7 days, comes back or occurs with a fever, rash, or persistent headache. These could be signs of a serious condition.

Keep out of reach of children. In case of overdose, get medical help or contact a Poison Control Center right away.

DIRECTIONS
- may be given every 6 to 8 hours. Do not give more than 4 doses in 24 hours unless directed by a doctor

Age	Dose
children under 4 years of age	**do not use**
children 4 to under 6 years of age	1 teaspoonful (5 mL)
children 6 to under 12 years of age	2 teaspoonfuls (10 mL)

OTHER INFORMATION
- **each teaspoonful contains:** sodium 7 mg
- protect from light
- store at controlled room temperature 20-25°C (68-77°F).

INACTIVE INGREDIENTS
benzoic acid, citric acid, dibasic sodium phosphate, edetate disodium, flavors, propylene glycol, purified water, sorbitol, sucrose

QUESTIONS OR COMMENTS?
Call **1-800-452-0051**

TRIPLE PASTE (zinc oxide)

Summers Laboratories, Inc.

DRUG FACTS

Active Ingredient(s)	Purpose(s)
Zinc oxide 12.8%	Skin protectant

USES
- helps treat and prevent diaper rash
- protects chafed skin due to diaper rash and helps protect from wetness

WARNINGS
- **For external use only**

WHEN USING THIS PRODUCT
- do not get into eyes

STOP USE AND ASK A DOCTOR IF
- if condition worsens or does not improve within 7 days

Keep out of reach of children. If swallowed, get medical help or contact a Poison Control Center right away.

DIRECTIONS
- Change wet and soiled diapers promptly
- Cleanse the diaper area and allow skin to dry
- Apply ointment liberally as often as necessary, with each diaper change, especially at bedtime or any time exposure to wet diapers may be prolonged

INACTIVE INGREDIENTS
white petrolatum, corn starch, anhydrous lanolin, stearyl alcohol, beeswax, bisabolol, cholesterol, water, glycerine, oat (avena sativa) kernel extract, polysorbate 80

TUCKS FAST RELIEF SPRAY (pramoxine hydrochloride)

McNeil-PPC, Inc.

DRUG FACTS

Active Ingredient(s)
Pramoxine HCL 1%

Purpose(s)
Pain reliever

USE
- temporary relieves these local symptoms associated with hemorrhoids:
  - pain
  - itching
  - discomfort

WARNINGS
For external use only

WHEN USING THIS PRODUCT
- do not use more than directed unless told to do so by a doctor
- do not put into the rectum by using fingers or any mechanical device or applicator

STOP USE AND ASK A DOCTOR IF
- allergic reaction occurs
- redness, irritation, swelling, pain, or other symptoms begin or increase

- rectal bleeding occurs
- condition worsens or does not improve within 7 days

Keep out of reach of children. If swallowed, get medical help or contact a Poison Control Center right away.

DIRECTIONS
- adults and children 12 years of age and older: apply to the affected area up to 5 times daily
  - when practical, cleanse the affected area with mild soap and warm water and rinse thoroughly
  - gently dry by patting or blotting with toilet tissue or a soft cloth before application
- children under 12 years of age: ask a doctor

OTHER INFORMATION
- store at 20 to 25°C (68-77°F)

INACTIVE INGREDIENTS
aloe barbadensis leaf juice, denatonium benzoate, ethyl alcohol, polysorbate 20, t-butyl alcohol, tocopheryl acetate, water

QUESTIONS OR COMMENTS?
call toll-free **800-223-0182** or **215-273-8755 (collect)**
Distributed by: Johnson & Johnson
Healthcare Products
Division of McNEIL-PPC, Inc.
Skillman, NJ 08558-9418
©McNEIL-PPC, Inc. 2012

TUCKS HEMORRHOIDAL OINTMENT (mineral oil, pramoxine hydrochloride, and zinc oxide)
McNeil-PPC, Inc.

DRUG FACTS

Active Ingredient(s)	Purpose(s)
Mineral Oil 46.6%	Protectant
Pramoxine HCl 1%	Pain reliever
Zinc oxide 12.5%	Protectant

USES
- temporarily relieves these local symptoms associated with hemorrhoids or anorectal inflammation:
  - pain
  - soreness
  - burning
  - itching
- temporarily forms a protective coating over the inflamed tissues to help prevent drying of tissues

WARNINGS
For external use only

WHEN USING THIS PRODUCT
- do not use more than directed unless told to do so by a doctor
- do not put into the rectum by using fingers or any mechanical device or applicator

STOP USE AND ASK A DOCTOR IF
- allergic reaction occurs
- rectal bleeding occurs
- redness, irritation, swelling, pain, or other symptoms begin or increase
- condition worsens or does not improve within 7 days

Keep out of reach of children. If swallowed, get medical help or contact a Poison Control Center right away.

DIRECTIONS
- adults: apply externally to the affected area up to 5 times daily
  - when practical, clean the affected area with mild soap and warm water and rinse thoroughly
  - gently dry by patting or blotting with toilet tissue or a soft cloth before applying
  - to use dispensing cap
  - attach it to tube, lubricate well, then gently insert part way into anus
  - squeeze tube to deliver medication
  - thoroughly cleanse dispensing cap after use
- children under 12 years of age: ask a doctor

OTHER INFORMATION
- store at 20° to 25°C (68° to 75°F)

INACTIVE INGREDIENTS
benzyl benzoate, calcium phosphate dibasic, cocoa butter, glyceryl monooleate, glyceryl monostearate, kaolin, peruvian balsam, and polyethylene wax

QUESTIONS OR COMMENTS?
call toll-free **800-223-0182,** weekdays, 9 AM- 5 PM EST
Distributed by:
McNEIL-PPC, Inc.
Skillman, NJ 08558 USA

TUCKS INTERNAL SOOTHERS HEMORRHOIDAL (starch)
McNeil-PPC, Inc.

DRUG FACTS

Active Ingredient(s)
Topical Starch 51%

Purpose(s)
Protectant

USE
- temporary relieves these local symptoms associated with hemorrhoids and other anorectal disorders:
  - pain
  - itching
  - discomfort
- temporarily forms a protective coating over inflamed tissues to help prevent drying of tissues
- temporarily protects the inflamed, irritated anorectal surface to help make bowel movement less painful

WARNINGS
For rectal use only

WHEN USING THIS PRODUCT
- do not use more than directed unless told to do so by a doctor

STOP USE AND ASK A DOCTOR IF
- rectal bleeding occurs
- condition worsens or does not improve within 7 days

If pregnant or breastfeeding, ask a healthcare professional before use.
Keep out of reach of children. If swallowed, get medical help or contact a Poison Control Center right away.

DIRECTIONS
- see bottom panel for directions for opening suppository wrapper
- adults: insert one (1) suppository rectally up to 6 times daily or after each bowel movement by following these steps:

- when practical, cleanse the affected area with mild soap and warm water and rinse thoroughly
- gently dry by patting or blotting with toilet tissue or a soft cloth before applying
- detach one (1) suppository from the strip of suppositories
- remove the wrapper before inserting into the rectum
- children under 12 years of age: ask a doctor

OTHER INFORMATION
- store at 68 to 77°F (20 to 25°C) to avoid melting

INACTIVE INGREDIENTS
benzyl alcohol, lecithin, partially hydrogenated palm kernel oil, tocopheryl acetate

QUESTIONS OR COMMENTS?
call toll-free **800-223-0182,** weekdays, 9 AM- 5 PM EST
Distributed by:
McNEIL-PPC, Inc.
Skillman, NJ 08558 USA

TUCKS MEDICATED COOLING PADS (witch hazel)

McNeil-PPC, Inc.

DRUG FACTS

Active Ingredient(s)
Witch Hazel 50%

Purpose(s)
Astringent

USE
- temporary relieves the local itching and discomfort associated with hemorrhoids
- aids in protecting irritated anorectal areas
- temporarily relieves itching and burning

WARNINGS
For external use only

WHEN USING THIS PRODUCT
- do not use more than directed unless told to do so by a doctor
- do not put into the rectum by using fingers or any mechanical device or applicator

STOP USE AND ASK A DOCTOR IF
- rectal bleeding occurs
- condition worsens or does not improve within 7 days

Keep out of reach of children. If swallowed, get medical help or contact a Poison Control Center right away.

DIRECTIONS
- adults:
  - when practical, cleanse the affected area with mild soap and warm water, and rinse thoroughly
  - gently dry by patting or blotting with toilet tissue or a soft cloth before applying
  - apply externally to the affected are up to 6 times daily or after each bowel movement
  - after application, discard pad
- children under 12 years of age: ask a doctor

OTHER INFORMATION
- store at 68 to 77°F (20 to 25°C)

INACTIVE INGREDIENTS
water, glycerin, alcohol, propylene glycol, sodium citrate, diazolidinyl urea, citric acid, methylparaben, proplyparaben

QUESTIONS OR COMMENTS?
call toll-free **800-223-0182,** weekdays, 9 AM- 5 PM EST
Distributed by: McNEIL-PPC, Inc.
Skillman, NJ 08558 USA

TUCKS TAKE ALONGS (witch hazel)

McNeil-PPC, Inc.

DRUG FACTS

Active Ingredient(s)	Purpose(s)
Witch hazel 50%	Astringent

USES
- temporarily relieves the local itching and discomfort associated with hemorrhoids
- aids in protecting irritated anorectal areas
- temporarily relieves irritation and burning

WARNINGS
For external use only

WHEN USING THIS PRODUCT
- do not use more than directed unless told to do so by a doctor
- do not put directly in the rectum by using fingers or any mechanical device or applicator

STOP USE AND ASK A DOCTOR IF
- rectal bleeding occurs
- condition worsens or does not improve within 7 days

Keep out of reach of children.
- If swallowed, get medical help or contact a Poison Control Center right away.

DIRECTIONS
Adults:
- when practical, clean the affected area with mild soap and warm water, and rinse thoroughly
- gently dry by patting or blotting with toilet tissue or a soft cloth before applying
- apply externally to the affected area up to 6 times daily or after each bowel movement
- after application, discard pad

Children under 12 years of age: ask a doctor

OTHER INFORMATION
- Store at 68° - 77°F (20° - 25°C)

INACTIVE INGREDIENTS
water, glycerin, alcohol, propylene gylcol, sodium citrate, diazolidinyl urea, citric acid, methylparaben, propylparaben

QUESTIONS OR COMMENTS?
call 1-800-223-0182 weekdays 9AM - 5PM EST

TUMS DUAL ACTION (famotidine, calcium carbonate, and magnesium hydroxide)

GlaxoSmithKline Consumer Healthcare LP

Active Ingredient(s) (in each chewable tablet)
Famotidine 10mg
Calcium carbonate 800mg
Magnesium hydroxide 165mg

Purpose(s)
Acid reducer
Antacid
Antacid

USE
relieves heartburn associated with acid indigestion and sour stomach

WARNINGS
Allergy alert:
Do not use if you are allergic to famotidine or other acid reducers

DO NOT USE
- if you have trouble or pain swallowing food, vomiting with blood, or bloody or black stools. These may be signs of a serious condition. See you doctor.
- with other acid reducers

ASK A DOCTOR BEFORE USE IF YOU HAVE
- had heartburn over 3 months. This may be a sign of a more serious condition.
- heartburn with **lightheadedness, sweating, or dizziness**
- chest pain or shoulder pain with shortness of breath; sweating; pain spreading to arms, neck or shoulders; or lightheadedness
- frequent **chest pain**
- frequent wheezing, particularly with heartburn
- unexplained weight loss
- nausea or vomiting
- stomach pain

ASK A DOCTOR OR PHARMACIST BEFORE USE IF YOU ARE
presently taking a prescription drug. Antacids may interact with certain prescription drugs.

STOP USE AND ASK A DOCTOR IF
- your heartburn continues or worsens
- you need to take this product for more than 14 days

If pregnant or breast-feeding,
ask a health professional before use.

Keep out of reach of children.
In case of overdose, get medical help or contact a Poison Control Center right away.

DIRECTIONS
- adults and children 12 years and over:
  - **do not swallow tablet whole: chew completely**
  - to relieve symptoms, **chew** 1 tablet before swallowing
  - do not use more than 2 chewable tablets in 24 hours
- children under 12 years: ask a doctor

OTHER INFORMATION
- each tablet contains: **calcium 320mg; magnesium 65mg**
- Phenylketonurics: Contains Phenylalanine 2.2mg per tablet
- read the directions and warnings before use
- read the bottle label. It contains important information.
- store at 20°-25°C (68°-77°F)
- protect from moisture

INACTIVE INGREDIENTS
aspartame, D&C red no. 7 calcium, dextrates, FD&C blue no. 1 lake, FD&C red no. 40 lake, flavor, glyceryl monostearate, lactose anhydrous, lactose monohydrate, magnesium stearate, microcrystalline cellulose, polyacrylate dispersion, polysorbate 80, povidone, pregelatinized starch, sodium starch glycolate, talc

QUESTIONS OR COMMENTS?
call toll-free **1-800-897-7535** (English/Spanish) weekdays

TUMS EX (calcium carbonate)

GlaxoSmithKline Consumer Heathcare LP

Active Ingredient(s) (per tablet)
Calcium carbonate USP 750 mg

Purpose(s)
Antacid

USES
relieves
- heartburn
- sour stomach
- acid indigestion
- upset stomach associated with these symptoms

WARNINGS

ASK A DOCTOR OR PHARMACIST BEFORE USE IF YOU ARE
taking a prescription drug. Antacids may interact with certain prescription drugs.

WHEN USING THIS PRODUCT
- do not take more than 10 tablets in 24 hours
- do not use the maximum dosage for more than 2 weeks

Keep out of reach of children.

WARNINGS SUGAR FREE ORANGE CREAM

ASK A DOCTOR OR PHARMACIST BEFORE USE IF YOU ARE
taking a prescription drug. Antacids may interact with certain prescription drugs.

WHEN USING THIS PRODUCT
- do not take more than 9 tablets in 24 hours
- do not use the maximum dosage for more than 2 weeks

Keep out of reach of children

DIRECTIONS
- chew 2 - 4 tablets as symptoms occur, or as directed by a doctor

OTHER INFORMATION
- for calcium and sodium content see Supplement Facts
- store below 30°C (86°F)

OTHER INFORMATION (ORANGE CREAM)
- for calcium content see Supplement Facts
- store below 25C (77F)

Phenylketonurics: Contains phenylalanine, less than 1mg per tablet.

INACTIVE INGREDIENTS ASSORTED FRUIT
sucrose, calcium carbonate, corn starch, talc, mineral oil, natural and artificial flavors, adipic acid, sodium polyphosphate, red 40 lake, yellow 6 lake, yellow 5 (tartrazine) lake, blue 1 lake

INACTIVE INGREDIENTS ASSORTED BERRIES
sucrose, calcium carbonate, corn starch, talc, mineral oil, adipic acid, artificial flavors, sodium polyphosphate, red 40 lake, blue 1 lake

INACTIVE INGREDIENTS SUGAR FREE ORANGE CREAM
calcium carbonate, sorbitol, acacia, natural and artificial flavors, calcium stearate, adipic acid, yellow 6 lake, aspartame

INACTIVE INGREDIENT ASSORTED TROPICAL FRUIT
sucrose, calcium carbonate, corn starch, talc, mineral oil, natural and artificial flavors, sodium polyphosphate, red 40 lake, yellow 6 lake, yellow 5 (tartrazine) lake

INACTIVE INGREDIENTS WINTERGREEN
sucrose, calcium carbonate, corn starch, talc, mineral oil, artificial flavor, sodium polyphosphate, yellow 5 (tartrazine) lake, blue 1 lake

INACTIVE INGREDIENTS CHERRY
sucrose, calcium carbonate, corn starch, talc, mineral oil, flavor, adipic acid, sodium polyphosphate, red 40 lake

QUESTIONS OR COMMENTS?
1-800-897-7535 weekdays

CALCIUM SUPPLEMENT

USES
As a daily source of extra calcium.

DIRECTIONS
Chew 2 tablets twice daily with a meal.
Supplement Facts
Serving Size: 2 Tablets
Servings Per Container: 48

Amount Per Serving	% Daily Value
Calories 10	
Sugars 2 g	
Calcium 600mg	60%
Sodium 5 mg	less than 1%

GlaxoSmithKline
Moon Twp, PA 15108
www.tums.com
Safety sealed - Do not use if printed inner seal beneath cap is missing or broken.
Supplement Facts (Orange Cream)
Serving Size: 2 Tablets
Servings Per Container: 40

Amount Per Serving	% Daily Value
Calories 5	
Sugars 1g	
Calcium 600mg	60%

TUMS FRESHERS (calcium carbonate)
GlaxoSmithKline Consumer Healthcare LP

Active Ingredient(s) (per tablet)
Calcium carbonate USP 500mg

Purpose(s)
Antacid

INDICATIONS AND USAGE

USES
relieves
• heartburn
• sour stomach
• acid indigestion
• upset stomach associated with these symptoms

WARNINGS

ASK A DOCTOR OR PHARMACIST BEFORE USE IF YOU ARE
taking a prescription drug. Antacids may interact with certain prescription drugs.

WHEN USING THIS PRODUCT
• do not take more than 15 tablets in 24 hours
• do not use the maximum dosage for more than 2 weeks
Keep Out of Reach of Children.

DIRECTIONS
• take 2-4 tablets as symptoms occur, or as directed by a doctor

OTHER INFORMATION
• **each tablet contains:** elemental calcium 200mg
• store below 25°C (77°F)

INACTIVE INGREDIENTS
calcium stearate, corn starch, FD&C blue #1, gum acacia, maltodextrin, natural & artificial flavor, sorbitol, sucralose, sucrose, tocopherols

QUESTIONS OR COMMENTS?
1-800-897-7535 (English/Spanish) weekdays

TUMS KIDS CHEWABLE TABLETS CHERRY BLAST (calcium carbonate)
GlaxoSmithKline Consumer Healthcare LP

DRUG FACTS

Active Ingredient(s) (in each chewable tablet)	Purpose(s)
Calcium carbonate USP 750mg	Antacid

SUPPLEMENT FACTS

Serving Size 1 Tablet

Each Serving Contains	Amount Per Serving	% DV Children 2-4 yrs of age	%DV Adults and Children over 4 yrs old
Calories	5		
Sugars	1 g		
Calcium	300 mg	38%	30%
Sodium	3 mg	*	Less than 1%
Magnesium	1 mg	Less than 1%	Less than 1%
*Daily Value not established			

USES
Relieves:
- Heartburn
- Sour stomach
- Acid indigestion
- Upset stomach associated with these symptoms

As a daily source of extra calcium

ASK A DOCTOR OR PHARMACIST BEFORE USE IF YOU ARE
- **taking a prescription drug. Antacids may interact with certain prescription drugs**

WHEN USING THIS PRODUCT
- do not take more than 2 tablets (2 - 4 year olds) or 4 tablets (5 - 11 year olds) in 24 hours or use the maximum dosage for more than 2 weeks except under the advice and supervision of a doctor.

Keep out of reach of children.

DIRECTIONS
As An Antacid
- Find the right dose on the chart below based on weight (preferred); otherwise use age. Chew 1/2 to 1 tablet as symptoms occur or as directed by a doctor.

Weight	Age	Dose
under 24 lbs	under 2 yrs	ask a doctor
24-47 lbs	2-4 yrs	½ tablet
over 48 lbs	over 4 yrs	1 tablet

As A Calcium Supplement
- 2-4 year olds: chew 1 tablet twice per day with a meal.
- Adults and children over 4 years old: chew 1 tablet three times a day with a meal.

OTHER INFORMATION
Store below 25°C (77°F)

INACTIVE INGREDIENTS
calcium carbonate, sorbitol, dextrose, sucrose, microcrystalline cellulose, magnesium stearate, adipic acid, natural and artificial flavors, maltodextrin, guar gum, red 40 lake, blue 1 lake

TUMS REGULAR (calcium carbonate)
GlaxoSmithKline Consumer Heathcare LP

Active Ingredient(s) (per tablet):
Calcium Carbonate USP 500mg

Purpose(s): Antacid

INACTIVE INGREDIENTS
Assorted Fruit:
sucrose, calcium carbonate, corn starch, talc, mineral oil, natural and artificial flavors, adipic acid, sodium polyphosphate, red 40 lake, yellow 6 lake, yellow 5 (tartrazine) lake, blue 1 lake.
Peppermint:
sucrose, calcium carbonate, corn starch, talc, mineral oil, natural flavors, sodium polyphosphate.

USES
Relieves:
Heartburn
Sour stomach
Acid indigestion
Upset stomach associated with these symptoms

WARNINGS

ASK A DOCTOR OR PHARMACIST BEFORE USE IF
you are taking a prescription drug.
Antacids may interact with certain prescription drugs.

WHEN USING THIS PRODUCT
Do not take more than 15 tablets in 24 hours.
Do not use the maximum dosage for more than 2 weeks.
Keep out of reach of children.

DIRECTIONS
Chew 2 - 4 tablets as symptoms occur, or as directed by a doctor.
As a Calcium Supplement:

USES
As a daily source of extra calcium

DIRECTIONS
Chew 2 tablets twice daily with a meal

SUPPLEMENT FACTS
Serving Size: 2 tablets

Amount Per Serving	% Daily Value
Calories: 5	
Sugars: 1g	
Calcium: 400mg	40%

OTHER INFORMATION
Store below 30°C (86°F)

TUMS SMOOTHIES (calcium carbonate)
GlaxoSmithKline Consumer Heathcare LP

Active Ingredient(s) (per tablet)
Calcium carbonate USP 750 mg

Purpose(s)
Antacid

USES
relieves
- heartburn
- sour stomach
- acid indigestion
- upset stomach associated with these symptoms

WARNINGS

ASK A DOCTOR OR PHARMACIST BEFORE USE IF YOU ARE
taking a prescription drug. Antacids may interact with certain prescription drugs.

WHEN USING THIS PRODUCT
- do not take more than 10 tablets in 24 hours
- do not use the maximum dosage for more than 2 weeks
Keep out of reach of children.

DIRECTIONS
- chew 2 - 4 tablets as symptoms occur, or as directed by a doctor

INACTIVE INGREDIENTS ASSORTED FRUIT
calcium carbonate, sorbitol, dextrose, sucrose, microcrystalline cellulose, magnesium stearate, adipic acid, corn starch, maltodextrin, guar gum, natural and artificial flavors, red 40 lake, yellow 6 lake, yellow 5 (tartrazine) lake, blue 1 lake. Contains milk

INACTIVE INGREDIENTS BERRY FUSION
calcium carbonate, sorbitol, dextrose, sucrose, microcrystalline cellulose, magnesium stearate, natural and artificial flavors, adipic acid, corn starch, guar gum, maltodextrin, red 40 lake, blue 1 lake. Contains soy

INACTIVE INGREDIENT ASSORTED TROPICAL FRUIT
calcium carbonate, sorbitol, dextrose, sucrose, microcrystalline cellulose, magnesium stearate, natural and artificial flavors, corn starch, guar gum, maltodextrin, adipic acid, yellow 6 lake, red 40 lake, blue 1 lake. Contains: soy

INACTIVE INGREDIENTS PEPPERMINT
calcium carbonate, sorbitol, dextrose, sucrose, microcrystalline cellulose, magnesium stearate, corn starch, guar gum, maltodextrin, natural and artificial flavors

INACTIVE INGREDIENTS COCOA AND CREME
calcium carbonate, sorbitol, dextrose, sucrose, cocoa powder, microcrystalline cellulose, natural and artificial flavors, magnesium stearate, corn starch, maltodextrin, guar gum, silicon dioxide. Contains: milk, soy

QUESTIONS OR COMMENTS?
1-800-897-7535 weekdays

OTHER INFORMATION
• for calcium/magnesium/sodium content see Supplement Facts
• store below 25ºC (77ºF). Keep the container tightly closed.

GlaxoSmithKline
Moon Twp, PA 15108
www.tums.com
Safety sealed - Do not use if printed inner seal beneath cap is missing or broken.
©2010 GSK

CALCIUM SUPPLEMENT

USES
As a daily source of extra calcium.

DIRECTIONS
Chew 2 tablets twice daily with a meal.
Supplement Facts
Serving Size: 2 Tablets
Servings Per Container: 30

Amount Per Serving	% Daily Value
Calories 10	
Sugars 2 g	
Calcium 600mg	60%
Sodium 5 mg	(less than 1%)
Magnesium 2mg	(less than 1%)

TUMS ULTRA STRENGTH (calcium carbonate)
GlaxoSmithKline Consumer Heathcare LP

Active Ingredient(s) (per tablet)
Calcium carbonate USP 1,000 mg

Purpose(s)
Antacid

USES
relieves
• heartburn
• sour stomach
• acid indigestion
• upset stomach associated with these symptoms

WARNINGS

ASK A DOCTOR OR PHARMACIST BEFORE USE IF YOU ARE
taking a prescription drug. Antacids may interact with certain prescription drugs.

WHEN USING THIS PRODUCT
• do not take more than 7 tablets in 24 hours
• do not use the maximum dosage for more than 2 weeks
Keep out of reach of children.

DIRECTIONS
• chew 2-3 tablets as symptoms occur, or as directed by a doctor

OTHER INFORMATION
• for calcium and sodium content see Supplement Facts
• store below 30ºC (86ºF)

INACTIVE INGREDIENTS (ASSORTED FRUIT)
sucrose, calcium carbonate, corn starch, talc, mineral oil, natural and artificial flavors, adipic acid, sodium polyphosphate, red 40 lake, yellow 6 lake, yellow 5 (tartrazine) lake, blue 1 lake

INACTIVE INGREDIENTS (ASSORTED TROPICAL FRUIT)
sucrose, calcium carbonate, corn starch, talc, mineral oil, natural and artificial flavors, sodium polyphosphate, red 40 lake, yellow 6 lake, yellow 5 (tartrazine) lake

INACTIVE INGREDIENTS (ASSORTED BERRY)
sucrose, calcium carbonate, corn starch, talc, mineral oil, adipic acid, artificial flavors, sodium polyphosphate, red 40 lake, blue 1 lake

INACTIVE INGREDIENT (PEPPERMINT)
sucrose, calcium carbonate, corn starch, talc, mineral oil, natural flavor, sodium polyphosphate

INACTIVE INGREDIENTS (PEPPERMINT TRI-COLOR)
sucrose, calcium carbonate, corn starch, talc, mineral oil, natural flavor, sodium polyphosphate, red 40 lake, yellow 5 (tartrazine) lake, blue 1 lake

QUESTIONS OR COMMENTS?
1-800-897-7535
weekdays

Gluten-Free
CALCIUM SUPPLEMENT

USES
As a daily source of extra calcium.

DIRECTIONS
Chew 2 tablets once or twice daily with a meal.

SUPPLEMENT FACTS
Serving Size: 2 Tablets
Servings Per Container: 36 **(For 72 count bottles)**
Servings Per Container: 43 **(For 86 count bottles)**

Amount Per Servings	%Daily Value
Calories 10	
Sugars 3g	
Calcium 800mg	80%
Sodium 10mg	less than 1%

Safety sealed- Do not use if printed inner seal beneath cap is missing or broken.

www.tums.com
GlaxoSmithKline
Moon Twp, PA 15108

INFANTS' TYLENOL ORAL SUSPENSION LIQUID (acetaminophen)

McNeil Consumer Healthcare Div. McNeil-PPC, Inc

DRUG FACTS

Active Ingredient(s) (in each 5 mL)	Purpose(s)
Acetaminophen 160 mg	Pain reliever/fever reducer

USES

temporarily reduces fever
temporarily relieves minor aches and pains due to:
• the common cold
• flu
• headache
• sore throat
• toothache

WARNINGS

Liver warning: This product contains acetaminophen. Severe liver damage may occur if your child takes
• more than 5 doses in 24 hours, which is the maximum daily amount
• with other drugs containing acetaminophen

Sore throat warning: if sore throat is severe, persists for more than 2 days, is accompanied or followed by fever, headache, rash, nausea, or vomiting, consult a doctor promptly.

DO NOT USE

• with any other drug containing acetaminophen (prescription or nonprescription). If you are not sure whether a drug contains acetaminophen, ask a doctor or pharmacist
• if your child is allergic to acetaminophen or any of the inactive ingredients in this product

ASK A DOCTOR BEFORE USE IF YOUR CHILD HAS

• liver disease

ASK A DOCTOR OR PHARMACIST BEFORE USE IF YOUR CHILD IS

• taking the blood thinning drug warfarin

WHEN USING THIS PRODUCT

• **do not exceed recommended dose (see overdose warning)**

STOP USE AND ASK A DOCTOR IF

• pain gets worse or lasts more than 5 days
• fever gets worse or lasts more than 3 days
• new symptoms occur
• redness or swelling is present

These could be signs of a serious condition.
Keep out of reach of children.

OVERDOSE WARNING

Overdose warning: In case of overdose, get medical help or contact a Poison Control Center right away. (1-800-222-1222). Quick medical attention is critical for adults as well as for children even if you do not notice any signs or symptoms.

DIRECTIONS

• **this product does not contain directions or complete warnings for adult use**
• **do not give more than directed (see overdose warning)**
• **shake well before using**
• mL = milliliter
• find the right dose on chart below. If possible, use weight to dose; otherwise, use age
• push air out of syringe. Firmly push syringe into the bottle opening
• turn bottle upside down and pull syringe to the correct dose
• dispense liquid slowly into child's mouth, toward inner cheek
• repeat dose every 4 hours while symptoms last
• do not give more than 5 times in 24 hours
• replace cap tightly to maintain child resistance

Weight (lb)	Age (yr)	Dose (mL)*
Under 24	Under 2 years	Ask a doctor
24-35	2-3 years	5 mL
*or as directed by a doctor		

Attention: Use only enclosed syringe specifically designed for use with this product. Do not use any other dosing device.

OTHER INFORMATION

store between 20-25°C (68-77°F)

INACTIVE INGREDIENTS

anhydrous citric acid, butylparaben, D&C red no.33, FD&C blue no.1, flavors, glycerin, high fructose corn syrup, microcrystalline cellulose and carboxymethylcellulose sodium, propylene glycol, purified water, sodium benzoate, sorbitol solution, sucralose, xanthan gum

QUESTIONS OR COMMENTS?

call **1-877-895-3665** (toll-free) or **215-273-8755** (collect)

JR. TYLENOL MELTAWAYS (acetaminophen)

McNeil Consumer Healthcare Div. McNeil-PPC, Inc

DRUG FACTS

Active Ingredient(s) (in each tablet)
Acetaminophen 160 mg

Purpose(s)
Pain reliever/fever reducer

USES

• temporarily relieves minor aches and pains due to:
  • the common cold
  • flu
  • headache
  • sore throat
• temporarily reduces fever

WARNINGS

Liver warning
This product contains acetaminophen. Severe liver damage may occur if your child takes
• more than 5 doses in 24 hours, which is the maximum daily amount
• with other drugs containing acetaminophen

Sore throat warning
if sore throat is severe, persists for more than 2 days, is accompanied or followed by fever, headache, rash, nausea, or vomiting, consult a doctor promptly.

DO NOT USE
- with any other drug containing acetaminophen (prescription or nonprescription).

If you are not sure whether a drug contains acetaminophen, ask a doctor or pharmacist.
- if your child is allergic to acetaminophen or any of the inactive ingredients in this product

ASK A DOCTOR BEFORE USE IF YOUR CHILD HAS
liver disease

ASK A DOCTOR OR PHARMACIST BEFORE USE IF YOUR CHILD IS
taking the blood thinning drug warfarin

WHEN USING THIS PRODUCT
do not exceed recommended dose (see overdose warning)

STOP USE AND ASK A DOCTOR IF
- pain gets worse or lasts more than 5 days
- fever gets worse or lasts more than 3 days
- new symptoms occur
- redness or swelling is present

These could be signs of a serious condition.
Keep out of reach of children.

OVERDOSE WARNING
Taking more than the recommended dose (overdose) may cause liver damage. In case of overdose, get medical help or contact a Poison Control Center right away. (1-800-222-1222) Quick medical attention is critical for adults as well as for children even if you do not notice any signs or symptoms.

DIRECTIONS
- **this product does not contain directions or complete warnings for adult use.**
- **do not give more than directed (see overdose warning)**
- find right dose on chart below. If possible, use weight to dose; otherwise, use age.
- chew before swallowing; this product will soften in mouth for ease of chewing
- repeat dose every 4 hours while symptoms last
- do not give more than 5 times in 24 hours

Weight (lb)	Age (yr)	Dose (tablets) *
under 48	under 6 years	ask a doctor
48-59	6-8 years	2 tablets
60-71	9-10 years	2½ tablets
72-95	11 years	3 tablets
*or as directed by a doctor		

OTHER INFORMATION
- store between 20-25°C (68-77°F). Avoid high humidity.
- **do not use if carton or blister unit is opened or broken**
- see side panel for lot number and expiration date

INACTIVE INGREDIENTS
anhydrous citric acid, cellulose acetate, crospovidone, D&C red no. 7 calcium lake, dextrose excipient, flavor, magnesium stearate, povidone, sucralose

QUESTIONS OR COMMENTS?
call **1-877-895-3665**

CHILDRENS TYLENOL MELTAWAYS
(acetaminophen)

McNeil Consumer Healthcare Div. McNeil-PPC, Inc

DRUG FACTS

Active Ingredient(s) (in each tablet)
Acetaminophen 80 mg

Purpose(s)
Pain reliever/fever reducer

USES
- temporarily relieves minor aches and pains due to:
  - the common cold
  - flu
  - headache
  - sore throat
  - toothache
- temporarily reduces fever

WARNINGS
Liver warning
This product contains acetaminophen. Severe liver damage may occur if your child takes
- more than 5 doses in 24 hours, which is the maximum daily amount
- with other drugs containing acetaminophen

Sore throat warning
if sore throat is severe, persists for more than 2 days, is accompanied or followed by fever, headache, rash, nausea, or vomiting, consult a doctor promptly.

DO NOT USE
- with any other drug containing acetaminophen (prescription or nonprescription). If you are not sure whether a drug contains acetaminophen, ask a doctor or pharmacist.
- if your child is allergic to acetaminophen or any of the inactive ingredients in this product

ASK A DOCTOR BEFORE USE IF YOUR CHILD HAS
liver disease

ASK A DOCTOR OR PHARMACIST BEFORE USE
if your child is taking the blood thinning drug warfarin

WHEN USING THIS PRODUCT
do not exceed recommended dose (see overdose warning)

STOP USE AND ASK A DOCTOR IF
- pain gets worse or lasts more than 5 days
- fever gets worse or lasts more than 3 days
- new symptoms occur
- redness or swelling is present

These could be signs of a serious condition.

Keep out of reach of children.

OVERDOSE WARNING
Taking more than the recommended dose (overdose) may cause liver damage. In case of overdose, get medical help or contact a Poison Control Center right away. (1-800-222-1222) Quick medical attention is critical for adults as well as for children even if you do not notice any signs or symptoms.

DIRECTIONS
- **this product does not contain directions or complete warnings for adult use.**
- **do not give more than directed (see overdose warning)**
- find right dose on chart below. If possible, use weight to dose; otherwise, use age.

- chew before swallowing; this product will soften in mouth for ease of chewing
- repeat dose every 4 hours while symptoms last
- do not give more than 5 times in 24 hours

Weight (lb)	Age (yr)	Dose (tablets)*
under 24	under 2 years	ask a doctor
24-35	2-3 years	2 tablets
36-47	4-5 years	3 tablets
48-59	6-8 years	4 tablets
60-71	9-10 years	5 tablets
72-95	11 years	6 tablets

*or as directed by a doctor

OTHER INFORMATION
- store between 20-25°C (68-77°F). Avoid high humidity.
- **do not use if carton is opened, or if neck wrap or foil inner seal imprinted with "SAFETY SEAL®" is broken or missing**
- see side panel for lot number and expiration date

INACTIVE INGREDIENTS
anhydrous citric acid, cellulose acetate, crospovidone, D&C red no. 7 calcium lake, dextrose excipient, flavor, magnesium stearate, povidone, sucralose

QUESTIONS OR COMMENTS?
call **1-877-895-3665**

CHILDREN'S TYLENOL SUSPENSION
(acetaminophen)

McNeil Consumer Healthcare Div. McNeil-PPC, Inc

DRUG FACTS

Active Ingredient(s) (in each 5 mL = 1 teaspoonful)
Acetaminophen 160 mg

Purpose(s)
Pain reliever/fever reducer

USES
temporarily:
- reduces fever
- relieves minor aches and pains due to:
  - the common cold
  - flu
  - headache
  - sore throat
  - toothache

WARNINGS
Liver warning
This product contains acetaminophen. Severe liver damage may occur if your child takes
- more than 5 doses in 24 hours, which is the maximum daily amount
- with other drugs containing acetaminophen

Sore throat warning
if sore throat is severe, persists for more than 2 days, is accompanied or followed by fever, headache, rash, nausea, or vomiting, consult a doctor promptly.

DO NOT USE
- with any other drug containing acetaminophen (prescription or nonprescription). If you are not sure whether a drug contains acetaminophen, ask a doctor or pharmacist.
- if your child is allergic to acetaminophen or any of the inactive ingredients in this product

ASK A DOCTOR BEFORE USE IF YOUR CHILD HAS
liver disease

ASK A DOCTOR OR PHARMACIST BEFORE USE IF YOUR CHILD IS
taking the blood thinning drug warfarin

WHEN USING THIS PRODUCT
do not exceed recommended dose (see overdose warning)

STOP USE AND ASK A DOCTOR IF
- pain gets worse or lasts more than 5 days
- fever gets worse or lasts more than 3 days
- new symptoms occur
- redness or swelling is present

These could be signs of a serious condition.
Keep out of reach of children.

OVERDOSE WARNING
Taking more than the recommended dose (overdose) may cause liver damage. In case of overdose, get medical help or contact a Poison Control Center right away. (1-800-222-1222) Quick medical attention is critical for adults as well as for children even if you do not notice any signs or symptoms.

DIRECTIONS
- **this product does not contain directions or complete warnings for adult use.**
- **do not give more than directed (see overdose warning)**
- **shake well before using**
- mL = milliliter; tsp = teaspoonful
- find right dose on chart below. If possible, use weight to dose; otherwise, use age.
- if needed, repeat dose every 4 hours while symptoms last
- do not give more than 5 times in 24 hours

Weight (lb)	Age (yr)	Dose (mL or tsp)*
under 24	under 2 years	ask a doctor
24-35	2-3 years	5 mL (1 tsp)
36-47	4-5 years	7.5 mL (1½ tsp)
48-59	6-8 years	10 mL (2 tsp)
60-71	9-10 years	12.5 mL (2½ tsp)
72-95	11 years	15 mL (3 tsp)

*or as directed by a doctor

Attention: use only enclosed dosing cup specifically designed for use with this product. Do not use any other dosing device.

OTHER INFORMATION
- **each 5 mL (1 tsp) contains:** sodium 2 mg
- store between 20-25°C (68-77°F)
- **do not use if neck wrap or foil inner seal imprinted with "SAFETY SEAL®" is broken or missing**
- see top panel for lot number and expiration date

INACTIVE INGREDIENTS
anhydrous citric acid, butylparaben, D&C red #33, FD&C blue #1, flavor, glycerin, high fructose corn syrup, microcrystalline cellulose and carboxymethylcellulose sodium, propylene glycol, purified water, sodium benzoate, sorbitol solution, xanthan gum

QUESTIONS OR COMMENTS?
call **1-877-895-3665**

CHILDREN'S TYLENOL PLUS COLD & COUGH (dextromethorphan hydrobromide, acetaminophen, and phenylephrine hydrochloride)
McNeil Consumer Healthcare Division

USES
For the temporary relief of the following cold/flu symptoms:
- Minor aches and pains.
- Headache.
- Sore throat.
- Cough.
- Stuffy nose.

Temporarily reduces fever.

AVAILABLE AS
For children ages 4 to 11 years:
Liquid
Dye-free grape flavor oral suspension

DIRECTIONS
- **This product does not contain directions or complete warnings for adult use.**
- **Do not give more then directed (see overdose warning).**
- **Shake well before using.**
- Find the right dose on chart below. If possible, use weight to dose; otherwise, use age.
- Use only enclosed dosing cup designed for use with this product. Do not use any other dosing device.
- If needed, repeat dose every 4 hours.
- Do not give more than 5 times in 24 hours

Weight (lb)	Age (yr)	Dose (tsp or mL)
Under 36 lbs	Under 4 years	Do not use
36-47 lbs	4-5 years	1 tsp or 5 mL
48-95 lbs	6-11 years	2 tsp or 10 mL

Attention: Use only enclosed dosing cup specifically designed for use with this product. Do not use any other dosing device.

INGREDIENTS
Active Ingredient(s): Acetaminophen
Purpose(s): Pain reliever/fever reducer
Active Ingredient(s): Dextromethorphan HBr
Purpose(s): Cough suppressant
Active Ingredient(s): Phenylephrine HCl
Purpose(s): Nasal decongestant

	Active Ingredients	Inactive Ingredients
Liquid - Grape Flavor	Acetaminophen 160 mg in each teaspoon (5 mL) Dextromethorphan HBr 5 mg in each teaspoon (5mL) Phenylephrine HCl 2.5 mg in each teaspoon (5 mL)	Anhydrous citric acid, butylparaben, flavors, glycerin, microcrystalline cellulose and carboxymethylcellulose sodium, propylene glycol, propylparaben, purified water, sodium citrate, sorbitol solution, sucralose, sucrose, xanthan gum

WARNINGS
Liver warning: This product contains acetaminophen. Severe liver damage may occur if your child takes
- more than 5 doses in 24 hours.
- with other drugs containing acetaminophen.

Caplet
Sore throat warning: If sore throat is severe, persists for more than 2 days, is accompanied or followed by fever, headache, rash, nausea or vomiting, consult a doctor promptly.

DO NOT USE
- with any other drug containing acetaminophen (prescription or nonprescription). If you are not sure whether a drug contains acetaminophen, ask a doctor or pharmacist.
- In a child who is taking a prescription monoamine oxidase inhibitor (MAOI) (certain drugs for depression, psychiatric, emotional conditions or Parkinson's disease), or for 2 weeks after stopping the MAOI drug. If you do not know if your child's prescription drug contains an MAOI, ask a doctor or pharmacist before giving this product.
- if your child has ever had an allergic reaction to this product or any of its ingredients

ASK A DOCTOR BEFORE USE IF YOU HAVE
- Liver disease.
- Heart disease.
- High blood pressure.
- Thyroid disease.
- Diabetes.
- Persistent or chronic cough such as occurs with asthma.
- Cough that occurs with too much phlegm (mucus).

ASK A DOCTOR OR PHARMACIST BEFORE USE IF YOUR CHILD IS
taking the blood thinning drug warfarin.

WHEN USING THIS PRODUCT
do not exceed recommended dose (see overdose warning).

STOP USE AND ASK A DOCTOR IF
- Nervousness, dizziness or sleeplessness occur.
- Pain, nasal congestion or cough gets worse or lasts more than 5 days.
- Fever gets worse or lasts more than 3 days.
- Redness or swelling is present.
- New symptoms occur.
- Cough comes back or occurs with rash or headache that lasts.

These could be signs of a serious condition.
Keep out of reach of children.

OVERDOSE WARNING
In case of overdose, get medical help or contact a Poison Control Center right away (1-800-222-1222). Quick medical attention is critical for adults as well as for children even if you do not notice any signs or symptoms.

STORAGE & PACKAGE SAFETY
- Store between 20-25° C (68-77° F).
- **Do not use if bottle wrap or foil inner seal imprinted "Safety Seal®" is broken or missing.**
- See package for lot number and expiration date.

QUESTIONS OR COMMENTS?
Call 1-877-TYLENOL (1-877-895-3665)

CHILDREN'S TYLENOL PLUS COLD
(acetaminophen, chlorpheniramine maleate, dextromethorphan hydrobromide, and phenylephrine hydrochloride)

McNeil Consumer Healthcare Division

USES
Temporarily relieves the following cold/flu symptoms:
- Minor aches and pains.
- Headache.
- Sore throat.
- Stuffy nose.
- Sneezing and runny nose.

Temporarily reduces fever.

AVAILABLE AS
For children ages 6 to 11 years:
Liquid
Grape Flavor

DIRECTIONS
- **This product does not contain directions or complete warnings for adult use.**
- **Do not give more than directed (see overdose warning).**
- **Shake well before using.**
- Find right dose on chart below. If possible, use weight to dose; otherwise, use age.
- Use only enclosed dosing cup designed for use with this product. Do not use any other dosing device.
- If needed, repeat dose every 4 hours.
- Do not give more than 5 times in 24 hours.

Weight (lb)	Age (yr)	Dose (tsp or mL)
Under 36 lbs	Under 4 years	Do not use
36-47 lbs	4-5 years	Do not use unless directed by a doctor
48-95 lbs	6-11 years	2 tsp or 10 mL

Attention: Use only enclosed dosing cup specifically designed for use with this product. Do not use any other dosing device.

INGREDIENTS
Active Ingredient(s): Acetaminophen
Purpose(s): Pain reliever/fever reducer
Active Ingredient(s): Chlorpheniramine maleate
Purpose(s): Antihistamine
Active Ingredient(s): Dextromethorphan HBr
Purpose(s): Cough suppressant
Active Ingredient(s): Phenylephrine HCl
Purpose(s): Nasal decongestant

	Active Ingredients	Inactive Ingredients
Grape Flavor	Acetaminophen 160 mg in each teaspoon (5 mL) Chlorpheniramine maleate 1 mg in each teaspoon (5 mL) Dextromethorphan HBr 5 mg in each teaspoon (5mL) Phenylephrine HCl 2.5 mg in each teaspoon (5 mL)	Anhydrous citric acid, D&C red #33, FD&C blue #1, FD&C red #40, flavors, glycerin, microcrystalline cellulose and carboxymethylcellulose sodium, purified water, sodium benzoate, sorbitol solution, sucrose, xanthan gum

WARNINGS
Liver warning: This product contains acetaminophen. Severe liver damage may occur if your child takes
- more than 5 doses in 24 hours.
- with other drugs containing acetaminophen.

Caplet
Sore throat warning: If sore throat is severe, persists for more than 2 days, is accompanied or followed by fever, headache, rash, nausea, or vomiting, consult a doctor promptly.

DO NOT USE
- with any other drug containing acetaminophen (prescription or nonprescription). If you are not sure whether a drug contains acetaminophen, ask a doctor or pharmacist.
- To make a child sleepy.
- In a child who is taking a prescription monoamine oxidase inhibitor (MAOI) (certain drugs for depression, psychiatric, or emotional conditions, or Parkinson's disease), or for 2 weeks after stopping the MAOI drug. If you do not know if your child's prescription drug contains an MAOI, ask a doctor or pharmacist before giving this product.
- if your child has ever had an allergic reaction to this product or any of its ingredients

ASK A DOCTOR BEFORE USE IF YOU HAVE
- Liver disease.
- Heart disease.
- High blood pressure.
- Thyroid disease.
- Diabetes.
- A breathing problem such as chronic bronchitis.
- Glaucoma.

ASK A DOCTOR OR PHARMACIST BEFORE USE IF YOUR CHILD IS
- taking the blood thinning drug warfarin
- taking sedatives or tranquilizers

WHEN USING THIS PRODUCT
- **Do not exceed recommended dose (see overdose warning).**
- Excitability may occur, especially in children.
- Marked drowsiness may occur.
- Sedatives and tranquilizers may increase drowsiness.

STOP USE AND ASK A DOCTOR IF
- Nervousness, dizziness or sleeplessness occur.
- Pain, nasal congestion or cough gets worse or lasts more than 5 days.
- Fever gets worse or lasts more than 3 days.
- Redness or swelling is present.
- New symptoms occur.
- Cough comes back or occurs with rash or headache that lasts.

These could be signs of a serious condition.
Keep out of reach of children.

OVERDOSE WARNING
In case of overdose, get medical help or contact a Poison Control Center right away (1-800-222-1222). Quick medical attention is critical for adults as well as for children even if you do not notice any signs or symptoms.

STORAGE & PACKAGE SAFETY
Store between 20—25°C (68—77°F).
Do not use if bottle wrap or foil inner seal imprinted with "Safety Seal®" is broken or missing.
See package for lot number and expiration date.

QUESTIONS OR COMMENTS?
Call 1-877-TYLENOL (1-877-895-3665)

CHILDREN'S TYLENOL PLUS COUGH & RUNNY NOSE (acetaminophen, chlorpheniramine maleate, and dextromethorphan hydrobromide)

McNeil Consumer Healthcare Division

USES
Temporarily relieves the following cold/flu symptoms:
• Minor aches and pains.
• Headache.
• Sore throat.
• Sneezing and runny nose.
• Cough.
Temporarily reduces fever.

AVAILABLE AS
For children ages 6 to 11 years:
Cherry Flavored Liquid

DIRECTIONS
• **This product does not contain directions or complete warnings for adult use.**
• **Do not give more than directed (see overdose warning).**
• **Shake well before using.**
• Find right dose on chart below. If possible, use weight to dose; otherwise, use age.
• Use only enclosed dosing cup designed for use with this product. Do not use any other dosing device.
• If needed, repeat dose every 4 hours
• Do not give more than 5 times in 24 hours.

Weight (lb)	Age (yr)	Dose (tsp or mL)
Under 36 lbs	Under 4 years	Do not use
36-47 lbs	4-5 years	Do not use unless directed by a doctor
48-95 lbs	6-11 years	2 tsp or 10 mL

Attention: Use only enclosed dosing cup specifically designed for use with this product. Do not use any other dosing device.

INGREDIENTS
Active Ingredient(s): Acetaminophen
Purpose(s): Pain reliever/fever reducer
Active Ingredient(s): Chlorpheniramine maleate
Purpose(s): Antihistamine
Active Ingredient(s): Dextromethorphan HBr
Purpose(s): Cough suppressant

	Active Ingredients	Inactive Ingredients
Liquid-Grape Flavor	Acetaminophen 160 mg in each teaspoon (5 mL) Chlorpheniramine maleate 1 mg in each teaspoon (5 mL) Dextromethorphan HBr 5 mg in each teaspoon (5mL)	Acesulfame potassium, anhydrous citric acid, D&C red #33, FD&C red #40, flavors, glycerin, high fructose corn syrup, microcrystalline cellulose and carboxymethylcellulose sodium, purified water, sodium benzoate, sorbitol solution, xanthan gum

WARNINGS
Liver warning: This product contains acetaminophen. Severe liver damage may occur if you take
• more than 5 doses in 24 hours
• with other drugs containing acetaminophen.

Caplet
Sore throat warning: If sore throat is severe, persists for more than 2 days, is accompanied or followed by fever, headache, rash, nausea, or vomiting, consult a doctor promptly.

DO NOT USE
• with any other drug containing acetaminophen (prescription or nonprescription). If you are not sure whether a drug contains acetaminophen, ask a doctor or pharmacist.
• To make a child sleepy.
• In a child who is taking a prescription monoamine oxidase inhibitor (MAOI) (certain drugs for depression, psychiatric or emotional conditions, or Parkinson's disease), or for 2 weeks after stopping the MAOI drug. If you do not know if your child's prescription drug contains an MAOI, ask a doctor or pharmacist before giving this product.
• if your child has ever had an allergic reaction to this product or any of its ingredients

ASK A DOCTOR BEFORE USE IF YOU HAVE
• Liver disease.
• A breathing problem such as chronic bronchitis
• Glaucoma.
• Persistent or chronic cough such as occurs with asthma.
• Cough that occurs with too much phlegm (mucus).

ASK A DOCTOR OR PHARMACIST BEFORE USE IF YOUR CHILD IS
• taking the blood thinning drug warfarin
• taking sedatives or tranquilizers

WHEN USING THIS PRODUCT
• **Do not exceed recommended dose (see overdose warning).**
• Excitability may occur, especially in children.
• Marked drowsiness may occur.
• Sedatives and tranquilizers may increase drowsiness.

STOP USE AND ASK A DOCTOR IF
• Fever gets worse or lasts more than 3 days.
• Redness or swelling is present.
• New symptoms occur.
• Cough comes back or occurs with rash or headache that lasts.

These could be signs of a serious condition.
Keep out of reach of children.

OVERDOSE WARNING
In case of overdose, get medical help or contact a Poison Control Center right away (1-800-222-1222). Quick medical attention is critical for adults as well as for children even if you do not notice any signs or symptoms.

STORAGE & PACKAGE SAFETY
• Store between 20-25° C (68-77° F).
• **Do not use if bottle wrap, or foil inner seal imprinted "Safety Seal®" is broken or missing.**
• See package for lot number and expiration date.

QUESTIONS OR COMMENTS?
Call 1-877-TYLENOL (1-877-895-3665)

CHILDREN'S TYLENOL PLUS COUGH & SORE THROAT (acetaminophen and dextromethorphan hydrobromide)

McNeil Consumer Healthcare Division

USES
Temporarily relieves the following cold/flu symptoms:
• Minor aches and pains.
• Headache.
• Sore throat.
• Cough.

Temporarily reduces fever.

AVAILABLE AS
For children ages 4 to 11 years:
Cherry Flavored Liquid

DIRECTIONS
• **This product does not contain directions or complete warnings for adult use.**
• **Do not give more than directed (see overdose warning).**
• **Shake well before using.**
• Find right dose on chart below. If possible, use weight to dose; otherwise, use age.
• Use only enclosed dosing cup designed for use with this product. Do not use any other dosing device.
• If needed, repeat dose every 4 hours.
• Do not give more than 5 times in 24 hours.

Weight (lb)	Age (yr)	Dose (tsp or mL)
Under 36 lbs	Under 4 years	Do not use
36-47 lbs	4-5 years	1 tsp or 5 mL
48-95 lbs	6-11 years	2 tsp or 10 mL

Attention: Use only enclosed dosing cup specifically designed for use with this product. Do not use any other dosing device.

INGREDIENTS
Active Ingredient(s): Acetaminophen
Purpose(s): Pain reliever/fever reducer
Active Ingredient(s): Dextromethorphan HBr
Purpose(s): Cough suppressant

	Active Ingredients	Inactive Ingredients
Liquid-Cherry Flavor	Acetaminophen 160 mg in each teaspoon (5 mL) Dextromethorphan HBr 5 mg in each teaspoon (5mL)	Acesulfame potassium, anhydrous citric acid, D&C red #33, FD&C red #40, flavors, glycerin, high fructose corn syrup, microcrystalline cellulose and carboxymethylcellulose sodium, purified water, sodium benzoate, sorbitol solution, xanthan gum

WARNINGS
Liver warning: This product contains acetaminophen. Severe liver damage may occur if your child takes
• more than 5 doses in 24 hours, which is the maximum daily amount.
• with other drugs containing acetaminophen.
Caplet
Sore throat warning: If sore throat is severe, persists for more than 2 days, is accompanied or followed by fever, headache, rash, nausea, or vomiting, consult a doctor promptly.

DO NOT USE
• with any other drug containing acetaminophen (prescription or nonprescription). If you are not sure whether a drug contains acetaminophen, ask a doctor or pharmacist.
• to make a child sleepy.
• in a child who is taking a prescription monoamine oxidase inhibitor (MAOI) (certain drugs for depression, psychiatric or emotional conditions, or Parkinson's disease), or for 2 weeks after stopping the MAOI drug. If you do not know if your child's prescription drug contains an MAOI, ask a doctor or pharmacist before giving this product.
• if your child has ever had an allergic reaction to this product or any of its ingredients

ASK A DOCTOR BEFORE USE IF THE CHILD HAS
• Liver disease.
• A persistent or chronic cough such as occurs with asthma.
• A cough that occurs with too much phlegm (mucus).

ASK A DOCTOR OR PHARMACIST BEFORE USE IF YOUR CHILD IS
taking the blood thinning drug warfarin.

WHEN USING THIS PRODUCT
do not exceed recommended dose (see overdose warning).

STOP USE AND ASK A DOCTOR IF
• Pain or cough gets worse or lasts more than 5 days.
• Fever gets worse or lasts more than 3 days.
• Redness or swelling is present.
• New symptoms occur.
• Cough comes back or occurs with rash or headache that lasts.

These could be signs of a serious condition.
Keep out of reach of children.

OVERDOSE WARNING
In case of overdose, get medical help or contact a Poison Control Center right away- (1-800-222-1222). Quick medical attention is critical for adults as well as for children even if you do not notice any signs or symptoms.

STORAGE & PACKAGE SAFETY
• Store between 20-25 C° (68-77° F).
• **Do not use if bottle wrap, or foil inner seal imprinted "Safety Seal®" is broken or missing.**
• See package for lot number and expiration date.

QUESTIONS OR COMMENTS?
Call 1-877-TYLENOL (1-877-895-3665)

CHILDREN'S TYLENOL PLUS FLU
(acetaminophen, chlorpheniramine maleate, dextromethorphan HBr, and phenylephrine HCl)

McNeil Consumer Healthcare Division

USES
Temporarily relieves the following cold/flu symptoms:
• Minor aches and pains.
• Headache.
• Sore throat.
• Sneezing and runny nose.
• Cough.
• Stuffy nose.

Temporarily reduces fever.

AVAILABLE AS
For children ages 6 to 11 years:
Liquid
Bubble Gum flavor

DIRECTIONS
- **This product does not contain directions or complete warnings for adult use.**
- **Do not give more than directed (see overdose warning).**
- **Shake well before using.**
- Find the right dose on chart below. If possible, use weight to dose; otherwise, use age.
- Use only enclosed dosing cup designed for use with this product. Do not use any other dosing device.
- If needed, repeat dose every 4 hours.
- Do not give more than 5 times in 24 hours.

Weight (lb)	Age (yr)	Dose (tsp or mL)
Under 36 lbs	Under 4 years	Do not use
36-47 lbs	4-5 years	Do not use unless directed by a doctor
48-95 lbs	6-11 years	2 tsp or 10 mL

Attention: Use only enclosed dosing cup specifically designed for use with this product. Do not use any other dosing device.

INGREDIENTS
Active Ingredient(s): Acetaminophen
Purpose(s): Pain reliever/fever reducer
Active Ingredient(s): Chlorpheniramine maleate
Purpose(s): Antihistamine
Active Ingredient(s): Dextromethorphan HBr
Purpose(s): Cough suppressant
Active Ingredient(s): Phenylephrine HCl
Purpose(s): Nasal decongestant

	Active Ingredients	Inactive Ingredients
Bubble gum flavor	Acetaminophen 160 mg in each teaspoon (5 mL) Chlorpheniramine maleate 1 mg in each teaspoon (5 mL) Dextromethorphan HBr 5 mg in each teaspoon (5mL) Phenylephrine HCl 2.5 mg in each teaspoon (5 mL)	Anhydrous citric acid, D&C red #33, FD&C red #40, flavors, glycerin, microcrystalline cellulose and carboxymethylcellulose sodium, purified water, sodium benzoate, sorbitol solution, sucrose, xanthan gum

WARNINGS
Liver warning: This product contains acetaminophen. Severe liver damage may occur if your child takes
- more than 5 doses in 24 hours, which is the maximum daily amount.
- with other drugs containing acetaminophen.

Caplet
Sore throat warning: If sore throat is severe, persists for more than 2 days, is accompanied or followed by fever, headache, rash, nausea or vomiting, consult a doctor promptly.

DO NOT USE
- with any other drug containing acetaminophen (prescription or nonprescription). If you are not sure whether a drug contains acetaminophen, ask a doctor or pharmacist.
- To make a child sleepy.
- In a child who is taking a prescription monoamine oxidase inhibitor (MAOI) (certain drugs for depression, psychiatric, emotional conditions or Parkinson's disease), or for 2 weeks after stopping the MAOI drug. If you do not know if your child's prescription drug contains an MAOI, ask a doctor or pharmacist before giving this product.

ASK A DOCTOR BEFORE USE IF YOU HAVE
- Liver disease.
- Heart disease.
- High blood pressure.
- Thyroid disease.
- Diabetes.
- Persistent or chronic cough such as occurs with asthma.
- Cough that occurs with too much phlegm (mucus).
- A breathing problem such as chronic bronchitis.
- Glaucoma.

ASK A DOCTOR OR PHARMACIST BEFORE USE IF YOUR CHILD IS
- taking the blood thinning drug warfarin
- taking sedatives or tranquilizers

WHEN USING THIS PRODUCT
- **Do not exceed recommended dose (see overdose warning).**
- Excitability may occur, especially in children.
- Marked Drowsiness may occur.
- Sedatives and tranquilizers may increase drowsiness.

STOP USE AND ASK A DOCTOR IF
- Nervousness, dizziness or sleeplessness occur.
- Pain, nasal congestion or cough gets worse or lasts more than 5 days.
- Fever gets worse or lasts more than 3 days.
- Redness or swelling is present.
- New symptoms occur.
- Cough comes back or occurs with rash or headache that lasts

These could be signs of a serious condition.
Keep out of reach of children.

OVERDOSE WARNING
In case of overdose, get medical help or contact a Poison Control Center right away (1-800-222-1222). Quick medical attention is critical for adults as well as for children even if you do not notice any signs or symptoms.

STORAGE & PACKAGE SAFETY
- Store between 20-25° C (68-77° F).
- **Do not use if bottle wrap, or foil inner seal imprinted "Safety Seal®" is broken or missing.**
- See package for lot number and expiration date.

QUESTIONS OR COMMENTS?
Call 1-877-TYLENOL (1-877-895-3665)

CHILDREN'S TYLENOL PLUS MULTI-SYMPTOM COLD (acetaminophen, chlorpheniramine maleate, dextromethorphan hydrobromide, and phenylephrine hydrochloride)
McNeil Consumer Healthcare Division

USES
Temporarily relieves the following cold/flu symptoms:
- Minor aches and pains.
- Headache.
- Sore throat.
- Cough.
- Stuffy nose.
- Sneezing and runny nose.

Temporarily reduces fever.

AVAILABLE AS
For children ages 6 to 11 years:
Honey Lemon Warming Liquid
Dye-free grape flavor oral suspension

DIRECTIONS
- **This product does not contain directions or complete warnings for adult use.**
- **Do not give more than directed (see overdose warning).**
- **Shake well before using.**
- Find right dose on chart below. If possible, use weight to dose; otherwise, use age.
- Use only enclosed dosing cup designed for use with this product. Do not use any other dosing device.
- If needed, repeat dose every 4 hours.
- Do not give more than 5 times in 24 hours.

Weight (lb)	Age (yr)	Dose (tsp or mL)
Under 36 lbs	Under 4 years	Do not use
36-47 lbs	4-5 years	Do not use unless directed by a doctor
48-95 lbs	6-11 years	2 tsp or 10 mL

Attention: Use only enclosed dosing cup specifically designed for use with this product. Do not use any other dosing device.

INGREDIENTS
Active Ingredient(s): Acetaminophen
Purpose(s): Pain reliever/fever reducer
Active Ingredient(s): Chlorpheniramine maleate
Purpose(s): Antihistamine
Active Ingredient(s): Dextromethorphan HBr
Purpose(s): Cough suppressant
Active Ingredient(s): Phenylephrine HCl
Purpose(s): Nasal decongestant

	Active Ingredients	Inactive Ingredients
Liquid— Grape Flavor	Acetaminophen 160 mg in each teaspoon (5 mL) Chlorpheniramine maleate 1 mg in each teaspoon (5 mL) Dextromethorphan HBr 5 mg in each teaspoon (5mL) Phenylephrine HCl 2.5 mg in each teaspoon (5 mL)	Anhydrous citric acid, D&C red #33, FD&C blue #1, FD&C red #40, flavors, glycerin, microcrystalline cellulose and carboxymethyl cellulose sodium, purified water, sodium benzoate, sorbitol solution, sucrose, xanthan gum
Liquid— Dye-Free Grape Flavor	Acetaminophen 160 mg in each teaspoon (5 mL) Chlorpheniramine maleate 1 mg in each teaspoon (5 mL) Dextromethorphan HBr 5 mg in each teaspoon (5mL) Phenylephrine HCl 2.5 mg in each teaspoon (5 mL)	Anhydrous citric acid, butylparaben, flavors, glycerin, microcrystalline cellulose and carboxymethyl cellulose sodium, propylene glycol, propylparaben, purified water, sodium citrate, sorbitol solution, sucralose, sucrose, xanthan gum

WARNINGS
Liver warning
This product contains acetaminophen. Severe liver damage may occur if you take
- more than 5 doses in 24 hours.
- with other drugs containing acetaminophen.

Sore throat warning
If sore throat is severe, persists for more than 2 days, is accompanied or followed by fever, headache, rash, nausea, or vomiting, consult a doctor promptly.

DO NOT USE
- with any other drug containing acetaminophen (prescription or nonprescription). If you are not sure whether a drug contains acetaminophen, ask a doctor or pharmacist.
- To make a child sleepy.
- In a child who is taking a prescription monoamine oxidase inhibitor (MAOI) (certain drugs for depression, psychiatric, or emotional conditions, or Parkinson's disease), or for 2 weeks after stopping the MAOI drug. If you do not know if your child's prescription drug contains an MAOI, ask a doctor or pharmacist before giving this product.
- if your child has ever had an allergic reaction to this product or any of its ingredients

ASK A DOCTOR BEFORE USE IF YOU HAVE
- Liver disease.
- Heart disease.
- High blood pressure.
- Thyroid disease.
- Diabetes.
- Persistent or chronic cough such as occurs with asthma.
- Cough that occurs with too much phlegm (mucus).
- A breathing problem such as chronic bronchitis.
- Glaucoma.

ASK A DOCTOR OR PHARMACIST BEFORE USE IF YOUR CHILD IS
- taking the blood thinning drug warfarin
- taking sedatives or tranquilizers

WHEN USING THIS PRODUCT
- **Do not exceed recommended dose (see overdose warning).**
- Excitability may occur, especially in children.
- Marked drowsiness may occur.
- Sedatives and tranquilizers may increase drowsiness.

STOP USE AND ASK A DOCTOR IF
- Nervousness, dizziness or sleeplessness occur.
- Pain, nasal congestion or cough gets worse or lasts more than 5 days.
- Fever gets worse or lasts more than 3 days.
- Redness or swelling is present.
- New symptoms occur.
- Cough comes back or occurs with rash or headache that lasts.

These could be signs of a serious condition.
Keep out of reach of children.

OVERDOSE WARNING
In case of overdose, get medical help or contact a Poison Control Center right away. (1-800-222-1222). Quick medical attention is critical for adults as well as for children even if you do not notice any signs or symptoms.

STORAGE & PACKAGE SAFETY
- Store between 20-25° C (68-77° F).
- **Do not use if bottle wrap, or foil inner seal imprinted with "Safety Seal®" is broken or missing.**
- See package for lot number and expiration date.

QUESTIONS OR COMMENTS?
Call 1-877-TYLENOL (1-877-895-3665)

TYLENOL 8 HOUR (acetaminophen)

McNeil Consumer Healthcare Div McNeil-PPC, Inc

OVERVIEW & USES
TYLENOL® 8 Hour silences body pain all day* without irritating your stomach the way that aspirin or even ibuprofen can.
TYLENOL® 8 Hour has one layer that dissolves quickly for fast relief and a second time-released layer that offers continuous relief for up to 8 hours.
*Up to 8 hours. Use as directed.

USES
Temporarily relieves minor aches and pains due to:
- Muscular aches
- Backache
- Headache
- Minor pain of arthritis

Temporarily reduces fever.
Available As
For adults & children 12 yrs & over:
Caplets

DIRECTIONS
Do not take more than directed (see overdose warning)
Adults & children 12 years & over:
- Take 2 caplets every 8 hours with water.
- Swallow whole-do not crush, chew, split, or dissolve.
- Do not take more than 6 caplets in 24 hours.
- Do not use for more than 10 days unless directed by a doctor.

Children under 12 years:
- Do not use.

INGREDIENTS
Active Ingredient(s): Acetaminophen
Purpose(s): Pain reliever/fever reducer

	Active ingredient	Inactive Ingredients
Caplet	Acetaminophen 650 mg in each caplet	Carnauba wax, corn starch, FD&C red #40, hydroxyethyl cellulose, hypromellose, magnesium stearate, microcrystalline cellulose, providone, powdered cellulose, pregelatinized starch, sodium starch, glycolate, sucralose, triacetin

WARNINGS
Liver warning: This product contains acetaminophen. Severe liver damage may occur if you take
- more than 6 caplets in 24 hours, which is the maximum daily amount
- with other drugs containing acetaminophen
- 3 or more alcoholic drinks every day while using this product

DO NOT USE
- with any other drug containing acetaminophen (prescription or nonprescription). If you are not sure whether a drug contains acetaminophen, ask a doctor or pharmacist
- if you are allergic to acetaminophen or any of the inactive ingredients in this product

ASK A DOCTOR BEFORE USE IF YOU HAVE
liver disease.

ASK A DOCTOR OR PHARMACIST BEFORE USE IF YOU ARE
taking the blood thinning drug warfarin.

STOP USE AND ASK A DOCTOR IF:
- Pain gets worse or lasts more than 10 days.
- Fever gets worse or lasts more than 3 days.
- New symptoms occur.
- Redness or swelling is present.

These could be signs of a serious condition.
If pregnant or breast-feeding, ask a health professional before use.
Keep out of reach of children.

OVERDOSE WARNING
In case of overdose, get medical help or contact a Poison Control Center right away. (1-800-222-1222). Quick medical attention is critical for adults as well as for children even if you do not notice any signs or symptoms.

OTHER INFORMATION
- Store at 20-25°C (68-77°F). Avoid excessive heat 40°C (104°F).

QUESTIONS OR COMMENTS?
Call **1-877-895-3665** (toll-free) or **215-273-8755** (collect)

TYLENOL ARTHRITIS PAIN (acetaminophen)

McNeil Consumer Healthcare Div McNeil-PPC, Inc

DRUG FACTS

Active Ingredient(s) (in each caplet)	Purpose(s)
Acetaminophen 650 mg	Pain reliever/fever reducer

USES
- temporarily relieves minor aches and pains due to:
  - arthritis
  - the common cold
  - headache
  - toothache
  - muscular aches
  - backache
  - menstrual cramps
- temporarily reduces fever

WARNINGS
Liver warning
This product contains acetaminophen. Severe liver damage may occur if you take
- more than 6 caplets in 24 hours, which is the maximum daily amount
- with other drugs containing acetaminophen
- 3 or more alcoholic drinks every day while using this product

DO NOT USE
with any other drug containing acetaminophen (prescription or nonprescription). If you are not sure whether a drug contains acetaminophen, ask a doctor or pharmacist.

ASK A DOCTOR BEFORE USE IF YOU HAVE
liver disease

ASK A DOCTOR OR PHARMACIST BEFORE USE IF YOU ARE
taking the blood thinning drug warfarin

STOP USE AND ASK A DOCTOR IF
• pain gets worse or lasts more than 10 days
• fever gets worse or lasts more than 3 days
• new symptoms occur
• redness or swelling is present

These could be signs of a serious condition.
If pregnant or breast-feeding, ask a health professional before use.
Keep out of reach of children.

OVERDOSE WARNING
Taking more than the recommended dose (overdose) may cause liver damage. In case of overdose, get medical help or contact a Poison Control Center right away. (1-800-222-1222) Quick medical attention is critical for adults as well as for children even if you do not notice any signs or symptoms.

DIRECTIONS
• **do not take more than directed (see overdose warning)**

adults	take 2 caplets every 8 hours with water swallow whole - do not crush, chew or dissolve do not take more than 6 caplets in 24 hours do not use for more than 10 days unless directed by a doctor
under 18 years of age	ask a doctor

OTHER INFORMATION
• store at 20-25°C (68-77°F). Avoid excessive heat 40°C (104°F).
• **do not use if carton is opened or neck wrap or foil inner seal imprinted with "Safety Seal®" is broken**
• see end panel for lot number and expiration date

INACTIVE INGREDIENTS
carnauba wax, corn starch, hydroxyethyl cellulose, hypromellose, magnesium stearate, microcrystalline cellulose, povidone, powdered cellulose, pregelatinized starch, sodium starch glycolate, titanium dioxide, triacetin

QUESTIONS OR COMMENTS?
call 1-877-895-3665 (English) or 1-888-466-8746 (Spanish)

TYLENOL COLD MULTI-SYMPTOM DAYTIME (acetaminophen, dextromethorphan hydrobromide, and phenylephrine hydrochloride)
McNeil Consumer Healthcare Div. McNeil-PPC, Inc

DRUG FACTS

Active Ingredient(s) (in each 15 mL = 1 tablespoon)	Purpose(s)
Acetaminophen 325 mg	Pain reliever/fever reducer
Dextromethorphan HBr 10 mg	Cough suppressant
Phenylephrine HCl 5 mg	Nasal decongestant

USES
• temporarily relieves these common cold/flu symptoms:
  • minor aches and pains
  • headache
  • sore throat
  • nasal congestion
  • cough
• sinus congestion and pressure
• helps clear nasal passages
• promotes nasal and sinus drainage
• temporarily reduces fever

WARNINGS
Liver warning
This product contains acetaminophen. Severe liver damage may occur if you take
• more than 12 tablespoons in 24 hours, which is the maximum daily amount
• with other drugs containing acetaminophen
• 3 or more alcoholic drinks every day while using this product

Sore throat warning
If sore throat is severe, persists for more than 2 days, is accompanied or followed by fever, headache, rash, nausea, or vomiting, consult a doctor promptly.

DO NOT USE
• with any other drug containing acetaminophen (prescription or nonprescription). If you are not sure whether a drug contains acetaminophen, ask a doctor or pharmacist.
• if you are now taking a prescription monoamine oxidase inhibitor (MAOI) (certain drugs for depression, psychiatric or emotional conditions, or Parkinson's disease), or for 2 weeks after stopping the MAOI drug. If you do not know if your prescription drug contains an MAOI, ask a doctor or pharmacist before taking this product.
• if you have ever had an allergic reaction to this product or any of its ingredients

ASK A DOCTOR BEFORE USE IF YOU HAVE
• liver disease
• heart disease
• high blood pressure
• thyroid disease
• diabetes
• trouble urinating due to an enlarged prostate gland
• persistent or chronic cough such as occurs with smoking, asthma or emphysema
• cough that occurs with too much phlegm (mucus)

ASK A DOCTOR OR PHARMACIST BEFORE USE IF YOU ARE
taking the blood thinning drug warfarin

WHEN USING THIS PRODUCT
do not exceed recommended dosage

STOP USE AND ASK A DOCTOR IF
• nervousness, dizziness, or sleeplessness occur
• pain, nasal congestion or cough gets worse or lasts more than 7 days
• fever gets worse or lasts more than 3 days
• redness or swelling is present
• new symptoms occur
• cough comes back or occurs with rash or headache that lasts

These could be signs of a serious condition.
If pregnant or breast-feeding, ask a health professional before use.
Keep out of reach of children.

OVERDOSE WARNING
Taking more than the recommended dose (overdose) may cause liver damage. In case of overdose, get medical help or contact a Poison Control Center right away. (1-800-222-1222) Quick medical attention is critical for adults as well as for children even if you do not notice any signs or symptoms.

DIRECTIONS
- **do not take more than directed (see overdose warning)**
- use only enclosed dosing cup designed for use with this product. Do not use any other dosing device.

adults and children 12 years and over	take 2 tablespoons (TBSP) or 30 mL in dose cup provided every 4 hours do not take more than 12 tablespoons (TBSP) or 180 mL in 24 hours
children under 12 years	ask a doctor

OTHER INFORMATION
- **each tablespoon contains:** sodium 5 mg
- store between 20-25°C (68-77°F). Do not refrigerate.
- **tamper evident statement**
- see back label for lot number and expiration date

INACTIVE INGREDIENTS
alcohol, anhydrous citric acid, FD&C yellow #6, flavors, glycerin, propylene glycol, purified water, sodium benzoate, sorbitol solution, sucralose

QUESTIONS OR COMMENTS?
call **1-877-895-3665**

TYLENOL COLD MULTI-SYMPTOM NIGHTTIME (acetaminophen, dextromethorphan hydrobromide, doxylamine succinate, and phenylephrine hydrochloride)

McNeil Consumer Healthcare Div McNeil-PPC, Inc

DRUG FACTS

Active Ingredient(s) (in each 15 mL = 1 tablespoon)	Purpose(s)
Acetaminophen 325 mg	Pain reliever/fever reducer
Dextromethorphan HBr 10 mg	Cough suppressant
Doxylamine succinate 6.25 mg	Antihistamine
Phenylephrine HCl 5 mg	Nasal decongestant

USES
- temporarily relieves these common cold/flu symptoms:
  - minor aches and pains
  - headache
  - sore throat
  - nasal congestion
  - runny nose and sneezing
  - cough
  - sinus congestion and pressure
- helps clear nasal passages
- relieves cough to help you sleep
- temporarily reduces fever

WARNINGS
Liver warning
This product contains acetaminophen. Severe liver damage may occur if you take
- more than 12 tablespoons in 24 hours, which is the maximum daily amount
- with other drugs containing acetaminophen
- 3 or more alcoholic drinks every day while using this product

Sore throat warning
If sore throat is severe, persists for more than 2 days, is accompanied or followed by fever, headache, rash, nausea, or vomiting, consult a doctor promptly.

DO NOT USE
- with any other drug containing acetaminophen (prescription or nonprescription). If you are not sure whether a drug contains acetaminophen, ask a doctor or pharmacist.
- if you are now taking a prescription monoamine oxidase inhibitor (MAOI) (certain drugs for depression, psychiatric or emotional conditions, or Parkinson's disease), or for 2 weeks after stopping the MAOI drug. If you do not know if your prescription drug contains an MAOI, ask a doctor or pharmacist before taking this product.
- if you have ever had an allergic reaction to this product or any of its ingredients

ASK A DOCTOR BEFORE USE IF YOU HAVE
- liver disease
- heart disease
- high blood pressure
- thyroid disease
- diabetes
- trouble urinating due to an enlarged prostate gland
- a breathing problem such as emphysema or chronic bronchitis
- glaucoma
- persistent or chronic cough such as occurs with smoking, asthma or emphysema
- cough that occurs with too much phlegm (mucus)

ASK A DOCTOR OR PHARMACIST BEFORE USE IF YOU ARE
- taking the blood thinning drug warfarin
- taking sedatives or tranquilizers

WHEN USING THIS PRODUCT
- **do not exceed recommended dosage**
- excitability may occur, especially in children
- marked drowsiness may occur
- alcohol, sedatives and tranquilizers may increase drowsiness
- avoid alcoholic drinks
- be careful when driving a motor vehicle or operating machinery

STOP USE AND ASK A DOCTOR IF
- nervousness, dizziness, or sleeplessness occur
- pain, nasal congestion or cough gets worse or lasts more than 7 days
- fever gets worse or lasts more than 3 days
- redness or swelling is present
- new symptoms occur
- cough comes back or occurs with rash or headache that lasts

These could be signs of a serious condition.
If pregnant or breast-feeding, ask a health professional before use.
Keep out of reach of children.

OVERDOSE WARNING
Taking more than the recommended dose (overdose) may cause liver damage. In case of overdose, get medical help or contact a Poison Control Center right away. (1-800-222-1222) Quick medical attention is critical for adults as well as for children even if you do not notice any signs or symptoms.

DIRECTIONS
- **do not take more than directed (see overdose warning)**
- use only enclosed dosing cup designed for use with this product. Do not use any other dosing device.

adults and children 12 years and over	take 2 tablespoons (tbsp) or 30 mL in dose cup provided every 4 hours do not take more than 12 tablespoons (tbsp) or 180 mL in 24 hours
children under 12 years	do not use this adult product in children under 12 years of age; this will provide more than the recommended dose (overdose) and may cause liver damage

OTHER INFORMATION
- each tablespoon contains: **sodium 5 mg**
- store between 20-25°C (68-77°F). Do not refrigerate.
- **do not use if plastic neck wrap or foil inner seal imprinted with "Safety Seal®" is broken or missing**
- see back label for lot number and expiration date

INACTIVE INGREDIENTS
anhydrous citric acid, ethyl alcohol, FD&C blue #1, flavor, glycerin, propylene glycol, purified water, sodium benzoate, sorbitol solution, sucralose

QUESTIONS OR COMMENTS?
call **1-877-895-3665**

TYLENOL COLD MULTI-SYMPTOM SEVERE
(acetaminophen, dextromethorphan hydrobromide, guaifenesin, and phenylephrine hydrochloride)
McNeil Consumer Healthcare Div McNeil-PPC, Inc

DRUG FACTS

Active Ingredient(s) (in each 15 mL = 1 tablespoon)	Purpose(s)
Acetaminophen 325 mg	Pain reliever/fever reducer
Dextromethorphan HBr 10 mg	Cough suppressant
Guaifenesin 200 mg	Expectorant
Phenylephrine HCl 5 mg	Nasal decongestant

USES
- for the temporary relief of the following cold/flu symptoms:
  - minor aches and pains
  - headache
  - sore throat
  - nasal congestion
  - cough
- helps loosen phlegm (mucus) and thin bronchial secretions to make coughs more productive
- temporarily reduces fever

WARNINGS
Liver warning
This product contains acetaminophen. Severe liver damage may occur if you take
- more than 12 tablespoons in 24 hours, which is the maximum daily amount
- with other drugs containing acetaminophen
- 3 or more alcoholic drinks every day while using this product

Sore throat warning
If sore throat is severe, persists for more than 2 days, is accompanied or followed by fever, headache, rash, nausea or vomiting, consult a doctor promptly.

DO NOT USE
- with any other drug containing acetaminophen (prescription or nonprescription). If you are not sure whether a drug contains acetaminophen, ask a doctor or pharmacist.
- if you are now taking a prescription monoamine oxidase inhibitor (MAOI) (certain drugs for depression, psychiatric or emotional conditions, or Parkinson's disease), or for 2 weeks after stopping the MAOI drug. If you do not know if your prescription drug contains an MAOI, ask a doctor or pharmacist before taking this product.
- if you have ever had an allergic reaction to this product or any of its ingredients

ASK A DOCTOR BEFORE USE IF YOU HAVE
- liver disease
- heart disease
- high blood pressure
- thyroid disease
- diabetes
- trouble urinating due to an enlarged prostate gland
- persistent or chronic cough such as occurs with smoking, asthma, chronic bronchitis, or emphysema
- cough that occurs with too much phlegm (mucus)

ASK A DOCTOR OR PHARMACIST BEFORE USE IF YOU ARE
taking the blood thinning drug warfarin

WHEN USING THIS PRODUCT
do not exceed recommended dosage

STOP USE AND ASK A DOCTOR IF
- nervousness, dizziness, or sleeplessness occur
- pain, nasal congestion or cough gets worse or lasts more than 7 days
- fever gets worse or lasts more than 3 days
- redness or swelling is present
- new symptoms occur
- cough comes back or occurs with rash or headache that lasts

These could be signs of a serious condition.
If pregnant or breast-feeding, ask a health professional before use.
Keep out of reach of children.

OVERDOSE WARNING
Taking more than the recommended dose (overdose) may cause liver damage. In case of overdose, get medical help or contact a Poison Control Center right away. (1-800-222-1222) Quick medical attention is critical for adults as well as for children even if you do not notice any signs or symptoms.

DIRECTIONS
- **do not take more than directed (see overdose warning)**
- use only enclosed dosing cup designed for use with this product. Do not use any other dosing device.

adults and children 12 years and over	take 2 tablespoons (TBSP) or 30 mL in dose cup provided every 4 hours do not take more than 12 tablespoons (TBSP) or 180 mL in 24 hours
children under 12 years	ask a doctor

OTHER INFORMATION
- **each tablespoon contains:** sodium 5 mg
- store between 20-25°C (68-77°F). Do not refrigerate.
- **do not use if plastic neck wrap or foil inner seal imprinted with "SAFETY SEAL®" is broken or missing**
- see back label for lot number and expiration date

INACTIVE INGREDIENTS
alcohol, anhydrous citric acid, FD&C blue #1, flavor, glycerin, propylene glycol, purified water, sodium benzoate, sorbitol solution, sucralose

QUESTIONS OR COMMENTS?
call 1-877-895-3665

TYLENOL EXTRA STRENGTH (acetaminophen)
McNeil Consumer Healthcare Div. McNeil-PPC, Inc

DRUG FACTS

Active Ingredient(s) (in each tablet)
Acetaminophen 500 mg

Purpose(s)
Pain reliever/fever reducer

USES
- temporarily relieves minor aches and pains due to:
  - headache
  - muscular aches
  - backache
  - minor pain of arthritis
  - the common cold
  - toothache
  - premenstrual and menstrual cramps
- temporarily reduces fever

WARNINGS
Liver warning
This product contains acetaminophen. Severe liver damage may occur if you take
- more than 8 tablets in 24 hours, which is the maximum daily amount
- with other drugs containing acetaminophen
- 3 or more alcoholic drinks every day while using this product

DO NOT USE
- with any other drug containing acetaminophen (prescription or nonprescription). If you are not sure whether a drug contains acetaminophen, ask a doctor or pharmacist.
- if you are allergic to acetaminophen or any of the inactive ingredients in this product

ASK A DOCTOR BEFORE USE IF YOU HAVE
liver disease

ASK A DOCTOR OR PHARMACIST BEFORE USE IF YOU ARE
taking the blood thinning drug warfarin

STOP USE AND ASK A DOCTOR IF
- pain gets worse or lasts more than 10 days
- fever gets worse or lasts more than 3 days
- new symptoms occur
- redness or swelling is present

These could be signs of a serious condition.
If pregnant or breast-feeding, ask a health professional before use.

Keep out of reach of children.

OVERDOSE WARNING
Taking more than the recommended dose (overdose) may cause liver damage. In case of overdose, get medical help or contact a Poison Control Center right away. (1-800-222-1222) Quick medical attention is critical for adults as well as for children even if you do not notice any signs or symptoms.

DIRECTIONS
- **do not take more than directed (see overdose warning)**

adults and children 12 years and over	take 2 tablets every 4 to 6 hours while symptoms last if needed, tablets may be crushed and should be taken immediately. Take the entire dose for best result. Crushing the tablets will result in a bitter taste. do not take more than 8 tablets in 24 hours do not use for more than 10 days unless directed by a doctor
children under 12 years	do not use this adult product in children under 12 years of age; this will provide more than the recommended dose (overdose) and may cause liver damage

OTHER INFORMATION
- store between 20-25°C (68-77°F)
- **do not use if carton is opened or neck wrap or foil inner seal imprinted with "Safety Seal®" is broken or missing**
- see end panel for lot number and expiration date

INACTIVE INGREDIENTS
corn starch, magnesium stearate, powdered cellulose, pregelatinized starch, sodium starch glycolate

QUESTIONS OR COMMENTS?
call 1-877-895-3665

TYLENOL PM EXTRA STRENGTH
(acetaminophen and diphenhydramine hydrochloride)
McNeil Consumer Healthcare Div McNeil-PPC, Inc

DRUG FACTS

Active Ingredient(s) (in each gelcap)	Purpose(s)
Acetaminophen 500 mg	Pain reliever
Diphenhydramine HCl 25 mg	Nighttime sleep aid

USES
temporary relief of occasional headaches and minor aches and pains with accompanying sleeplessness

WARNINGS
Liver warning
This product contains acetaminophen. Severe liver damage may occur if you take
- more than 4,000 mg of acetaminophen in 24 hours
- with other drugs containing acetaminophen
- 3 or more alcoholic drinks every day while using this product

DO NOT USE
- with any other drug containing acetaminophen (prescription or nonprescription). If you are not sure whether a drug contains acetaminophen, ask a doctor or pharmacist.
- with any other product containing diphenhydramine, even one used on skin

- in children under 12 years of age
- if you have ever had an allergic reaction to this product or any of its ingredients

ASK A DOCTOR BEFORE USE IF YOU HAVE
- liver disease
- a breathing problem such as emphysema or chronic bronchitis
- trouble urinating due to an enlarged prostate gland
- glaucoma

ASK A DOCTOR OR PHARMACIST BEFORE USE IF YOU ARE
- taking the blood thinning drug warfarin
- taking sedatives or tranquilizers

WHEN USING THIS PRODUCT
- drowsiness will occur
- avoid alcoholic drinks
- do not drive a motor vehicle or operate machinery

STOP USE AND ASK A DOCTOR IF
- sleeplessness persists continuously for more than 2 weeks. Insomnia may be a symptom of serious underlying medical illness.
- pain gets worse or lasts more than 10 days
- fever gets worse or lasts more than 3 days
- redness or swelling is present
- new symptoms occur

These could be signs of a serious condition.
If pregnant or breast-feeding, ask a health professional before use.
Keep out of reach of children.

OVERDOSE WARNING
Taking more than the recommended dose (overdose) may cause liver damage. In case of overdose, get medical help or contact a Poison Control Center right away. (1-800-222-1222) Quick medical attention is critical for adults as well as for children even if you do not notice any signs or symptoms.

DIRECTIONS
- **do not take more than directed (see overdose warning)**

| adults and children 12 years and over | take 2 gelcaps at bedtime do not take more than 2 gelcaps of this product in 24 hours |
| children under 12 years | do not use this adult product in children under 12 years of age; this will provide more than the recommended dose (overdose) and may cause liver damage |

OTHER INFORMATION
- store between 20-25°C (68-77°F). Avoid high humidity.
- **do not use if carton is opened or neck wrap or foil inner seal imprinted with "Safety Seal®" is broken or missing**
- see end panel for lot number and expiration date

INACTIVE INGREDIENTS
benzyl alcohol, black iron oxide, butylparaben, carboxymethylcellulose sodium, crospovidone, D&C red #28, edetate calcium disodium, FD&C blue #1, FD&C red #40, gelatin, hypromellose, magnesium stearate, methylparaben, microcrystalline cellulose, polyethylene glycol, polysorbate 80, powdered cellulose, pregelatinized starch, propylene glycol, propylparaben, red iron oxide, sodium citrate, sodium lauryl sulfate, sodium propionate, sodium starch glycolate, titanium dioxide, yellow iron oxide

QUESTIONS OR COMMENTS?
call 1-877-895-3665

TYLENOL PM SIMPLY SLEEP (diphenhydramine hydrochloride)
McNeil Consumer Healthcare Div. McNeil-PPC, Inc.

DRUG FACTS

Active ingredient(s) (in each caplet)	Purpose(s)
Diphenhydramine HCl 25 mg	Nighttime sleep aid

USES
for relief of occasional sleeplessness

DO NOT USE
- in children under 12 years of age
- with any other products containing diphenhydramine, even one used on skin

ASK A DOCTOR BEFORE USE IF YOU HAVE
- a breathing problem such as emphysema or chronic bronchitis
- glaucoma
- trouble urinating due to an enlarged prostate gland

ASK A DOCTOR OR PHARMACIST BEFORE USE IF YOU ARE
- taking sedatives or tranquilizers

WHEN USING THIS PRODUCT
- avoid alcoholic drinks
- drowsiness will occur
- do not drive a motor vehicle or operate machinery

STOP USE AND ASK A DOCTOR IF
- sleeplessness persists continuously for more than 2 weeks. Insomnia may be a symptom of a serious underlying medical illness.

If pregnant or breast-feeding, ask a health professional before use.
Keep out of reach of children.

OVERDOSE WARNING
In the case of overdose, get medical help or contact a Poison Control Center right away. (1-800-222-1222)

DIRECTIONS

| adults and children 12 years and over | take 2 caplets at bedtime if needed, or as directed by a doctor |
| children under 12 years | do not use |

OTHER INFORMATION
- **each caplet contains:** calcium 14 mg
- store between 20-25°C (68-77°F). Avoid high humidity. Protect from light.
- **do not use if carton is opened or carton tape and foil inner seal imprinted with "SAFETY SEAL®" are broken or missing**

INACTIVE INGREDIENTS
carnauba wax, croscarmellose sodium, dibasic calcium phosphate, FD&C blue no. 1 aluminum lake, hypromellose,

magnesium stearate, microcrystalline cellulose, polyethylene glycol, polysorbate 80, titanium dioxide

QUESTIONS OR COMMENTS?
call **1-877-895-3665** (toll-free) or **215-273-8755** (collect)

TYLENOL REGULAR STRENGTH

(acetaminophen)

McNeil Consumer Healthcare Div. McNeil-PPC, Inc

DRUG FACTS

Active Ingredient(s) (in each tablet)
Acetaminophen 325 mg

Purpose(s)
Pain reliever/fever reducer

USES
• temporarily relieves minor aches and pains due to:
  • headache
  • muscular aches
  • backache
  • minor pain of arthritis
  • the common cold
  • toothache
  • premenstrual and menstrual cramps
• temporarily reduces fever

WARNINGS
Liver warning
This product contains acetaminophen. The maximum daily dose of this product is 10 tablets (3,250 mg) in 24 hours for adults or 5 tablets (1,625 mg) in 24 hours for children. Severe liver damage may occur if
• adult takes more than 4,000 mg of acetaminophen in 24 hours
• child takes more than 5 doses in 24 hours, which is the maximum daily amount
• taken with other drugs containing acetaminophen
• adult has 3 or more alcoholic drinks every day while using this product

DO NOT USE
• with any other drug containing acetaminophen (prescription or nonprescription). If you are not sure whether a drug contains acetaminophen, ask a doctor or pharmacist.
• if you are allergic to acetaminophen or any of the inactive ingredients in this product

ASK A DOCTOR BEFORE USE IF THE USER HAS
liver disease

ASK A DOCTOR OR PHARMACIST BEFORE USE IF THE USER IS
taking the blood thinning drug warfarin

STOP USE AND ASK A DOCTOR IF
• pain gets worse or lasts more than 10 days in adults
• pain gets worse or lasts more than 5 days in children under 12 years
• fever gets worse or lasts more than 3 days
• new symptoms occur
• redness or swelling is present

These could be signs of a serious condition.
If pregnant or breast-feeding, ask a health professional before use.
Keep out of reach of children.

OVERDOSE WARNING
Taking more than the recommended dose (overdose) may cause liver damage. In case of overdose, get medical help or contact a Poison Control Center right away. (1-800-222-1222) Quick medical attention is critical for adults as well as for children even if you do not notice any signs or symptoms.

DIRECTIONS
• do not take more than directed (see overdose warning)

adults and children 12 years and over	take 2 tablets every 4 to 6 hours while symptoms last do not take more than 10 tablets in 24 hours do not use for more than 10 days unless directed by a doctor
children 6-11 years	take 1 tablet every 4 to 6 hours while symptoms last do not take more than 5 tablets in 24 hours do not use for more than 5 days unless directed by a doctor
children under 6 years	ask a doctor

OTHER INFORMATION
• store between 20-25°C (68-77°F)
• **do not use if carton is opened or neck wrap or foil inner seal imprinted with "SAFETY SEAL®" is broken or missing**

INACTIVE INGREDIENTS
corn starch, magnesium stearate, powdered cellulose, pregelatinized starch, sodium starch glycolate

QUESTIONS OR COMMENTS?
call **1-877-895-3665** (toll-free) or **215-273-8755** (collect)

TYLENOL SINUS CONGESTION AND PAIN DAYTIME (acetaminophen and phenylephrine hydrochloride)

McNeil Consumer Healthcare Div. McNeil-PPC, Inc

DRUG FACTS

Active Ingredient(s) (in each caplet)	Purpose(s)
Acetaminophen 325 mg	Pain reliever/fever reducer
Phenylephrine HCl 5 mg	Nasal decongestant

USES
• temporarily relieves these symptoms associated with hay fever or other respiratory allergies, and the common cold:
  • headache
  • sinus congestion and pressure
  • nasal congestion
  • minor aches and pains
• helps decongest sinus openings and passages
• promotes sinus drainage
• helps clear nasal passages
• temporarily reduces fever

WARNINGS
Liver warning
This product contains acetaminophen. The maximum daily dose of this product is 10 caplets (3,250 mg acetaminophen) in 24 hours. Severe liver damage may occur if you take
- more than 4,000 mg of acetaminophen in 24 hours
- with other drugs containing acetaminophen
- 3 or more alcoholic drinks every day while using this product

DO NOT USE
- with any other drug containing acetaminophen (prescription or nonprescription). If you are not sure whether a drug contains acetaminophen, ask a doctor or pharmacist.
- if you are now taking a prescription monoamine oxidase inhibitor (MAOI) (certain drugs for depression, psychiatric or emotional conditions, or Parkinson's disease), or for 2 weeks after stopping the MAOI drug. If you do not know if your prescription drug contains an MAOI, ask a doctor or pharmacist before taking this product.
- if you have ever had an allergic reaction to this product or any of its ingredients

ASK A DOCTOR BEFORE USE IF YOU HAVE
- liver disease
- heart disease
- high blood pressure
- thyroid disease
- diabetes
- trouble urinating due to an enlarged prostate gland

ASK A DOCTOR OR PHARMACIST BEFORE USE IF YOU ARE
taking the blood thinning drug warfarin

WHEN USING THIS PRODUCT
do not exceed recommended dose

STOP USE AND ASK A DOCTOR IF
- nervousness, dizziness, or sleeplessness occur
- pain or nasal congestion gets worse or lasts more than 7 days
- fever gets worse or lasts more than 3 days
- redness or swelling is present
- new symptoms occur

These could be signs of a serious condition.
If pregnant or breast-feeding, ask a health professional before use.
Keep out of reach of children.

OVERDOSE WARNING
In case of overdose, get medical help or contact a Poison Control Center right away. (1-800-222-1222) Quick medical attention is critical for adults as well as for children even if you do not notice any signs or symptoms.

DIRECTIONS
- **do not take more than directed (see overdose warning)**

adults and children 12 years and over	take 2 caplets every 4 hours swallow whole; do not crush, chew or dissolve do not take more than 10 caplets in 24 hours
children under 12 years	ask a doctor

OTHER INFORMATION
- store between 20-25°C (68-77°F)
- **do not use if carton is opened or if blister unit is broken**

INACTIVE INGREDIENTS
anhydrous citric acid, carnauba wax, corn starch, D&C yellow no. 10 aluminum lake, FD&C blue no. 1 aluminum lake, FD&C red no. 40 aluminum lake, flavors, hypromellose, magnesium stearate, microcrystalline cellulose, polyethylene glycol, polysorbate 80, potassium sorbate, powdered cellulose, pregelatinized starch, sodium benzoate, sodium citrate, sodium starch glycolate, sucralose, titanium dioxide

QUESTIONS OR COMMENTS?
call **1-877-895-3665** (toll-free) or **215-273-8755** (collect)

TYLENOL SINUS CONGESTION AND PAIN SEVERE (acetaminophen, guaifenesin, and phenylephrine hydrochloride)
McNeil Consumer Healthcare Div. McNeil-PPC, Inc

DRUG FACTS

Active Ingredient(s) (in each caplet)	Purpose(s)
Acetaminophen 325 mg	Pain reliever/fever reducer
Guaifenesin 200 mg	Expectorant
Phenylephrine HCl 5 mg	Nasal decongestant

USES
- temporarily relieves these symptoms associated with hay fever or other respiratory allergies, and the common cold:
  - sinus congestion and pressure
  - headache
  - nasal congestion
  - minor aches and pains
- helps loosen phlegm (mucus) and thin bronchial secretions to make coughs more productive
- temporarily reduces fever

WARNINGS
Liver warning
This product contains acetaminophen. The maximum daily dose of this product is 10 caplets (3,250 mg acetaminophen) in 24 hours. Severe liver damage may occur if you take
- more than 4,000 mg of acetaminophen in 24 hours
- with other drugs containing acetaminophen
- 3 or more alcoholic drinks every day while using this product

DO NOT USE
- with any other drug containing acetaminophen (prescription or nonprescription). If you are not sure whether a drug contains acetaminophen, ask a doctor or pharmacist.
- if you are now taking a prescription monoamine oxidase inhibitor (MAOI) (certain drugs for depression, psychiatric or emotional conditions, or Parkinson's disease), or for 2 weeks after stopping the MAOI drug. If you do not know if your prescription drug contains an MAOI, ask a doctor or pharmacist before taking this product.
- if you have ever had an allergic reaction to this product or any of its ingredients

ASK A DOCTOR BEFORE USE IF YOU HAVE
- liver disease
- heart disease
- high blood pressure
- thyroid disease
- diabetes
- trouble urinating due to an enlarged prostate gland
- persistent or chronic cough such as occurs with smoking, asthma, chronic bronchitis, or emphysema
- cough that occurs with too much phlegm (mucus)

ASK A DOCTOR OR PHARMACIST BEFORE USE IF YOU ARE
taking the blood thinning drug warfarin

WHEN USING THIS PRODUCT
do not exceed recommended dose

STOP USE AND ASK A DOCTOR IF
- nervousness, dizziness, or sleeplessness occur
- pain, nasal congestion or cough gets worse or lasts more than 7 days
- fever gets worse or lasts more than 3 days
- redness or swelling is present
- new symptoms occur
- cough comes back or occurs with rash or headache that lasts

These could be signs of a serious condition.

If pregnant or breast-feeding, ask a health professional before use.

Keep out of reach of children.

OVERDOSE WARNING
In case of overdose, get medical help or contact a Poison Control Center right away. (1-800-222-1222) Quick medical attention is critical for adults as well as for children even if you do not notice any signs or symptoms.

DIRECTIONS
- **do not take more than directed (see overdose warning)**

adults and children 12 years and over	• take 2 caplets every 4 hours • swallow whole - do not crush, chew or dissolve • do not take more than 10 caplets in 24 hours
children under 12 years	ask a doctor

OTHER INFORMATION
- **each caplet contains:** sodium 3 mg
- store between 20-25°C (68-77°F)
- **do not use if carton is opened or if blister unit is broken**

INACTIVE INGREDIENTS
carnauba wax, croscarmellose sodium, flavor, hydroxypropyl cellulose, hypromellose, magnesium stearate, microcrystalline cellulose, pregelatinized starch, sucralose, titanium dioxide, triacetin

QUESTIONS OR COMMENTS?
call **1-877-895-3665** (toll-free) or **215-273-8755** (collect)

UNISOM PM PAIN NIGHTTIME SLEEP-AID PLUS PAIN RELIEVER (acetaminophen and diphenhydramine hydrochloride)

Chattem, Inc.

DRUG FACTS

Active Ingredient(s)
(in each caplet)
Acetaminophen 325 mg

Purpose(s)
Pain reliever

Active Ingredient(s)
(in each caplet)
Diphenhydramine HCl 50 mg

Purpose(s)
Nighttime sleep-aid

USES
- for the temporary relief of occasional headaches and minor aches and pains with accompanying sleeplessness

WARNINGS
Liver warning:
This product contains acetaminophen. Severe liver damage may occur if you take
- more than 4,000 mg of acetaminophen in 24 hours
- with other drugs containing acetaminophen
- 3 or more alcoholic drinks every day while using this product

DO NOT USE
- with any other drug containing acetaminophen (prescription or nonprescription). If you are not sure whether a drug contains acetaminophen, ask a doctor or pharmacist.
- in children under 12 years of age
- with any other product containing diphenhydramine, even one used on skin
- if you have ever had an allergic reaction to this product or any of its ingredients

ASK A DOCTOR BEFORE USE IF YOU HAVE
- liver disease
- a breathing problem such as emphysema or chronic bronchitis
- trouble urinating due to an enlarged prostate gland
- glaucoma

ASK A DOCTOR OR PHARMACIST BEFORE USE IF YOU ARE
- taking the blood thinning drug warfarin
- taking sedatives or tranquilizers

WHEN USING THIS PRODUCT
- drowsiness will occur
- avoid alcoholic drinks
- do not drive a motor vehicle or operate machinery

STOP USE AND ASK A DOCTOR IF
- sleeplessness persists continuously for more than 2 weeks. Insomnia may be a symptom of serious medical illness.
- pain gets worse or lasts for more than 10 days
- fever gets worse or lasts for more than 3 days
- redness or swelling is present
- new symptoms occur

These could be signs of a serious condition.

If pregnant or breast-feeding,
ask a health professional before use.

Keep out of reach of children.

OVERDOSE WARNING
Taking more than the recommended dose (overdose) may cause liver damage. In case of overdose, get medical help or contact a Poison Control Center right away. Quick medical attention is critical for adults as well as for children even if you do not notice any signs or symptoms.

DIRECTIONS
- **do not take more than directed (see overdose warning)**
adults and children 12 years and older: • take 1 caplet at bedtime
- do not take more than 1 caplet of this product in 24 hours
children under 12 years: do not use this adult product in children under 12 years of age, this will provide more than the recommended dose (overdose) and may cause liver damage

INACTIVE INGREDIENTS
blue 1 lake, croscarmellose sodium, dicalcium phosphate, hydroxypropylcellulose, hypromellose, magnesium silicate,

magnesium stearate, microcrystalline cellulose, mineral oil, pregelatinized corn starch, PVP, silica, sodium carboxymethyl starch, stearic acid (283-056)

UNISOM SLEEPGELS (diphenhydramine hydrochloride)

Chattem, Inc.

DRUG FACTS

Active Ingredient(s) (in each softgel): Diphenhydramine HCl 50 mg

Purpose(s)
Nighttime sleep-aid

USE
For relief of occasional sleeplessness

WARNINGS

DO NOT USE
- *For children under 12 years of age*
- *With any other product containing diphenhydramine, even one used on skin*

ASK A DOCTOR BEFORE USE IF YOU HAVE
- *A breathing problem such as emphysema or chronic bronchitis*
- *Glaucoma*
- *Trouble urinating due to an enlarged prostate gland*

ASK A DOCTOR OR PHARMACIST BEFORE USE IF YOU ARE
- *Taking sedatives or tranquilizers*

WHEN USING THIS PRODUCT
- *Avoid alcoholic drinks*

STOP USE AND ASK DOCTOR IF
Sleeplessness persists continuously for more than 2 weeks. Insomnia may be a symptom of serious underlying medical illness.
If pregnant or breast-feeding, *ask a health professional before use.*
Keep out of reach of children.
In case of overdose, get medical help or contact a Poison Control Center right away.

DIRECTIONS
Adults and children 12 years of age and over: 1 softgel (50 mg) at bedtime if needed, or as directed by a doctor.

INACTIVE INGREDIENTS
blue 1, gelatin, glycerin, polyethylene glycol, polyvinyl acetate phthalate, propylene glycol, sorbitol, titanium dioxide and water.

UNISOM SLEEPMELTS (diphenhydramine hydrochloride)

Chattem, Inc.

DRUG FACTS

Active Ingredient(s)
(in each caplet)
Diphenhydramine HCl 25 mg

Purpose(s)
Nighttime sleep-aid

USES
- for relief of occasional sleeplessness

WARNINGS

DO NOT USE
- for children under 12 years of age
- with any other product containing diphenhydramine, even one used on skin

ASK A DOCTOR BEFORE USE IF YOU HAVE
- a breathing problem such as emphysema or chronic bronchitis
- glaucoma
- trouble urinating due to an enlarged prostate gland

ASK A DOCTOR OR PHARMACIST BEFORE USE IF YOU ARE
taking sedatives or tranquilizers

WHEN USING THIS PRODUCT
avoid alcoholic drinks

STOP USE AND ASK A DOCTOR IF
sleeplessness persists continuously for more than 2 weeks. Insomnia may be a symptom of serious underlying medical illness.

If pregnant or breast-feeding,
ask a health professional before use.

Keep out of reach of children.
In case of overdose, get medical help or contact a Poison Control Center right away.

DIRECTIONS
- adults and children 12 years of age and over: 2 sleep melts (25 mg each) at bedtime if needed, or as directed by a doctor
- place 2 tablets on tongue; tablets dissolve with or without water
- allow tablets to dissolve in mouth or chew before swallowing

INACTIVE INGREDIENTS
citric acid, ethylcellulose, flavor, hydroxypropyl cellulose, mannitol, microcrystalline cellulose, PVP, red 7, starch, sucralose, sucrose (245-236)
Dist. by: CHATTEM, Inc.
P.O. Box 2219, Chattanooga, TN 37409 USA
© 2008 Chattem Inc. www.chattem.com

UNISOM SLEEPTABS (doxylamine succinate)

Chattem, Inc.

DRUG FACTS

Active Ingredient(s) (in each tablet)
Doxylamine succinate 25 mg

Purpose(s)
Nighttime sleep-aid

USE
- helps to reduce difficulty in falling asleep

WARNINGS

ASK A DOCTOR BEFORE USE IF YOU HAVE
- a breathing problem such as asthma, emphysema or chronic bronchitis
- glaucoma
- trouble urinating due to an enlarged prostate gland

ASK A DOCTOR OR PHARMACIST BEFORE USE IF YOU
are taking any other drugs

WHEN USING THIS PRODUCT
- avoid alcoholic beverages
- take only at bedtime

STOP USE AND ASK A DOCTOR IF
- side effects occur. You may report side effects to FDA at 1-800-FDA-1088.
- sleeplessness persists continuously for more than two weeks. Insomnia may be a symptom of serious underlying medical illness.

If pregnant or breast-feeding,
ask a health professional before use.

Keep out of reach of children.
In case of overdose, get medical help or contact a Poison Control Center right away.

DIRECTIONS
- adults and children 12 years of age and over: take one tablet 30 minutes before going to bed; take once daily or as directed by a doctor
- children under 12 years of age: do not use

OTHER INFORMATION
- store at 20 - 25ºC (68 - 77ºF)

INACTIVE INGREDIENTS
dibasic calcium phosphate, FD&C blue no. 1 aluminum lake, magnesium stearate, microcrystalline cellulose, and sodium starch glycolate

---

VAGISTAT-1 VAGINAL OINTMENT (tioconazole)

Novartis Consumer Health, Inc.

DRUG FACTS

Active Ingredient(s) (in each applicator)	Purpose(s)
Tioconazole 300 mg (6.5%)	Vaginal antifungal

USES
- Treats vaginal yeast infections

WARNINGS
For vaginal use only

DO NOT USE
- If you have never had a vaginal yeast infection diagnosed by a doctor

ASK A DOCTOR BEFORE USE IF YOU HAVE
- **Vaginal itching and discomfort for the first time**
- **Lower abdominal, back or shoulder pain, fever, chills, nausea, vomiting, or foul-smelling vaginal discharge. You may have a more serious condition.**
- Vaginal yeast infections often (such as once a month or 3 in 6 months). You could be pregnant or have a serious underlying medical cause for your symptoms, including diabetes or a weakened immune system.
- Been exposed to human immunodeficiency virus (HIV) that causes AIDS.

WHEN USING THIS PRODUCT
- Do not use tampons, douches, spermicides, or other vaginal products. Condoms and diaphragms may be damaged and fail to prevent pregnancy or sexually transmitted disease (STDs).
- Do not have vaginal intercourse.
- Mild increase in vaginal burning, itching, or irritation may occur.
- If you do not get complete relief ask a doctor before using another product.

STOP USE AND ASK A DOCTOR IF
- **Symptoms do not get better after 3 days.**
- **Symptoms last more than 7 days.**
- **You get a rash or hives, abdominal pain, fever, chills, nausea, vomiting or foul-smelling vaginal discharge.**

If pregnant or breastfeeding, ask a health professional before use.
Keep out of reach of children. If swallowed, get medical help or contact a Poison Control Center right away.

DIRECTIONS
- Before using this product read the enclosed brochure and instructions on foil packet for complete directions and information
- Adults and children 12 years and over:
  - Open the foil packet just before use and remove blue cap.
  - Insert entire contents of applicator into the vagina at bedtime. Throw applicator away after use.
- Children under 12 years of age: ask a doctor.

OTHER INFORMATION
- This product is a 1-dose treatment; most women do not experience complete relief of their symptoms in just one day. Most women experience some relief within one day and complete relief of symptoms within 7 days.
- If you have questions about yeast infections, consult your doctor.
- Store at 15°-30°-C (59°--86°-F).
- See end flap of carton for lot number and expiration date.

INACTIVE INGREDIENTS BUTYLATED HYDROXYANISOLE, MAGNESIUM ALUMINUM SILICATE, WHITE PETROLATUM

QUESTIONS OR COMMENTS?
1-888-824-4782

VICKS DAYQUIL COLD & FLU (acetaminophen, dextromethorphan HBr, and phenylephrine HCl)

Procter & Gamble

DRUG FACTS

Active Ingredient(s) (in each 15 mL tablespoon)	Purpose(s)
Acetaminophen 325 mg	Pain reliever/fever reducer
Dextromethorphan HBr 10 mg	Cough suppressant
Phenylephrine HCl 5 mg	Nasal decongestant

USES
temporarily relieves common cold/flu symptoms:
- nasal congestion
- cough due to minor throat & bronchial irritation
- sore throat
- headache
- minor aches & pains
- fever

WARNINGS

LIVER WARNING

This product contains acetaminophen. Severe liver damage may occur if adult/child takes

- more than 4 doses in 24 hours, which is the maximum daily amount for this product
- with other drugs containing acetaminophen
- adult has 3 or more alcoholic drinks every day while using this product

SORE THROAT WARNING

If sore throat is severe, lasts for more than 2 days, occurs with or is followed by fever, headache, rash, nausea, or vomiting, see a doctor promptly.

DO NOT USE

- with any other drug containing acetaminophen (prescription or nonprescription). If you are not sure whether a drug contains acetaminophen, ask a doctor or pharmacist.
- if you are now taking a prescription monoamine oxidase inhibitor (MAOI) (certain drugs for depression, psychiatric or emotional conditions, or Parkinson's disease), or for 2 weeks after stopping the MAOI drug. If you do not know if your prescription drug contains an MAOI, ask a doctor or pharmacist before taking this product.

ASK A DOCTOR BEFORE USE IF YOU HAVE

- liver disease
- heart disease
- thyroid disease
- diabetes
- high blood pressure
- trouble urinating due to enlarged prostate gland
- cough that occurs with too much phlegm (mucus)
- persistent or chronic cough as occurs with smoking, asthma, or emphysema
- a sodium-restricted diet

ASK A DOCTOR OR PHARMACIST BEFORE USE IF YOU ARE

- taking the blood thinning drug warfarin.

WHEN USING THIS PRODUCT

- do not use more than directed.

STOP USE AND ASK A DOCTOR IF

- you get nervous, dizzy or sleepless
- symptoms get worse or last more than 5 days (children) or 7 days (adults)
- fever gets worse or lasts more than 3 days
- redness or swelling is present
- new symptoms occur
- cough comes back, or occurs with rash or headache that lasts.

These could be signs of a serious condition.

If pregnant or breast-feeding, ask a health professional before use.

Keep out of reach of children.

OVERDOSE WARNING

Taking more than directed can cause serious health problems. In case of overdose, get medical help or contact a Poison Control Center right away. Quick medical attention is critical for adults & for children even if you do not notice any signs or symptoms.

DIRECTIONS

- take only as directed - see **OVERDOSE WARNING**
- use dose cup or tablespoon (TBSP)
- do not exceed 4 doses per 24 hrs

adults & children 12 yrs & over	30 mL (2 TBSP) every 4 hrs
children 6 to under 12 yrs	15 mL (1 TBSP) every 4 hrs
children 4 to under 6 yrs	ask a doctor
children under 4 yrs	do not use

- **when using other DayQuil or NyQuil products, carefully read each label to insure correct dosing**

OTHER INFORMATION

- **each tablespoon contains:** sodium 50 mg
- store at room temperature

INACTIVE INGREDIENTS

carboxymethylcellulose sodium, citric acid, disodium EDTA, FD&C Yellow No. 6, flavor, glycerin, propylene glycol, purified water, saccharin sodium, sodium benzoate, sodium chloride, sodium citrate, sorbitol, sucralose

QUESTIONS OR COMMENTS?

1-800-251-3374
www.vicks.com

VICKS DAYQUIL COLD & FLU MULTI-SYMPTOM RELIEF (acetaminophen, dextromethorphan HBr, and phenylephrine HCl)

Procter & Gamble

DRUGS FACTS

Active Ingredient(s) (in each LiquiCap)	Purpose(s)
Acetaminophen 325 mg	Pain reliever/fever reducer
Dextromethorphan HBr 10 mg	Cough suppressant
Phenylephrine HCl 5 mg	Nasal decongestant

USES

temporarily relieves common cold/flu symptoms:
- nasal congestion
- cough due to minor throat & bronchial irritation
- sore throat
- headache
- minor aches & pains
- fever

WARNINGS

Liver warning

This product contains acetaminophen. Severe liver damage may occur if you take

- more than 4 doses in 24 hrs, which is the maximum daily amount for this product
- with other drugs containing acetaminophen
- 3 or more alcoholic drinks daily while using this product

Sore throat warning

If sore throat is severe, lasts for more than 2 days, occurs with or is followed by fever, headache, rash, nausea, or vomiting, see a doctor promptly.

DO NOT USE

- with any other drug containing acetaminophen (prescription or nonprescription). If you are not sure whether a drug contains acetaminophen, ask a doctor or pharmacist.
- if you are now taking a prescription monoamine oxidase inhibitor (MAOI) (certain drugs for depression, psychiatric or emotional conditions, or Parkinson's disease), or for 2 weeks after stopping the MAOI drug. If you do not know if your

prescription drug contains an MAOI, ask a doctor or pharmacist before taking this product.

ASK A DOCTOR BEFORE USE IF YOU HAVE
- liver disease
- heart disease
- thyroid disease
- diabetes
- high blood pressure
- trouble urinating due to enlarged prostate gland
- cough that occurs with too much phlegm (mucus)
- persistent or chronic cough as occurs with smoking, asthma, or emphysema

ASK A DOCTOR OR PHARMACIST BEFORE USE IF YOU ARE
- taking the blood thinning drug warfarin.

WHEN USING THIS PRODUCT
- do not use more than directed.

STOP USE AND ASK A DOCTOR IF
- you get nervous, dizzy or sleepless
- symptoms get worse or last more than 5 days (children) or 7 days (adults)
- fever gets worse or lasts more than 3 days
- redness or swelling is present
- new symptoms occur
- cough comes back, or occurs with rash or headache that lasts. These could be signs of a serious condition.

If pregnant or breast-feeding, ask a health professional before use.
Keep out of reach of children.

OVERDOSE WARNING
Taking more than directed can cause serious health problems. In case of overdose, get medical help or contact a Poison Control Center right away. Quick medical attention is critical for adults & for children even if you do not notice any signs or symptoms.

DIRECTIONS
- take only as directed - see **OVERDOSE WARNING**
- do not exceed 4 doses per 24 hrs

adults & children 12 yrs & over	2 LiquiCaps with water every 4 hrs
children 4 to under 12 yrs	ask a doctor
children under 4 yrs	do not use

- **when using other DayQuil or NyQuil products, carefully read each label to insure correct dosing**

OTHER INFORMATION
- store at room temperature

INACTIVE INGREDIENTS
FD&C Red No. 40, FD&C Yellow No. 6, gelatin, glycerin, polyethylene glycol, povidone, propylene glycol, purified water, sorbitol special, titanium dioxide

QUESTIONS OR COMMENTS?
Call 1-800-251-3374

VICKS FORMULA 44 CUSTOM CARE CHESTY COUGH MEDICINE (dextromethorphan hydrobromide and guaifenesin)
Procter & Gamble

DIRECTIONS
- Use dose cup, teaspoon (tsp), or tablespoon (TBSP).
- Do not exceed 6 doses per 24 hours.

Adults and children 12 years and over	15 mL (1 TBSP) every 4 hours
Children 6 to under 12 years	7-1/2 mL (1-1/2 tsp) every 4 hours
Children 4 to under 6 years	Ask a doctor.
Children under 4 years	Do not use.

INGREDIENTS
Active Ingredient(s) (in each 15 mL tablespoon) (Purpose(s))
Dextromethorphan HBr 20 mg (Cough suppressant)
Guaifenesin 200 mg (Expectorant)

INACTIVE INGREDIENTS
carboxymethylcellulose sodium, citric acid, FD&C red no. 40, flavor, high fructose corn syrup, propylene glycol, purified water, saccharin sodium, sodium benzoate, sodium citrate

OTHER INFORMATION
- **Each tablespoon contains** sodium 26 mg.
- Store at room temperature.

WARNINGS

DO NOT USE IF YOU ARE NOW TAKING A PRESCRIPTION MONOAMINE OXIDASE INHIBITOR (MAOI) (CERTAIN DRUGS FOR DEPRESSION, PSYCHIATRIC OR EMOTIONAL CONDITIONS, OR PARKINSON'S DISEASE), OR FOR 2 WEEKS AFTER STOPPING THE MAOI DRUG. IF YOU DO NOT KNOW IF YOUR PRESCRIPTION DRUG CONTAINS AN MAOI, ASK A DOCTOR OR PHARMACIST BEFORE TAKING THIS PRODUCT.

ASK A DOCTOR BEFORE USE IF YOU HAVE
- A sodium-restricted diet
- Persistent or chronic cough such as occurs with smoking, asthma, chronic bronchitis, or emphysema
- Cough that occurs with too much phlegm (mucus)

STOP USE AND ASK A DOCTOR IF
- Cough lasts more than 7 days, comes back, or occurs with fever, rash, or headache that lasts

These could be signs of a serious condition.
If pregnant or breast-feeding, ask a health professional before use.
Keep out of reach of children. In case of overdose, get medical help or contact a Poison Control Center right away.
Tamper evident: Do not use if printed shrinkband is missing or broken.

QUESTIONS OR COMMENTS?
Call 1-800-342-6844.

VICKS FORMULA 44 CUSTOM CARE COUGH & COLD PM (acetaminophen, chlorpheniramine maleate, and dextromethorphan hydrobromide)

Procter & Gamble

DIRECTIONS
- Take only as recommended—see Overdose warning.
- Use dose cup or tablespoon (TBSP).
- Do not exceed 4 doses per 24 hours.

Adults and children 12 years and over	15 mL (1 TBSP) every 6 hours
Children 4 to under 12 years	Ask a doctor.
Children under 4 years	Do not use.

INGREDIENTS
Active Ingredient(s) (in each 15 mL tablespoon) (Purpose(s))
Acetaminophen 650 mg (Pain reliever/fever reducer)
Chlorpheniramine maleate 4 mg (Antihistamine)
Dextromethorphan HBr 30 mg (Cough suppressant)

INACTIVE INGREDIENTS
- acesulfame potassium, carboxymethylcellulose sodium, citric acid, FD&C red no. 40, flavor, high fructose corn syrup, polyethylene glycol, propylene glycol, purified water, saccharin sodium, sodium benzoate, sodium citrate, sucralose

OTHER INFORMATION
- **Each tablespoon contains** sodium 26 mg.
- Store at room temperature.

WARNINGS
Liver warning: This product contains acetaminophen. Severe liver damage may occur if you take:
- More than 4 doses in 24 hours, which is the maximum daily amount for this product
- With other drugs containing acetaminophen
- 3 or more alcoholic drinks every day while using this product

Sore throat warning: If sore throat is severe, lasts for more than 2 days, occurs with or is followed by a fever, headache, rash, nausea, or vomiting, see a doctor promptly.

DO NOT USE
- With any other drug containing acetaminophen (prescription or nonprescription). If you are not sure whether a drug contains acetaminophen, ask a doctor or pharmacist.
- If you are now taking a prescription monoamine oxidase inhibitor (MAOI) (certain drugs for depression, psychiatric or emotional conditions, or Parkinson's disease), or for 2 weeks after stopping the MAOI drug. If you do not know if your prescription drug contains an MAOI, ask a doctor or pharmacist before taking this product.
- To make a child sleep

ASK A DOCTOR BEFORE USE IF YOU HAVE
- Liver disease
- Glaucoma
- Cough that occurs with too much phlegm (mucus)
- A breathing problem or chronic cough that lasts or as occurs with smoking, asthma, chronic bronchitis, or emphysema
- Trouble urinating due to enlarged prostate gland

ASK A DOCTOR OR PHARMACIST BEFORE USE IF YOU ARE
- Taking sedatives or tranquilizers
- Taking the blood-thinning drug warfarin

WHEN USING THIS PRODUCT
- **Do not use more than directed.**
- Excitability may occur, especially in children.
- Marked drowsiness may occur.
- Avoid alcoholic drinks.
- Be careful when driving a motor vehicle or operating machinery.
- Alcohol, sedatives, and tranquilizers may increase drowsiness.

STOP USE AND ASK A DOCTOR IF
- Pain or cough gets worse or lasts more than 7 days
- Fever gets worse or lasts more than 3 days
- Redness or swelling is present
- New symptoms occur
- Cough comes back, or occurs with rash or headache that lasts

These could be signs of a serious condition.
If pregnant or breast-feeding, ask a health professional before use.
Keep out of reach of children.

OVERDOSE WARNING
Taking more than directed can cause serious health problems. In case of overdose, get medical help or contact a Poison Control Center right away. Quick medical attention is critical for adults and for children even if you do not notice any signs or symptoms.
Tamper evident: Do not use if printed shrinkband is missing or broken.

QUESTIONS OR COMMENTS?
Call 1-800-342-6844.

VICKS FORMULA 44 CUSTOM CARE DRY COUGH SUPPRESSANT (dextromethorphan hydrobromide)

Procter & Gamble

DIRECTIONS
- Use dose cup, teaspoon (tsp), or tablespoon (TBSP).
- Do not exceed 4 doses per 24 hours.

Adults and children 12 years and over	15 mL (1 TBSP) every 6 to 8 hours
Children 6 to under 12 years	7-1/2 mL (1-1/2 tsp) every 6 to 8 hours
Children 4 to under 6 years	Ask a doctor.
Children under 4 years	Do not use.

INGREDIENTS
Active Ingredient(s) (in each 15 mL tablespoon) (Purpose(s))
Dextromethorphan HBr 30 mg (Cough suppressant)

INACTIVE INGREDIENTS
carboxymethylcellulose sodium, citric acid, FD&C red no. 40, flavor, high fructose corn syrup, propylene glycol, purified water, saccharin sodium, sodium benzoate, sodium citrate

OTHER INFORMATION
- **Each tablespoon contains** sodium 26 mg.
- Store at room temperature.

WARNINGS

DO NOT USE
if you are now taking a prescription monoamine oxidase inhibitor (MAOI) (certain drugs for depression, psychiatric or emotional conditions, or Parkinson's disease), or for 2 weeks after stopping the MAOI drug. If you do not know if your

prescription drug contains an MAOI, ask a doctor or pharmacist before taking this product.

ASK A DOCTOR BEFORE USE IF YOU HAVE
- Cough that occurs with too much phlegm (mucus)
- Persistent or chronic cough such as occurs with smoking, asthma, or emphysema

STOP USE AND ASK A DOCTOR IF
- Cough lasts more than 7 days, comes back, or occurs with fever, rash, or headache that lasts

These could be signs of a serious condition.
If pregnant or breast-feeding, ask a health professional before use.
Keep out of reach of children. In case of overdose, get medical help or contact a Poison Control Center right away.
Tamper evident: Do not use if printed shrinkband is missing or broken.

QUESTIONS OR COMMENTS?
Call 1-800-342-6844.

VICKS NATURE FUSION COLD & FLU NIGHTTIME RELIEF LIQUID (acetaminophen, dextromethorphan HBr, and doxylamine succinate)

The Procter & Gamble

DRUG FACTS

Active Ingredient(s) (in each 30 mL dose cup)	Purpose(s)
Acetaminophen 650 mg	Pain reliever/fever reducer
Dextromethorphan HBr 30 mg	Cough suppressant
Doxylamine succinate 7.5 mg	Antihistamine

USES
Temporarily relieves common cold and flu symptoms: cough due to minor throat and bronchial irritation, sore throat, headache, minor aches and pains, fever, runny nose/sneezing
- Runny Nose/Sneezing
- Cough
- Aches and Pain
- Sore Throat
- Fever

WARNINGS
Failure to follow these warnings could result in serious consequences.
Liver warning: This product contains acetaminophen. Severe liver damage may occur if you take:
- More than 4 doses in 24 hours, which is the maximum daily amount for this product
- With other drugs containing acetaminophen
- 3 or more alcoholic drinks daily while using this product

Sore throat warning: If sore throat is severe, lasts for more than 2 days, occurs with or is followed by fever, headache, rash, nausea, or vomiting, see a doctor promptly.

DO NOT USE
- With any other drug containing acetaminophen (prescription or nonprescription). If you are not sure whether a drug contains acetaminophen, ask a doctor or pharmacist.
- If you are now taking a prescription monoamine oxidase inhibitor (MAOI) (certain drugs for depression, psychiatric or emotional conditions, or Parkinson's disease), or for 2 weeks after stopping the MAOI drug. If you do not know if your prescription drug contains an MAOI, ask a doctor or pharmacist before taking this product.
- To make a child sleep.

ASK A DOCTOR BEFORE USE IF YOU HAVE
- Liver disease
- Glaucoma
- Cough that occurs with too much phlegm (mucus)
- A breathing problem or chronic cough that lasts or as occurs with smoking, asthma, chronic bronchitis, or emphysema
- Trouble urinating due to enlarged prostate gland
- A sodium-restricted diet

ASK A DOCTOR OR PHARMACIST BEFORE USE IF YOU ARE
- Taking sedatives or tranquilizers
- Taking the blood-thinning drug warfarin

WHEN USING THIS PRODUCT
- Do not use more than directed.
- Excitability may occur, especially in children.
- Marked drowsiness may occur.
- Avoid alcoholic drinks.
- Be careful when driving a motor vehicle or operating machinery.
- Alcohol, sedatives, and tranquilizers may increase drowsiness.

STOP USE AND ASK A DOCTOR IF
- Pain or cough gets worse or lasts more than 7 days
- Fever gets worse or lasts more than 3 days
- Redness or swelling is present
- New symptoms occur
- Cough comes back, or occurs with rash, fever, or headache that lasts

These could be signs of a serious condition.
If pregnant or breast-feeding, ask a health professional before use.
Keep out of reach of children.

OVERDOSE WARNING
Taking more than the recommended dose can cause serious health problems. In case of overdose, get medical help or contact a Poison Control Center right away. Quick medical attention is critical for adults as well as for children, even if you do not notice any signs or symptoms.
Tamper evident: Do not use if printed foil inner seal under bottle cap is broken or missing.

DIRECTIONS
- Take only as directed—see Overdose warning.
- Use dose cup or tablespoon (TBSP).
- Do not exceed 4 doses per 24 hours.

Adults and children 12 years and over	30 mL (2 TBSP) every 6 hours
Children under 12 years	Ask a doctor.

When using other Nature Fusion™ products, carefully read each label to ensure correct dosing.

OTHER INFORMATION
- Each 30 mL dose cup contains: sodium 36 mg.
- Store at room temperature.

INACTIVE INGREDIENTS
citric acid, flavor, glycerin, high fructose corn syrup, honey, polyethylene glycol, propylene glycol, purified water, sodium citrate

QUESTIONS OR COMMENTS?
Call 1-877-340-8824.

VICKS NATURE FUSION COLD & FLU RELIEF CAPLETS (acetaminophen, dextromethorphan HBr, and phenylephrine HCl)

The Procter & Gamble

DRUG FACTS

Active Ingredient(s) (in each caplet)	Purpose(s)
Acetaminophen 325 mg	Pain reliever/fever reducer
Dextromethorphan HBr 10 mg	Cough suppressant
Phenylephrine HCl 5 mg	Nasal decongestant

USES
Temporarily relieves common cold and flu symptoms: nasal congestion, cough due to minor throat and bronchial irritation, sore throat, headache, minor aches and pains, fever
- Nasal Congestion
- Cough
- Sore Throat
- Aches and Pain
- Fever

WARNINGS
Failure to follow these warnings could result in serious consequences.
Liver warning: This product contains acetaminophen. Severe liver damage may occur if you take:
- More than 4 doses in 24 hours, which is the maximum daily amount for this product
- With other drugs containing acetaminophen
- 3 or more alcoholic drinks daily while using this product

Sore throat warning: If sore throat is severe, lasts for more than 2 days, or occurs with or is followed by fever, headache, rash, nausea, or vomiting, see a doctor promptly.

DO NOT USE
- With any other drug containing acetaminophen (prescription or nonprescription). If you are not sure whether a drug contains acetaminophen, ask a doctor or pharmacist.
- If you are now taking a prescription monoamine oxidase inhibitor (MAOI) (certain drugs for depression, psychiatric or emotional conditions, or Parkinson's disease), or for 2 weeks after stopping the MAOI drug. If you do not know if your prescription drug contains an MAOI, ask a doctor or pharmacist before taking this product.

ASK A DOCTOR BEFORE USE IF YOU HAVE
- Liver disease
- Heart disease
- Thyroid disease
- Diabetes
- High blood pressure
- Trouble urinating due to enlarged prostate gland
- Cough that occurs with too much phlegm (mucus)
- Persistent or chronic cough as occurs with smoking, asthma, or emphysema

ASK A DOCTOR OR PHARMACIST BEFORE USE IF YOU ARE
- **taking the blood-thinning drug warfarin.**

WHEN USING THIS PRODUCT
- **do not use more than directed.**

STOP USE AND ASK A DOCTOR IF
- You get nervous, dizzy, or sleepless
- Symptoms get worse or last more than 7 days
- Fever gets worse or lasts more than 3 days
- Redness or swelling is present
- New symptoms occur
- Cough comes back, or occurs with rash, fever, or headache that lasts

These could be signs of a serious condition.
If pregnant or breast-feeding, ask a health professional before use.
Keep out of reach of children.

OVERDOSE WARNING
Taking more than directed can cause serious health problems. In case of overdose, get medical help or contact a Poison Control Center right away. Quick medical attention is critical for adults and for children, even if you do not notice any signs or symptoms.
Tamper evident: This package is safety sealed and child resistant. Use only if blisters are intact. If the package is difficult to open, use scissors.

DIRECTIONS
- Take only as directed—see Overdose warning.
- Do not exceed 4 doses per 24 hours.

Adults and children 12 years and over	2 caplets with water every 4 hours
Children under 12 years	Ask a doctor.

When using other Nature Fusion™ products, carefully read each label to ensure correct dosing.

OTHER INFORMATION
- Save carton for full directions and warnings.
- Store at room temperature.

INACTIVE INGREDIENTS
EDTA, honey, hydroxypropyl methylcellulose, magnesium stearate, maltodextrin, medium chain triglycerides, microcrystalline cellulose, natural flavor, polydextrose, polyvinyl pyrrolidone, propylene glycol, starch, stearic acid, sucralose, talc, titanium dioxide, yellow iron oxide

QUESTIONS OR COMMENTS?
Call 1-877-340-8824.

VICKS NATURE FUSION COLD & FLU RELIEF DAY AND NIGHT COMBO PACK
(acetaminophen, dextromethorphan HBr, doxylamine succinate, and phenylephrine HCl)

The Procter & Gamble

DRUG FACTS

Nature Fusion Cold & Flu Nighttime Relief

Active Ingredient(s) (in each 30 mL dose cup)	Purpose(s)
Acetaminophen 650 mg	Pain reliever/fever reducer
Dextromethorphan HBr 30 mg	Cough suppressant
Doxylamine succinate 7.5 mg	Antihistamine

Nature Fusion Cold & Flu Multi-Symptom Relief

Active Ingredient(s) (in each caplet)	Purpose(s)
Acetaminophen 325 mg	Pain reliever/fever reducer
Dextromethorphan HBr 10 mg	Cough suppressant
Phenylephrine HCl 5 mg	Nasal decongestant

USES
Nature Fusion Cold & Flu Nighttime Relief temporarily relieves common cold and flu symptoms: cough due to minor throat and bronchial irritation, sore throat, headache, minor aches and pains, fever, runny nose and sneezing
- Runny Nose/Sneezing
- Cough
- Aches and Pain
- Sore Throat
- Fever

Nature Fusion Cold & Flu Multi-Symptom Relief temporarily relieves common cold and flu symptoms: nasal congestion, cough due to minor throat and bronchial irritation, sore throat, headache, minor aches and pains, fever
- Nasal congestion
- Cough
- Sore throat
- Aches and Pains
- Fever

WARNINGS
Nature Fusion Cold & Flu Nighttime Relief
Failure to follow these warnings could result in serious consequences.
Liver warning: This product contains acetaminophen. Severe liver damage may occur if you take:
- More than 4 doses in 24 hours, which is the maximum daily amount for this product
- With other drugs containing acetaminophen
- 3 or more alcoholic drinks every day while using this product

Sore throat warning: If sore throat is severe, lasts for more than 2 days, or occurs with or is followed by fever, headache, rash, nausea, or vomiting, see a doctor promptly.
Nature Fusion Cold & Flu Multi-Symptom Relief
Failure to follow these warnings could result in serious consequences.
Liver warning: This product contains acetaminophen. Severe liver damage may occur if you take:
- More than 4 doses in 24 hours, which is the maximum daily amount for this product
- With other drugs containing acetaminophen
- 3 or more alcoholic drinks every day while using this product

Sore throat warning: If sore throat is severe, lasts for more than 2 days, or occurs with or is followed by fever, headache, rash, nausea, or vomiting, see a doctor promptly.

DO NOT USE
Nature Fusion Cold & Flu Nighttime Relief
- With any other drug containing acetaminophen (prescription or nonprescription). If you are not sure whether a drug contains acetaminophen, ask a doctor or pharmacist.
- If you are now taking a prescription monoamine oxidase inhibitor (MAOI) (certain drugs for depression, psychiatric or emotional conditions, or Parkinson's disease), or for 2 weeks after stopping the MAOI drug. If you do not know if your prescription drug contains an MAOI, ask a doctor or pharmacist before taking this product.
- To make a child sleep.

Nature Fusion Cold & Flu Multi-Symptom Relief
- With any other drug containing acetaminophen (prescription or nonprescription). If you are not sure whether a drug contains acetaminophen, ask a doctor or pharmacist.

- If you are now taking a prescription monoamine oxidase inhibitor (MAOI) (certain drugs for depression, psychiatric or emotional conditions, or Parkinson's disease), or for 2 weeks after stopping the MAOI drug. If you do not know if your prescription drug contains an MAOI, ask a doctor or pharmacist before taking this product.

ASK A DOCTOR BEFORE USE IF YOU HAVE
Nature Fusion Cold & Flu Nighttime Relief
- Liver disease
- Glaucoma
- Cough that occurs with too much phlegm (mucus)
- A breathing problem or chronic cough that lasts or as occurs with smoking, asthma, chronic bronchitis, or emphysema
- Trouble urinating due to enlarged prostate gland
- A sodium-restricted diet

Nature Fusion Cold & Flu Multi-Symptom Relief
- Liver disease
- Heart disease
- Thyroid disease
- Diabetes
- High blood pressure
- Trouble urinating due to enlarged prostate gland
- Cough that occurs with too much phlegm (mucus)
- Persistent or chronic cough as occurs with smoking, asthma, or emphysema

ASK A DOCTOR OR PHARMACIST BEFORE USE IF YOU ARE
Nature Fusion Cold & Flu Nighttime Relief
- Taking sedatives or tranquilizers
- Taking the blood-thinning drug warfarin

Nature Fusion Cold & Flu Multi-Symptom Relief
- **taking the blood-thinning drug warfarin.**

WHEN USING THIS PRODUCT
Nature Fusion Cold & Flu Nighttime Relief
- **Do not use more than directed.**
- Excitability may occur, especially in children.
- Marked drowsiness may occur.
- Avoid alcoholic drinks.
- Be careful when driving a motor vehicle or operating machinery.
- Alcohol, sedatives, and tranquilizers may increase drowsiness.

Nature Fusion Cold & Flu Multi-Symptom Relief
- **do not use more than directed.**

STOP USE AND ASK A DOCTOR IF
Nature Fusion Cold & Flu Nighttime Relief
- Pain or cough gets worse or lasts more than 7 days
- Fever gets worse or lasts more than 3 days
- Redness or swelling is present
- New symptoms occur
- Cough comes back, or occurs with rash, fever, or headache that lasts

These could be signs of a serious condition.
If pregnant or breast-feeding, ask a health professional before use.
Keep out of reach of children.
Nature Fusion Cold & Flu Multi-Symptom Relief
- You get nervous, dizzy, or sleepless
- Symptoms get worse or last more than 7 days
- Fever gets worse or lasts more than 3 days
- Redness or swelling is present
- New symptoms occur
- Cough comes back, or occurs with rash, fever, or headache that lasts

These could be signs of a serious condition.
If pregnant or breast-feeding, ask a health professional before use.
Keep out of reach of children.

OVERDOSE WARNING
Nature Fusion Cold & Flu Nighttime Relief
Taking more than the recommended dose can cause serious health problems. In case of overdose, get medical help or contact a Poison Control Center right away. Quick medical attention is critical for adults as well as for children, even if you do not notice any signs or symptoms.
Tamper evident: Do not use if printed foil inner seal under bottle cap is broken or missing.
Nature Fusion Cold & Flu Multi-Symptom Relief
Taking more than the recommended dose can cause serious health problems. In case of overdose, get medical help or contact a Poison Control Center right away. Quick medical attention is critical for adults and for children, even if you do not notice any signs or symptoms.
Tamper evident: This package is safety sealed and child resistant. Use only if blisters are intact. If the package is difficult to open, use scissors.

DIRECTIONS
Nature Fusion Cold & Flu Nighttime Relief
• Take only as directed—see Overdose warning.
• Use dose cup or tablespoon (TBSP).
• Do not exceed 4 doses per 24 hours.

| Adults and children 12 years and over | 30 mL (2 TBSP) every 6 hours |
| Children under 12 years | Ask a doctor. |

When using other Nature Fusion™ products, carefully read each label to ensure correct dosing.
Nature Fusion Cold & Flu Multi-Symptom Relief
• Take only as directed—see Overdose warning.
• Do not exceed 4 doses per 24 hours.

| Adults and children 12 years and over | 2 caplets with water every 4 hours |
| Children under 12 years | Ask a doctor. |

OTHER INFORMATION
Nature Fusion Cold & Flu Nighttime Relief
• Each 30 mL dose cup contains: sodium 36 mg.
• Store at room temperature.

Nature Fusion Cold & Flu Multi-Symptom Relief
• Save carton for full directions and warnings.
• Store at room temperature.

INACTIVE INGREDIENTS
Nature Fusion Cold & Flu Nighttime Relief
citric acid, flavor, glycerin, high fructose corn syrup, honey, polyethylene glycol, propylene glycol, purified water, sodium citrate
Nature Fusion Cold & Flu Multi-Symptom Relief
EDTA, honey, hydroxypropyl methylcellulose, magnesium stearate, maltodextrin, medium chain triglycerides, microcrystalline cellulose, natural flavor, polydextrose, polyvinyl pyrrolidone, propylene glycol, starch, stearic acid, sucralose, talc, titanium dioxide, yellow iron oxide

QUESTIONS OR COMMENTS?
Call **1-877-340-8824.**

VICKS NATURE FUSION COUGH MEDICINE
(dextromethorphan HBr)
The Procter & Gamble

DRUG FACTS

Active Ingredient(s) (in each 30 mL dose cup)	Purpose(s)
Dextromethorphan HBr 30 mg	Cough suppressant

USES
Temporarily relieves cough due to minor throat and bronchial irritation
• Cough

DO NOT USE
• If you are now taking a prescription monoamine oxidase inhibitor (MAOI) (certain drugs for depression, psychiatric or emotional conditions, or Parkinson's disease), or for 2 weeks after stopping the MAOI drug. If you do not know if your prescription drug contains an MAOI, ask a doctor or pharmacist before taking this product.

ASK A DOCTOR BEFORE USE IF YOU HAVE
• Cough that occurs with too much phlegm (mucus)
• Persistent or chronic cough as occurs with smoking, asthma, or emphysema
• A sodium-restricted diet

STOP USE AND ASK A DOCTOR IF
• If cough lasts more than 7 days, comes back, or occurs with fever, rash, or headache that lasts. These could be signs of a serious condition.
If pregnant or breast-feeding, ask a health professional before use.
Keep out of reach of children. In case of overdose, get medical help or contact a Poison Control Center right away.
Tamper evident: Do not use if printed foil inner seal under bottle cap is broken or missing.

DIRECTIONS
• Use dose cup or tablespoon (TBSP).
• Do not exceed 4 doses per 24 hours.

| Adults and children 12 years and over | 30 mL (2 TBSP) every 6-8 hours |
| Children under 12 years | Ask a doctor. |

When using other Nature Fusion™ products, carefully read each label to ensure correct dosing.

OTHER INFORMATION
• Each 30 mL dose cup contains: sodium 36 mg.
• Store at room temperature.

INACTIVE INGREDIENTS
citric acid, flavor, glycerin, high fructose corn syrup, honey, polyethylene glycol, propylene glycol, purified water, sodium citrate

QUESTIONS OR COMMENTS?
Call **1-877-340-8824.**

VICKS NATURE FUSION COUGH & CHEST CONGESTION LIQUID (dextromethorphan HBr and guaifenesin)

The Procter & Gamble

DRUG FACTS

Active Ingredient(s) (in each 30 mL dose cup)	Purpose(s)
Dextromethorphan HBr 20 mg	Cough suppressant
Guaifenesin 200 mg	Expectorant

USES
Temporarily relieves cough associated with the common cold and helps loosen phlegm and thin bronchial secretions to rid the bronchial passageways of bothersome mucus
- Cough
- Chest Congestion

DO NOT USE
- If you are now taking a prescription monoamine oxidase inhibitor (MAOI) (certain drugs for depression, psychiatric or emotional conditions, or Parkinson's disease), or for 2 weeks after stopping the MAOI drug. If you do not know if your prescription drug contains an MAOI, ask a doctor or pharmacist before taking this product.

ASK A DOCTOR BEFORE USE IF YOU HAVE
- Persistent or chronic cough such as occurs with smoking, asthma, chronic bronchitis, or emphysema
- Cough that occurs with too much phlegm (mucus)
- A sodium-restricted diet

STOP USE AND ASK A DOCTOR IF
- cough lasts more than 7 days, comes back, or occurs with fever, rash, or headache that lasts. These could be signs of a serious condition.

If pregnant or breast-feeding, ask a health professional before use.
Keep out of reach of children. In case of overdose, get medical help or contact a Poison Control Center right away.
Tamper evident: Do not use if printed foil inner seal under bottle cap is broken or missing.

DIRECTIONS
- Use dose cup or tablespoon (TBSP).
- Do not exceed 6 doses per 24 hours.

Adults and children 12 years and over	30 mL (2 TBSP) every 4 hours
Children under 12 years	Ask a doctor.

When using other Nature Fusion™ products, carefully read each label to ensure correct dosing.

OTHER INFORMATION
- Each 30 mL dose cup contains: sodium 36 mg.
- Store at room temperature.

INACTIVE INGREDIENTS
citric acid, flavor, glycerin, high fructose corn syrup, honey, polyethylene glycol, propylene glycol, purified water, sodium citrate

QUESTIONS OR COMMENTS?
Call 1-877-340-8824.

VISINE ORIGINAL REDNESS RELIEF
(tetrahydrozoline hydrochloride)

Johnson & Johnson Healthcare Products, Division of McNeil-PPC, Inc.

DRUG FACTS

Active Ingredient(s)
Tetrahydrozoline HCl 0.05%

Purpose(s)
Redness reliever

USE
- for the relief of redness of the eye due to minor eye irritations

WARNINGS

ASK A DOCTOR BEFORE USE IF YOU HAVE
narrow angle glaucoma.

WHEN USING THIS PRODUCT
- pupils may become enlarged temporarily
- overuse may cause more eye redness
- remove contact lenses before using
- do not use if this solution changes color or becomes cloudy
- do not touch tip of container to any surface to avoid contamination
- replace cap after each use

STOP USE AND ASK A DOCTOR IF
- you feel eye pain
- changes in vision occur
- redness or irritation of the eye lasts
- condition worsens or lasts more than 72 hours

If pregnant or breast-feeding, ask a health professional before use.
Keep out of reach of children. If swallowed, get medical help or contact a Poison Control Center right away.

DIRECTIONS
- put 1 to 2 drops in the affected eye(s) up to 4 times daily
- children under 6 years of age: ask a doctor

OTHER INFORMATION
- store at 15° to 25°C (59° to 77°F)

INACTIVE INGREDIENTS
benzalkonium chloride, boric acid, edetate disodium, purified water, sodium borate, sodium chloride

QUESTIONS OR COMMENTS?
call 1-888-734-7648
Dist: **Johnson & Johnson Healthcare Products** Division of McNEIL-PPC, Inc., Skillman, NJ 08558 USA

VISINE TEARS DRY EYE RELIEF (glycerin, hypromellose, and polyethylene glycol 400)

Johnson & Johnson Healthcare Products, Division of McNeil-PPC, Inc.

DRUG FACTS

Active Ingredient(s)	Purpose(s)
Glycerin 0.2%	Lubricant
Hypromellose 0.2%	Lubricant
Polyethylene glycol 400 1%	Lubricant

USES
- for temporary relief of burning and irritation due to dryness of the eye
- for protection against further irritation

WARNINGS

WHEN USING THIS PRODUCT
- remove contact lenses before using
- do not use if this solution changes color or becomes cloudy
- do not touch tip of container to any surface to avoid contamination
- replace cap after each use

STOP USE AND ASK A DOCTOR IF
- you feel eye pain
- changes in vision occur
- redness or irritation of the eye lasts
- condition worsens or lasts more than 72 hours

If pregnant or breast-feeding, ask a health professional before use.
Keep out of reach of children. If swallowed, get medical help or contact a Poison Control Center right away.

DIRECTIONS
- put 1 or 2 drops in the affected eye(s) as needed
- children under 6 years of age: ask a doctor

OTHER INFORMATION
- store at 15° to 25°C (59° to 77°F)

INACTIVE INGREDIENTS
ascorbic acid, benzalkonium chloride, boric acid, dextrose, disodium phosphate, glycine, magnesium chloride, potassium chloride, purified water, sodium borate, sodium chloride, sodium citrate, sodium lactate

QUESTIONS OR COMMENTS?
call **1-888-734-7648**
Dist: **Johnson & Johnson Healthcare Products** Division of McNEIL-PPC, Inc., Skillman, NJ 08558 USA

VISINE TEARS LONG LASTING DRY EYE RELIEF (glycerin, hypromellose, and polyethylene glycol 400)

Johnson & Johnson Healthcare Products, Division of McNeil-PPC, Inc.

DRUG FACTS

Active Ingredient(s)	Purpose(s)
Glycerin 0.2%	Lubricant
Hypromellose 0.36%	Lubricant
Polyethylene glycol 400 1%	Lubricant

USES
- for temporary relief of burning, irritation and discomfort due to dryness of the eye or exposure to wind or sun
- for protection against further irritation

WARNINGS

WHEN USING THIS PRODUCT
- remove contact lenses before using
- do not use if this solution changes color or becomes cloudy
- do not touch tip of container to any surface to avoid contamination
- replace cap after each use

STOP USE AND ASK A DOCTOR IF
- you feel eye pain
- changes in vision occur
- redness or irritation of the eye lasts
- condition worsens or lasts more than 72 hours

If pregnant or breast-feeding, ask a health professional before use.
Keep out of reach of children. If swallowed, get medical help or contact a Poison Control Center right away.

DIRECTIONS
- put 1 or 2 drops in the affected eye(s) as needed
- children under 6 years of age: ask a doctor

OTHER INFORMATION
- store at 15° to 25°C (59° to 77°F)

INACTIVE INGREDIENTS
ascorbic acid, benzalkonium chloride, boric acid, dextrose, glycine, magnesium chloride, potassium chloride, purified water, sodium borate, sodium chloride, sodium citrate, sodium lactate, sodium phosphate dibasic

QUESTIONS OR COMMENTS?
call **1-888-734-7648**

VISINE TIRED EYE RELIEF LUBRICANT
(glycerin, hypromellose, and polyethylene glycol 400)
Johnson & Johnson Healthcare Products, Division of McNeil-PPC, Inc.

DRUG FACTS

Active Ingredient(s)	Purpose(s)
Glycerin 0.2%	Lubricant
Hypromellose 0.36%	Lubricant
Polyethylene glycol 400 1%	Lubricant

USES
- for the temporary relief of burning, irritation, and discomfort due to dryness of the eye or exposure to wind or sun
- for protection against further irritation

WARNINGS

WHEN USING THIS PRODUCT
- remove contact lenses before using
- do not use if this solution changes color or becomes cloudy
- do not touch tip of container to any surface to avoid contamination
- replace cap after each use

STOP USE AND ASK A DOCTOR IF
- you feel eye pain
- changes in vision occur
- redness or irritation of the eye lasts
- condition worsens or lasts more than 72 hours

If pregnant or breast-feeding, ask a health professional before use.
Keep out of reach of children. If swallowed, get medical help or contact a Poison Control Center right away.

DIRECTIONS
- put 1 or 2 drops in the affected eye(s) as needed
- children under 6 years of age: ask a doctor

OTHER INFORMATION
- store at 15° and 25°C (59° to 77°F)

INACTIVE INGREDIENTS
ascorbic acid, benzalkonium chloride, boric acid, dextrose, glycine, magnesium chloride, potassium chloride, purified water, sodium borate, sodium chloride, sodium citrate, sodium lactate, sodium phosphate dibasic

QUESTIONS OR COMMENTS?
Call **1-888-734-7648**
Dist: **Johnson & Johnson Healthcare Products** Division of McNEIL-PPC, Inc., Skillman, NJ 08558 USA

VISINE TOTALITY MULTI-SYMPTOM RELIEF
(glycerin, hypromellose, polyethylene glycol 400, tetrahydrozoline hydrochloride, and zinc sulfate)
Johnson & Johnson Healthcare Products, Division of McNeil-PPC, Inc.

DRUG FACTS

Active Ingredient(s)	Purpose(s)
Glycerin 0.2%	Lubricant
Hypromellose 0.36%	Lubricant
Polyethylene glycol 400 1%	Lubricant
Tetrahydrozoline HCl 0.05%	Redness reliever
Zinc sulfate 0.25%	Astringent

USES
- for temporary relief of discomfort and redness of the eye due to minor eye irritations
- relieves dryness of the eye
- for the temporary relief of burning and irritation due to exposure to wind or sun
- for protection against further irritation

WARNINGS

ASK A DOCTOR BEFORE USE IF YOU HAVE
narrow angle glaucoma.

WHEN USING THIS PRODUCT
- pupils may become enlarged temporarily
- overuse may cause more eye redness
- remove contact lenses before using
- do not use if this solution changes color or becomes cloudy
- do not touch tip of container to any surface to avoid contamination
- replace cap after each use

STOP USE AND ASK A DOCTOR IF
- you feel eye pain
- changes in vision occur
- redness or irritation of the eye lasts
- condition worsens or lasts more than 72 hours

If pregnant or breast feeding, ask a health professional before use.
Keep out of reach of children. If swallowed, get medical help or contact a Poison Control Center right away.

DIRECTIONS
- put 1 to 2 drops in the affected eye(s) up to 4 times daily
- children under 6 years of age: ask a doctor

OTHER INFORMATION
- some users may experience a brief tingling sensation
- store at 20° to 25°C (68° to 77°F)

INACTIVE INGREDIENTS
benzalkonium chloride, boric acid, edetate disodium, purified water, sodium chloride, sodium citrate

QUESTIONS OR COMMENTS?
call **1-888-734-7648**
Dist: **Johnson & Johnson Healthcare Products** Division of McNEIL-PPC, Inc., Skillman, NJ 08558 USA

ZADITOR EYE ITCH RELIEF EYE DROPS
(ketotifen fumarate)
Novartis Pharmaceuticals Corporation

Active ingredient(s)
Ketotifen (0.025%)
(equivalent to ketotifen fumarate 0.035%)

Purpose(s)
Antihistamine

USE
Temporarily relieves itchy eyes due to pollen, ragweed, grass, animal hair and dander.

WARNINGS

DO NOT USE
- if solution changes color or becomes cloudy
- if you are sensitive to any ingredient in this product
- to treat contact lens related irritation

WHEN USING THIS PRODUCT
- do not touch tip of container to any surface to avoid contamination
- remove contact lenses before use
- wait at least 10 minutes before reinserting contact lenses after use
- replace cap after each use

STOP USE AND ASK A DOCTOR IF YOU
experience any of the following:
- eye pain
- changes in vision
- redness of the eye
- itching worsens or lasts for more than 72 hours

DIRECTIONS
- **Adults and children 3 years of age and older:** Put 1 drop in the affected eye(s) twice daily, every 8-12 hours, no more than twice per day.
- **Children under 3 years of age:** Consult a doctor.

OTHER INFORMATION
- Only for use in the eye.
- Store between 4°-25°C (39°-77°F).

INACTIVE INGREDIENTS
benzalkonium chloride 0.01%, glycerol, sodium hydroxide and/or hydrochloric acid, and purified water

QUESTIONS OR COMMENTS?
call toll-free
1-866-393-6336, weekdays,
8:30 AM - 5:00 PM EST.
Serious side effects associated with the use of this product may be reported to this number.

MAXIMUM STRENGTH ZANTAC 150
(ranitidine)
Boehringer Ingelheim Pharmaceuticals Inc.

DRUG FACTS

Active Ingredient(s) (in each tablet)	Purpose(s)
Ranitidine 150 mg (as ranitidine hydrochloride 168 mg)	Acid reducer

USES
- relieves heartburn associated with acid indigestion and sour stomach
- prevents heartburn associated with acid indigestion and sour stomach brought on by certain foods and beverages

WARNINGS
Allergy alert: Do not use if you are allergic to ranitidine or other acid reducers

DO NOT USE
- if you have trouble or pain swallowing food, vomiting with blood, or bloody or black stools. These may be signs of a serious condition. See your doctor.
- with other acid reducers
- if you have kidney disease, except under the advice and supervision of a doctor

ASK A DOCTOR BEFORE USE IF YOU HAVE
- frequent **chest pain** • frequent wheezing, particularly with heartburn • unexplained weight loss • nausea or vomiting • stomach pain • had heartburn over 3 months. This may be a sign of a more serious condition. • heartburn with **lightheadedness, sweating or dizziness** • chest pain or shoulder pain with shortness of breath; sweating; pain spreading to arms, neck or shoulders; or lightheadedness

STOP USE AND ASK A DOCTOR IF
- your heartburn continues or worsens • you need to take this product for more than 14 days
If pregnant or breast-feeding, ask a health professional before use.
Keep out of reach of children. In case of overdose, get medical help or contact a Poison Control Center right away.

DIRECTIONS
- adults and children 12 years and over:
  - to **relieve** symptoms, swallow 1 tablet with a glass of water
  - to **prevent** symptoms, swallow 1 tablet with a glass of water **30 to 60 minutes before** eating food or drinking beverages that cause heartburn
  - can be used up to twice daily (do not take more than 2 tablets in 24 hours)
- children under 12 years: ask a doctor

OTHER INFORMATION
- Blister: do not use if individual blister unit is open or torn Bottle: do not use if printed foil under bottle cap is open or torn
- store at 20°-25°C (68°-77°F)
- avoid excessive heat or humidity
- this product is sodium and sugar free

INACTIVE INGREDIENTS
hypromellose, magnesium stearate, microcrystalline cellulose, synthetic red iron oxide, titanium dioxide, triacetin

QUESTIONS OR COMMENTS?
Call **1-888-285-9159** or visit **www.zantacotc.com**

ZANTAC 150 MAXIMUM STRENGTH COOL MINT (ranitidine)

Boehringer Ingelheim Pharmaceuticals Inc.

DRUG FACTS

Active Ingredient(s) (in each tablet)	Purpose(s)
Ranitidine 150 mg (as ranitidine hydrochloride 168 mg)	Acid reducer

USES
- relieves heartburn associated with acid indigestion and sour stomach
- prevents heartburn associated with acid indigestion and sour stomach brought on by eating or drinking certain foods and beverages

WARNINGS
Allergy alert: Do not use if you are allergic to ranitidine or other acid reducers

DO NOT USE
- with other acid reducers
- if you have kidney disease, except under the advice and supervision of a doctor
- if you have trouble or pain swallowing food, vomiting with blood, or bloody or black stools.
  These may be signs of a serious condition. See your doctor.

ASK A DOCTOR BEFORE USE IF YOU HAVE
- nausea or vomiting
- stomach pain
- unexplained weight loss
- frequent **chest pain**
- frequent wheezing, particularly with heartburn
- had heartburn over 3 months. This may be a sign of a more serious condition.
- heartburn with **lightheadedness, sweating or dizziness**
- chest pain or shoulder pain with shortness of breath; sweating; pain spreading to arms, neck or shoulders; or lightheadedness

STOP USE AND ASK A DOCTOR IF
- your heartburn continues or worsens
- you need to take this product for more than 14 days
  If pregnant or breast-feeding, ask a health professional before use.
  Keep out of reach of children. In case of overdose, get medical help or contact a Poison Control Center right away.

DIRECTIONS
- adults and children 12 years and over:
  - to **relieve** symptoms, swallow 1 tablet with a glass of water
  - to **prevent** symptoms, swallow 1 tablet with a glass of water **30 to 60 minutes before** eating food or drinking beverages that cause heartburn
  - can be used up to twice daily (do not take more than 2 tablets in 24 hours)
  - do not chew tablet
- children under 12 years: ask a doctor

OTHER INFORMATION
- Blister: do not use if individual blister unit is open or torn
  Bottle: do not use if printed foil under bottle cap is open or torn
- store at 20°-25°C (68°-77°F)
- avoid excessive heat or humidity
- this product is sodium and sugar free

INACTIVE INGREDIENTS
carrageenan, FD&C blue no.1, flavors, hypromellose, magnesium stearate, microcrystalline cellulose, polyethylene glycol, polysorbate, sucralose, and titanium dioxide

QUESTIONS OR COMMENTS?
Call **1-888-285-9159** or visit **www.zantacotc.com**

ZANTAC 75 (ranitidine)

Boehringer Ingelheim Pharmaceuticals Inc.

DRUG FACTS

Active Ingredient(s) (in each tablet)
Ranitidine 75 mg (as ranitidine hydrochloride 84 mg)

Purpose(s)
Acid reducer

USES
- relieves heartburn associated with acid indigestion and sour stomach
- prevents heartburn associated with acid indigestion and sour stomach brought on by certain foods and beverages

WARNINGS
Allergy alert: Do not use if you are allergic to ranitidine or other acid reducers

DO NOT USE
- if you have trouble or pain swallowing food, vomiting with blood, or bloody or black stools. These may be signs of a serious condition. See your doctor.
- with other acid reducers

ASK A DOCTOR BEFORE USE IF YOU HAVE
- frequent **chest pain**
- frequent wheezing, particularly with heartburn
- unexplained weight loss
- nausea or vomiting
- stomach pain
- had heartburn over 3 months. This may be a sign of a more serious condition.
- heartburn with **lightheadedness, sweating or dizziness**
- chest pain or shoulder pain with shortness of breath; sweating; pain spreading to arms, neck or shoulders; or lightheadedness

STOP USE AND ASK A DOCTOR IF
- your heartburn continues or worsens
- you need to take this product for more than 14 days
- **If pregnant or breast-feeding**, ask a health professional before use.
  Keep out of reach of children. In case of overdose, get medical help or contact a Poison Control Center right away.

DIRECTIONS
- adults and children 12 years and over:
  - to **relieve** symptoms, swallow 1 tablet with a glass of water
  - to **prevent** symptoms, swallow 1 tablet with a glass of water **30 to 60 minutes before** eating food or drinking beverages that cause heartburn

- can be used up to twice daily (do not take more than 2 tablets in 24 hours)
- children under 12 years: ask a doctor

OTHER INFORMATION
- Blister: do not use if individual blister unit is open or torn Bottle: do not use if printed foil under bottle cap is open or torn
- store at 20°-25°C (68°-77°F)
- avoid excessive heat or humidity
- this product is sodium and sugar free

INACTIVE INGREDIENTS
hypromellose, magnesium stearate, microcrystalline cellulose, synthetic red iron oxide, titanium dioxide, triacetin

QUESTIONS OR COMMENTS?
Call **1-888-285-9159** or visit **www.zantacotc.com**

ZEASORB (miconazole)
Stiefel Laboratories, Inc

DRUG FACTS

Active Ingredient(s)	Purpose(s)
Miconazole nitrate 2%	Antifungal

USES
Athlete's Foot
- for the cure of most athlete's foot

Jock Itch
- for the cure of most jock itch

WARNINGS
For external use only

DO NOT USE
- on children under 2 years of age unless directed by a doctor.

Avoid contact with the eyes.

STOP USE AND ASK A DOCTOR IF
Athlete's Foot
- irritation occurs or there is no improvement within 4 weeks.

Jock Itch
- irritation occurs or there is no improvement within 2 weeks

Keep out of reach of children.
If swallowed, get medical help or contact a Poison Control Center right away.

DIRECTIONS
Athlete's Foot
- Clean the affected area and dry thoroughly.
- Apply a thin layer of the product over affected area twice daily (morning and night) or as directed by a doctor.
- Supervise children in the use of this product.
- Pay special attention to spaces between the toes; wear well-fitting, ventilated shoes, and change shoes and socks at least once daily.
- Use daily for 4 weeks.
- If condition persists longer, consult a doctor.
- This product is not effective on the scalp or nails.

Jock Itch
- Clean the affected area and dry thoroughly.
- Apply a thin layer of the product over affected area twice daily (morning and night) or as directed by a doctor.
- Supervise children in the use of this product.
- Use daily for 2 weeks.

- If condition persists longer, consult a doctor.
- This product is not effective on the scalp or nails.

OTHER INFORMATION
- Product settles during shipment. Package contains full net weight.

INACTIVE INGREDIENTS
acrylamide/sodium acrylate copolymer, aldioxa, chloroxylenol, fragrance, imidurea, microporous cellulose, talc. Contains no starch.

QUESTIONS OR COMMENTS?
call **1-888-438-7426.** Side effects should be reported to this number.

ZEGERID OTC (omeprazole and sodium bicarbonate)
MSD Consumer Care, Inc.

DRUG FACTS

Active Ingredient(s) (in each capsule)	Purpose(s)
Omeprazole 20 mg	Acid reducer
Sodium Bicarbonate 1100 mg	Allows absorption of this omeprazole product

USE
- treats frequent heartburn (occurs *2 or more* days a week)
- not intended for immediate relief of heartburn, this drug may take 1 to 4 days for full effect.

WARNINGS
Allergy alert
Do not use if you are allergic to omeprazole

DO NOT USE
if you have:
- trouble or pain swallowing food
- vomiting with blood
- bloody or black stools

These may be signs of a serious condition. See your doctor.

ASK A DOCTOR BEFORE USE IF YOU HAVE
- had heartburn over 3 months. This may be a sign of a more serious condition.
- heartburn with **lightheadedness, sweating or dizziness**
- chest pain or shoulder pain with shortness of breath; sweating; pain spreading to arms, neck or shoulders; or lightheadedness
- frequent **chest pain**
- frequent wheezing, particularly with heartburn
- unexplained weight loss
- nausea or vomiting
- stomach pain
- a sodium-restricted diet

ASK A DOCTOR OR PHARMACIST BEFORE USE IF YOU ARE
taking
- warfarin, clopidogrel or cilostazol (blood-thinning medicines)
- prescription antifungal or anti-yeast medicines
- diazepam (anxiety medicine)
- digoxin (heart medicine)
- tacrolimus (immune system medicine)
- prescription antiretrovirals (medicines for HIV infection)
- any other prescription drugs. Sodium bicarbonate may interact with certain prescription drugs

STOP USE AND ASK DOCTOR IF
- your heartburn continues or worsens
- you need to take this product for more than 14 days
- you need to take more than 1 course of treatment every 4 months

If pregnant or breast-feeding, ask a health professional before use.

Keep out of reach of children. In case of overdose, get medical help or contact a Poison Control Center right away.

DIRECTIONS
- for adults 18 years of age and older
- this product is to be used once a day (every 24 hours), every day for 14 days
- it may take 1 to 4 days for full effect, although some people get complete relief of symptoms within 24 hours
  - **14-Day Course of Treatment**
    - swallow 1 capsule with a glass of water at least 1 hour before eating in the morning
    - take every day for 14 days
    - do not take more than 1 capsule a day
    - do not chew or crush the capsule
    - do not open capsule and sprinkle on food
    - do not use for more than 14 days unless directed by your doctor
  - **Repeated 14-Day Courses (if needed)**
    - you may repeat a 14-day course every 4 months
    - **do not take for more than 14 days or more often than every 4 months unless directed by a doctor**
- children under 18 years of age: ask a doctor

Heartburn in children may sometimes be caused by a serious condition.

OTHER INFORMATION
- each capsule contains: **sodium 303 mg**
- read the directions, warnings and accompanying label information before use
- store at 20°-25°C (68°-77°F)
- tamper-evident: do not use if the blue band around the capsule is missing or broken. Do not use if foil under cap, printed with, "Sealed for your protection" is missing, open or broken.
- keep product out of high heat and humidity
- protect product from moisture

INACTIVE INGREDIENTS
croscarmellose sodium, FD&C blue no. 1, gelatin, magnesium stearate, pharmaceutical ink, polysorbate 80, titanium dioxide

QUESTIONS OR COMMENTS?
Call **1-888-ZEG-OTC (1-888-493-4682)** between 8:00AM and 5:00PM Central Standard Time, Monday through Friday or visit www.ZegeridOTC.com
© Copyright & Distributed by MSD Consumer Care, Inc., PO Box 377, Memphis, TN 38151 USA, a subsidiary of Merck & Co., Inc., Whitehouse Station, NJ USA.

ZICAM COLD REMEDY CHEWABLES (zincum aceticum and zincum gluconicum)

Matrixx Initiatives, Inc.

DRUG FACTS

Active Ingredient(s) (in each chewable)	Purpose(s)
Zincum Aceticum 2x	Reduces duration and severity of a cold
Zincum Gluconicum 2x	

USES
- Reduces duration of a cold
- Reduces severity of cold symptoms:
  - sore throat
  - stuffy nose
  - sneezing
  - coughing
  - congestion

WARNINGS

STOP USE AND ASK A DOCTOR
if symptoms persist or are accompanied by fever.
ZICAM® Cold Remedy was formulated to shorten the duration of a cold and is not known to be effective for flu or allergies.
If pregnant or breast-feeding, ask a health professional before use.
Keep out of reach of children.

DIRECTIONS
For best results, use at the first sign of a cold and continue to use for an additional 48 hours after symptoms subside.
- Adults and children 12 years of age and older:
  - Take 1 chewable square at the onset of symptoms. Chew thoroughly before swallowing.
  - Repeat every 3 hours until symptoms are gone.
  - To avoid minor stomach upset, do not take on an empty stomach.
  - Do not eat or drink for 15 minutes after use. Do not eat or drink citrus fruits or juices for 30 minutes before or after use. Otherwise, drink plenty of fluids.
- This product is not recommended for children under 12 years of age due to the hazard of choking.

INACTIVE INGREDIENTS
coconut oil, corn syrup, corn syrup solids, FD&C red no. 40, glycerin, natural and artificial flavors, purified water, soy lecithin, sucralose, sucrose, sugar

QUESTIONS? COMMENTS? SIDE EFFECTS?
Call 877-942-2626 toll free or visit us on the web at www.zicam.com

---

ZICAM COLD REMEDY LIQUI-LOZ (zincum aceticum and zincum gluconicum)

Matrixx Initiatives, Inc.

DRUG FACTS

Active Ingredient(s) (in each lozenge)	Purpose(s)
Zincum Aceticum 2x	Reduces duration and severity of the common cold
Zincum Gluconicum 2x	

USES
- Reduces duration of the common cold
- Reduces severity of cold symptoms:
  - sore throat
  - stuffy nose
  - sneezing
  - coughing
  - nasal congestion

ASK A DOCTOR BEFORE USE IF YOU HAVE
- a sensitivity to zinc or are allergic to zinc

WARNINGS

STOP USE AND ASK A DOCTOR
if symptoms persist or are accompanied by fever.
ZICAM® Cold Remedy was formulated to shorten the duration of the common cold and was not formulated to be effective for flu or allergies.
If pregnant or breast-feeding, ask a health professional before use.
Keep out of reach of children. In case of overdose, get medical help or contact a Poison Control Center right away.

DIRECTIONS

For best results, use at the first sign of a cold and continue to use for an additional 48 hours after symptoms subside.
• Adults and children 12 years of age and older:
  • Take 1 lozenge at the onset of symptoms. Completely dissolve lozenge in mouth. Do not chew. Do not swallow whole.
  • Repeat every 3 hours until symptoms are gone.
  • To avoid minor stomach upset, do not take on an empty stomach.
  • Do not eat or drink for 15 minutes after use. Do not eat or drink citrus fruits or juices for 30 minutes before or after use. Otherwise, drink plenty of fluids.
• children under 12 years of age: do not use due to the hazard of choking.

OTHER INFORMATION
• Store between 15° C-29° C (59° F-84° F)
• Avoid freezing and excessive heat.

INACTIVE INGREDIENTS
citric acid, corn syrup, FD&C blue no. 1, FD&C red no. 40, glycerin, natural and artificial flavors, peppermint oil, purified water, soy lecithin, sucralose, sucrose

QUESTIONS? COMMENTS? SIDE EFFECTS?
call 877-942-2626 toll free
or visit us on the web at
www.zicam.com

ZICAM COLD REMEDY PLUS ORAL MIST
(zincum aceticum and zincum gluconium)

Matrixx Initiatives, Inc.

DRUG FACTS

Active Ingredient(s)
Zincum Aceticum 2x
Zincum Gluconicum 1 x

Purpose(s)
Reduces duration and severity of the common cold

USES
• Reduces duration of the common cold
• Reduces severity of cold symptoms:
  • sore throat
  • stuffy nose
  • sneezing
  • coughing
  • congestion

WARNINGS
For oral use only.

WHEN USING THIS PRODUCT
• Avoid contact with eyes. In case of accidental contact with eyes, flush with water and immediately seek professional help.

STOP USE AND ASK A DOCTOR
if symptoms persist or are accompanied by fever.
Zicam® Cold Remedy Plus was formulated to shorten the duration of the common cold and was not formulated to be effective for flu or allergies.
If you are allergic or sensitive to zinc, consult a doctor before using.
If pregnant or breast-feeding, ask a health professional before use.
Keep out of reach of children.

DIRECTIONS
• **For best results, use at the first sign of a cold and continue to use until symptoms completely subside.**
  • Adults and children 12 years of age and older:
    • Spray 4 times in mouth at the onset of symptoms. Spray on inside of cheeks, roof of mouth and gums. Retain for 15 seconds. Swallow.
    • Repeat every 3 hours until symptoms are gone.
    • To avoid minor stomach upset, do not take on an empty stomach.
    • Do not eat or drink for 15 minutes after use. Do not eat or drink citrus fruits or juices for 30 minutes before or after use. Otherwise, drink plenty of fluids.
  • Children under 12 years of age: Ask a doctor before use.

OTHER INFORMATION
Store at room temperature 15° C-29° C (59° F-84° F)

INACTIVE INGREDIENTS
acesulfame potassium, artificial flavor, citric acid, glycerin, menthol, PEG-40 hydrogenated castor oil, potassium sorbate, purified water, sucralose

QUESTIONS? COMMENTS? SIDE EFFECTS?
call 877-942-2626 toll free or visit us on the web at
www.zicam.com
Distributed by Matrixx Initiatives, Inc.
Scottsdale, Arizona 85255

ZICAM COLD REMEDY RAPIDMELTS (zincum aceticum and zincum gluconicum)

Matrixx Initiatives, Inc.

DRUG FACTS

Active Ingredient(s) (in each tablet)
Zincum Aceticum 2x
Zincum Gluconicum 1x

Purpose(s)
Reduces duration and severity of the common cold

USES
• Reduces duration of the common cold
• Reduces severity of cold symptoms:
  • sore throat
  • stuffy nose
  • sneezing
  • coughing
  • congestion

WARNINGS

STOP USE AND ASK A DOCTOR
if symptoms persist or are accompanied by fever.
Zicam® Cold Remedy was formulated to shorten the duration of the common cold and was not formulated to be effective for flu or allergies.
If you are allergic or sensitive to zinc, consult a doctor before using.

If pregnant or breast-feeding, ask a health professional before use.

Keep out of reach of children.

DIRECTIONS

- **For best results, use at the first sign of a cold and continue to use until symptoms completely subside.**
  - Adults and children 12 years of age and older:
    - Take 1 tablet at the onset of symptoms.
    - Dissolve entire tablet in mouth. Do not chew. Do not swallow whole.
    - Repeat every 3 hours until symptoms are gone.
    - To avoid minor stomach upset, do not take on an empty stomach.
    - Do not eat or drink for 15 minutes after use. Do not eat or drink citrus fruits or juices for 30 minutes before or after use. Otherwise, drink plenty of fluids.
  - Children under 12 years of age: Ask a doctor before use.

OTHER INFORMATION

Store at room temperature 15° C-29° C (59° F-84° F)

INACTIVE INGREDIENTS

artifical flavor, crospovidone, FD&C red no. 40 aluminum lake, magnesium stearate, mannitol, mono-ammonium glycyrrhizinate, sodium starch glycolate, stearic acid, sucralose

QUESTIONS? COMMENTS? SIDE EFFECTS?

call 877-942-2626 toll free or visit us on the web at **www.zicam.com**
Distributed by Matrixx Initiatives, Inc.
Scottsdale, Arizona 85255

ZICAM COLD REMEDY ULTRA CRYSTALS

(zincum aceticum and zincum gluconicum)

Matrixx Initiatives, Inc.

DRUG FACTS

Active Ingredient(s) (in each packet)
Zincum Aceticum 2×
Zincum Gluconicum 1×

Purpose(s)
Reduces duration and severity of the common cold

USES

- Reduces duration of the common cold
- Reduces severity of cold symptoms:
  - sore throat
  - stuffy nose
  - sneezing
  - coughing
  - congestion

WARNINGS

STOP USE AND ASK A DOCTOR
if symptoms persist or are accompanied by fever.
Zicam® Cold Remedy was formulated to shorten the duration of the common cold and was not formulated to be effective for flu or allergies.
If you are allergive or sensitive to zinc, consult a doctor before using.
If pregnant or breast-feeding, ask a health professional before use.

Keep out of reach of children.

DIRECTIONS

- **For best results, use at the first sign of a cold and continue to use until symptoms completely subside.**

- Adults and children 12 years of age and older:
  - Take 1 packet at the onset of symptoms.
  - Dissolve contents of packet in mouth. Do not chew. Do not swallow whole.
  - Repeat every 4-6 hours, not to exceed 4 packets in 24 hours.
  - To avoid minor stomach upset, do not take on an empty stomach.
  - Do not eat or drink for 15 minutes after use. Do not eat or drink citrus fruits or juices for 30 minutes before or after use. Otherwise, drink plenty of fluids.
- Children under 12 years of age: Ask a doctor before use.

OTHER INFORMATION

Store at room temperature 15° C-29°C (59° F-84° F)

INACTIVE INGREDIENTS

butylated hydroxyanisole, citric acid, cocoa butter, confectioner's sugar, crospovidone, gum acacia, hypromellose, maltitol, maltodextrin, microcrystalline cellulose, polyethylene glycol, polysorbate, silicon dioxide, sodium lauryl sulfate, sorbitan monostearate, starch, sucralose, sugar

---

ZICAM COLD REMEDY ULTRA LOZENGE

(zincum aceticum and zincum gluconicum)

Matrixx Initiatives, Inc.

DRUG FACTS

Active Ingredient(s)
Zincum Aceticum 2×
Zincum Gluconicum 2×

Purpose(s)
Reduces duration and severity of the common cold

USES

- Reduces duration of the common cold
- Reduces severity of cold symptoms:
  - sore throat
  - stuffy nose
  - sneezing
  - coughing
  - congestion

WARNINGS

STOP USE AND ASK A DOCTOR
if symptoms persist or are accompanied by fever.
Zicam® ULTRA Cold Remedy was formulated to shorten the duration of the common cold and was not formulated to be effective for flu or allergies. Ask a doctor or pharmacist before use if you are allergic or sensitive to zinc.
If pregnant or breast-feeding, ask a health professional before use.

Keep out of reach of children.

DIRECTIONS

- **For best results, use at the first sign of a cold and continue to use until symptoms completely subside.**
- Adults and children 12 years of age and older:
  - Take 1 lozenge at the onset of symptoms.
  - Completely dissolve entire lozenge in mouth. Do not chew. Do not swallow whole.
  - Repeat every 4-6 hours, not to exceed 4 lozenges in 24 hours.
  - To avoid minor stomach upset, do not take on an empty stomach.
  - Do not eat or drink for 15 minutes after use. Do not eat or drink citrus fruits or juices for 30 minutes before or after use. Otherwise, drink plenty of fluids.
- Children under 12 years of age: Ask a doctor before use.

INACTIVE INGREDIENTS
citric acid, corn syrup, honey, natural color, natural flavors, purified water, sucrose

QUESTIONS? COMMENTS? SIDE EFFECTS?
call 877-942-2626 toll free or visit us on the web at www.zicam.com

---

ZILACTIN EARLY RELIEF COLD SORE GEL
(benzyl alcohol)

Blairex Laboratories, Inc.

Instructions & Usage

Active Ingredient(s)
Benzyl Alcohol 10%

USES
Temporarily relieves pain caused by:
• Cold sores/fever blisters
• Canker sores, mouth sores
• Gum irritations

WARNINGS
• **Flammable**
• Keep away from fire or flame
• Apply only to affected areas
• Do not exceed recommended dosage
• Avoid contact with the eyes
• Do not use for more than 7 days unless directed by a physician or dentist

STOP USE AND ASK A PHYSICIAN IF
• Sore mouth symptoms do not improve in 7 days
• Condition worsens or symptoms clear up and occur again within a few days
• Swelling, rash or fever develops
• Irritation, pain or redness persists or worsens

Keep out of reach of children. If swallowed, get medical help or contact a poison control center immediately.

DIRECTIONS
Adults and children 2 years and older. Dry affected area. Apply with cotton swab or clean finger up to 4 times daily. Allow to dry 30-60 seconds.

Children under 12 years
Adult supervision should be given in the use of this product

Children under 2 years
Do not use. Consult a physician or dentist

OTHER INFORMATION
• Do not peel off protective film. Attempting to peel off film may result in skin irritation or tenderness. To remove film, first apply another coat of Zilactin to film, and immediately wipe the area with a moist gauze pad or tissue.
• Contains alcohol 73% by volume
• Store at 15-20°C (59-86°F)

INACTIVE INGREDIENTS
boric acid, hydroxypropylcellulose, propylene glycol, purified water, salicylic acid, SD alcohol 37, tannic acid

---

ZILACTIN-B 6 HOUR CANKER & MOUTH SORE RELIEF (benzocaine)

Blairex Laboratories, Inc.

Instructions & Usage

Active Ingredient(s)
Benzocaine 10%

USES
Temporarily relieves pain caused by:
• Canker sores
• Minor mouth sores and gum irritations
• Denture and brace pain

WARNINGS
• Flammable
• Keep away from fire or flame
• Apply only to affected areas
• Do not exceed recommended dosage
• Avoid contact with the eyes
• Do not use for more than 7 days unless directed by a physician or dentist

STOP USE AND ASK A PHYSICIAN IF
• Sore mouth symptoms do not improve in 7 days
• Swelling, rash or fever develops
• Irritation, pain or redness persists or worsens

Keep out of reach of children. If swallowed, get medical help or contact a poison control center immediately.

DIRECTIONS
Adults and children 2 years and older. Dry affected area. Apply a thin coat of gel with cotton swab or clean finger up to 4 times daily. Allow to dry 30-60 seconds.

Children under 12
Adult supervision should be given in the use of this product.

Children under 2 years
Do not use. Consult a physician or dentist.

OTHER INFORMATION
• Do not peel off protective film. Attempting to peel off film may result in skin irritation or tenderness. To remove film, first apply another coat of Zilactin®-B to film and immediately wipe the area with a moist gauze pad or tissue.
• Contains alcohol 70% by volume
• Store at 15-20° (59-86°F)

INACTIVE INGREDIENTS
boric acid, hydroxypropylcellulose, propylene glycol, purified water, salicylic acid, SD alcohol 38-B, tannic acid

---

CHILDRENS ZYRTEC (cetirizine hydrochloride)
McNeil Consumer Healthcare Div McNeil-PPC, Inc

DRUG FACTS

Active Ingredient(s) (in each 5 mL teaspoonful)
Cetirizine HCl 5 mg

Purpose(s)
Antihistamine

USES
temporarily relieves these symptoms due to hay fever or other upper respiratory allergies:
• runny nose
• sneezing

- itchy, watery eyes
- itching of the nose or throat

WARNINGS

DO NOT USE

if you have ever had an allergic reaction to this product or any of its ingredients or to an antihistamine containing hydroxyzine.

ASK A DOCTOR BEFORE USE IF YOU HAVE

liver or kidney disease. Your doctor should determine if you need a different dose.

ASK A DOCTOR OR PHARMACIST BEFORE USE IF YOU ARE

taking tranquilizers or sedatives.

WHEN USING THIS PRODUCT

- drowsiness may occur
- avoid alcoholic drinks
- alcohol, sedatives, and tranquilizers may increase drowsiness
- be careful when driving a motor vehicle or operating machinery

STOP USE AND ASK A DOCTOR IF

an allergic reaction to this product occurs. Seek medical help right away.

If pregnant or breast-feeding:

- if breast-feeding: not recommended
- if pregnant: ask a health professional before use.

Keep out of reach of children. In case of overdose, get medical help or contact a Poison Control Center right away. (1-800-222-1222)

DIRECTIONS

- use only with enclosed dosing cup

adults and children 6 years and over	1 teaspoonful (5 mL) or 2 teaspoonfuls (10 mL) once daily depending upon severity of symptoms; do not take more than 2 teaspoonfuls (10 mL) in 24 hours.
adults 65 years and over	1 teaspoonful (5 mL) once daily; do not take more than 1 teaspoonful (5 mL) in 24 hours.
children 2 to under 6 years of age	1/2 teaspoonful (2.5 mL) once daily. If needed, dose can be increased to a maximum of 1 teaspoonful (5 mL) once daily or ½ teaspoonful (2.5 mL) every 12 hours. Do not give more than 1 teaspoonful (5 mL) in 24 hours.
children under 2 years of age	ask a doctor
consumers with liver or kidney disease	ask a doctor

OTHER INFORMATION

- store between 20° to 25°C (68° to 77°F)
- **do not use if carton is opened; or if bottle wrap or foil inner seal printed with "Safety Seal®" is broken or missing**
- see bottom panel for lot number and expiration date

INACTIVE INGREDIENTS

anhydrous citric acid, flavors, propylene glycol, purified water, sodium benzoate, sorbitol solution, sucralose

QUESTIONS OR COMMENTS?

call **1-800-343-7805**

ZYRTEC LIQUID GELS (cetirizine hydrochloride)
McNeil Consumer Healthcare Div McNeil-PPC, Inc

DRUG FACTS

Active Ingredient(s) (in each capsule)
Cetirizine HCl 10 mg

Purpose(s)
Antihistamine

USES

temporarily relieves these symptoms due to hay fever or other upper respiratory allergies:
- runny nose
- sneezing
- itchy, watery eyes
- itching of the nose or throat

WARNINGS

DO NOT USE

if you have ever had an allergic reaction to this product or any of its ingredients or to an antihistamine containing hydroxyzine.

ASK A DOCTOR BEFORE USE IF YOU HAVE

liver or kidney disease. Your doctor should determine if you need a different dose.

ASK A DOCTOR OR PHARMACIST BEFORE USE IF YOU ARE

taking tranquilizers or sedatives.

WHEN USING THIS PRODUCT

- drowsiness may occur
- avoid alcoholic drinks
- alcohol, sedatives, and tranquilizers may increase drowsiness
- be careful when driving a motor vehicle or operating machinery

STOP USE AND ASK A DOCTOR IF

an allergic reaction to this product occurs. Seek medical help right away.

If pregnant or breast-feeding:

- if breast-feeding: not recommended
- if pregnant: ask a health professional before use.

Keep out of reach of children. In case of overdose, get medical help or contact a Poison Control Center right away. (1-800-222-1222)

DIRECTIONS

adults and children 6 years and over	one 10 mg capsule once daily; do not take more than one 10 mg capsule in 24 hours. A 5 mg product may be appropriate for less severe symptoms.
adults 65 years and over	ask a doctor
children under 6 years of age	ask a doctor
consumers with liver or kidney disease	ask a doctor

OTHER INFORMATION
- store at 20° - 25°C (68° - 77°F)
- avoid high humidity and excessive heat above 40°C (104°F)
- protect from light
- **do not use if foil inner seal printed with "Safety Seal®" is broken or missing**

INACTIVE INGREDIENTS
gelatin, glycerin, mannitol, pharmaceutical ink, polyethylene glycol 400, purified water, sodium hydroxide, sorbitan, sorbitol

QUESTIONS OR COMMENTS?
call **1-800-343-7805**

ZYRTEC TABLETS (cetirizine hydrochloride)
McNeil Consumer Healthcare Div McNeil-PPC, Inc

DRUG FACTS

Active Ingredient(s) (in each tablet)
Cetirizine HCl 10 mg

Purpose(s)
Antihistamine

USES
temporarily relieves these symptoms due to hay fever or other upper respiratory allergies:
- runny nose
- sneezing
- itchy, watery eyes
- itching of the nose or throat

WARNINGS

DO NOT USE
if you have ever had an allergic reaction to this product or any of its ingredients or to an antihistamine containing hydroxyzine.

ASK A DOCTOR BEFORE USE IF YOU HAVE
liver or kidney disease. Your doctor should determine if you need a different dose.

ASK A DOCTOR OR PHARMACIST BEFORE USE IF YOU ARE
taking tranquilizers or sedatives.

WHEN USING THIS PRODUCT
- drowsiness may occur
- avoid alcoholic drinks
- alcohol, sedatives, and tranquilizers may increase drowsiness
- be careful when driving a motor vehicle or operating machinery

STOP USE AND ASK A DOCTOR IF
an allergic reaction to this product occurs. Seek medical help right away.

If pregnant or breast-feeding:
- if breast-feeding: not recommended
- if pregnant: ask a health professional before use.

Keep out of reach of children. In case of overdose, get medical help or contact a Poison Control Center right away. (1-800-222-1222)

DIRECTIONS

adults and children 6 years and over	one 10 mg tablet once daily; do not take more than one 10 mg tablet in 24 hours. A 5 mg product may be appropriate for less severe symptoms.
adults 65 years and over	ask a doctor
children under 6 years of age	ask a doctor
consumers with liver or kidney disease	ask a doctor

OTHER INFORMATION
- store between 20° to 25°C (68° to 77°F)
- **do not use if imprinted foil inner seal on bottle is broken or missing**

INACTIVE INGREDIENTS
carnauba wax, corn starch, hypromellose, lactose monohydrate, magnesium stearate, polyethylene glycol, povidone, titanium dioxide

QUESTIONS OR COMMENTS?
call **1-800-343-7805**

ZYRTEC-D ALLERGY AND CONGESTION
(cetirizine hydrochloride and pseudoephedrine hydrochloride)
McNeil Consumer Healthcare Div McNeil-PPC, Inc

DRUG FACTS

Active Ingredient(s) (in each extended release tablet)
Cetirizine HCl 5 mg
Pseudoephedrine HCl 120 mg

Purpose(s)
Antihistamine
Nasal decongestant

USES
- temporarily relieves these symptoms due to hay fever or other upper respiratory allergies:
  - runny nose
  - sneezing
  - itchy, watery eyes
  - itching of the nose or throat
  - nasal congestion
- reduces swelling of nasal passages
- temporarily relieves sinus congestion and pressure
- temporarily restores freer breathing through the nose

WARNINGS

DO NOT USE
- if you have ever had an allergic reaction to this product or any of its ingredients or to an antihistamine containing hydroxyzine.
- if you are now taking a prescription monoamine oxidase inhibitor (MAOI) (certain drugs for depression, psychiatric, or emotional conditions, or Parkinson's disease), or for 2 weeks after stopping the MAOI drug. If you do not know if your prescription drug contains an MAOI, ask a doctor or pharmacist before taking this product.

ASK A DOCTOR BEFORE USE IF YOU HAVE
- heart disease
- thyroid disease
- diabetes

- glaucoma
- high blood pressure
- trouble urinating due to an enlarged prostate gland
- liver or kidney disease. Your doctor should determine if you need a different dose.

ASK A DOCTOR OR PHARMACIST BEFORE USE IF YOU ARE
taking tranquilizers or sedatives.

WHEN USING THIS PRODUCT
- **do not use more than directed**
- drowsiness may occur
- avoid alcoholic drinks
- alcohol, sedatives, and tranquilizers may increase drowsiness
- be careful when driving a motor vehicle or operating machinery

STOP USE AND ASK A DOCTOR IF
- an allergic reaction to this product occurs. Seek medical help right away.
- you get nervous, dizzy, or sleepless
- symptoms do not improve within 7 days or are accompanied by fever

If pregnant or breast-feeding:
- if breast-feeding: not recommended
- if pregnant: ask a health professional before use.

Keep out of reach of children. In case of overdose, get medical help or contact a Poison Control Center right away. (1-800-222-1222)

DIRECTIONS
- do not break or chew tablet; swallow tablet whole

adults and children 12 years and over	take 1 tablet every 12 hours; do not take more than 2 tablets in 24 hours.
adults 65 years and over	ask a doctor
children under 12 years of age	ask a doctor
consumers with liver or kidney disease	ask a doctor

OTHER INFORMATION
- store between 20° to 25°C (68° to 77°F)
- **do not use if individual blister unit is open or torn**
- see back panel for lot number and expiration date

INACTIVE INGREDIENTS
colloidal silicon dioxide, croscarmellose sodium, hypromellose, lactose monohydrate, magnesium stearate, microcrystalline cellulose, polyethylene glycol, titanium dioxide

QUESTIONS OR COMMENTS?
call **1-800-343-7805**

APPENDIX A
POISON CONTROL CENTERS

The American Association of Poison Control Centers (AAPCC) uses a single, nationwide emergency number to automatically link callers with their regional poison center. This toll-free number, **800-222-1222**, also works for **teletype lines (TTY)** for the hearing-impaired and **telecommunication devices (TDD)** for individuals who are deaf. However, a few local poison centers and the ASPCA/Animal Poison Control Center are not part of this nationwide system and continue to use separate numbers.

Most of the centers listed below are accredited by the AAPCC. **Certified centers are marked by an asterisk after the name.** Each has to meet certain criteria. It must, for example, serve a large geographic area; it must be open 24 hours a day and provide direct-dial or toll-free access; it must be supervised by a medical director; and it must have registered pharmacists or nurses available to answer questions from the public.

Within each state, centers are listed alphabetically by city. Some state poison centers also list their original emergency numbers (including TDD/TTY) that only work within that state. For these listings, callers may use either the state number or the nationwide 800 number.

ALABAMA

BIRMINGHAM

Regional Poison Control Center (*)
Children's Hospital of Alabama

1600 7th Ave South
Birmingham AL 35233-1711
Business: 205-939-9201
Emergency: 800-222-1222
www.chsys.org

TUSCALOOSA

Alabama Poison Center (*)

2503 Phoenix Dr
Tuscaloosa AL 35405
Business: 205-345-0600
Emergency: 800-222-1222
              800-462-0800 (AL)
www.alapoisoncenter.org

ALASKA

(PORTLAND, OR)

Oregon Poison Center (*)
Oregon Health and Science University

3181 SW Sam Jackson Park Rd
Suite CB550
Portland OR 97239
Business: 503-494-8600
Emergency: 800-222-1222
www.ohsu.edu/xd/outreach/
oregon-poison-center

ARIZONA

PHOENIX

Banner Poison Control Center (*)
Banner Good Samaritan Medical Center

1111 E McDowell
Phoenix AZ 85006
Business: 602-495-6360
Emergency: 800-222-1222
              800-362-0101 (AZ)
              800-253-3334 (AZ)
www.bannerpoisoncontrol.com

TUCSON

Arizona Poison and Drug Information Center (*)
Arizona Health Sciences Center

1295 N Martin, Room B308
Tucson AZ 85721
Business: 520-626-7899
Emergency: 800-222-1222
www.pharmacy.arizona.edu/
outreach/poison

ARKANSAS

LITTLE ROCK

Arkansas Poison and Drug Information Center (*)
College of Pharmacy – UAMS

4301 W Markham St – MS 522-2
Little Rock AR 72205
Business: 501-686-5540
Emergency: 800-222-1222
              800-376-4766 (AR)
TDD/TTY: 800-641-3805
www.uams.edu/cop

ASPCA/ANIMAL POISON CONTROL CENTER

1717 S Philo Rd – Suite 36
Urbana IL 61802
Business: 217-337-5030
Emergency: 888-426-4435
                        800-548-2423
www.aspcapro.org/
animal-poison-control.php

CALIFORNIA

FRESNO/MADERA

**California Poison Control
System
Fresno/Madera Division (*)
Children's Hospital Central
California**

9300 Valley Children's Place –
MB 15
Madera CA 93636
Business: 559-622-2300
Emergency: 800-222-1222
                        800-876-4766 (CA)
TDD/TTY: 800-972-3323
www.calpoison.org

SACRAMENTO

**California Poison Control
System
Sacramento Division (*)
UC Davis Medical Center**

2315 Stockton Blvd
Room HSF 1024
Sacramento CA 95817
Business: 916-227-1400
Emergency: 800-222-1222
                        800-876-4766 (CA)
TDD/TTY: 800-972-3323
www.calpoison.org

SAN DIEGO

**California Poison Control
System
San Diego Division (*)
UC San Diego Medical Center**

200 W Arbor Dr
San Diego CA 92103-8925
Business: 858-715-6300
Emergency: 800-222-1222
                        800-876-4766 (CA)
TDD/TTY: 800-972-3323
www.calpoison.org

SAN FRANCISCO

**California Poison Control
System
San Francisco Division (*)**

UCSF Box 1369
San Francisco CA 94143
Business: 415-502-8600
Emergency: 800-222-1222
                        800-876-4766 (CA)
TDD/TTY: 800-972-3323
www.calpoison.org

COLORADO

DENVER

**Rocky Mountain Poison and
Drug Center (*)**

777 Bannock St – MC 0180
Denver CO 80204-4507
Business: 303-389-1100
Emergency: 800-222-1222
TDD/TTY: 303-739-1127 (CO)
www.rmpdc.org

CONNECTICUT

FARMINGTON

**Connecticut Poison Control
Center (*)
University of Connecticut
Health Center**

263 Farmington Ave
Farmington CT 06030-5365
Business: 860-679-4540
Emergency: 800-222-1222
TDD/TTY: 866-218-5372
http://poisoncontrol.uchc.edu

DELAWARE

(PHILADELPHIA, PA)

**The Poison Control Center (*)
Children's Hospital of
Philadelphia**

34th St & Civic Center Blvd
Philadelphia PA 19104-4399
Business: 215-590-2003
Emergency: 800-222-1222
                        800-722-7112 (DE)
TDD/TTY: 215-590-8789
www.chop.edu/service/
poison-control-center/home.html

DISTRICT OF COLUMBIA

WASHINGTON, DC

**National Capital Poison Center
(*)**

3201 New Mexico Ave NW
Suite 310
Washington DC 20016
Business: 202-362-3867
Emergency: 800-222-1222
www.poison.org

FLORIDA

JACKSONVILLE

Florida Poison Information Center-Jacksonville (*)
SHANDS Hospital

655 W 8th St, Box C23
Jacksonville FL 32209
Business: 904-244-4465
Emergency: 800-222-1222
http://fpicjax.org

MIAMI

Florida/USVI Poison Information Center-Miami (*)
University of Miami, Department of Pediatrics

Jackson Memorial Hospital
1611 NW 12th Ave
(R-131) Institute Annex,
3rd Floor
Miami FL 33136
Business: 305-585-5250
Emergency: 800-222-1222
www.med.miami.edu/
poisoncontrol

TAMPA

Florida Poison Information Center-Tampa (*)
Tampa Division

PO Box 1289
Tampa FL 33601-1289
Business: 813-844-7044
Emergency: 800-222-1222
www.poisoncentertampa.org

GEORGIA

ATLANTA

Georgia Poison Center (*)
Hughes Spalding Children's Hospital
Grady Health System

50 Hurt Plaza – Suite 600
PO Box 26066
Atlanta GA 30303
Business: 404-616-9237
Emergency: 800-222-1222
              404-616-9000
              (Atlanta)
TDD: 404-616-9287
www.georgiapoisoncenter.org

HAWAII

(DENVER, CO)

Rocky Mountain Poison and Drug Center (*)

777 Bannock St – MC 0180
Denver CO 80204-4507
Business: 303-389-1100
Emergency: 800-222-1222
www.rmpdc.org

IDAHO

(OMAHA, NE)

The Poison Control Center
Children's Hospital

8200 Dodge St
Omaha NE 68114
Business: 402-390-5555
Emergency: 800-222-1222
www.nebraskapoison.com

ILLINOIS

CHICAGO

Illinois Poison Center (*)

222 S Riverside Plaza –
Suite 1900
Chicago IL 60606
Business: 312-906-6136
Emergency: 800-222-1222
TDD/TTY: 312-906-6185
www.illinoispoisoncenter.org

INDIANA

INDIANAPOLIS

Indiana Poison Center (*)
Clarian Health Partners
Methodist Hospital

I-65 at 21st Street
Indianapolis, IN 46206-1367
Business: 317-962-2335
Emergency: 800-222-1222
              800-382-9097 (IN)
              317-962-2323
              (Indianapolis)
www.clarian.org/poisoncontrol

IOWA

SIOUX CITY

Iowa Statewide Poison Control Center (*)

401 Douglas St – Suite 40
Sioux City IA 51101
Business: 712-279-3710
Emergency: 800-222-1222
              712-277-2222 (IA)
www.iowapoison.org

KANSAS

KANSAS CITY

Mid-America Poison Control University of Kansas Medical Center

3901 Rainbow Blvd
Room B-400
Kansas City KS 66160-7231
Business: 913-588-6638
Emergency: 800-222-1222
                    800-332-6633 (KS)
TDD: 913-588-6639
www.kumed.com/poison

KENTUCKY

LOUISVILLE

Kentucky Regional Poison Center (*)

Medical Towers South
234 E Gray St – Suite 847
Louisville KY 40202
Business: 502-629-7264
Emergency: 800-222-1222
                    502-589-8222
                    (Louisville)
www.krpc.com

LOUISIANA

MONROE

Louisiana Drug and Poison Information Center (*) LSUHSC Shreveport Department of Emergency Medicine - Section of Clinical Toxicology

1455 Wilkinson St
Shreveport LA 71130
Business: 318-342-3648
Emergency: 800-222-1222
www.lapcc.org

MAINE

PORTLAND

Northern New England Poison Center (*)

Maine Medical Center
22 Bramhall St
Portland ME 04102
Business: 207-662-7220
Emergency: 800-222-1222
TDD/TTY   877-299-4447 (ME)
www.nnepc.org

MARYLAND

BALTIMORE

Maryland Poison Center (*) University of Maryland at Baltimore School of Pharmacy

220 Arch St, Office Level 1
Baltimore MD 21201
Business: 410-706-7604
Emergency: 800-222-1222
TDD: 410-706-1858
www.mdpoison.com

(WASHINGTON, DC)

National Capital Poison Center (*)

3201 New Mexico Ave NW
Suite 310
Washington DC 20016
Business: 202-362-3867
Emergency: 800-222-1222
www.poison.org

MASSACHUSETTS

BOSTON

Regional Center for Poison Control and Prevention (*)

300 Longwood Ave
Boston MA 02115
Business: 617-355-6609
Emergency: 800-222-1222
TDD/TTY   888-244-5313
www.maripoisoncenter.com

MICHIGAN

DETROIT

Regional Poison Control Center (*) VHS Children's Hospital of Michigan

4707 St Antoine – Suite 302
Detroit MI 48201
Business: 313-745-5335
Emergency: 800-222-1222
                    313-745-5711
                    (Detroit)
www.mitoxic.org/pcc

MINNESOTA

MINNEAPOLIS

Minnesota Poison Control System (*) Hennepin County Medical Center

701 Park Avenue, Mail Code RL
Minneapolis MN 55415
Business: 612-873-3144
Emergency: 800-222-1222
www.mnpoison.org

MISSISSIPPI

JACKSON

Mississippi Regional Poison Control Center University of Mississippi Medical Center

2500 N State St
Jackson MS 39216
Business: 601-984-1680
Emergency: 800-222-1222
http://poisoncontrol.umc.edu

MISSOURI

ST. LOUIS

Missouri Regional Poison Center (*)
Cardinal Glennon Children's Medical Center

7980 Clayton Rd – Suite 200
St. Louis MO 63117
Business: 314-577-5610
Emergency: 800-222-1222
www.cardinalglennon.com

MONTANA

(DENVER, CO)

Rocky Mountain Poison and Drug Center (*)

777 Bannock St – MC 0180
Denver CO 80204-4507
Business: 303-389-1100
Emergency: 800-222-1222
www.rmpdc.org

NEBRASKA

OMAHA

The Poison Center (*)
Children's Hospital

8200 Dodge St
Omaha NE 68114
Business: 402-390-5555
Emergency: 800-222-1222
www.nebraskapoison.com

NEVADA

(DENVER, CO)

Rocky Mountain Poison and Drug Center (*)

777 Bannock St – MC 0180
Denver CO 80204-4507
Business: 303-389-1100
Emergency: 800-222-1222
www.rmpdc.org

NEW HAMPSHIRE

(PORTLAND, ME)

Northern New England Poison Center (*)

22 Bramhall St
Portland ME 04102
Business: 207-662-7220
Emergency: 800-222-1222
www.nnepc.org

NEW JERSEY

NEWARK

New Jersey Poison Information and Education System (*)
UMDNJ

140 Bergen Street – PO Box 1709
Newark NJ 07107
Business: 973-972-9280
Emergency: 800-222-1222
TDD/TTY: 973-926-8008
www.njpies.org

NEW MEXICO

ALBUQUERQUE

New Mexico Poison and Drug Information Center (*)

1 University of New Mexico – MSC 09 5080
Albuquerque NM 87131-0001
Business: 505-272-4261
Emergency: 800-222-1222
http://hsc.unm.edu/pharmacy/poison

NEW YORK

NEW YORK CITY

New York City Poison Control Center (*)
NYC Bureau of Public Health

455 1st Ave – Room 123
Box 81
New York NY 10016
Business: 212-447-8152
English
Emergency: 800-222-1222
212-340-4494
212-POISONS
(212-764-7667)

Spanish
Emergency: 212-VENENOS
(212-836-3667)
www.nyc.gov/html/doh/html/poison/poison.shtml

SYRACUSE

Upstate New York Poison Center (*)
SUNY Upstate Medical University

750 E Adams St
Syracuse NY 13210
Business: 315-464-7078
Emergency: 800-222-1222
TTY: 315-464-5424
www.upstate.edu/poison/contactus

NORTH CAROLINA

CHARLOTTE

Carolinas Poison Center (*)
Carolinas Medical Center

PO Box 32861
Charlotte NC 28232
Business: 704-395-3795
Emergency: 800-222-1222
TDD: 800-735-8262
TYY: 800-735-2962
www.ncpoisoncenter.org

NORTH DAKOTA

(MINNEAPOLIS, MN)

Minnesota Poison Control System (*)
Hennepin County Medical Center

701 Park Avenue, Mail Code RL
Minneapolis MN 55415
Business: 612-873-3144
Emergency: 800-222-1222
www.mnpoison.org

OHIO

CINCINNATI

Cincinnati Drug and Poison Information Center (*)
Regional Poison Control System

3333 Burnett Ave
Vernon Place, 3rd Floor
Cincinnati OH 45229
Business: 513-636-5111
Emergency: 800-222-1222
TTY: 800-253-7955
www.cincinnatichildrens.org/dpic

CLEVELAND

Greater Cleveland Poison Control Center
University Hospitals

11100 Euclid Ave – B261
MP6007
Cleveland OH 44106
Business: 216-844-1573
Emergency: 800-222-1222
                  216-231-4455 (OH)
www.uhhospitals.org/rainbow
children/tabid/195/default.aspx

COLUMBUS

Central Ohio Poison Center (*)
Nationwide Children's Hospital

700 Children's Dr, Room L032
Columbus OH 43205
Business: 614-722-2635
Emergency: 800-222-1222
                  614-228-1323
                  937-222-2227
                  (Dayton region)
www.nationwidechildrens.org/
poison-center

OKLAHOMA

OKLAHOMA CITY

Oklahoma Poison Control Center (*)
Children's Hospital at OU Health Science Center

940 NE 13th St – Room 3510
Oklahoma City OK 73104
Business: 405-271-5062
Emergency: 800-222-1222
www.oklahomapoison.org

OREGON

PORTLAND

Oregon Poison Center (*)
Oregon Health and Science University

3181 SW Sam Jackson Park Rd
Suite CB550
Portland OR 97239
Business: 503-494-8600
Emergency: 800-222-1222
www.ohsu.edu/xd/outreach/
oregon-poison-center

PENNSYLVANIA

PHILADELPHIA

The Poison Control Center (*)
Children's Hospital of Philadelphia

34th St & Civic Center Blvd
Philadelphia PA 19104-4399
Business: 215-590-2003
Emergency: 800-222-1222
TDD/TTY: 215-590-8789
www.chop.edu/service/
poison-control-center

PITTSBURGH

Pittsburgh Poison Center (*)
University of Pittsburgh Medical Center

200 Lothrop Street
Pittsburgh PA 15213
Business: 412-390-3300
Emergency: 800-222-1222
                  412-681-6669
                  (Pittsburgh)
www.upmc.com/services/
poison-center

RHODE ISLAND

(BOSTON, MA)

Regional Center for Poison Control and Prevention (*)

300 Longwood Ave
Boston MA 02115
Business: 617-355-6609
Emergency: 800-222-1222
TDD/TTY   888-244-5313
www.maripoisoncenter.com

SOUTH CAROLINA

COLUMBIA

Palmetto Poison Center (*)
University of South Carolina
College of Pharmacy

USC
Columbia SC 29208
Business: 803-777-7909
Emergency: 800-222-1222
http://poison.sc.edu

SOUTH DAKOTA

(MINNEAPOLIS, MN)

Minnesota Poison Control
System (*)
Hennepin County Medical
Center

701 Park Ave, Mail Code RL
Minneapolis MN 55415
Business: 612-873-3144
Emergency: 800-222-1222
www.mnpoison.org

SIOUX FALLS

Sanford Poison Center
Sanford Health USD Medical
Center

1305 W 18th St – PO Box 5039
Sioux Falls SD 57117
Business: 605-333-6638
Emergency: 800-222-1222
www.sdpoison.org

TENNESSEE

NASHVILLE

Tennessee Poison Center (*)

1161 21st Ave South
501 Oxford House
Nashville TN 37232-4632
Business: 615-936-0760
Emergency: 800-222-1222
www.tnpoisoncenter.org

TEXAS

AMARILLO

Texas Panhandle Poison
Center (*)
Texas Poison Center Network

1501 S Coulter Dr
Amarillo TX 79106
Business: 806-354-1630
Emergency: 800-222-1222
www.poisoncontrol.org

DALLAS

North Texas Poison Center (*)
Texas Poison Center Network
Parkland Health & Hospital
System

5201 Harry Hines Blvd
Dallas TX 75235
Business: 214-589-0911
Emergency: 800-222-1222
www.poisoncontrol.org

EL PASO

West Texas Regional Poison
Center (*)
Thomason Hospital

4815 Alameda Ave
El Paso TX 79905
Business: 915-534-3802
Emergency: 800-222-1222
www.poisoncontrol.org

GALVESTON

Southeast Texas Poison
Center (*)
The University of Texas Medical
Branch

201 University Blvd
3.112 Trauma Bldg
Galveston TX 77555-1175
Business: 409-766-4403
Emergency: 800-222-1222
www.utmb.edu/setpc

SAN ANTONIO

South Texas Poison Center (*)
The University of Texas Health
Science Center-San Antonio

7703 Floyd Curl Dr – MSC 7849
Trauma Bldg
San Antonio TX 78229-3900
Business: 210-567-5762
Emergency: 800-222-1222
www.texaspoison.com

TEMPLE

Central Texas Poison Center (*)
Scott & White Memorial Hospital

2401 S 31st St
Temple TX 76508-0001
Business: 254-724-2111
Emergency: 800-222-1222
www.sw.org/poison-center/
poison-landing

UTAH

SALT LAKE CITY

Utah Poison Control Center (*)
University of Utah

585 Komas Dr – Suite 200
Salt Lake City UT 84108-1234
Business: 801-581-7504
Emergency: 800-222-1222
http://uuhsc.utah.edu/poison

VERMONT

(PORTLAND, ME)

Northern New England Poison
Center (*)
Maine Medical Center

22 Bramhall St
Portland ME 04102
Business: 207-662-7220
Emergency: 800-222-1222
www.nnepc.org

VIRGINIA

CHARLOTTESVILLE

Blue Ridge Poison Center (*)
University of Virginia School of Medicine

Jefferson Park Place
1222 Jefferson Park Ave
PO Box 800774
Charlottesville VA 22908-0774
Business: 434-982-3196
Emergency: 800-222-1222
             800-451-1418 (VA)
www.healthsystem.virginia.edu/
brpc

RICHMOND

Virginia Poison Center (*)
Virginia Commonwealth
University Medical Center

PO Box 980522
Richmond VA 23298-0522
Business: 804-828-4780
Emergency: 800-222-1222
             804-828-9123
TDD/TYY: 804-828-9123
www.poison.vcu.edu

(WASHINGTON, DC)

National Capital Poison
Center (*)

3201 New Mexico Ave NW
Suite 310
Washington DC 20016
Business: 202-362-3867
Emergency: 800-222-1222
www.poison.org

WASHINGTON

SEATTLE

Washington Poison Control
Center (*)

155 NE 100th St – Suite 100
Seattle WA 98125-8007
Business: 206-517-2350
Emergency: 800-222-1222
             206-517-2394 (WA)
TDD: 800-572-0638 (WA)
             206-517-2394
             (Seattle)
www.wapc.org

WEST VIRGINIA

CHARLESTON

West Virginia Poison Center (*)
WVU Robert C. Byrd Health
Sciences Center

3110 MacCorkle Ave SE
Charleston WV 25304
Business: 304-347-1212
Emergency: 800-222-1222
www.wvpoisoncenter.org

WISCONSIN

MILWAUKEE

Wisconsin Poison Center
Children's Hospital of
Wisconsin

PO Box 1997, Mail Station C660
Milwaukee WI 53201-1997
Business: 414-266-2630
Emergency: 800-222-1222
TDD/TYY: 414-964-3497
www.wisconsinpoison.org

WYOMING

(OMAHA, NE)

Nebraska Regional Poison
Center (*)

8401 W Dodge Rd – Suite 115
Omaha NE 68114
Business: 402-955-5555
Emergency: 800-222-1222
www.nebraskapoison.com

PRODUCT COMPARISON TABLES

This section offers a graphic overview of the most common over-the-counter (OTC) drugs for select categories or conditions, as well as information that may be helpful in selecting appropriate products. Always consult with your doctor or pharmacist if you have any questions on products listed in these tables.

- Acne Products
- Analgesic Products
- Antacid and Heartburn Products
- Antidiarrheal Products
- Antiflatulent Products
- Antifungal Products
- Antipyretic Products

- Commonly Used Herbal Products
- Contact Dermatitis Products
- Cough-Cold-Flu-Allergy Products
- Diaper Rash Products
- Hemorrhoidal Products
- Insomnia Products

Table 1. ACNE PRODUCTS

BRANDS	INGREDIENT(S)/STRENGTH(S)	DOSAGE
BENZOYL PEROXIDES		
Clean & Clear Advantage 3-in-1 Exfoliating Cleanser	Benzoyl peroxide 5%	Use qd to start, then increase to bid prn or ud.
Clean & Clear Continuous Control Acne Cleanser	Benzoyl peroxide 10%	Use bid (AM and PM).
Clean & Clear Persa-Gel 10 Maximum Strength	Benzoyl peroxide 10%	Apply a thin layer to affected area qd up to tid.
Clearasil Daily Clear Tinted Acne Treatment Cream	Benzoyl peroxide 10%	Apply a thin layer to affected area qd to start, then increase to bid-tid prn or ud.
Clearasil Daily Clear Vanishing Acne Treatment Cream	Benzoyl peroxide 10%	Apply a thin layer to affected area qd to start, then increase to bid-tid prn or ud.
Clearasil Ultra Rapid Action Vanishing Treatment Cream	Benzoyl peroxide 10%	Apply a thin layer to affected area qd to start, then increase to bid-tid prn or ud.
Neutrogena Clear Pore Cleanser/ Mask	Benzoyl peroxide 3.5%	**Cleanser:** Use qd or every other day. **Mask:** Apply even layer over skin and allow to dry up to 5 minutes. Do not exceed 2-3 times per week.
Neutrogena On-the-Spot Acne Treatment Vanishing Formula	Benzoyl peroxide 2.5%	Apply to affected area qd to start, then increase to bid-tid prn or ud.
Oxy Clinical Clearing Treatment	Benzoyl peroxide 5%	Apply a thin layer to affected area qd to start, then increase to bid-tid prn or ud.
Oxy Maximum Action Advanced Face Wash	Benzoyl peroxide 10%	Use qd to start, then increase to bid-tid prn or ud.
Oxy Maximum Action Spot Treatment	Benzoyl peroxide 10%	Apply a thin layer to affected area qd to start, then increase to bid-tid prn or ud.
PanOxyl 4% Acne Creamy Wash	Benzoyl peroxide 4%	Use qd to start, then increase to bid-tid prn or ud.
PanOxyl 10% Acne Cleansing Bar	Benzoyl peroxide 10%	Use qd to start, then increase to bid-tid prn or ud.
PanOxyl 10% Acne Foaming Wash	Benzoyl peroxide 10%	Use qd to start, then increase to bid-tid prn or ud.
Zapzyt Acne Treatment Gel	Benzoyl peroxide 10%	Apply to affected area qd up to tid.

(Continued)

BRANDS	INGREDIENT(S)/STRENGTH(S)	DOSAGE
SALICYLIC ACIDS		
Aveeno Clear Complexion Cleansing Bar	Salicylic acid 0.5%	Use qd ud.
Aveeno Clear Complexion Cream Cleanser	Salicylic acid 2%	Use qd ud.
Aveeno Clear Complexion Daily Cleansing Pads	Salicylic acid 0.5%	Use qd ud.
Aveeno Clear Complexion Daily Moisturizer	Salicylic acid 0.5%	Apply a thin layer to affected area qd to start, then increase to bid-tid prn or ud.
Aveeno Clear Complexion Foaming Cleanser	Salicylic acid 0.5%	Use qd ud.
Biore Blemish Fighting Ice Cleanser	Salicylic acid 2%	Use qd ud.
Biore Blemish Treating Astringent	Salicylic acid 2%	Apply to affected area qd to start, then increase to bid-tid prn or ud.
Biore Warming Anti-Blackhead Cleanser	Salicylic acid 2%	Use qd ud.
Bye Bye Blemish Drying Lotion	Salicylic acid 2%	Apply to affected area and leave on overnight ud.
Clean & Clear Advantage Acne Cleanser	Salicylic acid 2%	Use qd ud.
Clean & Clear Advantage Acne Control Moisturizer	Salicylic acid 0.5%	Apply a thin layer to affected area qd up to tid.
Clean & Clear Advantage Acne Spot Treatment	Salicylic acid 2%	Apply a thin layer to affected area qd to start, then increase to bid-tid prn or ud.
Clean & Clear Advantage Mark Treatment	Salicylic acid 2%	Apply a thin layer to affected area qd to start, then increase to bid-tid prn or ud.
Clean & Clear Blackhead Eraser Cleansing Mask	Salicylic acid 0.5%	Apply a thin layer and let dry for 5 minutes or until mask turns white. Use 1-2 times per week.
Clean & Clear Blackhead Eraser Scrub	Salicylic acid 2%	Use qd ud.
Clean & Clear Essentials Deep Cleaning Astringent	Salicylic acid 2%	Apply a thin layer to affected area qd to start, then increase to bid-tid prn or ud.

BRANDS	INGREDIENT(S)/STRENGTH(S)	DOSAGE
SALICYLIC ACIDS *(Continued)*		
Clean & Clear Essentials Deep Cleaning Toner	Salicylic acid 0.5%	Apply a thin layer to affected area qd to start, then increase to bid-tid prn or ud.
Clean & Clear Essentials Dual Action Moisturizer	Salicylic acid 0.5%	Apply a thin layer to affected area qd to start, then increase to bid-tid prn or ud.
Clearasil Daily Clear Daily Facial Scrub	Salicylic acid 2%	Use qd to start, then increase to bid-tid prn or ud.
Clearasil Daily Clear Daily Pore Cleansing Pads	Salicylic acid 2%	Apply to affected area qd to start, then increase to bid-tid prn or ud.
Clearasil Daily Clear Oil-Free Daily Face Wash	Salicylic acid 2%	Use qd to start, then increase to bid-tid prn or ud.
Clearasil Daily Clear Oil-Free Daily Face Wash Sensitive	Salicylic acid 2%	Use qd to start, then increase to bid-tid prn or ud.
Clearasil PerfectaWash Automatic Face Wash Dispenser & Refills	Salicylic acid 2%	Use bid ud.
Clearasil PerfectaWash Automatic Face Wash Refill Soothing Plant Extracts	Salicylic acid 2%	Use bid ud.
Clearasil PerfectaWash Automatic Face Wash Refill Superfruit Splash	Salicylic acid 2%	Use bid ud.
Clearasil Ultra Acne + Marks Spot Lotion	Salicylic acid 2%	Apply a thin layer to affected area qd to start, then increase to bid-tid prn or ud.
Clearasil Ultra Acne + Marks Wash and Mask	Salicylic acid 2%	**Wash:** Use qd to start, then increase to bid-tid prn or ud. **Mask:** Apply to damp skin and leave on for 1 minute. Use up to 3 times per week.
Clearasil Ultra Overnight Scrub	Salicylic acid 2%	Use at night time ud.
Clearasil Ultra Overnight Wash	Salicylic acid 2%	Use qd to start, then increase to bid-tid prn or ud.
Clearasil Ultra Rapid Action Daily Face Wash	Salicylic acid 2%	Use qd to start, then increase to bid-tid prn or ud.
Clearasil Ultra Rapid Action Face Scrub	Salicylic acid 2%	Use qd to start, then increase to bid-tid prn or ud.
Clearasil Ultra Rapid Action Pads	Salicylic acid 2%	Apply to affected area qd to start, then increase to bid-tid prn or ud.

(Continued)

Brands	Ingredient(s)/Strength(s)	Dosage
SALICYLIC ACIDS *(Continued)*		
Clearasil Ultra Rapid Action Seal-to-Clear Gel	Salicylic acid 2%	Apply a thin layer to affected area qd to start, then increase to bid-tid prn or ud.
Clearasil Ultra Rapid Action Treatment Gel	Salicylic acid 2%	Apply a thin layer to affected area qd to start, then increase to bid-tid prn or ud.
L'Oreal Go 360° Clean Anti-Breakout Facial Cleanser	Salicylic acid 2%	Use bid ud.
Neutrogena All-in-1 Acne Control Daily Scrub	Salicylic acid 2%	Use bid ud.
Neutrogena All-in-1 Acne Control Facial Treatment	Salicylic acid 1%	Apply a thin layer to affected area qd to start, then increase to bid-tid prn or ud.
Neutrogena Blackhead Eliminating Cleanser Mask	Salicylic acid 2%	**Cleanser:** Use qd or every other day. **Mask:** Apply even layer over skin and allow to dry up to 5 minutes. Do not exceed 2-3 times per week.
Neutrogena Blackhead Eliminating Daily Scrub	Salicylic acid 2%	Use qd ud.
Neutrogena Body Clear Body Scrub	Salicylic acid 2%	Use ud.
Neutrogena Clear Pore Oil-Eliminating Astringent	Salicylic acid 2%	Use qd-tid ud.
Neutrogena Men Skin Clearing Acne Wash	Salicylic acid 2%	Use bid ud.
Neutrogena Oil-Free Acne Stress Control 3-in-1 Hydrating Acne Treatment	Salicylic acid 2%	Apply a thin layer to affected area qd to start, then increase to bid-tid prn or ud.
Neutrogena Oil-Free Acne Stress Control Power-Clear Scrub	Salicylic acid 2%	Use qd ud.
Neutrogena Oil-Free Acne Stress Control Power-Foam Wash	Salicylic acid 0.5%	Use qd ud.
Neutrogena Oil-Free Acne Wash	Salicylic acid 2%	Use bid ud.
Neutrogena Oil-Free Acne Wash Cleansing Cloths	Salicylic acid 2%	Use qd ud.
Neutrogena Oil-Free Acne Wash Cream Cleanser	Salicylic acid 2%	Use bid ud.

Brands	Ingredient(s)/Strength(s)	Dosage
SALICYLIC ACIDS (Continued)		
Neutrogena Oil-Free Anti-Acne Moisturizer	Salicylic acid 2%	Apply a thin layer qd-tid.
Neutrogena Rapid Clear 2-in-1 Fight & Fade Gel	Salicylic acid 2%	Apply a thin layer to affected area qd to start, then increase to bid-tid prn or ud.
Neutrogena Rapid Clear Acne Defense Face Lotion	Salicylic acid 2%	Apply a thin layer to affected area qd to start, then increase to bid-tid prn or ud.
Neutrogena Rapid Clear Acne Eliminating Spot Gel	Salicylic acid 2%	Apply a thin layer to affected area qd to start, then increase to bid-tid prn or ud.
Neutrogena Rapid Clear Foaming Scrub	Salicylic acid 2%	Use bid ud.
Noxzema Clean Blemish Control Daily Scrub	Salicylic acid 1%	Use qd ud.
Noxzema Clean Blemish Control Foaming Wash	Salicylic acid 1%	Use qd ud.
Noxzema Triple Clean Anti-Blemish Pads	Salicylic acid 2%	Apply to affected area qd to start, then increase to bid-tid prn or ud.
Olay Acne Control Face Wash	Salicylic acid 2%	Use 1 to 2 pumps bid ud.
Olay Blackhead Clearing Scrub	Salicylic acid 2%	Use qd ud.
Olay Pro-X Clear Acne Protocol	**Cleanser:** Salicylic acid 1.8% **Treatment:** Salicylic acid 1.5%	Use bid ud.
Olay Total Effects Blemish Control Salicylic Acid Acne Cleanser	Salicylic acid 2%	Use qd-tid ud.
Oxy Clinical Advanced Face Wash	Salicylic acid 2%	Use bid ud.
Oxy Clinical Advanced Treatment Pads	Salicylic acid 2%	Apply to affected area qd to start, then increase to bid-tid prn or ud.
Oxy Clinical Foaming Face Wash	Salicylic acid 2%	Use qd to start, then increase to bid prn or ud.
Oxy Daily Defense Cleansing Pads	Salicylic acid 2%	Apply to affected area qd to start, then increase to bid-tid prn or ud.
Oxy Exfoliating Body Scrub	Salicylic acid 1%	Use ud.
Oxy Hydrating Body Wash	Salicylic acid 2%	Use ud.

(Continued)

Brands	Ingredient(s)/Strength(s)	Dosage
SALICYLIC ACIDS *(Continued)*		
Oxy Maximum Purifying Face Scrub	Salicylic acid 2%	Use qd ud.
Phisoderm Anti-Blemish Body Wash	Salicylic acid 2%	Use ud.
St. Ives Naturally Clear Blemish & Blackhead Control Apricot Scrub	Salicylic acid 2%	Use 3-4 times per week ud.
Stridex Essential Pads	Salicylic acid 1%	Apply to affected area qd to start, then increase to bid-tid prn or ud.
Stridex Maximum Pads	Salicylic acid 2%	Apply to affected area qd to start, then increase to bid-tid prn or ud.
Stridex Natural Control Pads	Salicylic acid 1%	Apply to affected area qd to start, then increase to bid-tid prn or ud.
Stridex Sensitive Pads	Salicylic acid 0.5%	Apply to affected area qd to start, then increase to bid-tid prn or ud.
Zapzyt Acne Wash	Salicylic acid 2%	Use bid (AM and PM).
Zapzyt Pore Clearing Scrub	Salicylic acid 2%	Use qd ud.
TRICLOSANS		
Clean & Clear Essential Foaming Facial Cleanser	Triclosan 0.25%	Use qd ud.
Noxzema Triple Clean Anti-Bacterial Lathering Cleanser	Triclosan 0.3%	Use qd ud.
COMBINATION PRODUCTS		
Clearasil Daily Clear Adult Tinted Treatment Cream	Resorcinol/Sulfur 2%-8%	Apply a thin layer to affected area qd to start, then increase to bid-tid prn or ud.

Table 2. ANALGESIC PRODUCTS

Brand	Ingredient(s)/Strength(s)	Dosage
ACETAMINOPHENS		
FeverAll Children's Suppositories	Acetaminophen 120mg	**Peds 3-6 yrs:** 1 supp q4-6h. **Max:** 5 doses/24h.
FeverAll Infants' Suppositories	Acetaminophen 80mg	**Peds 6-11 months:** 1 supp q6h. **Max:** 4 doses/24h. **12-36 months:** 1 supp q4-6h. **Max:** 5 doses/24h.
FeverAll Jr. Strength Suppositories	Acetaminophen 325mg	**Adults & Peds ≥12 yrs:** 2 supp q4-6h. **Max:** 6 doses/24h. **Peds 6-12 yrs:** 1 supp q4-6h. **Max:** 5 doses/24h.
Tylenol 8 Hour Caplets†	Acetaminophen 650mg	**Adults & Peds ≥12 yrs:** 2 tabs q8h prn. **Max:** 6 tabs/24h.
Tylenol Arthritis Pain Caplets†	Acetaminophen 650mg	**Adults:** 2 tabs q8h prn. **Max:** 6 tabs/24h.
Tylenol Arthritis Pain Gelcaps†	Acetaminophen 650mg	**Adults:** 2 caps q8h prn. **Max:** 6 caps/24h.
Tylenol Children's Meltaways Chewable Tablets*	Acetaminophen 80mg	**Peds 2-3 yrs (24-35 lbs):** 2 tabs. **4-5 yrs (36-47 lbs):** 3 tabs. **6-8 yrs (48-59 lbs):** 4 tabs. **9-10 yrs (60-71 lbs):** 5 tabs. **11 yrs (72-95 lbs):** 6 tabs. May repeat q4h. **Max:** 5 doses/24h.
Tylenol Children's Oral Suspension*	Acetaminophen 160mg/5mL	**Peds 2-3 yrs (24-35 lbs):** 1 tsp (5mL). **4-5 yrs (36-47 lbs):** 1.5 tsp (7.5mL). **6-8 yrs (48-59 lbs):** 2 tsp (10mL). **9-10 yrs (60-71 lbs):** 2.5 tsp (12.5mL). **11 yrs (72-95 lbs):** 3 tsp (15mL). May repeat q4h. **Max:** 5 doses/24h.
Tylenol Extra Strength Caplets	Acetaminophen 500mg	**Adults & Peds ≥12 yrs:** 2 tabs q6h prn. **Max:** 6 tabs/24h.
Tylenol Extra Strength EZ Tablets†	Acetaminophen 500mg	**Adults & Peds ≥12 years:** 2 tabs q4-6h prn. **Max:** 8 tabs/24h.
Tylenol Extra Strength Rapid Blast Liquid	Acetaminophen 500mg/15mL	**Adults & Peds ≥12 yrs:** 2 tbsp (30mL) q6h prn. **Max:** 6 tbsp (90mL)/24h.
Tylenol Extra Strength Rapid Release Gelcaps	Acetaminophen 500mg	**Adults & Peds ≥12 yrs:** 2 caps q6h prn. **Max:** 6 caps/24h.

(Continued)

BRAND	INGREDIENT(S)/STRENGTH(S)	DOSAGE
ACETAMINOPHENS *(Continued)*		
Tylenol Infants' Oral Suspension†	Acetaminophen 160mg/5mL	**Peds 2-3 yrs (24-35 lbs):** 5mL q4h prn. **Max:** 5 doses/24h.
Tylenol Jr. Meltaways Chewable Tablets*	Acetaminophen 160mg	**Peds 6-8 yrs (48-59 lbs):** 2 tabs. **9-10 yrs (60-71 lbs):** 2.5 tabs. **11 yrs (72-95 lbs):** 3 tabs. May repeat q4h. **Max:** 5 doses/24h.
Tylenol Regular Strength Tablets	Acetaminophen 325mg	**Adults & Peds ≥12 yrs:** 2 tabs q4-6h prn. **Max:** 10 tabs/24h. **Peds 6-11 yrs:** 1 tab q4-6h prn. **Max:** 5 tabs/24h.
ACETAMINOPHEN COMBINATIONS		
Excedrin Back & Body Caplets	Acetaminophen/Aspirin buffered 250mg-250mg	**Adults & Peds ≥12 yrs:** 2 tabs q6h prn. **Max:** 8 tabs/24h.
Excedrin Extra Strength Caplets	Acetaminophen/Aspirin/Caffeine 250mg-250mg-65mg	**Adults & Peds ≥12 yrs:** 2 tabs q6h prn. **Max:** 8 tabs/24h.
Excedrin Extra Strength Express Gels	Acetaminophen/Aspirin/Caffeine 250mg-250mg-65mg	**Adults & Peds ≥12 yrs:** 2 caps q6h prn. **Max:** 8 caps/24h.
Excedrin Extra Strength Geltabs	Acetaminophen/Aspirin/Caffeine 250mg-250mg-65mg	**Adults & Peds ≥12 yrs:** 2 tabs q6h prn. **Max:** 8 tabs/24h.
Excedrin Extra Strength Tablets	Acetaminophen/Aspirin/Caffeine 250mg-250mg-65mg	**Adults & Peds ≥12 yrs:** 2 tabs q6h prn. **Max:** 8 tabs/24h.
Excedrin Menstrual Complete Express Gels	Acetaminophen/Aspirin/Caffeine 250mg-250mg-65mg	**Adults & Peds ≥12 yrs:** 2 caps q4-6h prn. **Max:** 8 caps/24h.
Excedrin Migraine Coated Caplets	Acetaminophen/Aspirin/Caffeine 250mg-250mg-65mg	**Adults:** 2 tabs prn. **Max:** 2 tabs/24h.
Excedrin Sinus Headache Caplets	Acetaminophen/Phenylephrine HCI 325mg-5mg	**Adults & Peds ≥12 yrs:** 2 tabs q4h prn. **Max:** 12 tabs/24h.
Excedrin Sinus Headache Tablets	Acetaminophen/Phenylephrine HCI 325mg-5mg	**Adults & Peds ≥12 yrs:** 2 tabs q4h. **Max:** 12 tabs/24h.
Excedrin Tension Headache Caplets	Acetaminophen/Caffeine 500mg-65mg	**Adults & Peds ≥12 yrs:** 2 tabs q6h prn. **Max:** 8 tabs/24h.
Excedrin Tension Headache Express Gels	Acetaminophen/Caffeine 500mg-65mg	**Adults & Peds ≥12 yrs:** 2 caps q6h prn. **Max:** 8 caps/24h.
Excedrin Tension Headache Geltabs	Acetaminophen/Caffeine 500mg-65mg	**Adults & Peds ≥12 yrs:** 2 tabs q6h prn. **Max:** 8 tabs/24h.
Goody's Back & Body Pain Powder	Acetaminophen/Aspirin 325mg-500mg	**Adults & Peds ≥12 yrs:** Place 1 powder on tongue q6h prn. **Max:** 4 powders/24h.

Brand	Ingredient(s)/Strength(s)	Dosage
ACETAMINOPHEN COMBINATIONS *(Continued)*		
Goody's Cool Orange Powder	Acetaminophen/Aspirin/Caffeine 325mg-500mg-65mg	**Adults & Peds ≥12 yrs:** Place 1 powder on tongue q6h prn. **Max:** 4 powders/24h.
Goody's Extra Strength Caplets	Acetaminophen/Aspirin/Caffeine 250mg-250mg-65mg	**Adults & Peds ≥12 yrs:** 2 tabs q6h. **Max:** 8 tabs/24h.
Goody's Extra Strength Headache Powder	Acetaminophen/Aspirin/Caffeine 260mg-500mg-32.5mg	**Adults & Peds ≥12 yrs:** Place 1 powder on tongue q6h prn. **Max:** 4 powders/24h.
Goody's Migraine Relief Caplets	Acetaminophen/Aspirin/Caffeine 250mg-250mg-65mg	**Adults:** 2 tabs. **Max:** 2 tabs/24h.
Midol Complete Caplets	Acetaminophen/Caffeine/Pyrilamine maleate 500mg-60mg-15mg	**Adults & Peds ≥12 yrs:** 2 tabs q6h prn. **Max:** 6 tabs/24h.
Midol Complete Gelcaps	Acetaminophen/Caffeine/Pyrilamine maleate 500mg-60mg-15mg	**Adults & Peds ≥12 yrs:** 2 caps q6h prn. **Max:** 6 caps/24h.
Midol Teen Formula Caplets	Acetaminophen/Pamabrom 500mg-25mg	**Adults & Peds ≥12 yrs:** 2 tabs q6h prn. **Max:** 6 tabs/24h.
Pamprin Cramp Caplets	Acetaminophen/Magnesium salicylate/Pamabrom 250mg-250mg-25mg	**Adults & Peds ≥12 yrs:** 2 tabs q4-6h prn. **Max:** 8 tabs/24h.
Pamprin Max Caplets	Acetaminophen/Aspirin/Caffeine 250mg-250mg-65mg	**Adults & Peds ≥12 yrs:** 2 tabs q4-6h prn. **Max:** 8 tabs/24h.
Pamprin Multi-Symptom Caplets	Acetaminophen/Pamabrom/Pyrilamine maleate 500mg-25mg-15mg	**Adults & Peds ≥12 yrs:** 2 tabs q4-6h prn. **Max:** 8 tabs/24h.
Premsyn PMS Caplets	Acetaminophen/Pamabrom/Pyrilamine maleate 500mg-25mg-15mg	**Adults & Peds ≥12 yrs:** 2 tabs q4-6h prn. **Max:** 8 tabs/24h.
Vanquish Caplets	Acetaminophen/Aspirin/Caffeine 194mg-227mg-33mg	**Adults & Peds ≥12 yrs:** 2 tabs q6h prn. **Max:** 8 tabs/24h.
ACETAMINOPHENS/SLEEP AIDS		
Excedrin PM Caplets	Acetaminophen/Diphenhydramine citrate 500mg-38mg	**Adults & Peds ≥12 yrs:** 2 tabs hs prn. **Max:** 2 tabs/24h.
Excedrin PM Express Gels	Acetaminophen/Diphenhydramine citrate 500mg-38mg	**Adults & Peds ≥12 yrs:** 2 caps hs prn. **Max:** 2 caps/24h.
Goody's PM Powder	Acetaminophen/Diphenhydramine citrate 500mg-38mg	**Adults & Peds ≥12 yrs:** 2 powders hs prn.

(Continued)

BRAND	INGREDIENT(S)/STRENGTH(S)	DOSAGE
ACETAMINOPHENS/SLEEP AIDS *(Continued)*		
Midol PM Caplets	Acetaminophen/Diphenhydramine citrate 500mg-38mg	**Adults & Peds ≥12 yrs:** 2 tabs hs prn.**Max:** 8 tabs/24h.
Tylenol PM Caplets†	Acetaminophen/Diphenhydramine HCl 500mg-25mg	**Adults & Peds ≥12 yrs:** 2 tabs hs prn. **Max:** 2 tabs/24h.
Tylenol PM Geltabs†	Acetaminophen/Diphenhydramine HCl 500mg-25mg	**Adults & Peds ≥12 yrs:** 2 tabs hs prn. **Max:** 2 tabs/24h.
Tylenol PM Rapid Release Gels†	Acetaminophen/Diphenhydramine HCl 500mg-25mg	**Adults & Peds ≥12 yrs:** 2 caps hs prn. **Max:** 2 caps/24h.
NONSTEROIDAL ANTI-INFLAMMATORY DRUGS (NSAIDS)		
Advil Caplets	Ibuprofen 200mg	**Adults & Peds ≥12 yrs:** 1-2 tabs q4-6h prn. **Max:** 6 tabs/24h.
Advil Children's Suspension*	Ibuprofen 100mg/5mL	**Peds 2-3 yrs (24-35 lbs):** 1 tsp (5mL). **4-5 yrs (36-47 lbs):** 1.5 tsp (7.5mL). **6-8 yrs (48-59 lbs):** 2 tsp (10mL). **9-10 yrs (60-71 lbs):** 2.5 tsp (12.5mL). **11 yrs (72-95 lbs):** 3 tsp (15mL). May repeat q6-8h. **Max:** 4 doses/24h.
Advil Gel Caplets	Ibuprofen 200mg	**Adults & Peds ≥12 yrs:** 1-2 tabs q4-6h prn. **Max:** 6 tabs/24h.
Advil Infants' Concentrated Drops	Ibuprofen 50mg/1.25mL	**Peds 6-11 months (12-17 lbs):** 1.25mL. **12-23 months (18-23 lbs):** 1.875mL. May repeat q6-8h. **Max:** 4 doses/24h.
Advil Junior Strength Chewable Tablets	Ibuprofen 100mg	**Peds 6-8 yrs (48-59 lbs):** 2 tabs. **9-10 yrs (60-71 lbs):** 2.5 tabs. **11 yrs (72-95 lbs):** 3 tabs. May repeat q6-8h. **Max:** 4 doses/24h.
Advil Junior Strength Tablets	Ibuprofen 100mg	**Peds 6-10 yrs (48-71 lbs):** 2 tabs. **11 yrs (72-95 lbs):** 3 tabs. May repeat q6-8h. **Max:** 4 doses/24h.
Advil Liqui-Gels	Ibuprofen 200mg	**Adults & Peds ≥12 yrs:** 1-2 caps q4-6h prn. **Max:** 6 caps/24h.
Advil Migraine Capsules	Ibuprofen 200mg	**Adults:** 2 caps prn. **Max:** 2 caps/24h.
Advil Tablets	Ibuprofen 200mg	**Adults & Peds ≥12 yrs:** 1-2 tabs q4-6h prn. **Max:** 6 tabs/24h.

Brand	Ingredient(s)/Strength(s)	Dosage
NONSTEROIDAL ANTI-INFLAMMATORY DRUGS (NSAIDS) *(Continued)*		
Aleve Caplets	Naproxen sodium 220mg	**Adults & Peds ≥12 yrs:** 1 tab q8-12h. May take 1 additional tab within 1h of first dose. **Max:** 2 tabs/8-12h or 3 tabs/24h.
Aleve Gelcaps	Naproxen sodium 220mg	**Adults & Peds ≥12 yrs:** 1 cap q8-12h. May take 1 additional cap within 1h of first dose. **Max:** 2 caps/8-12h or 3 caps/24h.
Aleve Liquid Gels	Naproxen sodium 220mg	**Adults & Peds ≥12 yrs:** 1 cap q8-12h. May take 1 additional cap within 1h of first dose. **Max:** 2 caps/8-12h or 3 caps/24h.
Aleve Tablets	Naproxen sodium 220mg	**Adults & Peds ≥12 yrs:** 1 tab q8-12h. May take 1 additional tab within 1h of first dose. **Max:** 2 tabs/8-12h or 3 tabs/24h.
Midol Liquid Gels	Ibuprofen 200mg	**Adults & Peds ≥12 yrs:** 1-2 caps q4-6h prn. **Max:** 6 caps/24h.
Midol Extended Relief Caplets	Naproxen sodium 220mg	**Adults & Peds ≥12 yrs:** 1 tab q8-12h. May take 1 additional tab within 1h of first dose. **Max:** 2 tabs/8-12h or 3 tabs/24h.
Motrin Children's Oral Suspension	Ibuprofen 100mg/5mL	**Peds 2-3 yrs (24-35 lbs):** 1 tsp (5mL). **4-5 yrs (36-47 lbs):** 1.5 tsp (7.5mL). **6-8 yrs (48-59 lbs):** 2 tsp (10mL). **9-10 yrs (60-71 lbs):** 2.5 tsp (12.5mL). **11 yrs (72-95 lbs):** 3 tsp (15mL). May repeat q6-8h. **Max:** 4 doses/24h.
Motrin IB Caplets	Ibuprofen 200mg	**Adults & Peds ≥12 yrs:** 1-2 tabs q4-6h prn. **Max:** 6 tabs/24h.
Motrin Infants' Concentrated Drops	Ibuprofen 50mg/1.25mL	**Peds 6-11 months (12-17 lbs):** 1.25mL. **12-23 months (18-23 lbs):** 1.875mL. May repeat q6-8h. **Max:** 4 doses/24h.
Motrin Junior Strength Caplets†	Ibuprofen 100mg	**Peds 6-8 yrs (48-59 lbs):** 2 tabs. **9-10 yrs (60-71 lbs):** 2.5 tabs. **11 yrs (72-95 lbs):** 3 tabs. May repeat q6-8h. **Max:** 4 doses/24h.

(Continued)

BRAND	INGREDIENT(S)/STRENGTH(S)	DOSAGE
NONSTEROIDAL ANTI-INFLAMMATORY DRUGS (NSAIDS) *(Continued)*		
Motrin Junior Strength Chewable Tablets*†	Ibuprofen 100mg	**Peds 2-3 yrs (24-35 lbs):** 1 tab. **4-5 yrs (36-47 lbs):** 1.5 tabs. **6-8 yrs (48-59 lbs):** 2 tabs. **9-10 yrs (60-71 lbs):** 2.5 tabs. **11 yrs (72-95 lbs):** 3 tabs. May repeat q6-8h. **Max:** 4 doses/24h.
Pamprin All Day Caplets	Naproxen sodium 220mg	**Adults & Peds ≥12 yrs:** 1 tab q8-12h. May take 1 additional tab within 1h of first dose. **Max:** 2 tabs/8-12h or 3 tabs/24h.
NSAID SLEEP AIDS		
Advil PM Caplets	Ibuprofen/Diphenhydramine citrate 200mg-38mg	**Adults & Peds ≥12 yrs:** 2 tabs hs prn. **Max:** 2 tabs/24h.
Advil PM Liqui-Gels	Ibuprofen/Diphenhydramine HCl 200mg-25mg	**Adults & Peds ≥12 yrs:** 2 caps hs prn. **Max:** 2 caps/24h.
Motrin PM Caplets	Ibuprofen/Diphenhydramine citrate 200mg-38mg	**Adults & Peds ≥12 yrs:** 2 tabs hs prn. **Max:** 2 tabs/24h.
SALICYLATES		
Bayer Aspirin Extra Strength Caplets	Aspirin 500mg	**Adults & Peds ≥12 yrs:** 1-2 tabs q4-6h. **Max:** 8 tabs/24h.
Bayer Aspirin Safety Coated Caplets	Aspirin 325mg	**Adults & Peds ≥12 yrs:** 1-2 tabs q4h. **Max:** 12 tabs/24h.
Bayer Genuine Aspirin Tablets	Aspirin 325mg	**Adults & Peds ≥12 yrs:** 1-2 tabs q4h or 3 tabs q6h. **Max:** 12 tabs/24h.
Bayer Low Dose Aspirin Chewable Tablets*	Aspirin 81mg	**Adults & Peds ≥12 yrs:** 4-8 tabs q4h. **Max:** 48 tabs/24h.
Bayer Low Dose Aspirin Safety Coated Tablets	Aspirin 81mg	**Adults & Peds ≥12 yrs:** 4-8 tabs q4h. **Max:** 48 tabs/24h.
Ecotrin Low Strength Tablets	Aspirin 81mg	**Adults & Peds ≥12 yrs:** 4-8 tabs q4h. **Max:** 48 tabs/24h.
Ecotrin Regular Strength Tablets	Aspirin 325mg	**Adults & Peds ≥12 yrs:** 1-2 tabs q4h. **Max:** 12 tabs/24h.
Halfprin 81mg Tablets	Aspirin 81mg	**Adults & Peds ≥12 yrs:** 4-8 tabs q4h. **Max:** 48 tabs/24h.
Halfprin 162mg Tablets	Aspirin 162mg	**Adults & Peds ≥12 yrs:** 2-4 tabs q4h. **Max:** 24 tabs/24h.

Brand	Ingredient(s)/Strength(s)	Dosage
SALICYLATES *(Continued)*		
St. Joseph Aspirin Chewable Tablets	Aspirin 81mg	**Adults & Peds ≥12 yrs:** 4-8 tabs q4h. **Max:** 48 tabs/24h.
St. Joseph Regular Strength Safety Coated Tablets	Aspirin 325mg	**Adults & Peds ≥12 yrs:** 1-2 tabs q4h. **Max:** 12 tabs/24h.
St. Joseph Safety Coated Tablets	Aspirin 81mg	**Adults & Peds ≥12 yrs:** 4-8 tabs q4h. **Max:** 48 tabs/24h.
SALICYLATES, BUFFERED		
Alka-Seltzer Extra Strength Tablets	Aspirin/Citric acid/Sodium bicarbonate 500mg-1000mg-1985mg	**Adults ≥60 yrs:** 2 tabs q6h. **Max:** 3 tabs/24h. **Adults & Peds ≥12 yrs:** 2 tabs q6h. **Max:** 7 tabs/24h.
Alka-Seltzer Lemon Lime Tablets	Aspirin/Citric acid/Sodium bicarbonate 325mg-1000mg-1700mg	**Adults ≥60 yrs:** 2 tabs q4h. **Max:** 4 tabs/24h. **Adults & Peds ≥12 yrs:** 2 tabs q4h. **Max:** 8 tabs/24h.
Alka-Seltzer Original Tablets	Aspirin/Citric acid/Sodium bicarbonate 325mg-1000mg-1916mg	**Adults ≥60 yrs:** 2 tabs q4h. **Max:** 4 tabs/24h. **Adults & Peds ≥12 yrs:** 2 tabs q4h. **Max:** 8 tabs/24h.
Ascriptin Maximum Strength Caplets[†]	Aspirin 500mg buffered with Aluminum hydroxide/Calcium carbonate/ Magnesium hydroxide	**Adults & Peds ≥12 yrs:** 2 tabs q6h. **Max:** 8 tabs/24h.
Ascriptin Regular Strength Tablets[†]	Aspirin 325mg buffered with Aluminum hydroxide/Calcium carbonate/ Magnesium hydroxide	**Adults & Peds ≥12 yrs:** 2 tabs q4h. **Max:** 12 tabs/24h.
Bayer Aspirin Extra Strength Plus Caplets	Aspirin 500mg buffered with Calcium carbonate	**Adults & Peds ≥12 yrs:** 1-2 tabs q4-6h. **Max:** 8 tabs/24h.
Bayer Women's Low Dose Aspirin Caplets	Aspirin 81mg buffered with Calcium carbonate 777mg	**Adults & Peds ≥12 yrs:** 4-8 tabs q4h. **Max:** 10 tabs/24h.
Bufferin Low Dose Tablets[†]	Aspirin 81mg buffered with Calcium carbonate/Magnesium carbonate/ Magnesium oxide	**Adults & Peds ≥12 yrs:** 4-8 tabs q4h. **Max:** 48 tabs/24h.
SALICYLATE COMBINATIONS		
Anacin Caplets	Aspirin/Caffeine 400mg-32mg	**Adults & Peds ≥12 yrs:** 2 tabs q6h. **Max:** 8 tabs/24h.
Anacin Max Strength Tablets	Aspirin/Caffeine 500mg-32mg	**Adults & Peds ≥12 yrs:** 2 tabs q6h. **Max:** 8 tabs/24h.
Anacin Tablets	Aspirin/Caffeine 400mg-32mg	**Adults & Peds ≥12 yrs:** 2 tabs q6h. **Max:** 8 tabs/24h.

(Continued)

BRAND	INGREDIENT(S)/STRENGTH(S)	DOSAGE
SALICYLATE COMBINATIONS *(Continued)*		
Bayer AM Extra Strength Tablets	Aspirin/Caffeine 500mg-65mg	**Adults & Peds ≥12 yrs:** 2 tabs q6h. **Max:** 8 tabs/24h.
Bayer Back & Body Extra Strength Caplets	Aspirin/Caffeine 500mg-32.5mg	**Adults & Peds ≥12 yrs:** 2 tabs q6h. **Max:** 8 tabs/24h.
BC Arthritis Strength Powder	Aspirin/Caffeine 1000mg-65mg	**Adults & Peds ≥12 yrs:** Place 1 powder on tongue q6h. **Max:** 4 powders/24h.
BC Original Formula Powder	Aspirin/Caffeine 845mg-65mg	**Adults & Peds ≥12 yrs:** Place 1 powder on tongue q6h. **Max:** 4 powders/24h.
SALICYLATES/SLEEP AIDS		
Bayer PM Caplets	Aspirin/Diphenhydramine citrate 500mg-38.3mg	**Adults & Peds ≥12 yrs:** 2 tabs hs prn.

†Product currently on recall or temporarily unavailable from manufacturer, but generic forms may be available.
*Multiple flavors available.

Table 3. ANTACID AND HEARTBURN PRODUCTS

BRAND	INGREDIENT(S)/STRENGTH(S)	DOSAGE
ANTACIDS		
Alka-Seltzer Extra-Strength Tablets	Aspirin/Citric acid/Sodium bicarbonate 500mg-1000mg-1985mg	**Adults ≥60 yrs:** 2 tabs dissolved in 4 oz water q6h. **Max:** 3 tabs/24h. **Adults & Peds ≥12 yrs:** 2 tabs dissolved in 4 oz water q6h. **Max:** 7 tabs/24h.
Alka-Seltzer Gold Tablets	Citric acid/Potassium bicarbonate/ Sodium bicarbonate 1000mg-344mg-1050mg	**Adults ≥60 yrs:** 2 tabs dissolved in 4 oz water q4h prn. **Max:** 6 tabs/24h. **Adults & Peds ≥12 yrs:** 2 tabs dissolved in 4 oz water q4h prn. **Max:** 8 tabs/24h. **Peds <12 yrs:** 1 tab dissolved in 4 oz water q4h prn. **Max:** 4 tabs/24h.
Alka-Seltzer Heartburn Relief Tablets	Citric acid/Sodium bicarbonate 1000mg-1940mg	**Adults ≥60 yrs:** 2 tabs dissolved in 4 oz water q4h prn. **Max:** 4 tabs/24h.**Adults & Peds ≥12 yrs:** 2 tabs dissolved in 4 oz water q4h prn. **Max:** 8 tabs/24h.
Alka-Seltzer Lemon Lime Tablets	Aspirin/Citric acid/Sodium bicarbonate 325mg-1000mg-1700mg	**Adults ≥60 yrs:** 2 tabs dissolved in 4 oz water q4h. **Max:** 4 tabs/24h. **Adults & Peds ≥12 yrs:** 2 tabs dissolved in 4 oz water q4h. **Max:** 8 tabs/24h.
Alka-Seltzer Original Tablets	Aspirin/Citric acid/Sodium bicarbonate 325mg-1000mg-1916mg	**Adults ≥60 yrs:** 2 tabs dissolved in 4 oz water q4h. **Max:** 4 tabs/24h. **Adults & Peds ≥12 yrs:** 2 tabs dissolved in 4 oz water q4h. **Max:** 8 tabs/24h.
Brioschi Children's Foil Packs	Sodium bicarbonate/Tartaric acid 1.05g-1.28g/pack	**Peds 5-12 yrs:** 1 pack (4g) dissolved in 4-6 oz water q1h. **Max:** 6 doses/24h.
Brioschi Foil Packs	Sodium bicarbonate/Tartaric acid 1.80g-1.62g/pack	**Adults ≥60 yrs:** 1 pack (6g) dissolved in 4-6 oz water q1h. **Max:** 3 doses/24h. **Adults & Peds ≥12 yrs:** 1 pack (6g) dissolved in 4-6 oz water q1h. **Max:** 6 doses/24h.

(Continued)

BRAND	INGREDIENT(S)/STRENGTH(S)	DOSAGE
ANTACIDS *(Continued)*		
Brioschi Powder	Sodium bicarbonate/Tartaric acid 1.80g-1.62g/dose	**Adults ≥60 yrs:** 1 capful (6g) dissolved in 4-6 oz water q1h. **Max:** 3 doses/24h. **Adults & Peds ≥12 yrs:** 1 capful (6g) dissolved in 4-6 oz water q1h. **Max:** 6 doses/24h.
Gaviscon Extra Strength Chewable Tablets	Aluminum hydroxide/Magnesium carbonate 160mg-105mg	**Adults:** 2-4 tabs qid. **Max:** 16 tabs/24h.
Gaviscon Extra Strength Liquid	Aluminum hydroxide/Magnesium carbonate 254mg-237.5mg/5mL	**Adults:** 2-4 tsp (10-20mL) qid. **Max:** 16 tsp (80mL)/24h.
Gaviscon Regular Strength Chewable Tablets	Aluminum hydroxide/Magnesium trisilicate 80mg-14.2mg	**Adults:** 2-4 tabs qid. **Max:** 16 tabs/24h.
Gaviscon Regular Strength Liquid	Aluminum hydroxide/Magnesium carbonate 95mg-358mg/15mL	**Adults:** 1-2 tbl (15-30mL) qid. **Max:** 8 tbl (120mL)/24h.
Maalox Children's Relief Chewable Tablets	Calcium carbonate 400mg	**Peds 6-11 yrs (48-95 lbs):** 2 tabs prn. **Max:** 6 tabs/24h. **Peds 2-5 yrs (24-47 lbs):** 1 tab prn. **Max:** 3 tabs/24h.
Maalox Regular Strength Chewable Tablets	Calcium carbonate 600mg	**Adults:** 1-2 tabs prn. **Max:** 12 tabs/24h.
Mylanta Supreme Liquid	Calcium carbonate/Magnesium hydroxide 400mg-135mg/5mL	**Adults:** 2-4 tsp (10-20mL) between meals & at hs. **Max:** 18 tsp (90mL)/24h.
Mylanta Ultimate Strength Liquid	Aluminum hydroxide/Magnesium hydroxide 500mg-500mg/5mL	**Adults & Peds ≥12 yrs:** 2-4 tsp (10-20mL) between meals & at hs. **Max:** 9 tsp (45mL)/24h.
Pepto Bismol Children's Pepto Chewable Tablets	Calcium carbonate 400mg	**Peds 6-11 yrs (48-95 lbs):** 2 tabs prn. **Max:** 6 tabs/24h. **Peds 2-5 yrs (24-47 lbs):** 1 tab prn. **Max:** 3 tabs/24h.
Rolaids Extra Strength Chewable Tablets	Calcium carbonate/Magnesium hydroxide 675mg-135mg	**Adults:** 2-4 tabs q1h prn. **Max:** 12 tabs/24h.
Rolaids Extra Strength Softchews	Calcium carbonate 1177mg	**Adults:** 2-3 chews q1h prn. **Max:** 6 chews/24h.
Rolaids Regular Strength Chewable Tablets	Calcium carbonate/Magnesium hydroxide 550mg-110mg	**Adults:** 2-4 tabs q1h prn. **Max:** 12 tabs/24h.
Tums Extra Strength 750 Chewable Tablets	Calcium carbonate 750mg	**Adults:** 2-4 tabs prn. **Max:** 10 tabs/24h.
Tums Extra Strength 750 Sugar Free Chewable Tablets	Calcium carbonate 750mg	**Adults:** 2-4 tabs prn. **Max:** 15 tabs/24h.

BRAND	INGREDIENT(S)/STRENGTH(S)	DOSAGE
ANTACIDS (Continued)		
Tums Kids Chewable Tablets	Calcium carbonate 750mg	**Peds >4 yrs (>48 lbs):** 1 tab prn. **Max:** 4 tabs/24h. **Peds 2-4 yrs (24-47 lbs):** 1/2 tab prn. **Max:** 2 tabs/24h.
Tums Regular Strength Chewable Tablets	Calcium carbonate 500mg	**Adults:** 2-4 tabs prn. **Max:** 15 tabs/24h.
Tums Smoothies Chewable Tablets	Calcium carbonate 750mg	**Adults:** 2-4 tabs prn. **Max:** 10 tabs/24h.
Tums Ultra Strength 1000 Chewable Tablets	Calcium carbonate 1000mg	**Adults:** 2-3 tabs prn. **Max:** 7 tabs/24h.
ANTACIDS/ANTIFLATULENTS		
Gelusil Chewable Tablets	Aluminum hydroxide/Magnesium hydroxide/Simethicone 200mg-200mg-25mg	**Adults:** 2-4 tabs q1h prn. **Max:** 12 tabs/24h.
Maalox Advanced Maximum Strength Chewable Tablets	Calcium carbonate/Simethicone 1000mg-60mg	**Adults & Peds ≥12 yrs:** 1-2 tabs prn. **Max:** 8 tabs/24h.
Maalox Advanced Maximum Strength Liquid	Aluminum hydroxide/Magnesium hydroxide/Simethicone 400mg-400mg-40mg/5mL	**Adults & Peds ≥12 yrs:** 2-4 tsp (10-20mL) bid. **Max:** 8 tsp (40mL)/24h.
Maalox Advanced Regular Strength Liquid	Aluminum hydroxide/Magnesium hydroxide/Simethicone 200mg-200mg-20mg/5mL	**Adults & Peds ≥12 yrs:** 2-4 tsp (10-20mL) qid. **Max:** 16 tsp (80mL)/24h.
Maalox Junior Relief Chewable Tablets	Calcium carbonate/Simethicone 400mg-24mg	**Peds 6-11 yrs:** 2 tabs prn. **Max:** 6 tabs/24h.
Mylanta Maximum Strength Liquid	Aluminum hydroxide/Magnesium hydroxide/Simethicone 400mg-400mg-40mg/5mL	**Adults & Peds ≥12 yrs:** 2-4 tsp (10-20mL) between meals and at hs. **Max:** 12 tsp (60mL)/24h.
Mylanta Regular Strength Liquid	Aluminum hydroxide/Magnesium hydroxide/Simethicone 200mg-200mg-20mg/5mL	**Adults & Peds ≥12 yrs:** 2-4 tsp (10-20mL) between meals and at hs. **Max:** 24 tsp (120mL)/24h.
Rolaids Extra Strength Plus Gas Relief Softchews	Calcium carbonate/Simethicone 1177mg-80mg	**Adults:** 2-3 chews q1h prn. **Max:** 6 chews/24h.
Rolaids Multi-Symptom Chewable Tablets	Calcium carbonate/Magnesium hydroxide/Simethicone 675mg-135mg-60mg	**Adults:** 2-4 tabs q1h prn. **Max:** 8 tabs/24h.
BISMUTH SUBSALICYLATES		
Maalox Total Relief Maximum Strength Liquid	Bismuth subsalicylate 525mg/15mL	**Adults & Peds ≥12 yrs:** 2 tbl (30mL) q1h prn. **Max:** 8 tbl (120mL)/24h.

(Continued)

Brand	Ingredient(s)/Strength(s)	Dosage
BISMUTH SUBSALICYLATES *(Continued)*		
Pepto Bismol Caplets	Bismuth subsalicylate 262mg	**Adults & Peds ≥12 yrs:** 2 tabs q½-1h prn. **Max:** 8 doses (16 tabs)/24h.
Pepto Bismol Chewable Tablets	Bismuth subsalicylate 262mg	**Adults & Peds ≥12 yrs:** 2 tabs q½-1h prn. **Max:** 8 doses (16 tabs)/24h.
Pepto Bismol InstaCool Chewable Tablets	Bismuth subsalicylate 262mg	**Adults & Peds ≥12 yrs:** 2 tabs q½-1h prn. **Max:** 8 doses (16 tabs)/24h.
Pepto Bismol Liquid	Bismuth subsalicylate 262mg/15mL	**Adults & Peds ≥12 yrs:** 2 tbl (30mL) q½-1h prn. **Max:** 8 doses (16 tbl or 240mL)/24h.
Pepto Bismol Max Strength Liquid	Bismuth subsalicylate 525mg/15mL	**Adults & Peds ≥12 yrs:** 2 tbl (30mL) q1h prn. **Max:** 4 doses (8 tbl or 120mL)/24h.
H₂-RECEPTOR ANTAGONISTS		
Pepcid AC Maximum Strength EZ Chews	Famotidine 20mg	**Adults & Peds ≥12 yrs:** 1 tab prn. **Max:** 2 tabs/24h.
Pepcid AC Maximum Strength Tablets	Famotidine 20mg	**Adults & Peds ≥12 yrs:** 1 tab prn. **Max:** 2 tabs/24h.
Pepcid AC Original Strength Tablets	Famotidine 10mg	**Adults & Peds ≥12 yrs:** 1 tab prn. **Max:** 2 tabs/24h.
Tagamet HB 200 Tablets	Cimetidine 200mg	**Adults & Peds ≥12 yrs:** 1 tab prn. **Max:** 2 tabs/24h.
Zantac 75 Tablets	Ranitidine 75mg	**Adults & Peds ≥12 yrs:** 1 tab prn. **Max:** 2 tabs/24h.
Zantac 150 Tablets	Ranitidine 150mg	**Adults & Peds ≥12 yrs:** 1 tab prn. **Max:** 2 tabs/24h.
H₂-RECEPTOR ANTAGONISTS/ANTACIDS		
Pepcid Complete Chewable Tablets	Famotidine/Calcium carbonate/ Magnesium hydroxide 10mg-800mg-165mg	**Adults & Peds ≥12 yrs:** 1 tab prn. **Max:** 2 tabs/24h.
Tums Dual Action Chewable Tablets	Famotidine/Calcium carbonate/ Magnesium hydroxide 10mg-800mg-165mg	**Adults & Peds ≥12 yrs:** 1 tab prn. **Max:** 2 tabs/24h.

Brand	Ingredient(s)/Strength(s)	Dosage
PROTON PUMP INHIBITORS		
Prevacid 24 HR Capsules	Lansoprazole 15mg	**Adults:** 1 cap qd x 14 days. May repeat 14-day course q4 months.
Prilosec OTC Tablets	Omeprazole 20mg	**Adults:** 1 tab qd x 14 days. May repeat 14-day course q4 months.
Zegerid OTC Capsules	Omeprazole/Sodium bicarbonate 20mg-1100mg	**Adults:** 1 cap qd x 14 days. May repeat 14-day course q4 months.

Table 4. ANTIDIARRHEAL PRODUCTS

BRAND	INGREDIENT(S)/STRENGTH(S)	DOSAGE
ABSORBENTS		
Equalactin Chewable Tablets	Calcium Polycarbophil 625mg	**Adults & Peds ≥12 yrs:** 2 tabs prn up to 8 tabs/day. **Peds 6-<12 yrs:** 1 tab prn up to 4 tabs/day. **Peds 2-<6 yrs:** 1 tab prn up to 2 tabs/day.
Fibercon Caplets	Calcium Polycarbophil 625mg	**Adults & Peds ≥12 yrs:** 2 tabs up to qid.
Konsyl Fiber Caplets	Calcium Polycarbophil 625mg	**Adults:** 2 tabs qd-qid. **Max:** 8 tabs/day. **Peds 6-12 yrs:** 1 tab qd-tid.
ANTIPERISTALTICS		
Imodium A-D Caplets	Loperamide HCl 2mg	**Adults & Peds ≥12 yrs:** 2 tabs after first loose stool; 1 tab after each subsequent loose stool. **Max:** 4 tabs/24h. **Peds 9-11 yrs (60-95 lbs):** 1 tab after first loose stool; ½ tab after each subsequent loose stool. **Max:** 3 tabs/24h. **Peds 6-8 yrs (48-59 lbs):** 1 tab after first loose stool; ½ tab after each subsequent loose stool. **Max:** 2 tabs/24h.
Imodium A-D EZ Chews	Loperamide HCl 2mg	**Adults & Peds ≥12 yrs:** 2 tabs after first loose stool; 1 tab after each subsequent loose stool. **Max:** 4 tabs/24h. **Peds 9-11 yrs (60-95 lbs):** 1 tab after first loose stool; ½ tab after each subsequent loose stool. **Max:** 3 tabs/24h. **Peds 6-8 yrs (48-59 lbs):** 1 tab after first loose stool; ½ tab after each subsequent loose stool. **Max:** 2 tabs/24h.

(Continued)

BRAND	INGREDIENT(S)/STRENGTH(S)	DOSAGE
ANTIPERISTALTICS *(Continued)*		
Imodium A-D Liquid (Mint Flavor)	Loperamide HCl 1mg/7.5mL	**Adults & Peds ≥12 yrs:** 4 tsp (20mL) after first loose stool; 2 tsp (10mL) after each subsequent loose stool. **Max:** 8 tsp (40mL)/24h. **Peds 9-11 yrs (60-95 lbs):** 2 tsp (10mL) after first loose stool; 1 tsp (5mL) after each subsequent loose stool. **Max:** 6 tsp (30mL)/24h. **Peds 6-8 yrs (48-59 lbs):** 2 tsp (10mL) after first loose stool; 1 tsp (5mL) after each subsequent loose stool. **Max:** 4 tsp (20mL)/24h.
Imodium A-D Liquid for Use In Children (Mint Flavor)	Loperamide HCl 1mg/7.5mL	**Adults & Peds ≥12 yrs:** 6 tsp (30mL) after first loose stool; 3 tsp (15mL) after each subsequent loose stool. **Max:** 12 tsp (60mL)/24h. **Peds 9-11 yrs (60-95 lbs):** 3 tsp (15mL) after first loose stool; 1½ tsp (7.5mL) after each subsequent loose stool. **Max:** 9 tsp (45mL)/24h. **Peds 6-8 yrs (48-59 lbs):** 3 tsp (15mL) after first loose stool; 1½ tsp (7.5mL) after each subsequent loose stool. **Max:** 6 tsp (30mL)/24h.
ANTIPERISTALTICS/ANTIFLATULENTS		
Imodium Multi-Symptom Relief Caplets	Loperamide HCl/Simethicone 2mg-125mg	**Adults & Peds ≥12 yrs:** 2 tabs after first loose stool; 1 tab after each subsequent loose stool. **Max:** 4 tabs/24h. **Peds 9-11 yrs (60-95 lbs):** 1 tab after first loose stool; ½ tab after each subsequent loose stool. **Max:** 3 tabs/24h. **Peds 6-8 yrs (48-59 lbs):** 1 tab after first loose stool; ½ tab after each subsequent loose stool. **Max:** 2 tabs/24h.

Brand	Ingredient(s)/Strength(s)	Dosage
ANTIPERISTALTICS/ANTIFLATULENTS *(Continued)*		
Imodium Multi-Symptom Relief Chewable Tablets	Loperamide HCl/Simethicone 2mg-125mg	**Adults & Peds ≥12 yrs:** 2 tabs with 4-8 oz water after first loose stool; 1 tab with 4-8 oz water after each subsequent loose stool. **Max:** 4 tabs/24h. **Peds 9-11 yrs (60-95 lbs):** 1 tab with 4-8 oz water after first loose stool; ½ tab with 4-8 oz water after each subsequent loose stool. **Max:** 3 tabs/24h. **Peds 6-8 yrs (48-59 lbs):** 1 tab with 4-8 oz water after first loose stool; ½ tab with 4-8 oz water after each subsequent loose stool. **Max:** 2 tabs/24h.
BISMUTH SUBSALICYLATES		
Kaopectate Extra Strength Liquid (Peppermint Flavor)	Bismuth Subsalicylate 525mg/15mL	**Adults & Peds ≥12 yrs:** 2 tbl (30mL) q1h prn. **Max:** 4 doses (8 tbl)/24h.
Kaopectate Liquid (Peppermint Flavor)	Bismuth Subsalicylate 262mg/15mL	**Adults & Peds ≥12 yrs:** 2 tbl (30mL) q1h prn. **Max:** 4 doses (8 tbl)/24h.
Kaopectate Liquid (Vanilla Flavor; Cherry Flavor)	Bismuth Subsalicylate 262mg/15mL	**Adults & Peds ≥12 yrs:** 2 tbl (30mL) q½-1h prn. **Max:** 8 doses (16 tbl)/24h.
Maalox Total Relief Liquid	Bismuth Subsalicylate 525mg/15mL	**Adults & Peds ≥12 yrs:** 2 tbl (30mL) q1h prn. **Max:** 4 doses (8 tbl)/24h.
Pepto Bismol Caplets	Bismuth Subsalicylate 262mg	**Adults & Peds ≥12 yrs:** 2 tabs q½-1h prn. **Max:** 8 doses (16 tabs)/24h.
Pepto Bismol Chewable Tablets	Bismuth Subsalicylate 262mg	**Adults & Peds ≥12 yrs:** 2 tabs q½-1h prn. **Max:** 8 doses (16 tabs)/24h.
Pepto Bismol InstaCool Chewable Tablets	Bismuth Subsalicylate 262mg	**Adults & Peds ≥12 yrs:** 2 tabs q½-1h prn. **Max:** 8 doses (16 tabs)/24h.
Pepto Bismol Liquid	Bismuth Subsalicylate 525mg/30mL	**Adults & Peds ≥12 yrs:** 2 tbl (30mL) q½-1h prn. **Max:** 8 doses (16 tbl)/24h.
Pepto Bismol Max Strength Liquid	Bismuth Subsalicylate 1050mg/30mL	**Adults & Peds ≥12 yrs:** 2 tbl (30mL) q1h prn. **Max:** 4 doses (8 tbl)/24h.

Table 5. ANTIFLATULENT PRODUCTS

BRAND	INGREDIENT(S)/STRENGTH(S)	DOSAGE
ALPHA-GALACTOSIDASES		
Beano Meltaways Tablets	Alpha-galactosidase 300 GALU	**Adults:** Take 1 tab before meals.
Beano Tablets	Alpha-galactosidase enzyme 300 GALU	**Adults:** Take 2-3 tabs before meals.
ANTACIDS/ANTIFLATULENTS		
PLEASE REFER TO ANTACID AND HEARTBURN PRODUCTS CHART		
SIMETHICONE/SIMETHICONE COMBINATIONS		
Baby Gas-X Infant Drops	Simethicone 20mg/0.3mL	**Peds >2 yrs (>24 lbs):** 0.6mL prn after meals and at hs. **Peds <2 yrs (<24 lbs):** 0.3mL prn after meals and at hs. **Max:** 6 doses/24h.
Gas-X Chewable Tablets	Simethicone 80mg	**Adults:** Chew 1 or 2 tabs prn after meals and at hs. **Max:** 6 tabs/24h.
Gas-X Extra Strength Chewable Tablets	Simethicone 125mg	**Adults:** Chew 1 or 2 tabs prn after meals and at hs. **Max:** 4 tabs/24h.
Gas-X Extra Strength Chewable Tablets with Maalox	Simethicone/Calcium carbonate 125mg-500mg	**Adults:** Chew 1-2 tabs prn. **Max:** 4 tabs/24h.
Gas-X Extra Strength Softgels	Simethicone 125mg	**Adults:** Take 1 or 2 caps prn after meals and at hs. **Max:** 4 caps/24h.
Gas-X Thin Strips	Simethicone 62.5mg	**Adults:** Allow 2-4 strips to dissolve prn after meals and at hs. **Max:** 8 strips/24h.
Gas-X Ultra Strength Softgels	Simethicone 180mg	**Adults:** Take 1 or 2 caps prn after meals and at hs. **Max:** 2 caps/24h.
Infants' Mylicon Gas Relief Drops	Simethicone 20mg/0.3mL	**Peds >2 yrs (>24 lbs):** 0.6mL prn after meals and at hs. **Peds <2 yrs (<24 lbs):** 0.3mL prn after meals and at hs. **Max:** 12 doses/24h.
Little Remedies for Tummys Gas Relief Drops	Simethicone 20mg/0.3mL	**Peds ≥2 yrs (≥24 lbs):** 0.6mL prn after meals and at hs. **Peds <2 yrs (<24 lbs):** 0.3mL prn after meals and at hs. **Max:** 12 doses/24h.

(Continued)

BRAND	INGREDIENT(S)/STRENGTH(S)	DOSAGE
SIMETHICONE/SIMETHICONE COMBINATIONS *(Continued)*		
Mylanta Gas Maximum Strength Chewable Tablets	Simethicone 125mg	**Adults:** Chew 1-2 tabs prn after meals and at hs. **Max:** 4 tabs/24h.
PediaCare Infants Gas Relief Drops	Simethicone 20mg/0.3mL	**Peds ≥2 yrs (≥24 lbs):** 0.6mL prn after meals and at hs. **Peds <2 yrs (<24 lbs):** 0.3mL prn after meals and at hs. **Max:** 12 doses/24h.

Table 6. ANTIFUNGAL PRODUCTS

BRAND	INGREDIENT(S)/STRENGTH(S)	DOSAGE
BUTENAFINES		
Lotrimin Ultra Athlete's Foot Cream	Butenafine HCl 1%	**Adults & Peds ≥12 yrs:** **Athlete's Foot:** Apply bid for 1 week or qd for 4 weeks. **Jock Itch/Ringworm:** Apply qd for 2 weeks.
Lotrimin Ultra Jock Itch Cream	Butenafine HCl 1%	**Adults & Peds ≥12 yrs:** Apply qd for 2 weeks.
CLOTRIMAZOLES		
FungiCure Intensive Liquid	Clotrimazole 1%	**Adults & Peds ≥2 yrs:** **Athlete's Foot/Ringworm:** Apply bid for 4 weeks. **Jock Itch:** Apply bid for 2 weeks.
FungiCure Maximum Strength Manicure & Pedicure	Clotrimazole 1%	**Adults & Peds ≥2 yrs:** **Athlete's Foot/Ringworm:** Apply bid for 4 weeks.
Lotrimin AF Athlete's Foot Cream	Clotrimazole 1%	**Adults & Peds ≥2 yrs:** **Athlete's Foot/Ringworm:** Apply bid for 4 weeks. **Jock Itch:** Apply bid for 2 weeks.
Lotrimin AF Jock Itch Cream	Clotrimazole 1%	**Adults & Peds ≥2 yrs:** Apply bid for 2 weeks.
Lotrimin AF Ringworm Cream	Clotrimazole 1%	**Adults & Peds ≥2 yrs:** Apply bid for 4 weeks.
MICONAZOLES		
Clearly Confident Antifungal Cream	Miconazole nitrate 2%	**Adults & Peds ≥2 yrs:** Apply bid for 4 weeks.
Desenex Liquid Spray	Miconazole nitrate 2%	**Adults & Peds ≥2 yrs:** Apply bid for 4 weeks.
Desenex Powder	Miconazole nitrate 2%	**Adults & Peds ≥2 yrs:** Apply bid for 4 weeks.
Desenex Spray Powder	Miconazole nitrate 2%	**Adults & Peds ≥2 yrs:** Apply bid for 4 weeks.
Lotrimin AF Athlete's Foot Deodorant Powder Spray	Miconazole nitrate 2%	**Adults & Peds ≥2 yrs:** **Athlete's Foot/Ringworm:** Apply bid for 4 weeks. **Jock Itch:** Apply bid for 2 weeks.

(Continued)

Brand	Ingredient(s)/Strength(s)	Dosage
MICONAZOLES *(Continued)*		
Lotrimin AF Athlete's Foot Liquid Spray	Miconazole nitrate 2%	**Adults & Peds ≥2 yrs:** **Athlete's Foot/Ringworm:** Apply bid for 4 weeks. **Jock Itch:** Apply bid for 2 weeks.
Lotrimin AF Athlete's Foot Powder	Miconazole nitrate 2%	**Adults & Peds ≥2 yrs:** **Athlete's Foot/Ringworm:** Apply bid for 4 weeks. **Jock Itch:** Apply bid for 2 weeks.
Lotrimin AF Athlete's Foot Powder Spray	Miconazole nitrate 2%	**Adults & Peds ≥2 yrs:** **Athlete's Foot/Ringworm:** Apply bid for 4 weeks. **Jock Itch:** Apply bid for 2 weeks.
Lotrimin AF Jock Itch Powder Spray	Miconazole nitrate 2%	**Adults & Peds ≥2 yrs:** Apply bid for 2 weeks.
Micatin Cream	Miconazole nitrate 2%	**Adults & Peds ≥2 yrs:** **Athlete's Foot/Ringworm:** Apply bid for 4 weeks. **Jock Itch:** Apply bid for 2 weeks.
Miranel AF Cream	Miconazole nitrate 2%	**Adults & Peds ≥12 yrs:** **Athlete's Foot/Ringworm:** Apply bid for 4 weeks.
Ting AF Spray Powder	Miconazole nitrate 2%	**Adults & Peds ≥2 yrs:** **Athlete's Foot/Ringworm:** Apply bid for 4 weeks. **Jock Itch:** Apply bid for 2 weeks.
Zeasorb Super Absorbent Powder	Miconazole nitrate 2%	**Adults & Peds ≥2 yrs:** **Athlete's Foot:** Apply bid for 4 weeks. **Jock Itch:** Apply bid for 2 weeks.
TERBINAFINES		
Lamisil AT Cream	Terbinafine HCl 1%	**Adults & Peds ≥12 yrs:** **Athlete's Foot (between toes):** Apply bid for 1 week. **Athlete's Foot (on side or bottom of foot):** Apply bid for 2 weeks. **Jock Itch/Ringworm:** Apply qd for 1 week.
Lamisil AT Cream for Jock Itch	Terbinafine HCl 1%	**Adults & Peds ≥12 yrs:** Apply qd for 1 week.

Brand	Ingredient(s)/Strength(s)	Dosage
TERBINAFINES *(Continued)*		
Lamisil AT Gel	Terbinafine 1%	**Adults & Peds ≥12 yrs:** **Athlete's Foot (between toes):** Apply qhs for 1 week. **Jock Itch/Ringworm:** Apply qd for 1 week.
Lamisil AT Spray	Terbinafine HCl 1%	**Adults & Peds ≥12 yrs:** **Athlete's Foot (between toes):** Apply bid for 1 week. **Jock Itch/Ringworm:** Apply qd for 1 week.
Lamisil AT Spray for Jock Itch	Terbinafine HCl 1%	**Adults & Peds ≥12 yrs:** Apply qd for 1 week.
TOLNAFTATES		
Flexitol Medicated Foot Cream	Tolnaftate 1%	**Adults & Peds ≥2 yrs:** Apply bid for 4 weeks. **Prevention:** Apply qd or bid.
Lamisil AF Defense Shake Powder; Lamisil AF Defense Spray Powder	Tolnaftate 1%	**Adults & Peds ≥2 yrs:** Apply bid for 4 weeks. **Prevention:** Apply qd or bid.
Nailene Maximum Strength Antifungal Treatment	Tolnaftate 1%	**Adults & Peds ≥2 yrs:** Apply bid for 4 weeks.
Odor-Eaters Foot & Sneaker Spray Powder	Tolnaftate 1%	**Adults & Peds ≥2 yrs:** **Prevention:** Apply qd or bid.
ProClearz Maximum Strength Fungal Shield	Tolnaftate 1%	**Adults & Peds ≥2 yrs:** **Athlete's Foot/Ringworm:** Apply bid for 4 weeks. **Jock Itch:** Apply bid for 2 weeks.
Tinactin Athlete's Foot Cream	Tolnaftate 1%	**Adults & Peds ≥2 yrs:** Apply bid for 4 weeks. **Prevention:** Apply qd or bid.
Tinactin Athlete's Foot Deodorant Powder Spray	Tolnaftate 1%	**Adults & Peds ≥2 yrs:** Apply bid for 4 weeks. **Prevention:** Apply qd or bid.
Tinactin Athlete's Foot Liquid Spray	Tolnaftate 1%	**Adults & Peds ≥2 yrs:** Apply bid for 4 weeks. **Prevention:** Apply qd or bid.
Tinactin Athlete's Foot Powder Spray	Tolnaftate 1%	**Adults & Peds ≥2 yrs:** Apply bid for 4 weeks. **Prevention:** Apply qd or bid.

(Continued)

Brand	Ingredient(s)/Strength(s)	Dosage
TOLNAFTATES (Continued)		
Tinactin Athlete's Foot Super Absorbent Powder	Tolnaftate 1%	**Adults & Peds ≥2 yrs:** Apply bid for 4 weeks. **Prevention:** Apply qd or bid.
Tinactin Jock Itch Cream	Tolnaftate 1%	**Adults & Peds ≥2 yrs:** Apply bid for 2 weeks.
Tinactin Jock Itch Powder Spray	Tolnaftate 1%	**Adults & Peds ≥2 yrs:** Apply bid for 2 weeks.
Ting Cream	Tolnaftate 1%	**Adults & Peds ≥2 yrs:** **Athlete's Foot/Ringworm:** Apply bid for 4 weeks. **Jock Itch:** Apply bid for 2 weeks.
Ting Spray Liquid	Tolnaftate 1%	**Adults & Peds ≥2 yrs:** Apply bid for 4 weeks.
UNDECYLENIC ACIDS		
DiabetiDerm Antifungal Cream	Undecylenic acid 10%	**Adults & Peds ≥2 yrs:** **Athlete's Foot/Ringworm:** Apply bid for 4 weeks. **Jock Itch:** Apply bid for 2 weeks.
Flexitol Anti-Fungal Liquid	Undecylenic acid 25%	**Adults & Peds ≥2 yrs:** **Athlete's Foot/Ringworm:** Apply bid for 4 weeks.
Fungi Nail Anti-Fungal Solution	Undecylenic acid 25%	**Adults & Peds ≥2 yrs:** **Athlete's Foot/Ringworm:** Apply bid for 4 weeks.
Fungi Nail Anti-Fungal Solution Pen Brush Applicator	Undecylenic acid 25%	**Adults & Peds ≥2 yrs:** **Athlete's Foot/Ringworm:** Apply bid for 4 weeks.
Fungi Nail Toe & Foot Ointment	Zinc undecylenate/ Undecylenic acid 20%-5%	**Adults & Peds ≥2 yrs:** **Athlete's Foot/Ringworm:** Apply bid for 4 weeks. **Toe Fungus:** Apply under nail and around cuticle area bid.
FungiCure Maximum Strength Liquid	Undecylenic acid 25%	**Adults & Peds ≥2 yrs:** **Athlete's Foot/Ringworm:** Apply bid for 4 weeks.
Tineacide Antifungal Cream	Undecylenic acid 10%	**Adults & Peds ≥2 yrs:** **Athlete's Foot/Ringworm:** Apply bid for 4 weeks. **Jock Itch:** Apply bid for 2 weeks.

Table 7. ANTIPYRETIC PRODUCTS

BRAND	INGREDIENT(S)/STRENGTH(S)	DOSAGE
ACETAMINOPHENS		
FeverAll Children's Suppositories	Acetaminophen 120mg	**Peds 3-6 yrs:** 1 supp q4-6h. **Max:** 5 doses/24h.
FeverAll Infants' Suppositories	Acetaminophen 80mg	**Peds 6-11 months:** 1 supp q6h. **Max:** 4 doses/24h. **12-36 months:** 1 supp q4-6h. **Max:** 5 doses/24h.
FeverAll Jr. Strength Suppositories	Acetaminophen 325mg	**Adults & Peds ≥12 yrs:** 2 supp q4-6h. **Max:** 6 doses/24h. **Peds 6-12 yrs:** 1 supp q4-6h. **Max:** 5 doses/24h.
PediaCare Children Fever Reducer/ Pain Reliever Acetaminophen Oral Suspension	Acetaminophen 160mg/5mL	**Peds 2-3 yrs (24-35 lbs):** 1 tsp (5mL). **4-5 yrs (36-47 lbs):** 1.5 tsp (7.5mL). **6-8 yrs (48-59 lbs):** 2 tsp (10mL). **9-10 yrs (60-71 lbs):** 2.5 tsp (12.5mL). **11 yrs (72-95 lbs):** 3 tsp (15mL). May repeat q4h. **Max:** 5 doses/24h.
PediaCare Infants Fever Reducer/ Pain Reliever Acetaminophen Oral Suspension	Acetaminophen 160mg/5mL	**Peds 2-3 yrs (24-35 lbs):** 5mL. May repeat q4h. **Max:** 5 doses/24h.
Triaminic Children's Fever Reducer Pain Reliever Syrup*†	Acetaminophen 160mg/5mL	**Peds 2-3 yrs (24-35 lbs):** 1 tsp (5mL). **4-5 yrs (36-47 lbs):** 1.5 tsp (7.5mL). **6-8 yrs (48-59 lbs):** 2 tsp (10mL). **9-10 yrs (60-71 lbs)** 2.5 tsp (12.5mL). **11 yrs (72-95 lbs):** 3 tsp (15mL). May repeat q4h. **Max:** 5 doses/24h.
Triaminic Infants' Fever Reducer Pain Reliever Syrup*†	Acetaminophen 160mg/5mL	**Peds 2-3 yrs (24-35 lbs):** 1 tsp (5mL). May repeat q4h. **Max:** 5 doses/24h.
Tylenol 8 Hour Caplets†	Acetaminophen 650mg	**Adults & Peds ≥12 yrs:** 2 tabs q8h prn. **Max:** 6 tabs/24h.
Tylenol Arthritis Pain Caplets†	Acetaminophen 650mg	**Adults:** 2 tabs q8h prn. **Max:** 6 tabs/24h.
Tylenol Arthritis Pain Gelcaps†	Acetaminophen 650mg	**Adults:** 2 caps q8h prn. **Max:** 6 caps/24h.

(Continued)

Brand	Ingredient(s)/Strength(s)	Dosage
ACETAMINOPHENS (Continued)		
Tylenol Children's Meltaways Chewable Tablets*	Acetaminophen 80mg	**Peds 2-3 yrs (24-35 lbs):** 2 tabs. **4-5 yrs (36-47 lbs):** 3 tabs. **6-8 yrs (48-59 lbs):** 4 tabs. **9-10 yrs (60-71 lbs):** 5 tabs. **11 yrs (72-95 lbs):** 6 tabs. May repeat q4h. **Max:** 5 doses/24h.
Tylenol Children's Oral Suspension*	Acetaminophen 160mg/5mL	**Peds 2-3 yrs (24-35 lbs):** 1 tsp (5mL). **4-5 yrs (36-47 lbs):** 1.5 tsp (7.5mL). **6-8 yrs (48-59 lbs):** 2 tsp (10mL). **9-10 yrs (60-71 lbs):** 2.5 tsp (12.5mL). **11 yrs (72-95 lbs):** 3 tsp (15mL). May repeat q4h. **Max:** 5 doses/24h.
Tylenol Extra Strength Caplets	Acetaminophen 500mg	**Adults & Peds ≥12 yrs:** 2 tabs q6h prn. **Max:** 6 tabs/24h.
Tylenol Extra Strength EZ Tablets†	Acetaminophen 500mg	**Adults & Peds ≥12 yrs:** 2 tabs q4-6h prn. **Max:** 8 tabs/24h.
Tylenol Extra Strength Rapid Blast Liquid	Acetaminophen 500mg/15mL	**Adults & Peds ≥12 yrs:** 2 tbsp (30mL) q6h prn. **Max:** 6 tbsp (90mL)/24h.
Tylenol Extra Strength Rapid Release Gelcaps	Acetaminophen 500mg	**Adults & Peds ≥12 yrs:** 2 caps q6h prn. **Max:** 6 caps/24h.
Tylenol Jr. Meltaways Chewable Tablets*	Acetaminophen 160mg	**Peds 6-8 yrs (48-59 lbs):** 2 tabs. **9-10 yrs (60-71 lbs):** 2.5 tabs. **11 yrs (72-95 lbs):** 3 tabs. May repeat q4h. **Max:** 5 doses/24h.
Tylenol Regular Strength Tablets	Acetaminophen 325mg	**Adults & Peds ≥12 yrs:** 2 tabs q4-6h prn. **Max:** 10 tabs/24h. **Peds 6-11 yrs:** 1 tab q4-6h prn. **Max:** 5 tabs/24h.
NONSTEROIDAL ANTI-INFLAMMATORY DRUGS (NSAIDS)		
Advil Caplets	Ibuprofen 200mg	**Adults & Peds ≥12 yrs:** 1-2 tabs q4-6h prn. **Max:** 6 tabs/24h.

Brand	Ingredient(s)/Strength(s)	Dosage
NONSTEROIDAL ANTI-INFLAMMATORY DRUGS (NSAIDS) *(Continued)*		
Advil Children's Suspension*	Ibuprofen 100mg/5mL	**Peds 2-3 yrs (24-35 lbs):** 1 tsp (5mL). **4-5 yrs (36-47 lbs):** 1.5 tsp (7.5mL). **6-8 yrs (48-59 lbs):** 2 tsp (10mL). **9-10 yrs (60-71 lbs):** 2.5 tsp (12.5mL). **11 yrs (72-95 lbs):** 3 tsp (15mL). May repeat q6-8h. **Max:** 4 doses/24h.
Advil Gel Caplets	Ibuprofen 200mg	**Adults & Peds ≥12 yrs:** 1-2 tabs q4-6h prn. **Max:** 6 tabs/24h.
Advil Infants' Concentrated Drops	Ibuprofen 50mg/1.25mL	**Peds 6-11 months (12-17 lbs):** 1.25mL. **12-23 months (18-23 lbs):** 1.875mL. May repeat q6-8h. **Max:** 4 doses/24h.
Advil Junior Strength Chewable Tablets	Ibuprofen 100mg	**Peds 6-8 yrs (48-59 lbs):** 2 tabs. **9-10 yrs (60-71 lbs):** 2.5 tabs. **11 yrs (72-95 lbs):** 3 tabs. May repeat q6-8h. **Max:** 4 doses/24h.
Advil Junior Strength Tablets	Ibuprofen 100mg	**Peds 6-10 yrs (48-71 lbs):** 2 tabs. **11 yrs (72-95 lbs):** 3 tabs. May repeat q6-8h. **Max:** 4 doses/24h.
Advil Liqui-Gels	Ibuprofen 200mg	**Adults & Peds ≥12 yrs:** 1-2 caps q4-6h prn. **Max:** 6 caps/24h.
Advil Tablets	Ibuprofen 200mg	**Adults & Peds ≥12 yrs:** 1-2 tabs q4-6h prn. **Max:** 6 tabs/24h.
Aleve Caplets	Naproxen sodium 220mg	**Adults & Peds ≥12 yrs:** 1 tab q8-12h. May take 1 additional tab within 1h of first dose. **Max:** 2 tabs/8-12h or 3 tabs/24h.
Aleve Gelcaps	Naproxen sodium 220mg	**Adults & Peds ≥12 yrs:** 1 cap q8-12h. May take 1 additional cap within 1h of first dose. **Max:** 2 caps/8-12h or 3 caps/24h.
Aleve Liquid Gels	Naproxen sodium 220mg	**Adults & Peds ≥12 yrs:** 1 cap q8-12h. May take 1 additional cap within 1h of first dose. **Max:** 2 caps/8-12h or 3 caps/24h.

(Continued)

BRAND	INGREDIENT(S)/STRENGTH(S)	DOSAGE
NONSTEROIDAL ANTI-INFLAMMATORY DRUGS (NSAIDS) *(Continued)*		
Aleve Tablets	Naproxen sodium 220mg	**Adults & Peds ≥12 yrs:** 1 tab q8-12h. May take 1 additional tab within 1h of first dose. **Max:** 2 tabs/8-12h or 3 tabs/24h.
Motrin Children's Oral Suspension	Ibuprofen 100mg/5mL	**Peds 2-3 yrs (24-35 lbs):** 1 tsp (5mL). **4-5 yrs (36-47 lbs):** 1.5 tsp (7.5mL). **6-8 yrs (48-59 lbs):** 2 tsp (10mL). **9-10 yrs (60-71 lbs):** 2.5 tsp (12.5mL). **11 yrs (72-95 lbs):** 3 tsp (15mL). May repeat q6-8h. **Max:** 4 doses/24h.
Motrin IB Caplets	Ibuprofen 200mg	**Adults & Peds ≥12 yrs:** 1-2 tabs q4-6h prn. **Max:** 6 tabs/24h.
Motrin Infants' Concentrated Drops	Ibuprofen 50mg/1.25mL	**Peds 6-11 months (12-17 lbs):** 1.25mL. **12-23 months (18-23 lbs):** 1.875mL. May repeat q6-8h. **Max:** 4 doses/24h.
Motrin Junior Strength Caplets†	Ibuprofen 100mg	**Peds 6-8 yrs (48-59 lbs):** 2 tabs. **9-10 yrs (60-71 lbs):** 2.5 tabs. **11 yrs (72-95 lbs):** 3 tabs. May repeat q6-8h. **Max:** 4 doses/24h.
Motrin Junior Strength Chewable Tablets*†	Ibuprofen 100mg	**Peds 2-3 yrs (24-35 lbs):** 1 tab. **4-5 yrs (36-47 lbs):** 1.5 tabs. **6-8 yrs (48-59 lbs):** 2 tabs. **9-10 yrs (60-71 lbs):** 2.5 tabs. **11 yrs (72-95 lbs):** 3 tabs. May repeat q6-8h. **Max:** 4 doses/24h.
PediaCare Children Pain Reliever/ Fever Reducer IB Ibuprofen Oral Suspension	Ibuprofen 100mg/5mL	**Peds 2-3 yrs (24-35 lbs):** 1 tsp (5mL). **4-5 yrs (36-47 lbs):** 1.5 tsp (7.5mL). **6-8 yrs (48-59 lbs):** 2 tsp (10mL). **9-10 yrs (60-71 lbs):** 2.5 tsp (12.5mL). **11 yrs (72-95 lbs):** 3 tsp (15mL). May repeat q6-8h. **Max:** 4 doses/24h.
PediaCare Infants Pain Reliever/ Fever Reducer IB Ibuprofen Concentrated Oral Suspension	Ibuprofen 50mg/1.25mL	**Peds: 6-11 months (12-17 lbs):** 1.25mL. **12-23 months (18-23 lbs):** 1.865mL. May repeat q6-8h. **Max:** 4 doses/24h.

Brand	Ingredient(s)/Strength(s)	Dosage
SALICYLATES		
Bayer Aspirin Extra Strength Caplets	Aspirin 500mg	**Adults & Peds ≥12 yrs:** 1-2 tabs q4-6h. **Max:** 8 tabs/24h.
Bayer Aspirin Safety Coated Caplets	Aspirin 325mg	**Adults & Peds ≥12 yrs:** 1-2 tabs q4h. **Max:** 12 tabs/24h.
Bayer Genuine Aspirin Tablets	Aspirin 325mg	**Adults & Peds ≥12 yrs:** 1-2 tabs q4h or 3 tabs q6h. **Max:** 12 tabs/24h.
Bayer Low Dose Aspirin Chewable Tablets*	Aspirin 81mg	**Adults & Peds ≥12 yrs:** 4-8 tabs q4h. **Max:** 48 tabs/24h.
Bayer Low Dose Aspirin Safety Coated Tablets	Aspirin 81mg	**Adults & Peds ≥12 yrs:** 4-8 tabs q4h. **Max:** 48 tabs/24h.
Ecotrin Low Strength Tablets	Aspirin 81mg	**Adults & Peds ≥12 yrs:** 4-8 tabs q4h. **Max:** 48 tabs/24h.
Ecotrin Regular Strength Tablets	Aspirin 325mg	**Adults & Peds ≥12 yrs:** 1-2 tabs q4h. **Max:** 12 tabs/24h.
Halfprin 81mg Tablets	Aspirin 81mg	**Adults & Peds ≥12 yrs:** 4-8 tabs q4h. **Max:** 48 tabs/24h.
Halfprin 162mg Tablets	Aspirin 162mg	**Adults & Peds ≥12 yrs:** 2-4 tabs q4h. **Max:** 24 tabs/24h.
St. Joseph Aspirin Chewable Tablets	Aspirin 81mg	**Adults & Peds ≥12 yrs:** 4-8 tabs q4h. **Max:** 48 tabs/24h.
St. Joseph Regular Strength Safety Coated Tablets	Aspirin 325mg	**Adults & Peds ≥12 yrs:** 1-2 tabs q4h. **Max:** 12 tabs/24h.
St. Joseph Safety Coated Tablets	Aspirin 81mg	**Adults & Peds ≥12 yrs:** 4-8 tabs q4h. **Max:** 48 tabs/24h.
SALICYLATES, BUFFERED		
Bayer Aspirin Extra Strength Plus Caplets	Aspirin 500mg Buffered with Calcium carbonate	**Adults & Peds ≥12 yrs:** 1-2 tabs q4-6h. **Max:** 8 tabs/24h.
Bayer Women's Low Dose Aspirin Caplets	Aspirin 81mg Buffered with Calcium carbonate 777mg	**Adults & Peds ≥12 yrs:** 4-8 tabs q4h. **Max:** 10 tabs/24h.
Bufferin Low Dose Tablets†	Aspirin 81mg Buffered with Calcium carbonate/Magnesium oxide/ Magnesium carbonate	**Adults & Peds ≥12 yrs:** 4-8 tabs q4h. **Max:** 48 tabs/24h.

*Multiple flavors available.

†Product currently on recall or temporarily unavailable from manufacturer, but generic forms may be available.

Table 8. COMMONLY USED HERBAL PRODUCTS

Name	Accepted Uses	Unproven Uses	Interactions
Aloe vera	**Topical:** Resolution of psoriatic plaques, reduce desquamation, erythema, and infiltration **Oral:** Constipation	**Topical:** Burns, frostbite, herpes simplex, wound healing **Oral:** Diabetes, ulcerative colitis, hyperlipidemia	Antidiabetics, digoxin, diuretics, sevoflurane, stimulant laxatives, warfarin
Black cohosh	Menopausal symptoms (eg, hot flashes)	Labor induction, osteoporosis	Atorvastatin, cisplatin, drugs metabolized by the liver (CYP2D6 substrates), hepatotoxic drugs
Black psyllium	Constipation, hypercholesterolemia	Cancer, diarrhea, irritable bowel syndrome	Antidiabetics, carbamazepine, digoxin, lithium
Capsicum	**Topical:** Pain, fibromyalgia, prurigo nodularis **Intranasal:** Cluster headache, perennial rhinitis (nonallergic, noninfectious)	**Oral:** Dyspepsia, peptic ulcers, swallowing dysfunction **Intranasal:** Migraine headaches, sinonasal polyposis, allergic rhinitis	Cocaine, ACE inhibitors, anticoagulants, antiplatelets, theophylline, coca
Chamomile	Colic, dyspepsia, oral mucositis	Restlessness, insomnia, menstrual cramps, diarrhea, fibromyalgia	Benzodiazepines, CNS depressants, contraceptives, drugs metabolized by the liver (CYP1A2, CYP3A4 substrates), estrogens, tamoxifen, warfarin
Cranberry	Urinary tract infections	Benign prostatic hyperplasia, urine deodorant	Drugs metabolized by the liver (CYP2C9 substrates), warfarin
Echinacea	**Oral:** Common cold, vaginal candidiasis **Topical:** Superficial wounds, burns	Influenza, leukopenia	Caffeine, drugs metabolized by the liver (CYP1A2, CYP3A4 substrates), immunosuppressants, midazolam
Eucalyptus		Asthma, upper respiratory tract inflammation, wounds, burns, congestion, ulcers, acne, bleeding gums, bladder disease, diabetes, fever, flu, loss of appetite, arthritis pain, liver/gallbladder problems	Drugs metabolized by the liver (CYP1A2, CYP2C19, CYP2C9, CYP3A4 substrates), antidiabetics, herbs that contain hepatotoxic pyrrolizidine alkaloids
Evening primrose oil	**Oral:** Mastalgia, osteoporosis	Rheumatoid arthritis, Sjogren's syndrome, chronic fatigue syndrome	Anesthesia, anticoagulants, antiplatelets, phenothiazines

(Continued)

Name	Accepted Uses	Unproven Uses	Interactions
Feverfew	Migraine headaches	Fever, menstrual irregularities, arthritis, psoriasis, allergies, asthma, dizziness, nausea, vomiting, earache, cancer, common cold	Drugs metabolized by the liver (CYP1A2, CYP2C19, CYP2C9, CYP3A4 substrates), anticoagulants, antiplatelets
Flaxseed	Diabetes, hypercholesterolemia, menopausal symptoms, systemic lupus erythematosus nephritis	Breast cancer, cardiovascular disease, colorectal cancer, constipation, endometrial cancer, lung cancer, mastalgia, prostate cancer	Acetaminophen, antibiotics, anticoagulants, antiplatelets, antidiabetics, estrogens, furosemide, ketoprofen, metoprolol, decreased absorption of oral medications
Garlic	**Oral:** Atherosclerosis, gastric cancer, hypertension, tick bites **Topical:** Tinea corporis (ringworm), tinea cruris (jock itch), tinea pedis (athlete's foot)	Benign prostatic hyperplasia, common cold, corns, preeclampsia, prostate cancer, warts	Anticoagulants, antiplatelets, contraceptives, cyclosporine, drugs metabolized by the liver (CYP2E1, CYP3A4 substrates), isoniazid, non-nucleoside reverse transcriptase inhibitors, saquinavir, warfarin
Ginger	Dysmenorrhea, morning sickness, osteoarthritis, postoperative nausea and vomiting, vertigo	Chemotherapy-induced nausea and vomiting, migraine headache, myalgia, rheumatoid arthritis	Anticoagulants, antiplatelets, antidiabetics, calcium channel blockers, phenprocoumon, warfarin
Ginkgo	Age-related memory impairment, cognitive function, dementia, diabetic retinopathy, glaucoma, peripheral vascular disease, premenstrual syndrome, Raynaud's syndrome, vertigo	Age-related macular degeneration, anxiety, ADHD, colorectal cancer, fibromyalgia, hearing loss, ovarian cancer, radiation exposure, schizophrenia, stroke, vitiligo	Alprazolam, anticoagulants, antiplatelets, anticonvulsants, antidiabetics, buspirone, drugs metabolized by the liver (CYP1A2, CYP2C19, CYP2C9, CYP2D6, CYP3A4 substrates), efavirenz, fluoxetine, hydrochlorothiazide, ibuprofen, omeprazole, seizure threshold-lowering drugs, trazodone, St John's wort, warfarin
Ginseng	Diabetes, respiratory tract infections	ADHD, breast cancer	Antidiabetics, monoamine oxidase inhibitors, warfarin
Licorice	Dyspepsia	Atopic dermatitis, hepatitis, muscle cramps, peptic ulcers, weight loss	Cardiac glycoside-containing herbs (eg, digitalis), stimulant laxative herbs (eg, aloe), antihypertensives, corticosteroids, drugs metabolized by the liver (CYP2B6, CYP2C9, CYP3A4 substrates), digoxin, diuretics, estrogens, ethacrynic acid, furosemide, warfarin, grapefruit juice, salt

Name	Accepted Uses	Unproven Uses	Interactions
Milk thistle	Diabetes, dyspepsia	Alcohol-related liver disease, *amanita* mushroom poisoning, hepatitis B or C, toxin-induced liver damage	Drugs metabolized by the liver (CYP2C9 substrates), estrogens, drugs that undergo glucuronidation (eg, metronidazole), HMG-CoA reductase inhibitors ("statins"), tamoxifen
Peppermint	Barium enema-related colonic spasm, dyspepsia, irritable bowel syndrome, tension headache	**Topical:** Postherpetic neuralgia	Antacids, cyclosporine, drugs metabolized by the liver (CYP1A2, CYP2C19, CYP2C9, CYP3A4 substrates), H_2-blockers, proton pump inhibitors
Saw palmetto	Benign prostatic hyperplasia	Androgenic alopecia, prostate cancer, prostatitis and chronic pelvic pain syndrome	Anticoagulants, antiplatelets, contraceptives, estrogens
Senna	Constipation, bowel preparation	Hemorrhoids, irritable bowel syndrome, weight loss	Digoxin, diuretics, warfarin, horsetail, licorice, stimulant laxatives
St John's wort	Depression, menopausal symptoms, somatization disorder, wound healing	Obsessive-compulsive disorder, premenstrual syndrome, seasonal affective disorder	Numerous medications
Valerian	Insomnia	Anxiety, dyssomnia	Alcohol, alprazolam, drugs metabolized by the liver (CYP3A4 substrates), benzodiazepines, CNS depressants, herbs and supplements with sedative properties

Source: Natural Medicines Comprehensive Database.

Table 9. CONTACT DERMATITIS PRODUCTS

BRAND	INGREDIENT(S)/STRENGTH(S)	DOSAGE
ANTIHISTAMINES		
Benadryl Extra Strength Itch Stopping Gel	Diphenhydramine HCl 2%	**Adults & Peds ≥2 yrs:** Apply to affected area ≤ tid-qid.
ANTIHISTAMINE COMBINATIONS		
Benadryl Extra Strength Itch Relief Stick	Diphenhydramine HCl/Zinc acetate 2%-0.1%	**Adults & Peds ≥2 yrs:** Apply to affected area ≤ tid-qid.
Benadryl Extra Strength Itch Stopping Cream	Diphenhydramine HCl/Zinc acetate 2%-0.1%	**Adults & Peds ≥2 yrs:** Apply to affected area ≤ tid-qid.
Benadryl Extra Strength Spray	Diphenhydramine HCl/Zinc acetate 2%-0.1%	**Adults & Peds ≥2 yrs:** Apply to affected area ≤ tid-qid.
Benadryl Original Strength Itch Stopping Cream	Diphenhydramine HCl/Zinc acetate 1%-0.1%	**Adults & Peds ≥2 yrs:** Apply to affected area ≤ tid-qid.
Benadryl Readymist Itch Stopping Spray	Diphenhydramine HCl/Zinc acetate 2%-0.1%	**Adults & Peds ≥2 yrs:** Apply to affected area ≤ tid-qid.
Calagel Maximum Strength Anti-Itch Gel	Diphenhydramine HCl/Zinc acetate/Benzethonium chloride 2%-0.215%-0.15%	**Adults & Peds ≥2 yrs:** Apply to affected area ≤ tid.
Ivarest Maximum Strength Poison Ivy Itch Cream	Diphenhydramine HCl/Benzyl alcohol/Calamine 2%-10.5%-14%	**Adults & Peds ≥2 yrs:** Apply to affected area ≤ tid-qid.
ASTRINGENTS		
Domeboro Astringent Solution Powder Packets	Aluminum acetate (combination of Calcium acetate 952mg and Aluminum sulfate 1347mg)	Dissolve 1-3 pkts in 16 oz of water and soak affected area for 15-30 min tid or apply as compress/wet dressing to affected area for 15-30 min as needed.
ASTRINGENT COMBINATIONS		
Aveeno Anti-Itch Concentrated Lotion	Calamine/Pramoxine HCl 3%-1%	**Adults & Peds ≥2 yrs:** Apply to affected area ≤ qid.
Aveeno Calamine & Pramoxine HCl Anti-Itch Cream	Calamine/Pramoxine HCl 3%-1%	**Adults & Peds ≥2 yrs:** Apply to affected area ≤ qid.
Caladryl Anti-Itch Lotion	Calamine/Pramoxine HCl 8%-1%	**Adults & Peds ≥2 yrs:** Apply to affected area ≤ tid-qid.
Caladryl Clear Anti-Itch Lotion	Zinc acetate/Pramoxine HCl 0.1%-1%	**Adults & Peds ≥2 yrs:** Apply to affected area ≤ tid-qid.
Calamine Lotion (generic)	Calamine/Zinc oxide 8%-8%	Apply to affected area prn.
Ivy-Dry Cream	Benzyl alcohol/Camphor/Menthol 10%-0.6%-0.4%	**Adults & Peds ≥2 yrs:** Apply to affected area ≤ tid.

(Continued)

BRAND	INGREDIENT(S)/STRENGTH(S)	DOSAGE
ASTRINGENT COMBINATIONS *(Continued)*		
Ivy-Dry Super Spray	Benzyl alcohol/Camphor/ Menthol 10%-0.5%-0.25%	**Adults & Peds ≥6 yrs:** Apply to affected area ≤ tid.
CLEANSERS		
Ivarest Medicated Poison Ivy Cleansing Foam	Menthol 1%	**Adults & Peds ≥2 yrs:** Gently rub into affected area and rinse under running water ≤ tid-qid.
CORTICOSTEROIDS		
Aveeno 1% Hydrocortisone Anti-Itch Cream	Hydrocortisone 1%	**Adults & Peds ≥2 yrs:** Apply to affected area ≤ tid-qid.
Cortaid 12-Hour Advanced Anti-Itch Cream	Hydrocortisone 1%	**Adults & Peds ≥2 yrs:** Apply to affected area ≤ tid-qid.
Cortaid Intensive Therapy Cooling Spray	Hydrocortisone 1%	**Adults & Peds ≥2 yrs:** Apply to affected area ≤ tid-qid.
Cortaid Maximum Strength Cream	Hydrocortisone 1%	**Adults & Peds ≥2 yrs:** Apply to affected area ≤ tid-qid.
Corticool 1% Hydrocortisone Anti-Itch Gel	Hydrocortisone 1%	**Adults & Peds ≥2 yrs:** Apply to affected area ≤ tid-qid.
Cortizone-10 Cooling Relief Gel	Hydrocortisone 1%	**Adults & Peds ≥2 yrs:** Apply to affected area ≤ tid-qid.
Cortizone-10 Creme	Hydrocortisone 1%	**Adults & Peds ≥2 yrs:** Apply to affected area ≤ tid-qid.
Cortizone-10 Easy Relief Applicator Liquid	Hydrocortisone 1%	**Adults & Peds ≥2 yrs:** Apply to affected area ≤ tid-qid.
Cortizone-10 Hydratensive Eczema Formula	Hydrocortisone 1%	**Adults & Peds ≥2 yrs:** Apply to affected area ≤ tid-qid.
Cortizone-10 Hydratensive Healing Formula	Hydrocortisone 1%	**Adults & Peds ≥2 yrs:** Apply to affected area ≤ tid-qid.
Cortizone-10 Intensive Healing Eczema Lotion	Hydrocortisone 1%	**Adults & Peds ≥2 yrs:** Apply to affected area ≤ tid-qid.
Cortizone-10 Intensive Healing Formula Creme	Hydrocortisone 1%	**Adults & Peds ≥2 yrs:** Apply to affected area ≤ tid-qid.
Cortizone-10 Ointment	Hydrocortisone 1%	**Adults & Peds ≥2 yrs:** Apply to affected area ≤ tid-qid.
Cortizone-10 Plus Creme	Hydrocortisone 1%	**Adults & Peds ≥2 yrs:** Apply to affected area ≤ tid-qid.
Cortizone-10 Quick Shot 360° Continuous Spray	Hydrocortisone 1%	**Adults & Peds ≥2 yrs:** Apply to affected area ≤ tid-qid.

Brand	Ingredient(s)/Strength(s)	Dosage
LOCAL ANESTHETICS		
Aveeno Skin Relief Medicated Anti-Itch Treatment	Pramoxine HCl 0.5%	**Adults & Peds ≥2 yrs:** Apply to affected area ≤ tid-qid.
Solarcaine Cool Aloe Burn Relief Gel	Lidocaine HCl 0.5%	**Adults & Peds ≥2 yrs:** Apply to affected area ≤ tid-qid.
Solarcaine Cool Aloe Burn Relief Spray	Lidocaine HCl 0.5%	**Adults & Peds ≥2 yrs:** Apply to affected area ≤ tid-qid.
LOCAL ANESTHETIC COMBINATIONS		
Bactine Original First Aid Liquid	Lidocaine HCl/Benzalkonium chloride 2.5%-0.13%	**Adults & Peds ≥2 yrs:** Apply to affected area qd-tid.
Bactine Pain Relieving Cleansing Spray	Lidocaine HCl/Benzalkonium chloride 2.5%-0.13%	**Adults & Peds ≥2 yrs:** Apply to affected area qd-tid.
Gold Bond Maximum Relief Medicated Anti-Itch Cream	Pramoxine HCl/Menthol 1%-1%	**Adults & Peds ≥2 yrs:** Apply to affected area ≤ tid-qid.
Lanacane First Aid Spray	Benzocaine/Benzethonium chloride 20%-0.2%	**Adults & Peds ≥2 yrs:** Apply to affected area ≤ qd-tid.
Lanacane Maximum Strength Anti-Itch Cream	Benzocaine/Benzethonium chloride 20%-0.2%	**Adults & Peds ≥2 yrs:** Apply to affected area ≤ qd-tid.
SKIN PROTECTANTS		
Aveeno Skin Relief 24-Hour Moisturizing Lotion	Dimethicone 1.3%	Apply prn.
Aveeno Skin Relief Overnight Cream	Dimethicone 1.3%	Apply prn.
SKIN PROTECTANT COMBINATIONS		
Gold Bond Cornstarch Plus Medicated Baby Powder	Cornstarch/Kaolin/Zinc oxide 79%-4%-15%	**Adults & Peds ≥2 yrs:** Apply to affected area ≤ tid-qid.
Gold Bond Extra Strength Medicated Body Lotion	Dimethicone/Menthol 5%-0.5%	**Adults & Peds ≥2 yrs:** Apply to affected area tid-qid.
Gold Bond Extra Strength Medicated Body Powder	Zinc oxide/Menthol 5%-0.8%	**Adults & Peds ≥2 yrs:** Apply to affected area ≤ tid-qid.
Gold Bond Intensive Healing Anti-Itch Skin Protectant Cream	Dimethicone/Pramoxine HCl 6%-1%	**Adults & Peds ≥2 yrs:** Apply to affected area ≤ tid-qid.
Gold Bond Intensive Relief Medicated Anti-Itch Lotion	Dimethicone/Menthol/Pramoxine HCl 5%-0.5%-1%	**Adults & Peds ≥2 yrs:** Apply to affected area tid-qid.
Gold Bond Original Strength Medicated Body Lotion	Dimethicone/Menthol 5%-0.15%	**Adults & Peds ≥2 yrs:** Apply to affected area tid-qid.
Gold Bond Original Strength Medicated Body Powder	Zinc oxide/Menthol 1%-0.15%	**Adults & Peds ≥2 yrs:** Apply to affected area ≤ tid-qid.

Table 10. COUGH-COLD-FLU-ALLERGY PRODUCTS

BRAND NAME	ANALGESIC	ANTIHISTAMINE	DECONGESTANT	COUGH SUPPRESSANT	EXPECTORANT	DOSAGE
ANTIHISTAMINES						
Alavert For Kids 6+ Orally Disintegrating Tablets		Loratadine 10mg				**Adults & Peds ≥6 yrs:** 1 tab qd. **Max:** 1 tab/24h.
Alavert Orally Disintegrating Tablets*		Loratadine 10mg				**Adults & Peds ≥6 yrs:** 1 tab qd. **Max:** 1 tab/24h.
Benadryl Allergy Dye-Free Liqui-Gels†		Diphenhydramine HCl 25mg				**Adults & Peds ≥12 yrs:** 1-2 caps q4-6h. **Peds 6-<12 yrs:** 1 cap q4-6h. **Max:** 6 doses/24h.
Benadryl Allergy Ultratab Tablets		Diphenhydramine HCl 25mg				**Adults & Peds ≥12 yrs:** 1-2 tabs q4-6h. **Peds 6-<12 yrs:** 1 tab q4-6h. **Max:** 6 doses/24h.
Children's Benadryl Allergy Fastmelt Tablets†		Diphenhydramine HCl 12.5mg				**Adults & Peds ≥12 yrs:** 2-4 tabs q4-6h. **Peds 6-<12 yrs:** 1-2 tabs q4-6h. **Max:** 6 doses/24h.
Children's Benadryl Allergy Liquid		Diphenhydramine HCl 12.5mg/5mL				**Peds 6-11 yrs:** 1-2 tsp (5-10mL) q4-6h. **Max:** 6 doses/24h.
Children's Benadryl Allergy Perfect Measure Pre-Filled Single Use Spoons†		Diphenhydramine HCl 12.5mg/5mL spoon				**Adults & Peds ≥12 yrs:** 2-4 prefilled spoons (10-20mL) q4-6h. **Peds 6-11 yrs:** 1-2 prefilled spoons (5-10mL) q4-6h. **Max:** 6 doses/24h.
Children's Benadryl Dye-Free Allergy Liquid†		Diphenhydramine HCl 12.5mg/5mL				**Peds 6-11 yrs:** 1-2 tsp (5-10mL) q4-6h. **Max:** 6 doses/24h.

(Continued)

Brand Name	Analgesic	Antihistamine	Decongestant	Cough Suppressant	Expectorant	Dosage
ANTIHISTAMINES *(Continued)*						
Children's Claritin Chewables		Loratadine 5mg				**Adults & Peds ≥6 yrs:** 2 tabs qd. **Max:** 2 tabs/24h. **Peds 2-<6 yrs:** 1 tab qd. **Max:** 1 tab/24h.
Children's Claritin Syrup		Loratadine 5mg/5mL				**Adults & Peds ≥6 yrs:** 2 tsp (10mL) qd. **Max:** 2 tsp (10mL)/24h. **Peds 2-<6 yrs:** 1 tsp (5mL) qd. **Max:** 1 tsp (5mL)/24h.
Children's Zyrtec Allergy Syrup†		Cetirizine HCl 5mg/5mL				**Adults ≥65 yrs:** 1 tsp (5mL) qd. **Max:** 1 tsp (5mL)/24h. **Adults <65 yrs & Peds ≥6 yrs:** 1-2 tsp (5-10mL) qd. **Max:** 2 tsp (10mL)/24h. **Peds 2-<6 yrs:** ½-1 tsp (2.5-5mL) qd or ½ tsp (2.5mL) q12h. **Max:** 1 tsp (5mL)/24h.
Claritin Liqui-Gels		Loratadine 10mg				**Adults & Peds ≥6 yrs:** 1 cap qd. **Max:** 1 cap/24h.
Claritin RediTabs 12-Hour		Loratadine 5mg				**Adults & Peds ≥6 yrs:** 1 tab q12h. **Max:** 2 tabs/24h.
Claritin RediTabs 24-Hour		Loratadine 10mg				**Adults & Peds ≥6 yrs:** 1 tab qd. **Max:** 1 tab/24h.
Claritin RediTabs 12-Hour Ages 6 Years & Older		Loratadine 5mg				**Adults & Peds ≥6 yrs:** 1 tab q12h. **Max:** 2 tabs/24h.
Claritin RediTabs 24-Hour Ages 6 Years & Older		Loratadine 10mg				**Adults & Peds ≥6 yrs:** 1 tab qd. **Max:** 1 tab/24h.
Claritin Tablets		Loratadine 10mg				**Adults & Peds ≥6 yrs:** 1 tab qd. **Max:** 1 tab/24h.

ANTIHISTAMINES (Continued)

Brand Name	Analgesic	Antihistamine	Decongestant	Cough suppressant	Expectorant	Dosage
PediaCare Children Allergy		Diphenhydramine HCl 12.5mg/5mL				**Peds 6-11 yrs (48-95 lbs):** 1 tsp (5mL) q4h. **Max:** 6 doses/24h.
PediaCare Children's 24 Hour Allergy		Cetirizine HCl 5mg/5mL				**Adults ≥65 yrs:** 1 tsp (5mL) qd. **Max:** 1 tsp (5mL)/24h. **Adults <65 & Peds ≥6 yrs:** 1-2 tsp (5-10mL) qd. **Max:** 2 tsp (10mL)/24h. **Peds 2-<6 yrs:** ½-1 tsp (2.5-5mL) qd or ½ tsp (2.5mL) q12h. **Max:** 1 tsp (5mL)/24h.
Zyrtec Liquid Gels		Cetirizine HCl 10mg				**Adults <65 yrs & Peds ≥6 yrs:** 1 cap qd. **Max:** 1 cap/24h.
Zyrtec Tablets		Cetirizine HCl 10mg				**Adults <65 yrs & Peds ≥6 yrs:** 1 tab qd. **Max:** 1 tab/24h.

ANTIHISTAMINES + DECONGESTANTS

Brand Name	Analgesic	Antihistamine	Decongestant	Cough suppressant	Expectorant	Dosage
Alavert Allergy & Sinus D-12 Hour Tablets		Loratadine 5mg	Pseudoephedrine sulfate 120mg			**Adults & Peds ≥12 yrs:** 1 tab q12h. **Max:** 2 tabs/24h.
Allerest PE Tablets		Chlorpheniramine maleate 4mg	Phenylephrine HCl 10mg			**Adults & Peds ≥12 yrs:** 1 tab q4h. **Peds 6-<12 yrs:** ½ tab q4h. **Max:** 6 doses/24h.
Benadryl-D Allergy Plus Sinus Tablets†		Diphenhydramine HCl 25mg	Phenylephrine HCl 10mg			**Adults & Peds ≥12 yrs:** 1 tab q4h. **Max:** 6 tabs/24h.
Children's Benadryl-D Allergy & Sinus Liquid		Diphenhydramine HCl 12.5mg/5mL	Phenylephrine HCl 5mg/5mL			**Adults & Peds ≥12 yrs:** 2 tsp (10mL) q4h. **Peds 6-11 yrs:** 1 tsp (5mL) q4h. **Max:** 6 doses/24h.

(Continued)

ANTIHISTAMINES + DECONGESTANTS (Continued)

Brand Name	Analgesic	Antihistamine	Decongestant	Cough Suppressant	Expectorant	Dosage
Children's Delsym Night Time Cough & Cold Liquid		Diphenhydramine HCl 6.25mg/5mL	Phenylephrine HCl 2.5mg/5mL			**Peds 6–<12 yrs:** 2 tsp (10mL) q4h. **Max:** 6 doses/24h.
Children's Dimetapp Cold & Allergy Chewable Tablets		Brompheniramine maleate 1mg	Phenylephrine HCl 2.5mg			**Adults & Peds ≥12 yrs:** 4 tabs q4h. **Peds 6–<12 yrs:** 2 tabs q4h. **Max:** 6 doses/24h.
Children's Dimetapp Cold & Allergy Syrup		Brompheniramine maleate 1mg/5mL	Phenylephrine HCl 2.5mg/5mL			**Adults & Peds ≥12 yrs:** 4 tsp (20mL) q4h. **Peds 6–<12 yrs:** 2 tsp (10mL) q4h. **Max:** 6 doses/24h.
Children's Dimetapp Nighttime Cold & Congestion Syrup		Diphenhydramine HCl 6.25mg/5mL	Phenylephrine HCl 2.5mg/5mL			**Adults & Peds ≥12 yrs:** 4 tsp (20mL) q4h. **Peds 6–<12 yrs:** 2 tsp (10mL) q4h. **Max:** 6 doses/24h.
Claritin-D 12 Hour Tablets		Loratadine 5mg	Pseudoephedrine sulfate 120mg			**Adults & Peds ≥12 yrs:** 1 tab q12h. **Max:** 2 tabs/24h.
Claritin-D 24 Hour Tablets		Loratadine 10mg	Pseudoephedrine sulfate 240mg			**Adults & Peds ≥12 yrs:** 1 tab qd. **Max:** 1 tab/24h.
Delsym Night Time Cough & Cold Liquid		Diphenhydramine HCl 6.25mg/5mL	Phenylephrine HCl 2.5mg/5mL			**Adults & Peds ≥12 yrs:** 4 tsp (20mL) q4h. **Peds 6–<12 yrs:** 2 tsp (10mL) q4h. **Max:** 6 doses/24h.
Sudafed PE Sinus+Allergy Tablets†		Chlorpheniramine maleate 4mg	Phenylephrine HCl 10mg			**Adults & Peds ≥12 yrs:** 1 tab q4h. **Max:** 6 tabs/24h.
Triaminic Cold & Allergy Syrup		Chlorpheniramine maleate 1mg/5mL	Phenylephrine HCl 2.5mg/5mL			**Peds 6–<12 yrs:** 2 tsp (10mL) q4h. **Max:** 6 doses/24h.

ANTIHISTAMINES + DECONGESTANTS (Continued)

Brand Name	Analgesic	Antihistamine	Decongestant	Cough Suppressant	Expectorant	Dosage
Triaminic Night Time Cold & Cough Syrup		Diphenhydramine HCl 6.25mg/5mL	Phenylephrine HCl 2.5mg/5mL			**Peds 6-<12 yrs:** 2 tsp (10mL) q4h. **Max:** 6 doses/24h.
Zyrtec-D Tablets		Cetirizine HCl 5mg	Pseudoephedrine HCl 120mg			**Adults <65 & Peds ≥12 yrs:** 1 tab q12h. **Max:** 2 tabs/24h.

ANTIHISTAMINES + DECONGESTANTS + ANALGESICS

Brand Name	Analgesic	Antihistamine	Decongestant	Cough Suppressant	Expectorant	Dosage
Advil Allergy Sinus Caplets	Ibuprofen 200mg	Chlorpheniramine maleate 2mg	Pseudoephedrine HCl 30mg			**Adults & Peds ≥12 yrs:** 1 tab q4-6h. **Max:** 6 tabs/24h.
Alka-Seltzer Plus Cold Formula Effervescent Tablets*	Aspirin 325mg	Chlorpheniramine maleate 2mg	Phenylephrine bitartrate 7.8mg			**Adults & Peds ≥12 yrs:** 2 tabs q4h. **Max:** 8 tabs/24h.
Benadryl Allergy Plus Cold Kapgels†	Acetaminophen 325mg	Diphenhydramine HCl 12.5mg0	Phenylephrine HCl 5mg			**Adults & Peds ≥12 yrs:** 2 caps q4h. **Max:** 12 caps/24h.
Benadryl Allergy Plus Sinus Headache Kapgels†	Acetaminophen 325mg	Diphenhydramine HCl 12.5mg	Phenylephrine HCl 5mg			**Adults & Peds ≥12 yrs:** 2 caps q4h. **Max:** 12 caps/24h.
Benadryl Severe Allergy Plus Sinus Headache Caplets†	Acetaminophen 325mg	Diphenhydramine HCl 25mg	Phenylephrine HCl 5mg			**Adults & Peds ≥12 yrs:** 2 tabs q4h. **Max:** 12 tabs/24h.
Children's Tylenol Plus Cold Liquid†	Acetaminophen 160mg/5mL	Chlorpheniramine maleate 1mg/5mL	Phenylephrine HCl 2.5mg/5mL			**Peds 6-11 yrs (48-95 lbs):** 2 tsp (10mL) q4h. **Max:** 5 doses/24h.
Dristan Cold Multi-Symptom Formula Tablets	Acetaminophen 325mg	Chlorpheniramine maleate 2mg	Phenylephrine HCl 5mg			**Adults & Peds ≥12 yrs:** 2 tabs q4h. **Max:** 12 tabs/24h.

(Continued)

ANTIHISTAMINES + DECONGESTANTS + ANALGESICS (Continued)

Brand Name	Analgesic	Antihistamine	Decongestant	Cough Suppressant	Expectorant	Dosage
Robitussin Peak Cold Nighttime Multi-Symptom Cold CF	Acetaminophen 160mg/5mL	Diphenhydramine HCl 6.25mg/5mL	Phenylephrine HCl 2.5mg/5mL			**Adults & Peds ≥12 yrs:** 4 tsp (20mL) q4h. **Max:** 6 doses/24h.
Robitussin Peak Cold Nighttime Cold Nasal Relief	Acetaminophen 325mg	Chlorpheniramine maleate 2mg	Phenylephrine HCl 5mg			**Adults & Peds ≥12 yrs:** 2 tabs q4h. **Max:** 12 tabs/24h.
Sudafed PE Severe Cold Caplets†	Acetaminophen 325mg	Diphenhydramine HCl 12.5mg	Phenylephrine HCl 5mg			**Adults & Peds ≥12 yrs:** 2 tabs q4h. **Max:** 12 tabs/24h.
Theraflu Cold & Sore Throat Powder Packets	Acetaminophen 325mg/packet	Pheniramine maleate 20mg/packet	Phenylephrine HCl 10mg/packet			**Adults & Peds ≥12 yrs:** 1 pkt q4h. **Max:** 6 pkts/24h.
Theraflu Flu & Sore Throat Powder Packets	Acetaminophen 650mg/packets	Pheniramine maleate 20mg/packet	Phenylephrine HCl 10mg/packet			**Adults & Peds ≥12 yrs:** 1 pkt q4h. **Max:** 6 pkts/24h.
Theraflu Nighttime Severe Cold & Cough Powder Packets	Acetaminophen 650mg/packet	Diphenhydramine HCl 25mg/packet	Phenylephrine HCl 10mg/packet			**Adults & Peds ≥12 yrs:** 1 pkt q4h. **Max:** 6 pkts/24h.
Theraflu Sinus & Cold Powder Packets	Acetaminophen 325mg/packet	Pheniramine maleate 20mg/packet	Phenylephrine HCl 10mg/packet			**Adults & Peds ≥12 yrs:** 1 pkt q4h. **Max:** 6 pkts/24h.
Theraflu Sugar-Free Nighttime Severe Cold & Cough Powder Packets	Acetaminophen 650mg/packet	Diphenhydramine HCl 25mg/packet	Phenylephrine HCl 10mg/packet			**Adults & Peds ≥12 yrs:** 1 pkt q4h. **Max:** 6 pkts/24h.
Theraflu Warming Relief Flu & Sore Throat Syrup	Acetaminophen 325mg/15mL	Diphenhydramine HCl 12.5mg/15mL	Phenylephrine HCl 5mg/15mL			**Adults & Peds ≥12 yrs:** 2 tbl (30mL) q4h. **Max:** 6 doses (12 tbl or 180mL)/24h.

Brand Name	Analgesic	Antihistamine	Decongestant	Cough Suppressant	Expectorant	Dosage
ANTIHISTAMINES + DECONGESTANTS + ANALGESICS *(Continued)*						
Theraflu Warming Relief Nighttime Severe Cold & Cough Syrup	Acetaminophen 325mg/15mL	Diphenhydramine HCl 12.5mg/15mL	Phenylephrine HCl 5mg/15mL			**Adults & Peds ≥12 yrs:** 2 tbl (30mL) q4h. **Max:** 6 doses (12 tbl or 180mL)/24h.
Theraflu Warming Relief Sinus & Cold Syrup	Acetaminophen 325mg/15mL	Diphenhydramine HCl 12.5mg/15mL	Phenylephrine HCl 5mg/15mL			**Adults & Peds ≥12 yrs:** 2 tbl (30mL) q4h. **Max:** 6 doses (12 tbl or 180mL)/24h.
Vicks NyQuil Sinex Nighttime Sinus Relief LiquiCaps	Acetaminophen 325mg	Doxylamine succinate 6.25mg	Phenylephrine HCl 5mg			**Adults & Peds ≥12 yrs:** 2 caps q4h. **Max:** 4 doses/24h.
COUGH SUPPRESSANTS						
Children's Delsym 12 Hour Cough Relief Liquid*				Dextromethorphan HBr 30mg/5mL		**Adults & Peds ≥12 yrs:** 2 tsp (10mL) q12h. **Max:** 4 tsp (20mL)/24h. **Peds 6-<12 yrs:** 1 tsp (5mL) q12h. **Max:** 2 tsp (10mL)/24h. **Peds 4-<6 yrs:** ½ tsp (2.5mL) q12h. **Max:** 1 tsp (5mL)/24h.
Children's Robitussin Cough Long-Acting				Dextromethorphan HBr 7.5mg/5mL		**Adults & Peds ≥12 yrs:** 4 tsp (20mL) q6-8h. **Peds 6-<12 yrs:** 2 tsp (10mL) q6-8h. **Peds 4-<6 yrs:** 1 tsp (5mL) q6-8h. **Max:** 4 doses/24h.

(Continued)

COUGH SUPPRESSANTS (Continued)

BRAND NAME	ANALGESIC	ANTIHISTAMINE	DECONGESTANT	COUGH SUPPRESSANT	EXPECTORANT	DOSAGE
Delsym 12 Hour Cough Relief Liquid*				Dextromethorphan HBr 30mg/5mL		**Adults & Peds ≥12 yrs:** 2 tsp (10mL) q12h. **Max:** 4 tsp (20mL)/24h. **Peds 6-<12 yrs:** 1 tsp (5mL) q12h. **Max:** 2 tsp (10mL)/24h. **Peds 4-<6 yrs:** ½ tsp (2.5mL) q12h. **Max:** 1 tsp (5mL)/24h.
Robitussin Lingering Cold Long-Acting Cough				Dextromethorphan HBr 15mg/5mL		**Adults & Peds ≥12 yrs:** 2 tsp (10mL) q6-8h. **Max:** 4 doses/24h.
Robitussin Lingering Cold Long-Acting CoughGels				Dextromethorphan HBr 15mg		**Adults & Peds ≥12 yrs:** 2 caps q6-8h. **Max:** 8 caps/24h.
Triaminic Long-Acting Cough Syrup				Dextromethorphan HBr 7.5mg/5mL		**Peds 6-<12 yrs:** 2 tsp (10mL) q6-8h. **Peds 4-<6 yrs:** 1 tsp (5mL) q6-8h. **Max:** 4 doses/24h.
Vicks BabyRub Soothing Aroma Ointment				Petrolatum, fragrance, aloe extract, eucalyptus oil, lavender oil, rosemary oil		**Peds ≥3 months:** Gently massage on the chest, neck, and back to help soothe and comfort.
Vicks DayQuil Cough Liquid				Dextromethorphan HBr 15mg/15mL		**Adults & Peds ≥12 yrs:** 2 tbl (30mL) q6-8h. **Peds 6-<12 yrs:** 1 tbl (15mL) q6-8h. **Max:** 4 doses/24h.
Vicks Formula 44 Custom Care Dry Cough Suppressant Liquid				Dextromethorphan HBr 30mg/15mL		**Adults & Peds ≥12 yrs:** 1 tbl (15mL) q6-8h. **Peds 6-<12 yrs:** 1½ tsp (7.5mL) q6-8h. **Max:** 4 doses/24h.

Brand name	Analgesic	Antihistamine	Decongestant	Cough suppressant	Expectorant	Dosage
COUGH SUPPRESSANTS *(Continued)*						
Vicks VapoDrops*				Menthol 1.7mg (cherry); Menthol 3.3mg (menthol)		**Adults & Peds ≥5 yrs:** 3 drops (cherry). **Adults & Peds ≥5 yrs:** 2 drops (menthol).
Vicks VapoRub Topical Ointment				Camphor 4.8%, Menthol 2.6%, Eucalyptus oil 1.2%		**Adults & Peds ≥2 yrs:** Apply to chest and throat. **Max:** 3 times/24h.
Vicks VapoSteam				Camphor 6.2%		**Adults & Peds ≥2 yrs:** 1 tbl/quart of water or 1½ tsp/pint of water (for use in a hot steam vaporizer). **Max:** 3 times/24h.
COUGH SUPPRESSANTS + ANTIHISTAMINES						
Children's Dimetapp Long Acting Cough Plus Cold Syrup		Chlorpheniramine maleate 1mg/5mL		Dextromethorphan HBr 7.5mg/5mL		**Adults & Peds ≥12 yrs:** 4 tsp (20mL) q6h. **Peds 6-<12 yrs:** 2 tsp (10mL) q6h. **Max:** 4 doses/24h.
Children's Robitussin Cough & Cold Long-Acting		Chlorpheniramine maleate 1mg/5mL		Dextromethorphan HBr 7.5mg/5mL		**Adults & Peds ≥12 yrs:** 4 tsp (20mL) q6h. **Peds 6-<12 yrs:** 2 tsp (10mL) q6h. **Max:** 4 doses/24h.
Coricidin HBP Cough & Cold		Chlorpheniramine maleate 4mg		Dextromethorphan HBr 30mg		**Adults & Peds ≥12 yrs:** 1 tab q6h. **Max:** 4 tabs/24h.
Vicks Children's NyQuil Cold & Cough Liquid		Chlorpheniramine maleate 2mg/15mL		Dextromethorphan HBr 15mg/15mL		**Adults & Peds ≥12 yrs:** 2 tbl (30mL) q6h. **Peds 6-11 yrs:** 1 tbl (15mL) q6h. **Max:** 4 doses/24h.
Vicks NyQuil Cough Liquid		Doxylamine succinate 12.5mg/30mL		Dextromethorphan HBr 30mg/30mL		**Adults & Peds ≥12 yrs:** 2 tbl (30mL) q6h. **Max:** 4 doses/24h.

(Continued)

Brand Name	Analgesic	Antihistamine	Decongestant	Cough Suppressant	Expectorant	Dosage
COUGH SUPPRESSANTS + ANALGESICS						
PediaCare Children Cough & Sore Throat Plus Acetaminophen	Acetaminophen 160mg/5mL			Dextromethorphan HBr 5mg/5mL		**Peds 6-11 yrs (48-95 lbs):** 2 tsp (10mL) q4h. **Max:** 5 times/24h.
Triaminic Cough & Sore Throat Syrup	Acetaminophen 160mg/5mL			Dextromethorphan HBr 5mg/5mL		**Peds 6-<12 yrs:** 2 tsp (10mL) q4h. **Peds 4-<6 yrs:** 1 tsp (5mL) q4h. **Max:** 5 doses/24h.
COUGH SUPPRESSANTS + ANTIHISTAMINES + ANALGESICS						
Children's Tylenol Plus Cough & Runny Nose Liquid†	Acetaminophen 160mg/5mL	Chlorpheniramine maleate 1mg/5mL		Dextromethorphan HBr 5mg/5mL		**Peds 6-11 yrs (48-95 lbs):** 2 tsp (10mL) q4h. **Max:** 5 doses/24h.
Coricidin HBP Day & Night Multi-Symptom Cold	Acetaminophen 500mg (nighttime dose only)	Chlorpheniramine maleate 2mg (nighttime dose only)		Dextromethorphan HBr 10mg (daytime dose), 15mg (nighttime dose)	Guaifenesin 200mg (daytime dose only)	(Day) **Adults & Peds ≥12 yrs:** 1-2 softgels q4h. **Max:** 6 caps/12h. (Night) **Adults & Peds ≥12 yrs:** 2 tabs hs and q6h. **Max:** 4 tabs/12h.
Coricidin HBP Maximum Strength Flu	Acetaminophen 500mg	Chlorpheniramine maleate 2mg		Dextromethorphan HBr 15mg		**Adults & Peds ≥12 yrs:** 2 tabs q6h. **Max:** 8 tabs/24h.
Coricidin HBP Nighttime Multi-Symptom Cold Liquid	Acetaminophen 500mg/15mL (10 fl oz bottle), Acetaminophen 325mg/15mL (12 fl oz bottle)	Doxylamine succinate 6.25mg/15mL		Dextromethorphan HBr 15mg/15mL		**Adults & Peds ≥12 yrs:** 2 tbl (30mL) q6h. **Max:** 4 doses/24h.
Delsym Night Time Multi-Symptom Liquid	Acetaminophen 325mg/15mL	Doxylamine succinate 6.25mg/15mL		Dextromethorphan HBr 15mg/15mL		**Adults & Peds ≥12 yrs:** 2 tbl (30mL) q6h. **Max:** 4 doses/24h.

COUGH SUPPRESSANTS + ANTIHISTAMINES + ANALGESICS (Continued)

Brand Name	Analgesic	Antihistamine	Decongestant	Cough Suppressant	Expectorant	Dosage
PediaCare Children Cough & Runny Nose Plus Acetaminophen	Acetaminophen 160mg/5mL	Chlorpheniramine maleate 1mg/5mL		Dextromethorphan HBr 5mg/5mL		**Peds 6-11 yrs (48-95 lbs):** 2 tsp (10mL) q4h. **Max:** 5 times/24h.
Triaminic Multi-Symptom Fever Syrup	Acetaminophen 160mg/5mL	Chlorpheniramine maleate 1mg/5mL		Dextromethorphan HBr 7.5mg/5mL		**Peds 6-<12 yrs:** 2 tsp (10mL) q6h. **Max:** 4 doses/24h.
Vicks Alcohol Free NyQuil Cold & Flu Relief Liquid	Acetaminophen 650mg/30mL	Chlorpheniramine maleate 4mg/30mL		Dextromethorphan HBr 30mg/30mL		**Adults & Peds ≥12 yrs:** 2 tbl (30mL) q6h. **Max:** 4 doses/24h.
Vicks Formula 44 Custom Care Cough & Cold PM Liquid	Acetaminophen 650mg/15mL	Chlorpheniramine maleate 4mg/15mL		Dextromethorphan HBr 30mg/15mL		**Adults & Peds ≥12 yrs:** 1 tbl (15mL) q6h. **Max:** 4 doses/24h.
Vicks NyQuil Cold & Flu Relief LiquiCaps	Acetaminophen 325mg	Doxylamine succinate 6.25mg		Dextromethorphan HBr 15mg		**Adults & Peds ≥12 yrs:** 2 caps q6h. **Max:** 4 doses/24h.
Vicks NyQuil Cold & Flu Relief Liquid	Acetaminophen 650mg/30mL	Doxylamine succinate 12.5mg/30mL		Dextromethorphan HBr 30mg/30mL		**Adults & Peds ≥12 yrs:** 2 tbl (30mL) q6h. **Max:** 4 doses/24h.

COUGH SUPPRESSANTS + ANTIHISTAMINES + ANALGESICS + DECONGESTANTS

Brand Name	Analgesic	Antihistamine	Decongestant	Cough Suppressant	Expectorant	Dosage
Alka-Seltzer Plus Cold & Cough Formula Effervescent Tablets	Aspirin 325mg	Chlorpheniramine maleate 2mg	Phenylephrine bitartrate 7.8mg	Dextromethorphan HBr 10mg		**Adults & Peds ≥12 yrs:** 2 tabs q4h. **Max:** 8 tabs/24h.
Alka-Seltzer Plus Cold & Cough Formula Liquid Gels	Acetaminophen 325mg	Chlorpheniramine maleate 2mg	Phenylephrine HCl 5mg	Dextromethorphan HBr 10mg		**Adults & Peds ≥12 yrs:** 2 caps q4h. **Max:** 10 caps/24h.
Alka-Seltzer Plus Night Cold Formula Effervescent Tablets	Aspirin 500mg	Doxylamine succinate 6.25mg	Phenylephrine bitartrate 7.8mg	Dextromethorphan HBr 10mg		**Adults & Peds ≥12 yrs:** 2 tabs q4- 6h. **Max:** 8 tabs/24h.

(Continued)

COUGH SUPPRESSANTS + ANTIHISTAMINES + ANALGESICS + DECONGESTANTS (Continued)

Brand Name	Analgesic	Antihistamine	Decongestant	Cough Suppressant	Expectorant	Dosage
Alka-Seltzer Plus Night Cold & Flu Formula Liquid Gels	Acetaminophen 325mg	Doxylamine succinate 6.25mg	Phenylephrine HCl 5mg	Dextromethorphan HBr 10mg		**Adults & Peds ≥12 yrs:** 2 caps q4h. **Max:** 10 caps/24h.
Alka-Seltzer Plus Severe Cold & Flu Formula Effervescent Tablets	Acetaminophen 250mg	Chlorpheniramine maleate 2mg	Phenylephrine HCl 5mg	Dextromethorphan HBr 10mg		**Adults & Peds ≥12 yrs:** 2 tabs q4h. **Max:** 8 tabs/24h.
Children's Dimetapp MultiSymptom Cold & Flu Syrup	Acetaminophen 160mg/5mL	Chlorpheniramine maleate 1mg/5mL	Phenylephrine HCl 2.5mg/5mL	Dextromethorphan HBr 5mg/5mL		**Adults & Peds ≥12 yrs:** 4 tsp (20mL) q4h. **Peds 6-<12 yrs:** 2 tsp (10mL) q4h. **Max:** 5 doses/24h.
Children's Tylenol Plus Flu Liquid†	Acetaminophen 160mg/5mL	Chlorpheniramine maleate 1mg/5mL	Phenylephrine HCl 2.5mg/5mL	Dextromethorphan HBr 5mg/5mL		**Peds 6-11 yrs (48-95 lbs):** 2 tsp (10mL) q4h. **Max:** 5 times/24h.
Children's Tylenol Plus Multi-Symptom Cold Liquid†	Acetaminophen 160mg/5mL	Chlorpheniramine maleate 1mg/5mL	Phenylephrine HCl 2.5mg/5mL	Dextromethorphan HBr 5mg/5mL		**Peds 6-11 yrs (48-95 lbs):** 2 tsp (10mL) q4h. **Max:** 5 doses/24h.
PediaCare Children Flu Plus Acetaminophen	Acetaminophen 160mg/5mL	Chlorpheniramine maleate 1mg/5mL	Phenylephrine HCl 2.5mg/5mL	Dextromethorphan HBr 5mg/5mL		**Peds 6-11 yrs (48-95 lbs):** 2 tsp (10mL) q4h. **Max:** 5 times/24h.
PediaCare Children Multi-Symptom Cold Plus Acetaminophen	Acetaminophen 160mg/5mL	Chlorpheniramine maleate 1mg/5mL	Phenylephrine HCl 2.5mg/5mL	Dextromethorphan HBr 5mg/5mL		**Peds 6-11 yrs (48-95 lbs):** 2 tsp (10mL) q4h. **Max:** 5 times/24h.
Theraflu Warming Relief Nighttime Multi-Symptom Cold Caplets	Acetaminophen 325mg	Chlorpheniramine maleate 2mg	Phenylephrine HCl 5mg	Dextromethorphan HBr 10mg		**Adults & Peds ≥12 yrs:** 2 tabs q4h. **Max:** 12 tabs/24h.
Tylenol Cold Multi-Symptom Nighttime Liquid*	Acetaminophen 325mg/15mL	Doxylamine succinate 6.25mg/15mL	Phenylephrine HCl 5mg/15mL	Dextromethorphan HBr 10mg/15mL		**Adults & Peds ≥12 yrs:** 2 tbl (30mL) q4h. **Max:** 12 tbl (180mL)/24h.

Brand Name	Analgesic	Antihistamine	Decongestant	Cough Suppressant	Expectorant	Dosage
COUGH SUPPRESSANTS + ANTIHISTAMINES + DECONGESTANTS						
Children's Dimetapp Cold & Cough Syrup		Brompheniramine maleate 1mg/5mL	Phenylephrine HCl 2.5mg/5mL	Dextromethorphan HBr 5mg/5mL		**Adults & Peds ≥12 yrs:** 4 tsp (20mL) q4h. **Peds 6-<12 yrs:** 2 tsp (10mL) q4h. **Max:** 6 doses/24h.
COUGH SUPPRESSANTS + DECONGESTANTS						
Children's Sudafed PE Cold & Cough Liquid			Phenylephrine HCl 2.5mg/5mL	Dextromethorphan HBr 5mg/5mL		**Peds 6-11 yrs:** 2 tsp (10mL) q4h. **Peds 4-5 yrs:** 1 tsp (5mL) q4h. **Max:** 6 doses/24h.
PediaCare Children Daytime Multi-Symptom Cold			Phenylephrine HCl 2.5mg/5mL	Dextromethorphan HBr 5mg/5mL		**Peds 6-11 yrs (48-95 lbs):** 2 tsp (10mL) q4h. **Peds 4-5 yrs (36-47 lbs):** 1 tsp (5mL) q4h. **Max:** 6 doses/24h.
PediaCare Children Nighttime Multi-Symptom Cold			Phenylephrine HCl 2.5mg/5mL	Diphenhydramine HCl 6.25mg/5mL		**Peds 6-11 yrs:** 2 tsp (10mL) q4h. **Max:** 6 doses q24h.
Triaminic Day Time Cold & Cough Syrup			Phenylephrine HCl 2.5mg/5mL	Dextromethorphan HBr 5mg/5mL		**Peds 6-<12 yrs:** 2 tsp (10mL) q4h. **Peds 4-<6 yrs:** 1 tsp (5mL) q4h. **Max:** 6 doses/24h.
COUGH SUPPRESSANTS + DECONGESTANTS + ANALGESICS						
Alka-Seltzer Plus Day & Night Cold & Flu Formula Liquid Gels	Acetaminophen 325mg	Doxylamine succinate 6.25mg (nighttime dose only)	Phenylephrine HCl 5mg	Dextromethorphan HBr 10mg		**Adults & Peds ≥12 yrs:** 2 caps q4h. **Max:** 10 caps/24h.
Alka-Seltzer Plus Day & Night Multi-Symptom Cold Formula Effervescent Tablets	Aspirin 325mg (day); Aspirin 500mg (night)	Doxylamine succinate 6.25mg (nighttime dose only)	Phenylephrine bitartrate 7.8mg	Dextromethorphan HBr 10mg		(Day) **Adults & Peds ≥12 yrs:** 2 tabs q4h. **Max:** 8 tabs/24h. (Night) **Adults & Peds ≥12 yrs:** 2 tabs q4-6h. **Max:** 8 tabs/24h.

(Continued)

COUGH SUPPRESSANTS + DECONGESTANTS + ANALGESICS (Continued)

Brand Name	Analgesic	Antihistamine	Decongestant	Cough Suppressant	Expectorant	Dosage
Alka-Seltzer Plus Day Non–Drowsy Cold & Flu Formula Liquid Gels	Acetaminophen 325mg		Phenylephrine HCl 5mg	Dextromethorphan HBr 10mg		**Adults & Peds ≥12 yrs:** 2 caps q4h. **Max:** 10 caps/24h.
Children's Tylenol Plus Cold & Cough Liquid†	Acetaminophen 160mg/5mL		Phenylephrine HCl 2.5mg/5mL	Dextromethorphan HBr 5mg/5mL		**Peds 6-11 yrs (48-95 lbs):** 2 tsp (10mL) q4h. **Peds 4-5 yrs (36-47 lbs):** 1 tsp (5mL) q4h. **Max:** 5 doses/24h.
Theraflu Daytime Severe Cold & Cough Powder Packets	Acetaminophen 650mg/packet		Phenylephrine HCl 10mg/packet	Dextromethorphan HBr 20mg/packet		**Adults & Peds ≥12 yrs:** 1 pkt q4h. **Max:** 6 pkts/24h.
Theraflu Multi-Symptom Severe Cold with Lipton Green Tea & Honey Lemon Flavors Powder Packets	Acetaminophen 500mg/packet		Phenylephrine HCl 10mg/packet	Dextromethorphan HBr 20mg/packet		**Adults & Peds ≥12 yrs:** 1 pkt q4h. **Max:** 6 pkts/24h.
Theraflu Warming Relief Daytime Multi-Symptom Cold Caplets	Acetaminophen 325mg		Phenylephrine HCl 5mg	Dextromethorphan HBr 10mg		**Adults & Peds ≥12 yrs:** 2 tabs q4h. **Max:** 12 tabs/24h.
Theraflu Warming Relief Daytime Severe Cold & Cough Syrup	Acetaminophen 325mg/15mL		Phenylephrine HCl 5mg/15mL	Dextromethorphan HBr 10mg/15mL		**Adults & Peds ≥12 yrs:** 2 tbl (30mL) q4h. **Max:** 6 doses/24h.
Tylenol Cold Multi-Symptom Daytime Caplets	Acetaminophen 325mg		Phenylephrine HCl 5mg	Dextromethorphan HBr 10mg		**Adults & Peds ≥12 yrs:** 2 caps q4h. **Max:** 10 caps/24h.

Brand Name	Analgesic	Antihistamine	Decongestant	Cough Suppressant	Expectorant	Dosage
COUGH SUPPRESSANTS + DECONGESTANTS + ANALGESICS *(Continued)*							
Tylenol Cold Multi-Symptom Daytime Liquid	Acetaminophen 325mg/15mL		Phenylephrine HCl 5mg/15mL	Dextromethorphan HBr 10mg/15mL		**Adults & Peds ≥12 yrs:** 2 tbl (30mL) q4h. **Max:** 12 tbl (180mL)/24h.
Vicks DayQuil Cold & Flu Relief LiquiCaps	Acetaminophen 325mg		Phenylephrine HCl 5mg	Dextromethorphan HBr 10mg		**Adults & Peds ≥12 yrs:** 2 caps q4h. **Max:** 4 doses/24h.
Vicks DayQuil Cold & Flu Relief Liquid	Acetaminophen 325mg/15mL		Phenylephrine HCl 5mg/15mL	Dextromethorphan HBr 10mg/15mL		**Adults & Peds ≥12 yrs:** 2 tbl (30mL) q4h. **Peds 6-<12 yrs:** 1 tbl (15mL) q4h. **Max:** 4 doses/24h.
COUGH SUPPRESSANTS + DECONGESTANTS + EXPECTORANTS							
Children's Mucinex Multi-Symptom Cold Liquid			Phenylephrine 2.5mg/5mL	Dextromethorphan HBr 5mg/5mL	Guaifenesin 100mg/5mL	**Peds 6-<12 yrs:** 2 tsp (10mL) q4h. **Peds 4-<6 yrs:** 1 tsp (5mL) q4h. **Max:** 6 doses/24h.
Children's Robitussin Cough & Cold CF			Phenylephrine HCl 2.5mg/5mL	Dextromethorphan HBr 5mg/5mL	Guaifenesin 50mg/5mL	**Adults & Peds ≥12 yrs:** 4 tsp (20mL) q4h. **Peds 6-<12 yrs:** 2 tsp (10mL) q4h. **Peds 4-<6 yrs:** 1 tsp (5mL) q4h. **Max:** 6 doses/24h.
Entex PAC (Entex T tabs + Entex S liquid)			Pseudoephedrine HCl 60mg (tabs)	Dextromethorphan HBr 20mg/5mL (liquid)	Guaifenesin 375mg (tabs)	(Tabs) **Adults & Peds ≥12 yrs:** 1 tab q4-6h. **Peds 6-<12 yrs:** ½ tab q4-6h. **Max:** 4 doses/24h. (Liquid) **Adults & Peds ≥12 yrs:** 1 tsp (5mL) q4h. **Peds 6-<12 yrs:** ½ tsp (2.5mL) q4h. **Max:** 4 doses/24h.

(Continued)

Brand Name	Analgesic	Antihistamine	Decongestant	Cough Suppressant	Expectorant	Dosage
COUGH SUPPRESSANTS + DECONGESTANTS + EXPECTORANTS *(Continued)*						
Mucinex Maximum Strength Fast-Max Severe Congestion & Cough Liquid			Phenylephrine HCl 10mg/20mL	Dextromethorphan HBr 20mg/20mL	Guaifenesin 400mg/20mL	**Adults & Peds ≥12 yrs:** 4 tsp (20mL) q4h. **Max:** 6 doses/24h.
Robitussin Peak Cold Multi-Symptom Cold CF			Phenylephrine HCl 5mg/5mL	Dextromethorphan HBr 10mg/5mL	Guaifenesin 100mg/5mL	**Adults & Peds ≥12 yrs:** 2 tsp (10mL) q4h. **Max:** 6 doses/24h.
COUGH SUPPRESSANTS + DECONGESTANTS + EXPECTORANTS + ANALGESICS						
Children's Mucinex Cold, Cough & Sore Throat Liquid	Acetaminophen 325mg/10mL		Phenylephrine HCl 5mg/10mL	Dextromethorphan HBr 10mg/10mL	Guaifenesin 200mg/10mL	**Peds 6-<12 yrs:** 2 tsp (10mL) q4h. **Max:** 5 doses/24h.
Children's Mucinex Multi-Symptom Cold & Fever Liquid	Acetaminophen 325mg/10mL		Phenylephrine HCl 5mg/10mL	Dextromethorphan HBr 10mg/10mL	Guaifenesin 200mg/10mL	**Peds 6-<12 yrs:** 2 tsp (10mL) q4h. **Max:** 5 doses/24h.
Mucinex Maximum Strength Fast-Max Cold, Flu & Sore Throat Liquid	Acetaminophen 650mg/20mL		Phenylephrine HCl 10mg/20mL	Dextromethorphan HBr 20mg/20mL	Guaifenesin 400mg/20mL	**Adults & Peds ≥12 yrs:** 4 tsp (20mL) q4h. **Max:** 6 doses/24h.
Sudafed PE Cold & Cough Caplets†	Acetaminophen 325mg		Phenylephrine HCl 5mg	Dextromethorphan HBr 10mg	Guaifenesin 100mg	**Adults & Peds ≥12 yrs:** 2 tabs q4h. **Max:** 12 tabs/24h.
Theraflu Max-D Severe Cold & Flu Powder Packets	Acetaminophen 1000mg/packet		Pseudoephedrine HCl 60mg/packet	Dextromethorphan HBr 30mg/packet	Guaifenesin 400mg/packet	**Adults & Peds ≥12 yrs:** 1 pkt q6h. **Max:** 4 pkts/24h.
Tylenol Cold & Flu Severe Caplets	Acetaminophen 325mg		Phenylephrine HCl 5mg	Dextromethorphan HBr 10mg	Guaifenesin 200mg	**Adults & Peds ≥12 yrs:** 2 tabs q4h. **Max:** 10 tabs/24h.
Tylenol Cold & Flu Severe Liquid	Acetaminophen 325mg/15mL		Phenylephrine HCl 5mg/15mL	Dextromethorphan HBr 10mg/15mL	Guaifenesin 200mg/15mL	**Adults & Peds ≥12 yrs:** 2 tbl (30mL) q4h. **Max:** 12 tbl (180mL)/24h.

Brand Name	Analgesic	Antihistamine	Decongestant	Cough Suppressant	Expectorant	Dosage
COUGH SUPPRESSANTS + DECONGESTANTS + EXPECTORANTS + ANALGESICS *(Continued)*						
Tylenol Cold Multi-Symptom Severe Liquid	Acetaminophen 325mg/15mL		Phenylephrine HCl 5mg/15mL	Dextromethorphan HBr 10mg/15mL	Guaifenesin 200mg/15mL	**Adults & Peds ≥12 yrs:** 2 tbl (30mL) q4h. **Max:** 12 tbl (180mL)/24h.
COUGH SUPPRESSANTS + EXPECTORANTS						
Alka-Seltzer Plus Mucus & Congestion Break Up Formula Liquid Gels				Dextromethorphan HBr 10mg	Guaifenesin 200mg	**Adults & Peds ≥12 yrs:** 2 caps q4h. **Max:** 12 caps/24h.
Children's Mucinex Cough Liquid				Dextromethorphan HBr 5mg/5mL	Guaifenesin 100mg/5mL	**Peds 6-<12 yrs:** 1-2 tsp (5-10mL) q4h. **Peds 4-<6 yrs:** ½-1 tsp (2.5-5mL) q4h. **Max:** 6 doses/24h.
Coricidin HBP Chest Congestion & Cough				Dextromethorphan HBr 10mg	Guaifenesin 200mg	**Adults & Peds ≥12 yrs:** 1-2 caps q4h. **Max:** 12 caps/24h.
Mucinex Cough Mini-Melts				Dextromethorphan HBr 5mg/packet	Guaifenesin 100mg/packet	**Adults & Peds ≥12 yrs:** 2-4 pkts q4h. **Peds 6-<12 yrs:** 1-2 pkts q4h. **Peds 4-<6 yrs:** 1 pkt q4h. **Max:** 6 doses/24h.
Mucinex DM				Dextromethorphan HBr 30mg	Guaifenesin 600mg	**Adults & Peds ≥12 yrs:** 1-2 tabs q12h. **Max:** 4 tabs/24h.
Mucinex DM Maximum Strength				Dextromethorphan HBr 60mg	Guaifenesin 1200mg	**Adults & Peds ≥12 yrs:** 1 tab q12h. **Max:** 2 tabs/24h.
Mucinex Maximum Strength Fast-Max DM Max Liquid				Dextromethorphan HBr 20mg/20mL	Guaifenesin 400mg/20mL	**Adults & Peds ≥12 yrs:** 4 tsp (20mL) q4h. **Max:** 6 doses/24h.

(Continued)

Brand Name	Analgesic	Antihistamine	Decongestant	Cough Suppressant	Expectorant	Dosage
COUGH SUPPRESSANTS + EXPECTORANTS *(Continued)*						
PediaCare Children Cough & Congestion				Dextromethorphan HBr 5mg/5mL	Guaifenesin 100mg/5mL	**Peds 6-11 yrs (48-95 lbs):** 1-2 tsp (5-10mL). **Peds 4-6 yrs (36-47 lbs):** ½-1 tsp (2.5-5mL). **Max:** 6 doses/24h.
Robitussin Peak Cold Cough + Chest Congestion DM				Dextromethorphan HBr 10mg/5mL	Guaifenesin 100mg/5mL	**Adults & Peds ≥12 yrs:** 2 tsp (10mL) q4h. **Max:** 6 doses/24h.
Robitussin Peak Cold Maximum Strength Cough + Chest Congestion DM				Dextromethorphan HBr 10mg/5mL	Guaifenesin 200mg/5mL	**Adults & Peds ≥12 yrs:** 2 tsp (10mL) q4h. **Max:** 6 doses/24h.
Robitussin Peak Cold Sugar-Free Cough + Chest Congestion DM				Dextromethorphan HBr 10mg/5mL	Guaifenesin 100mg/5mL	**Adults & Peds ≥12 yrs:** 2 tsp (10mL) q4h. **Max:** 6 doses/24h.
Vicks DayQuil Mucus Control DM Liquid				Dextromethorphan HBr 10mg/15mL	Guaifenesin 200mg/15mL	**Adults & Peds ≥12 yrs:** 2 tbl (30mL) q4h. **Peds 6-<12 yrs:** 1 tbl (15mL) q4h. **Max:** 6 doses/24h.
Vicks Formula 44 Custom Care Chesty Cough Liquid				Dextromethorphan HBr 20mg/15mL	Guaifenesin 200mg/15mL	**Adults & Peds ≥12 yrs:** 1 tbl (15mL) q4h. **Peds 6-<12 yrs:** 1½ tsp (7.5mL) q4h. **Max:** 6 doses/24h.
DECONGESTANTS						
Children's Sudafed Nasal Decongestant Liquid			Pseudoephedrine HCl 15mg/5mL			**Peds 6-11 yrs:** 2 tsp (10mL) q4-6h. **Peds 4-5 yrs:** 1 tsp (5mL) q4-6h. **Max:** 4 doses/24h.

DECONGESTANTS (Continued)

Brand Name	Analgesic	Antihistamine	Decongestant	Cough Suppressant	Expectorant	Dosage
Children's Sudafed PE Nasal Decongestant Liquid			Phenylephrine HCl 2.5mg/5mL			**Peds 6-11 yrs:** 2 tsp (10mL) q4h. **Peds 4-5 yrs:** 1 tsp (5mL) q4h. **Max:** 6 doses/24h.
Mucinex Sinus-Max Full Force Nasal Spray			Oxymetazoline HCl 0.05%			**Adults & Peds ≥6 yrs:** 2-3 sprays in each nostril q10-12h. **Max:** 2 doses/24h.
Mucinex Sinus-Max Moisture Smart Nasal Spray			Oxymetazoline HCl 0.05%			**Adults & Peds ≥6 yrs:** 2-3 sprays in each nostril q10-12h. **Max:** 2 doses/24h.
PediaCare Children's Decongestant			Phenylephrine HCl 2.5mg/5mL			**Peds 6-11 yrs:** 2 tsp (10mL) q4h. **Peds 4-5 yrs:** 1 tsp (5mL) q4h. **Max:** 6 doses/24h.
Sudafed 12-Hour Tablets			Pseudoephedrine HCl 120mg			**Adults & Peds ≥12 yrs:** 1 tab q12h. **Max:** 2 tabs/24h.
Sudafed 24-Hour Tablets			Pseudoephedrine HCl 240mg			**Adults & Peds ≥12 yrs:** 1 tab/24h. **Max:** 1 tab/24h.
Sudafed Congestion Caplets			Pseudoephedrine HCl 30mg			**Adults & Peds ≥12 yrs:** 2 tabs q4-6h. **Max:** 8 tabs/24h. **Peds 6-11 yrs:** 1 tab q4-6h. **Max:** 4 tabs/24h.
Sudafed PE Congestion Tablets†			Phenylephrine HCl 10mg			**Adults & Peds ≥12 yrs:** 1 tab q4h. **Max:** 6 tabs/24h.

(Continued)

Brand Name	Analgesic	Antihistamine	Decongestant	Cough Suppressant	Expectorant	Dosage
DECONGESTANTS (*Continued*)						
Vicks Sinex 12-Hour Decongestant Nasal Spray			Oxymetazoline HCl 0.05%			**Adults & Peds ≥6 yrs:** 2-3 sprays in each nostril q10-12h. **Max:** 2 doses/24h.
Vicks Sinex 12-Hour Decongestant UltraFine Mist Nasal Spray			Oxymetazoline HCl 0.05%			**Adults & Peds ≥6 yrs:** 2-3 sprays in each nostril q10-12h. **Max:** 2 doses/24h.
Vicks VapoInhaler			Levmetamfetamine 50mg			**Adults & Peds ≥12 yrs:** 2 inhalations in each nostril q2h. **Peds 6-<12 yrs:** 1 inhalation in each nostril q2h.
DECONGESTANTS + ANALGESICS						
Advil Cold & Sinus Caplets/ Liqui-Gels	Ibuprofen 200mg		Pseudoephedrine HCl 30mg			**Adults & Peds ≥12 yrs:** 1-2 caps q4-6h. **Max:** 6 caps/24h.
Advil Congestion Relief Tablets	Ibuprofen 200mg		Phenylephrine HCl 10mg			**Adults & Peds ≥12 yrs:** 1 tabs q4h. **Max:** 6 tabs/24h.
Alka-Seltzer Plus Sinus Formula Effervescent Tablets	Aspirin 325mg		Phenylephrine bitartrate 7.8mg			**Adults & Peds ≥12 yrs:** 2 tabs q4h. **Max:** 8 tabs/24h.
Contac Cold + Flu Maximum Strength Non-Drowsy Caplets	Acetaminophen 500mg		Phenylephrine HCl 5mg			**Adults & Peds ≥12 yrs:** 2 tabs q6h. **Max:** 8 tabs/24h.
Robitussin Peak Cold Nasal Relief	Acetaminophen 325mg		Phenylephrine HCl 5mg			**Adults & Peds ≥12 yrs:** 2 tabs q4h. **Max:** 12 tabs/24h.

Brand Name	Analgesic	Antihistamine	Decongestant	Cough Suppressant	Expectorant	Dosage
DECONGESTANTS + ANALGESICS *(Continued)*						
Sudafed 12-Hour Pressure + Pain Caplets	Naproxen sodium 220mg		Pseudoephedrine HCl 120mg			**Adults & Peds ≥12 yrs:** 1 tab q12h. **Max:** 2 tabs/24h.
Sudafed PE Pressure + Pain Caplets	Acetaminophen 325mg		Phenylephrine HCl 5mg			**Adults & Peds ≥12 yrs:** 2 tabs q4h. **Max:** 10 tabs/24h.
Tylenol Sinus Congestion & Pain Daytime Caplets	Acetaminophen 325mg		Phenylephrine HCl 5mg			**Adults & Peds ≥12 yrs:** 2 caps q4h. **Max:** 10 caps/24h.
DECONGESTANTS + EXPECTORANTS						
Children's Mucinex Stuffy Nose & Cold Liquid			Phenylephrine HCl 2.5mg/5mL		Guaifenesin 100mg/5mL	**Peds 6-<12 yrs:** 2 tsp (10mL) q4h. **Peds 4-<6 yrs:** 1 tsp (5mL) q4h. **Max:** 6 doses/24h.
Entex T			Pseudoephedrine HCl 60mg		Guaifenesin 375mg	**Adults & Peds ≥12 yrs:** 1 tab q4h. **Peds 6-<12 yrs:** ½ tab q4h. **Max:** 4 doses/24h.
Mucinex D			Pseudoephedrine HCl 60mg		Guaifenesin 600mg	**Adults & Peds ≥12 yrs:** 2 tabs q12h. **Max:** 4 tabs/24h.
Mucinex D Maximum Strength			Pseudoephedrine HCl 120mg		Guaifenesin 1200mg	**Adults & Peds ≥12 yrs:** 1 tab q12h. **Max:** 2 tabs/24h.
Sudafed PE Non-Drying Sinus Caplets†			Phenylephrine HCl 5mg		Guaifenesin 200mg	**Adults & Peds ≥12 yrs:** 2 tabs q4h. **Max:** 12 tabs/24h.
Triaminic Chest & Nasal Congestion Syrup			Phenylephrine HCl 2.5mg/5mL		Guaifenesin 50mg/5mL	**Peds 6-<12 yrs:** 2 tsp (10mL) q4h. **Peds 4-<6 yrs:** 1 tsp (5mL) q4h. **Max:** 6 doses/24h.

(Continued)

DECONGESTANTS + EXPECTORANTS + ANALGESICS

Brand Name	Analgesic	Antihistamine	Decongestant	Cough Suppressant	Expectorant	Dosage
Mucinex Maximum Strength Fast-Max Cold & Sinus Liquid	Acetaminophen 650mg/20mL		Phenylephrine HCl 10mg/20mL		Guaifenesin 400mg/20mL	**Adults & Peds ≥12 yrs:** 4 tsp (20mL) q4h. **Max:** 6 doses/24h.
Sudafed Triple Action Caplets†	Acetaminophen 325mg		Pseudoephedrine HCl 30mg		Guaifenesin 200mg	**Adults & Peds ≥12 yrs:** 2 tabs q4-6h. **Max:** 8 tabs/24h.
Theraflu Warming Relief Cold & Chest Congestion Liquid	Acetaminophen 325mg/15mL		Phenylephrine HCl 5mg/15mL		Guaifenesin 200mg/15mL	**Adults & Peds ≥12 yrs:** 2 tbl (30mL) q4h. **Max:** 6 doses/24h.
Tylenol Sinus Congestion & Pain Severe Caplets	Acetaminophen 325mg		Phenylephrine HCl 5mg		Guaifenesin 200mg	**Adults & Peds ≥12 yrs:** 2 tabs q4h. **Max:** 10 tabs/24h.

EXPECTORANTS

Brand Name	Analgesic	Antihistamine	Decongestant	Cough Suppressant	Expectorant	Dosage
Children's Mucinex Chest Congestion Liquid					Guaifenesin 100mg/5mL	**Peds 6-<12 yrs:** 1-2 tsp (5-10mL) q4h. **Peds 4-<6 yrs:** ½-1 tsp (2.5-5mL) q4h. **Max:** 6 doses/24h.
Mucinex					Guaifenesin 600mg	**Adults & Peds ≥12 yrs:** 1-2 tabs q12h. **Max:** 4 tabs/24h.
Mucinex Maximum Strength					Guaifenesin 1200mg	**Adults & Peds ≥12 yrs:** 1 tab q12h. **Max:** 2 tabs/24h.
Mucinex Mini-Melts (Bubble Gum Flavor)					Guaifenesin 100mg/packet	**Adults & Peds ≥12 yrs:** 2-4 pkts q4h. **Peds 6-<12 yrs:** 1-2 pkts q4h. **Peds 4-<6 yrs:** 1 pkt q4h. **Max:** 6 doses/24h.
Mucinex Mini-Melts (Grape Flavor)					Guaifenesin 50mg/packet	**Peds 6-<12 yrs:** 2-4 pkts q4h. **Peds 4-<6 yrs:** 1-2 pkts q4h. **Max:** 6 doses/24h.

Brand Name	Analgesic	Antihistamine	Decongestant	Cough Suppressant	Expectorant	Dosage
EXPECTORANTS + ANALGESICS						
Theraflu Flu & Chest Congestion Powder Packets	Acetaminophen 1000mg/packet				Guaifenesin 400mg/packet	**Adults & Peds ≥12 yrs:** 1 pkt q6h. **Max:** 4 pkts/24h.
ANTIHISTAMINES + ANALGESICS						
Advil PM Caplets	Ibuprofen 200mg	Diphenhydramine citrate 38mg				**Adults & Peds ≥12 yrs:** 2 tabs hs. **Max:** 2 tabs/24h.
Advil PM Liqui-Gels	Ibuprofen 200mg	Diphenhydramine HCl 25mg				**Adults & Peds ≥12 yrs:** 2 caps hs. **Max:** 2 caps/24h.
Coricidin HBP Cold & Flu	Acetaminophen 325mg	Chlorpheniramine maleate 2mg				**Adults & Peds ≥12 yrs:** 2 tabs q4-6h. **Max:** 12 tabs/24h. **Peds 6-<12 yrs:** 1 tab q4-6h. **Max:** 5 tabs/24h.
Motrin PM Caplets	Ibuprofen 200mg	Diphenhydramine citrate 38mg				**Adults & Peds ≥12 yrs:** 2 tabs hs. **Max:** 2 tabs/24h.
Tylenol Severe Allergy Caplets†	Acetaminophen 500mg	Diphenhydramine HCl 12.5mg				**Adults & Peds ≥12 yrs:** 2 tabs q4-6h. **Max:** 8 tabs/24h.

*Multiple flavors available.
†Product currently on recall or temporarily unavailable from manufacturer, but generic forms may be available.

Table 11. DIAPER RASH PRODUCTS

Brand	Ingredient(s)/Strength(s)	Dosage
CALAMINE POWDERS		
Baby Anti Monkey Butt Diaper Rash Powder with Calamine	Calamine Powder 8%	**Children ≥2 yrs:** Apply freely up to 3 or 4 times daily. **Peds:** Apply prn.
WHITE PETROLATUMS		
Aquaphor Healing Ointment	White Petrolatum 41%	**Peds:** Apply prn.
Balmex Multi-Purpose Healing Ointment	White Petrolatum 51.1%	**Peds:** Apply prn.
Desitin Multi-Purpose Ointment	White Petrolatum 60.4%	**Peds:** Apply prn.
Vaseline Petroleum Jelly	White Petrolatum 99.96%	**Peds:** Apply prn.
ZINC OXIDES		
Aveeno Baby Soothing Relief Diaper Rash Cream	Zinc Oxide 13%	**Peds:** Apply prn.
Balmex Diaper Rash Cream Stick	Zinc Oxide 11.3%	**Peds:** Apply prn.
Balmex Diaper Rash Cream with ActivGuard	Zinc Oxide 11.3%	**Peds:** Apply prn.
Boudreaux's Butt Paste, Diaper Rash Ointment	Zinc Oxide 16%	**Peds:** Apply prn.
Boudreaux's Butt Paste, Diaper Rash Ointment – All Natural	Zinc Oxide 16%	**Peds:** Apply prn.
Boudreaux's Butt Paste, Diaper Rash Ointment – Maximum Strength	Zinc Oxide 40%	**Peds:** Apply prn.
California Baby Calming Diaper Rash Cream	Zinc Oxide 12%	**Peds:** Apply prn.
California Baby Super Sensitive Diaper Rash Cream	Zinc Oxide 12%	**Peds:** Apply prn.
Canus Li'l Goat's Milk Ointment	Zinc Oxide 40%	**Peds:** Apply prn.
Desitin Maximum Strength Original Paste	Zinc Oxide 40%	**Peds:** Apply prn.
Desitin Rapid Relief Cream	Zinc Oxide 13%	**Peds:** Apply prn.
Earth Friendly Baby Natural Red Clover Diaper Care Cream	Zinc Oxide 12%	**Peds:** Apply prn.
Johnson's No More Rash Diaper Rash Cream with Zinc Oxide	Zinc Oxide 13%	**Peds:** Apply prn.
Mustela Bebe Vitamin Barrier Cream	Zinc Oxide 10%	**Peds:** Apply prn.
Triple Paste Medicated Ointment	Zinc Oxide 12.8%	**Peds:** Apply prn.

(Continued)

BRAND	INGREDIENT(S)/STRENGTH(S)	DOSAGE
COMBINATION PRODUCTS		
A+D Original Ointment	Petrolatum/Lanolin 53.4%-15.5%	**Peds:** Apply prn.
A+D Zinc Oxide Cream	Dimethicone/Zinc Oxide 1%-10%	**Peds:** Apply prn.
Baby Anti Monkey Butt Diaper Rash Cream with Calamine	Zinc Oxide/Calamine Powder 12%-2%	**Peds:** Apply prn.
Johnson's Baby Powder Medicated Zinc Oxide Skin Protectant	Zinc Oxide 10%/Cornstarch	**Peds:** Apply prn.
Lansinoh Diaper Rash Ointment	Dimethicone/USP Modified Lanolin/Zinc Oxide 5.0%-15.5%-5.5%	**Peds:** Apply prn.
Palmer's Cocoa Butter Formula Bottom Butter	Dimethicone/Petrolatum 1%-30%	**Peds:** Apply prn.
Palmer's Cocoa Butter Formula Bottom Butter Zinc Oxide Formula	Zinc Oxide/Dimethicone 10%-1%	**Peds:** Apply prn.

Table 12. HEMORRHOIDAL PRODUCTS

BRAND	INGREDIENT(S)/STRENGTH(S)	DOSAGE
ANESTHETICS/ANESTHETIC COMBINATIONS		
HemAway Cream	Lidocaine/Phenylephrine HCl 5%-0.25%	**Adults & Peds ≥12 yrs:** Apply externally to affected area up to 4 times a day.
Preparation H Maximum Strength Pain Relief Cream	Glycerin/Phenylephrine HCl/ Pramoxine HCl/White petrolatum 14.4%-0.25%-1%-15%	**Adults & Peds ≥12 yrs:** Apply externally to affected area up to 4 times a day.
Tronolane Cream	Pramoxine HCl/Zinc oxide 1%-5%	**Adults & Peds ≥12 yrs:** Apply externally to affected area up to 5 times a day.
Tucks Fast Relief Spray	Pramoxine HCl 1%	**Adults & Peds ≥12 yrs:** Apply to affected area up to 5 times a day.
Tucks Hemorrhoidal Ointment	Pramoxine HCl/Zinc oxide/ Mineral oil 1%-12.5%-46.6%	**Adults & Peds ≥12 yrs:** Apply externally to affected area up to 5 times a day.
HYDROCORTISONES		
Preparation H Anti-Itch Cream	Hydrocortisone 1%	**Adults & Peds ≥12 yrs:** Apply to affected area not more than tid-qid.
WITCH HAZEL/WITCH HAZEL COMBINATIONS		
Preparation H Cooling Gel	Phenylephrine HCl/ Witch hazel 0.25%-50%	**Adults & Peds ≥12 yrs:** Apply externally to affected area up to 4 times a day.
Preparation H Medicated Wipes	Witch hazel 50%	**Adults & Peds ≥12 yrs:** Apply to affected area up to 6 times a day.
T.N. Dickinson's Witch Hazel Hemorrhoidal Pads	Witch hazel 50%	**Adults & Peds ≥12 yrs:** Apply to affected area up to 6 times a day.
Tucks Medicated Cooling Pads	Witch hazel 50%	**Adults & Peds ≥12 yrs:** Apply externally to affected area up to 6 times a day.
Tucks Take Alongs Medicated Cooling Towelettes	Witch hazel 50%	**Adults & Peds ≥12 yrs:** Apply externally to affected area up to 6 times a day.

(Continued)

BRAND	INGREDIENT(S)/STRENGTH(S)	DOSAGE
MISCELLANEOUS		
Calmol 4 Suppositories	Cocoa butter/Zinc oxide 76%-10%	**Adults & Peds ≥12 yrs:** Insert 1 supp up to 6 times a day.
Medicone Ointment	Camphor/Phenol/Tannic acid/Zinc oxide 3%-2.5%-2.2%-6.6%	**Adults & Peds ≥12 yrs:** Apply externally to affected area up to 3 times a day.
Medicone Suppositories	Hard fat/Phenylephrine HCl 88.7%-0.25%	**Adults & Peds ≥12 yrs:** Insert 1 supp up to 4 times a day.
Preparation H Ointment	Mineral oil/Petrolatum/Phenylephrine HCl/ 14%-74.9%-0.25%	**Adults & Peds ≥12 yrs:** Apply to affected area up to 4 times a day.
Preparation H Suppositories	Cocoa butter/Phenylephrine HCl/ 88.44%-0.25%	**Adults & Peds ≥12 yrs:** Insert 1 supp up to 4 times a day.
Tronolane Suppositories	Hard fat/Phenylephrine HCl 88.7%-0.25%	**Adults & Peds ≥12 yrs:** Insert 1 supp up to 4 times a day.
Tucks Internal Soothers Suppositories	Topical starch 51%	**Adults & Peds ≥12 yrs:** Insert 1 supp up to 6 times a day.

*Please refer to the *Laxative Products* chart for stool softeners or bulk-forming laxatives adjunct therapies.

Table 13. INSOMNIA PRODUCTS

BRAND	INGREDIENT(S)/STRENGTH(S)	DOSAGE
DIPHENHYDRAMINES		
Compoz Maximum Strength Soft Gel Liquid Capsules	Diphenhydramine 50mg	**Adults & Peds ≥12 yrs:** 1 cap hs prn.
Nytol QuickCaps	Diphenhydramine 25mg	**Adults & Peds ≥12 yrs:** 2 tabs hs prn.
Simply Sleep Caplets	Diphenhydramine 25mg	**Adults & Peds ≥12 yrs:** 2 tabs hs prn.
Sleepinal Capsules	Diphenhydramine 50mg	**Adults & Peds ≥12 yrs:** 1 cap hs prn.
Sominex Maximum Strength Caplets	Diphenhydramine 50mg	**Adults & Peds ≥12 yrs:** 1 tab hs prn.
Sominex Original Formula Tablets	Diphenhydramine 25mg	**Adults & Peds ≥12 yrs:** 2 tabs hs prn.
Unisom SleepGels	Diphenhydramine 50mg	**Adults & Peds ≥12 yrs:** 1 cap hs prn.
Unisom SleepMelts	Diphenhydramine 25mg	**Adults & Peds ≥12 yrs:** 2 tabs on tongue hs prn.
ZzzQuil Liquid	Diphenhydramine 50mg per 30mL dose cup (2 tbsp)	**Adults & Peds ≥12 yrs:** 30mL (2 tbsp) hs prn.
ZzzQuil LiquiCaps	Diphenhydramine 25mg	**Adults & Peds ≥12 yrs:** 2 caps hs prn.
DIPHENHYDRAMINE COMBINATIONS		
Advil PM Caplets	Ibuprofen/Diphenhydramine Citrate 200mg-38mg	**Adults & Peds ≥12 yrs:** 2 tabs hs. **Max:** 2 tabs/24 hrs.
Advil PM Liqui-Gels	Ibuprofen/Diphenhydramine HCl 200mg-25mg	**Adults & Peds ≥12 yrs:** 2 caps hs. **Max:** 2 caps/24 hrs.
Bayer PM Caplets	Aspirin/Diphenhydramine Citrate 500mg-38.3mg	**Adults & Peds ≥12 yrs:** 2 tabs hs prn.
Excedrin PM Caplets	Acetaminophen/Diphenhydramine Citrate 500mg-38mg	**Adults & Peds ≥12 yrs:** 2 tabs hs prn. **Max:** 2 tabs/24 hrs.
Excedrin PM Express Gels	Acetaminophen/Diphenhydramine Citrate 500mg-38mg	**Adults & Peds ≥12 yrs:** 2 caps hs prn. **Max:** 2 caps/24 hrs.

(Continued)

BRAND	INGREDIENT(S)/STRENGTH(S)	DOSAGE
DIPHENHYDRAMINE COMBINATIONS (Continued)		
Goody's PM Powder	Acetaminophen/Diphenhydramine Citrate 500mg-38mg per powder	**Adults & Peds ≥12 yrs:** 2 powders hs prn with a full glass of water, or may stir powders into water or other liquid.
Motrin PM Caplets	Ibuprofen/Diphenhydramine Citrate 200mg-38mg	**Adults & Peds ≥12 yrs:** 2 tabs hs. **Max:** 2 tabs/24 hrs.
Tylenol PM Caplets	Acetaminophen/Diphenhydramine HCl 500mg-25mg	**Adults & Peds ≥12 yrs:** 2 tabs hs. **Max:** 2 tabs/24 hrs.
Tylenol PM Geltabs	Acetaminophen/Diphenhydramine HCl 500mg-25mg	**Adults & Peds ≥12 yrs:** 2 tabs hs. **Max:** 2 tabs/24 hrs.
Unisom PM Pain SleepCaps	Acetaminophen/Diphenhydramine HCl 325mg-50mg	**Adults & Peds ≥12 yrs:** 1 tab hs. **Max:** 1 tab/24 hrs.
DOXYLAMINES		
Unisom SleepTabs	Doxylamine Succinate 25mg	**Adults & Peds ≥12 yrs:** 1 tab 30 minutes before hs.

INDICES

PRODUCT NAME INDEX

GENERIC NAME INDEX

B

C

F

N

O

P